The Oxford Handbook of Down Syndrome and Development

OXFORD LIBRARY OF PSYCHOLOGY

AREA EDITORS:

Clinical Psychology
David H. Barlow

Cognitive Neuroscience
Kevin N. Ochsner and Stephen M. Kosslyn

Cognitive Psychology
Daniel Reisberg

Counseling Psychology
Elizabeth M. Altmaier and Jo-Ida C. Hansen

Developmental Psychology
Philip David Zelazo

Health Psychology
Howard S. Friedman

History of Psychology
David B. Baker

Methods and Measurement
Todd D. Little

Neuropsychology
Kenneth M. Adams

Organizational Psychology
Steve W. J. Kozlowski

Personality and Social Psychology
Kay Deaux and Mark Snyder

OXFORD LIBRARY OF PSYCHOLOGY

The Oxford Handbook of Down Syndrome and Development

Edited by

Jacob A. Burack, Jamie Edgin, and Leonard Abbeduto

OXFORD
UNIVERSITY PRESS

OXFORD
UNIVERSITY PRESS

Oxford University Press is a department of the University of Oxford. It furthers the University's objective of excellence in research, scholarship, and education by publishing worldwide. Oxford is a registered trade mark of Oxford University Press in the UK and certain other countries.

Published in the United States of America by Oxford University Press
198 Madison Avenue, New York, NY 10016, United States of America.

Library of Congress Cataloging-in-Publication Data
Names: Burack, Jacob A., editor. | Edgin, Jamie, editor. | Abbeduto, Leonard, 1954– editor.
Title: The Oxford handbook of Down syndrome and development /
edited by Jacob A. Burack, Jamie Edgin, & Leonard Abbeduto.
Other titles: Oxford library of psychology.
Description: New York, NY : Oxford University Press, [2023] |
Series: Oxford library of psychology series | Includes bibliographical references and index. |
Identifiers: LCCN 2022051683 (print) | LCCN 2022051684 (ebook) |
ISBN 9780190645441 (hardback) | ISBN 9780190645465 | ISBN 9780190672614 (epub)
Subjects: MESH: Down Syndrome | Growth and Development—physiology | Patient Advocacy
Classification: LCC RC571 (print) | LCC RC571 (ebook) | NLM WS 107 |
DDC 616.85/8842—dc23/eng/20230118
LC record available at https://lccn.loc.gov/2022051683
LC ebook record available at https://lccn.loc.gov/2022051684

DOI: 10.1093/oxfordhb/9780190645441.001.0001

Printed by Sheridan Books, Inc., United States of America

We dedicate this volume to the memories of Janet Carr and Josephine Mills, who each in their own way contributed immensely to the understanding and well-being of persons with Down syndrome and their families through a remarkable and longstanding commitment to research, advocacy, and empowerment.

CONTENTS

Section 5 Interventions and Future Directions

ACKNOWLEDGMENTS

We thank the many authors for their wonderful contributions to this volume. They have been exceptionally generous in sharing their expertise in this venture and particularly patient in completing this task that was considerably delayed for a variety of reasons, most of which were linked to the COVID-19 pandemic. We are particularly grateful to the contributors to our "Voices" epilogue for sharing their lived experiences. They have contributed considerable insights and clarity to the work presented here and, more importantly, to the research not yet undertaken. We thank Monica Gomez and her mother, Mary, for allowing us to use Monica's beautiful artwork on the cover. We thank ArtWorks Studio and the Mary T. Paulin Gallery from the University of Arizona Sonoran Center for Excellence in Disabilities for connecting us with Monica. We are also grateful to the many folks involved in the production of the volume. We thank Adina Gazith for her assistance in organizing, collecting, and editing proofs for the print version of our volume. From Newgen Knowledge Works, we thank our production managers Afrose A for the gentle persistence in following up on the various chapter revisions and Jaishree Srijan for putting the final touches on the publication of the hard copy. Our support from the editors at Oxford University Press was, as always, fantastic—we thank Andrea Zekus for her enthusiastic recruitment of the volume and her guidance in shaping it, Abby Gross for her helpful oversight for a short period of time, and Katie Pratt who for the past few years has been a nonstop source of encouragement and goodwill through the process of completing the volume.

FOREWORD

I consider it a privilege to be invited to write a Foreword for this Handbook. I believe it makes a unique contribution towards improving the lives of individuals with Down syndrome and their families. Unique because, while many of the chapters provide comprehensive and insightful reviews of academic research focusing on specific aspects of development, these are set in the context of a developmental approach and with the perspective of the history and progress made over the past 50 years.

The first chapter, setting out the history, also identifies that parents and parent organizations at local, national, and international levels have influenced beliefs, attitudes, and services for individuals with Down syndrome from birth to old age.

The second chapter acknowledges the work of pioneers. It explains the way in which Janet Carr's longitudinal study, begun in 1963, not only charted development of individuals with Down syndrome from birth, but also looked at the whole person, the quality of their lives, and the influence of environmental factors on their progress. This is reflected in the chapters with a focus on families and parenting.

The Editors have brought together an impressive group of international experts to provide up-to-date reviews of the research in their area. In addition to the chapters focusing on a specific area of development, they have included chapters to illustrate different methodological approaches. This includes chapters on brain development and on animal models, which highlight the complexities, potential benefits, and limitations of this research. They also include chapters on comorbid conditions which need to be addressed and may impact development and daily functioning.

I was pleased to see that chapters covering adult issues and aging are included, giving a life span approach, but highlighting that the majority of research has focused on children and we have limited research on adult life and adult issues.

The developmental approach of Zigler and Cicchetti transformed the study of infants and children with Down syndrome. In the 1960s, research into the development of typical children was almost nonexistent but it began to progress rapidly. It began to show us the dynamic nature of development, the processes that underpinned development, and the factors which might accelerate or hinder progress. This then allowed researchers to see how these processes may be influenced or altered by having Down syndrome. The research in typical development also showed that brain structure and function is driven by experience, input, activity, and learning—environments and opportunities to learn matter. Brain development is not fixed at birth for any child, including those with an extra chromosome.

Most of the chapters in this Handbook show researchers applying this developmental approach for a specific aspect of development. It is important, going forward, to acknowledge that development in one area influences another so there are limits to this focus. For example, it is noted that language influences executive function, motor development influences cognitive, language and social development and we need methods which can encapsulate this complexity. We also need to note that tasks used in research studies may not reflect function in daily lives with familiar people, in familiar environments. For example, communication and social emotional competence may be significantly influenced by the setting and the sensitivity of the partner.

It is clear, from the content of this volume, that we lack intervention research. It highlights that we know, in increasing detail, about the challenges—about how having Down syndrome may impact the child's progress across all developmental areas. Once we can identify a challenge, such as in executive function, then we should be designing and evaluating interventions to improve executive function. If research shows us that verbal short-term memory challenges are apparent in teenagers and young adults, we should be asking how does verbal short-term memory develop in infancy and how can we intervene early to change the trajectory and reduce the differences. The lack of intervention research means we are not using research to inform practice and improve lives. The lack of research on effective education is an urgent issue to be addressed.

There is still too little understanding of the impact that the child's daily experiences at home and school is having on development—environmental factors. This concern is addressed in Chapter 2 which does stress the need to see the whole child, embedded in their family and community, but as a research community I think we are only just beginning to tackle this. Some of the chapters do bring this out, including those on language, parenting, and families.

At the community level, the ways in which community beliefs about disability influence how parents adjust to their baby are highlighted. Studies of how parents adjust have tended to focus on the negatives, the added stresses, though that is changing. We have few studies which highlight how families influence positive progress, both in the ways they interact daily with their children and the ways they fight for education, services, community inclusion, and employment. Parents and parent associations could tell us this which brings me to another point, how do we capture the wisdom and experience of parents and of therapists and practitioners?

Some authors rightly draw attention to the fact that research studies do not recruit fully representative samples. Those who volunteer to take part in studies are often advantaged in education and resources. Volunteers may not include families who struggle and whose lives are impacted more severely. They may not join support groups but be in more need of support. More delayed children and adults are not included in many studies.

The last chapter shares the views of individuals with Down syndrome and illustrates hopes, successes, and ambitions. We are beginning to include the voices of individuals with Down syndrome in research but need to do more to capture their lived experience.

This book shows how far we have come in the lifetime of my daughter and my professional practice but also illustrates how far we still have to go to bring together all the knowledge from all sections of our community to really transform the lives of those with Down syndrome and their families.

Professor Sue Buckley OBE
Director for Science and Research, Down Syndrome Education International
Emeritus Professor of Developmental Disability, Department of Psychology,
University of Portsmouth

ABOUT THE EDITORS

Jacob A. Burack is Professor of School/Applied Child Psychology and Human Development in the Department of Educational and Counselling Psychology at McGill University. He is the Director of the McGill Youth Study Team (MYST) and the Scientific Director of the Summit Center for Education, Research, and Training (SCERT).

Jamie Edgin is an Associate Professor and Director of the Cognition and Neural Systems Program in the Department of Psychology at the University of Arizona. Dr. Edgin currently directs the University of Arizona Public Policy Fellowship in the Sonoran UCEDD, focused on policy development and advocacy for persons with developmental disabilities.

Leonard Abbeduto is the Director of the MIND Institute, the Tsakopoulos-Vismara Endowed Chair, and Professor of Psychiatry and Behavioral Sciences at the University of California, Davis. He is the Director of the NICHD-funded MIND Institute Intellectual and Developmental Disabilities Research Center, and he co-directs the UC Davis Redwood SEED Scholars program, which is a 4-year, residential, inclusive college program for individuals with intellectual disabilities.

LIST OF CONTRIBUTORS

Natalia Arias-Trejo
Universidad Nacional Autónoma de México (UNAM)

Nathaniel E. Arnold
Arizona State University

Nadine M. Aziz
Boston University

Armando Bertone
McGill University

Nancy Brady
University of Kansas

Shelley L. Bredin-Oja
Minot State University

Roy I. Brown
University of Calgary and Flinders University

Ellen G. Casale
Western Kentucky University

Chih-Chia Chen
Mississippi State University

Monica Cuskelly
University of Tasmania

Lisa A. Daunhauer
Colorado State University

Dean D'Souza
City, University of London

Hana D'Souza
University of Cambridge & Cardiff University

Deborah J. Fidler
Colorado State University

Linda Gilmore
Queensland University of Technology

Jacalyn Guy
MRC Cognition and Brain Sciences Unit

Laura J. Hahn
University of Illinois at Urbana-Champaign

Taralee Hamner
Nationwide Children's Hospital

Penny Hauser-Cram
Boston College

Tarik F. Haydar
Children's National Hospital

Elizabeth Head
University of California, Irvine

Alex Helman
University of Kentucky

Robert M. Hodapp
Vanderbilt University

Simon D. Holzapfel
Arizona State University

Katharine Hughes
Goldsmiths College

Christopher Jarrold
University of Bristol

Elizabeth A. Kaplan-Kahn
Syracuse University

Connie L. Kasari
University of California, Los Angeles

Payal Khosla
University of Arizona

Justin B. Kopec
University of Pittsburgh

Margaret R. Kyrkou
Flinders University

Jessica Lai
McGill University
Oriane Landry
Bendigo Community Health Services
Nancy Raitano Lee
Drexel University
Corinna Lopez
Arizona State University
Christina Marcone
Concordia University
Erin Matsuba
Syracuse University
Elizabeth P. McKernan
Syracuse University
Maria Mello
St John's University
Anna J. Moyer
Johns Hopkins University
Kahyun Nam
Arizona State University
Amanda D. Nunnally
University of California, Davis
Lina Patel
University of Colorado
Lauren Pisani
University of Arizona
Jessica Ramos-Sanchez
Radboud University
Roger H. Reeves
Johns Hopkins University
Shannon D. R. Ringenbach
Arizona State University
Natalie Russo
Syracuse University
Kelli A. Sanderson
California State University
Long Beach
Frederick A. Schmitt
University of Kentucky
Emily Schworer
University of Wisconsin, Madison
Cory Shulman
The Hebrew University of Jerusalem
Elizabeth A. Smith
Cardiff University
Laura del Hoyo Soriano
University of California Davis
MIND Institute
Goffredina Spanò
The University of Arizona
Carla M. Startin
University of Roehampton
Jillian Stewart
McGill University
André Strydom
Kings College London
Emily Stubbert
McGill University
Monica Szeto
Arizona State University
Angela John Thurman
University of California, Davis
Manisha D. Udhnani
The Ohio State University
Kathryn Van Pelt
University of Kentucky
Steven F. Warren
University of Kansas
Karen Watchman
University of Stirling
Ashley C. Woodman
University of Massachusetts, Amherst
Shahid H. Zaman
University of Cambridge

SECTION 1

Historic and Contemporary Scientific Approaches

CHAPTER 1

A Brief History of Down Syndrome: Key Moments and Reflections

Roy I. Brown, Margaret R. Kyrkou, Karen Watchman, *and* Robert M. Hodapp

Abstract

The chapter traces some key historical developments in the study of individuals with Down syndrome. After describing general issues of classification in intellectual disabilities, we describe Langdon Down's identification of the syndrome in the 1860s; the movement to name the syndrome after Down; the identification of trisomy 21 as the syndrome's cause; and the beginnings of sustained research attention to the syndrome. We end with a glimpse into the future, discussing issues of longer life spans, more integrated lives, and the roles of families, organizations, and self-advocates. Working together, researchers, practitioners, and individuals and their families can all continue to advance the lives of persons with Down syndrome.

Key Words: Down syndrome, history, research studies, practical application, developmental challenges, parents and families

For many centuries, researchers have been interested in individuals with Down syndrome, including its history, treatment, and causes. In his history of the syndrome, Stratford (1989) reported on a wide range of artifacts from the Olmecs living near the Gulf of Mexico around 1500 BC to 300 AD. These artifacts include figurines and wall paintings, some of which Stratford noted are obviously children with Down syndrome. Similarly in European history, paintings from the 15th to 18th centuries appear to depict or be associated with the syndrome. Among these are paintings by the Flemish painter Jacob Jordaens (1593–1678) who frequently painted portraits of his wife and daughter, with the latter showing clear features of Down syndrome.

An additional perspective relates to the care of individuals with Down syndrome. In Europe from the mid-18th to the mid-20th centuries, increasing societal concern led to the development of formal care and institutionalization (Tredgold, 1914). Such concerns arose at a time when, within many industrialized countries, increasing concern for people with disabilities and for social impoverishment occurred on a much more extensive scale. From 1950 onwards, there has been a proliferation of health and educational practitioners focused on persons with Down syndrome, along with the development of multidisciplinary activities in both research and practice.

In this chapter, we highlight key moments in the history of the study of individuals with Down syndrome, with special attention to the years up to and including the early 21st century. Although wide-ranging and filled with colorful anecdotes, this history remains mostly unknown, including to Down syndrome researchers, practitioners, and even family members and individuals with Down syndrome themselves. Like so many aspects of the syndrome, this story too deserves to become better known to the world at large. We highlight only four of these issues: the classification-identification of Down syndrome; the discovery of trisomy 21; the change of name to Down syndrome; and modern behavioral studies.

Classification and Identification of Down syndrome

A first issue involves the basic issue of classification, including how Down syndrome came to be identified as a unique condition causing intellectual disability (ID). As described by Burack (1990), the 19th and early 20th centuries saw the emergence of various classification systems toward persons with intellectual disabilities. In the United Kingdom, government institutions first described persons with intellectual disability ID as "idiots" and "imbeciles," but definitions for these outdated and now derogatory terms were at first vague (see U.K. Education Act, 1870). Gradually, degrees of impairment and support needs associated with ID began to be recognized, along with the idea of differing potential to benefit from education. In the U.K. Mental Deficiency Acts of 1913 (which, though later amended, remained in effect until the middle of the 20th century), idiocy was seen as the severest form of ID. Those in this category were thought unable to guard themselves against common physical dangers. Langdon Down believed most persons with Down syndrome functioned in this category. The category above idiot was imbecile, with individuals who were slightly higher functioning classified as feeble minded (Clarke & Clarke, 1958). The reader should note that the foregoing terms did not have the pejorative connotations then that they carry today.

Despite the predominant thinking, Clarke and Clarke (1958) argued that individuals with Down syndrome could improve in their ability to function in daily life, an important shift in the understanding of Down syndrome. Such development formed part of the story of Down syndrome in the last half of the 20th century onwards, gradually fostering the idea that individuals with Down syndrome were capable of growing in a variety of ways. Borthwick (1996) underscored this view, questioning the overriding belief that genetics prevented cognitive growth in Down syndrome. She argued that the impact of environment was a critical factor and that the "genetics view" was only one aspect of the story. In a contemporary extension of this view from the 1990s onward, researchers emphasize the treatment potential and high variability of outcomes in this population.

Dr. Langdon Down and Mongolism

Throughout early Western history, people with Down syndrome were grouped with other forms of disability and mental illness. Only in the late 19th century were people with the syndrome identified as a separate group. Although less often noted, certain aspects of Down syndrome had been independently noted by the French psychiatrist Jean-Étienne Dominique Esquirol (in 1838; Vardhan, 2011), and by the French-born American psychiatrist and educator Édouard Séguin (1866; Brockett, 1880).

More complete and sustained explorations, however, were undertaken by Langdon Down (Ward, 1999). After completing his medical studies at the London Hospital, Down noted similarities among groups of patients in the London clinic, as well as among patients at the Royal Earlswood Hospital, where he was appointed superintendent (Ward, 1999). In his paper, "Observations on an Ethnic Classification of Idiots," Down (1866) provided a comprehensive description of the visible features commonly observed in individuals with the syndrome. He noted that these patients had a broad, flat face and no prominences, a small nose, and roundish wide cheeks. Obliquely placed eyes were wider apart than in most people, with smaller palpebral fissures (i.e., narrow skin folds on the inner side of the upper eyelid). The forehead had transverse wrinkles due to the impact of the occipito-frontalis muscle assisting the levatores palpebrum to open the eyes. The lips were large and thick with crevices, and the skin lacked elasticity, appearing too big for the body. Down also noted a slightly yellowish tinge to the skin.

In addition to facial characteristics, Down also highlighted several behavioral and other characteristics. Although many individuals, he noted, were able to speak, their speech was often difficult to understand because of the long, thick, and rough tongue. Some were good imitators, with a sense of humor. Motor coordination was poor but could be improved with training. Their circulation was feeble, and intellectual progress was better in the warmer weather, regressing during winter, Down thought. As noted by one of his sons (who later qualified in medicine), a single palmar crease was another characteristic identified by Down.

One omission from Down's initial description was the flat back of the head. This omission is surprising in that Down regularly measured head sizes; he subsequently corrected this omission in his first Lettsomian Lecture. Although the precise number of people seen by Dr. Down presenting with the syndrome remains unknown, Down himself indicated that, "The Mongolian type of idiocy occurs in more than ten per cent of the cases which are presented to me" (Ward, 1999). Down (1866) believed that such individuals could be classified by ethnicity, which added to a generally negative view of people with the syndrome (as Down believed that children with so-called Mongolism were regressive examples of human beings, associated with less developed parts of the world).

While at Royal Earlswood, the first institution in the UK for people with ID, Down was supported by his wife, Mary who, as a volunteer, met parents and families and provided them with support. Mary's work although apparently unpaid, described in the records of the Langdon Down Museum, signals a critical change in the role of women in terms of administrative and family support in the field of disability. Ironically, Langdon Down's grandson, born in 1905, had Down syndrome and lived at Normansfield until he died at age 65 years (Ward, 1999).

When the Board of Earlswood learned that some patients boarded with staff members, they called Down to account, challenging Mary's volunteer administrative role. Down immediately resigned and he and his wife bought Normansfield in 1868 to be a place of care for those with intellectual disability. Most patients at Normansfield appeared to come from reasonably affluent families, able to financially contribute to their care and support. Building on the work they had started at Royal Earlswood, Down and his wife developed a progressive system of intervention, offering people with Down syndrome more than incarceration and care. The Downs espoused the importance of a healthy physical environment, and some patients had inclusive living opportunities in the local community.

The Race to Discover the Genetic Structure of Down Syndrome

A second interesting historical account concerns the genetics discovery of trisomy 21 as the cause of most cases of Down syndrome. As Carter (2002) noted, between 1932 and 1939 four researchers independently conjectured that Down syndrome might be a form of nondisjunction—Waardenburg (1932), Davenport (1932), Bleyer (1934), and Fanconi (1939). In separate papers around the same time, Turpin et al., (1937), Southwick (1939), and Penrose (1939) all proposed that Down syndrome could be due to a chromosomal anomaly, although none mentioned nondisjunction. In 1951, Dr. Jerome Lejeune (Strippoli et al., 2013 a physician and geneticist who dedicated his life to children with intellectual disability and their families, began to study patients with Down syndrome as the protégé of and assistant to Turpin, who was the Head of the Paediatric Unit at Armand Trousseau Hospital and had had a long-term interest in human genetic syndromes, particularly Down syndrome.

Beginning in September 1955, the pediatrician Marthe Gautier spent a year in Boston, where she learned to prepare cell cultures, a key technique for discerning chromosomal structure and number (Gautier & Harper, 2009). On returning to Paris, she accepted a position in Professor Turpin's Laboratory, in a separate section from Lejeune. Lacking a laboratory or the training to produce cell cultures, Turpin accepted Gautier's offer to set up a laboratory, in turn offering to provide her with tissue samples from people with Down syndrome. Gautier's equipment was old, and because she had no funding, she even purchased equipment with her own funds. When the tissue sample arrived on May 22, 1958, she reported distinguishing 47 chromosomes, including 3 small chromosomes. Unable to identify or photograph them for presentation, she accepted Lejeune's offer to take her slides to a better laboratory for photographing. After six months of silence, she learned that Lejeune and Turpin had written up the discovery, about to be published, including Gautier as the second author, with her name spelt incorrectly (as "Gauthier"). Although Gautier asserts that she had done most of the experimental work and was the first to identify an extra chromosome, Lejeune had identified it as chromosome 21. Presenting the slides at the International Conference of Human Genetics in Montreal, August 1958, Lejeune reported he had discovered the cause of Down syndrome.

On 26th January 1959, the Turpin laboratory announced the results of an analysis of their slides in the Proceedings of the Academy of Sciences. At that time, the Turpin group was rushing to beat the English researchers, including Jacobs and Penrose, and the international community had also realized the significance of the discovery. On March 16, 1959, the Turpin team reported nine cases of Down syndrome, and on April 4, 1959, an English Team consisting of Jacobs, Baikie, Court Brown, and Strong, working completely independently, published a paper corroborating the findings from the Turpin team. The trisomy appeared to be number 21, but was not named as such until the 1960 Denver Conference (Gautier & Harper, 2009).

Although the initial findings recognized all three scientists—Lejeune, Gautier, and Turpin—as being involved in the discovery, first Gautier then Turpin were gradually no longer included in various histories of Down syndrome research. Ultimately, to the outside world, it appeared that the discovery of trisomy 21 was solely the work of Lejeune. Over time, Lejeune, a staunch Catholic, was distressed to realize his discovery of trisomy 21 was resulting in prenatal identification of fetuses with Down syndrome and thus leading to abortions. Although Lejeune was expected to win a Nobel Prize for the discovery, he believed his strong public stance against abortion and contraception led to him not being awarded the Prize. Various accounts indicated that Lejeune took solace in the belief that his discovery helped remove the societal shame previously felt by families of people with Down syndrome.

Lejeune and Turpin are no longer alive to speak to their side of this story of the discovery of trisomy 21, but Marthe Gautier's account makes it clear that this discovery should be attributed to her significantly more than history has allowed. This story also emphasizes that science's systemic bias against women and minority researchers was also greatly felt in the field of Down syndrome. Although the almost equal mix of male and female contributors to this volume suggests one step forward toward progress, addressing these inequities likely has a long road ahead. Acknowledging these limitations and stories such as Gautier's is an important first step to a more inclusive science of persons with Down syndrome.

Changing Names: From Mongolism to Down syndrome

A third historical incident concerns the movement to the term Down syndrome, which is today used in most parts of the globe. From the early 1960s until today, many persons—professionals and laypersons alike—complained about the use of the term "Mongolism" first coined by Langdon Down. In 1961, the editor of *The Lancet* received a letter of concern signed by a number of eminent biomedical researchers, requesting a change of name from Mongolism to Down's syndrome (Allen et al., 1961). In 1965, a delegation from Mongolia informally requested that the World Health Organization (WHO) desist from using the names Mongol and Mongoloid.

Reacting to these concerns, the name was changed to Down's syndrome and announced when the WHO awarded Lionel Penrose a prize for his work in this field

(Wright, 2011). Penrose's book, *The Biology of Mental Defect*, published in multiple editions over several decades (1949–1966), was a seminal contribution that devoted considerable space to the syndrome (called Mongolism). Among many discoveries, Penrose examined the relative effects of maternal and paternal age on risk for Down syndrome. Penrose recognized chromosomal translocation in people with the syndrome and their relatives as well as triploid cell cultures from a macerated fetus (1961). Since then, parent coalitions and advocacy groups have preferred certain terms to refer to their loved ones with Down syndrome. At the writing of this volume, people-first language is preferred in this population ("persons with Down syndrome") and the term "intellectual disability" has replaced the earlier diagnostic term "mental retardation."

Behavioral Research and Intervention in Down Syndrome

Although different researchers will disagree as to the first "modern" publication in the behavioral study of persons with intellectual disability, many would point to the book *Mental Deficiency: The Changing Outlook* by Anne and Alan Clarke (1958). The Clarkes began by recounting the early history of the field of intellectual disability (called "mental deficiency" during this period), going on to detail the research, practice, and policy carried out since the end of World War II. They essentially deal with persons with intellectual disability, with limited reference to people with Down syndrome. The text also notes, however, that there was no certain knowledge of the etiology of Down syndrome, but it referred to Penrose's (1949a,b) observation that maternal age at the birth of a child with the syndrome was on average higher than mothers who gave birth to children without it. Those with Down syndrome were still thought to be very limited in their skills, but Clarke and Clarke (1958) noted that there were occasionally individuals assessed who showed higher levels of functioning than typically ascribed to individuals with the syndrome (see, for example, the case described by Cant et al., 1953).

Between December 1963 and November 1964, Janet Carr began a 50-year longitudinal study of individuals with Down syndrome. Repeatedly testing persons with DS over the years, Carr employed a wide range of standardized tests. These tests were consistent with the growing information about the use of appropriate assessment tools. Carr's work thus provided information regarding skills such as language and cognition, but also separately described the challenges facing parents. The results showed both positive and negative features, but overall the results indicated an increasingly optimistic outlook for individuals with Down syndrome (Carr, 1995; Carr & Collins, 2014; also, see Burack et al., this volume)

As the field entered the 1970s, change in research and practice accelerated. This rapid increase in knowledge is reflected in the need by 1974 for an updated third edition of Clarke and Clarke. In this revised third edition, a number of changes are apparent. The subject index now listed 25 entries for Down syndrome, compared with 9 in the book's first edition; such entries were now placed under the heading of Down's syndrome (not Mongolism).

There was increasing recognition that there needed to be some distinction with the category of intellectual disability so as to recognize the unique etiology and characteristics associated with Down syndrome. And, although studies of adverse parenting practices were recognized in the first edition, Clarke and Clarke now recognized that issues of family and other social circumstances have a direct impact on the behavior and development of people with various conditions, including those with Down syndrome (see Brown, 1976).

Also by the 1970s, Down syndrome had been recognized by a wider range of professionals as a complex condition requiring multidisciplinary study and application (Gunzburg, 1974). Research began to stress that individuals with Down syndrome, just as they vary from individual to individual in their physical and medical conditions, also show a wide range of variation in their behaviors (O'Connor & Hermelin, 1974).

Such findings also have important implications for intervention. In 1960, Lyle noted that children whose parents kept them at home, rather than placing them in institutions, seemed to function much more effectively (Tizard, 1964). Lyle identified a range of motor challenges and difficulties in DS that needed to receive greater attention in terms of research, which could then be applied to learning and performance. Cunningham (1996) raised issues surrounding early intervention, especially the differences between young children with Down syndrome who received it and those who did not. Although Cunningham (1987) noted immediate gains in behavior as a result of such intervention, later follow-up suggested that these gains did not appear to be maintained over the long term (Brinkworth, 1973). Wishart (1996) also carried out research into early intervention programs, some of which had shown gains in a wide range of behaviors (e.g., Hayden & Dmitriev, 1975), but at that time the long-term results appeared mixed in terms of what caused the gains (e.g., improved health, management of the child, child baseline abilities). More updated reviews of intervention research and the potential for lasting impacts can be found in many other chapters in this volume.

Interventions were also being examined for specific aspects of behavior in persons with Down syndrome. Speech and language, viewed as important aspects of behavior, develop somewhat differently in Down syndrome from other groups of people with ID. For example, differences in craniofacial and oromotor development in many individuals with Down syndrome hampers speech development and therefore the development of language. Compensation for some of these aspects of speech and language might then be enhanced through strengthening of visual motor skills, including the use of gesture (McCarthy, 1965). With the need for speech therapy came the simultaneous realization that other frontline professionals, such as health visitors and social workers, also needed to have greater knowledge and experience in working with children with Down syndrome (Penwill, 1958). Again, reviews of the current research on speech and language intervention can be found in the chapter by Warren et al. in this volume.

In the United Kingdom, followed by the United States, some of the first major policy and practice changes took place leading to a clearer understanding of ID, including of individuals with Down syndrome. These included the placement of people into training centers, with a few adults even gaining paid employment. Tizard (1964) and Baumeister (1968) carried out research into behavioral studies. Methodology in psychology had become more clearly defined, requiring the use of comparison groups and a clarification of the goals of research. Practical applications occurred that included behavioral training oriented and directed to useful work by adults with Down syndrome (e.g., solder assembly of parts for TV sets).

Recognizing the need for a specialized review, David Gibson (1978) wrote one of the first comprehensive and multifaceted accounts of research, policy, and practice in the Down syndrome field. Gibson noted that the range of intelligence across individuals was wider than had been previously thought, a view later confirmed by Borthwick (1996). Gibson also noted the noticeable effects of auditory distraction in individuals with Down syndrome (compared with people with ID but not Down syndrome). His work underscores the varied performance of people with Down syndrome, ranging from very low levels to occasionally low-average levels of performance, sometimes greater. Gibson also noted that people with DS in institutions performed at lower levels than those living in the community. Such results argued for greater exploration within the Down syndrome population by genetic structure, but also the importance of carrying out comparative studies with individuals who do not have any disabilities.

Gibson (1978) also provided detailed accounts of research in language, motor behavior, and modality effects in learning, reporting studies that provided different and sometimes opposing results and interpretations. Some of these studies contrast Down syndrome with other conditions. Gibson highlighted the need for advanced techniques relating to technology and the need to have more critical research in terms of neurological functions. Gibson (1978) also pointed out that "The DS literature is characteristic of the gap between basic and applied study in Mental Deficiency, and between the biological and the social sciences at the level of remediation" (p. 321). Identical issues persist today, namely the need for greater numbers of evidence-based practices (Mitchell, 2017).

The Changing World for People With Down syndrome

Inspired by this research and policy history, we end by reflecting on the future of persons with Down syndrome. Although more detailed considerations go beyond this chapter and are covered in many of the other chapters in this volume, we highlight issues that most relate to individuals with the syndrome.

Increasing Lifespans and the Movement Toward Healthy Aging

In 1929, a physician caring for a baby with Down syndrome would have realized that the baby's life expectancy was only about 9 years of age (Brown, 1996), increasing to 12 years by 1951 (Penrose & Smith, 1966). By 1975, Carr (1975) reported that the oldest adult in her sample was 63 years of age, and Dalton and Wisniewski (1990) reported three people with Down syndrome who had reached between 74 and 86 years. Overall, the median life expectancy in the syndrome has now reached 58 years (Torr et al., 2010) and is expected to go on increasing. In the economically developed world, there are now more adults than children with Down syndrome (Capie et al., 2006).

Even in the face of increasing life spans, persons with Down syndrome still live, on average, 5 or so years less than do others with ID (Glover et al., 2017), and they experience numerous health problems during later adult years. The expression "accelerated aging" has been used to describe adults with Down syndrome, meaning that in their 40s and 50s these individuals experience certain conditions more commonly seen in much older people. Families as well often report noticeable cognitive declines in their relative in the late 40s or 50s (see Helman et al., this volume).

Consequently, the challenge remains of how accelerated aging can be integrated with "aging well" for someone with the syndrome. Although, in many countries, the lack of studies compromises the ability of agencies and providers to plan for this older population, more people with Down syndrome are living for longer, a situation offering both opportunities and challenges to parent-driven advocacy organizations. One such organization, the National Association for Down Syndrome, USA, long ago took up this challenge, resulting in the development of the first Down syndrome clinic at Lutheran General Hospital in the suburbs of Chicago (Chicoine et al., 1994). This clinic has now been joined by over 50 Down syndrome clinics across the United States (National Down Syndrome Society, 2020), with additional clinics throughout the world.

With the increasing number of children with Down syndrome living into adulthood came the associated need for comprehensive health care and health screening for older adults with Down syndrome. This increasingly large population provided an opportunity to develop services on a long-term (rather than ad hoc) basis, particularly around changing health. Historically, these special needs have been best met when parents are effectively mobilized and multidisciplinary professionals work alongside families to design and pilot proposals for support and intervention (Hassold & Patterson, 1999). Such a specialist facility also avoids the challenge elsewhere that relatively small numbers of people with Down syndrome lead to needs being overlooked or overshadowed, particularly physical or mental health changes. Bigby et al. (2004) recognized that both health and social care support services need to be individualized and that it is important to compensate for loss of skill or function by making adjustments in environmental supports. The emphasis is on adapting the environment to compensate for losses associated with aging, bringing in additional supports where required and available.

Normalization, Inclusive Education, Work, and Community Living

A related issue concerns the movement toward integration that has occurred over the past five decades. In the west and increasingly in low- and middle-income (LAMI) countries, a major change for people with Down syndrome relates to how they have become integrated into home life and community across the life span. Begun in several countries in the late 1960s and early 1970s (Nirje, 1969; Wolfensberger, 1970), the normalization movement has greatly influenced persons with Down syndrome. Such influences—and their connections to Down syndrome—have occurred throughout the world, but especially in the United States, United Kingdom, Australia, and New Zealand.

A first major movement related to Down syndrome-specific educational approaches. Following from early behavioral interventions by Gold (1980), Brown (1976), and Parmenter (1976), specialized education for young children with Down syndrome started first in the United States focused on the preschool years, followed by primary and secondary education. However, such education was still not implemented in all countries, and "special schools" and privately funded schools became part of education provision in many countries. Funding came, in part from associations for persons with ID, and other groups of individuals with ID.

Burgoyne, Baxter, and Buckley (2014) and Moni and Jobling (2010) advocated for detailed education about Down syndrome for teaching personnel, involving not only knowledge of relevant research in literacy and reading but including the movement of research into practice. Although progress is being made, challenges still remain; only recently have some subjects been tackled, such as research into numeracy and mathematics (Faragher & Clarke, 2014).

Upon leaving school, many young adults with Down syndrome struggle in terms of work options. In Rome, for example, young people with Down syndrome have been included in mainstream (regular) education but, after leaving school, have difficulty obtaining meaningful employment, with many remaining at home with parents (doing little) or attending sheltered workshops (Bertoli et al., 2011). Such findings illustrate the challenges of transition, including leaving secondary school education for tertiary education, and adult inclusive living, a topic explored by Hughson and Uditsky (2007) in terms of college and university education and the positive opportunities for social experience.

When people with Down syndrome enter into adulthood, questions of partnership and marriage also arise. Although numbers are increasing, few adults with the syndrome marry or live with a partner, though, as Brown (1996) noted, the partners are typically both loving and supportive. Brown recorded interviews with people with Down syndrome who had married, and the accounts of "Pat and Jim" and "Gretchen and Joe" provide examples demonstrating how lives can be enhanced by such partnerships.

Throughout the young adulthood period, young adults with Down syndrome can also benefit greatly from social support. In a 6-year longitudinal study, Brown (1994) noted modest gains in social performance amongst young adults with Down syndrome, especially once they had additional support and intervention. In addition, those individuals whose parents felt positive about support-based intervention on quality of life (QOL) principles performed better than those whose parents believed their children would never improve. Such intervention had been denied in a care model and not considered in terms of greater opportunities for personal choices and support enabling an individual to increase self-image (Brown & Brown, 2003). Unfortunately, QOL initially focused on adolescents and adults and only entered the education realm for children with Down syndrome as an approach in the late 20th and early 21st centuries (see Brown & Shearer, 1999; Faragher et al., 2014).

Parents, Families, Organizations, and Individuals With Down Syndrome

Offspring with Down syndrome, of whatever age, are greatly influenced by their families. During the last half of the 20th century onwards, there has been considerable growth of parent organizations concerned with Down syndrome. Collectively, parents of children with Down syndrome have formed local parent support groups, which subsequently develop into state, provincial, and even national organizations. In the United Kingdom, the Down Syndrome Association (DSA) was founded in 1970, and from this and other national groups arose Down Syndrome International (DSI) in 1993. A similar progression occurred in the United States, with groups such as the National Down Syndrome Congress (NDSC, founded in 1973) and the National Down Syndrome Society (NDSS; founded 1979) both exceptionally influential. Parent-led organizations that inform and assist parents and their children are now available in many countries.

These parent groups frequently involve professionals at all levels, some of whom are also parents of a child with Down syndrome themselves. Many parents of children with Down syndrome have become educators and researchers, as well as advisers and chairs of government committees. One such pioneering example is Down Syndrome Education International (DSEI), started in 1979 in Portsmouth, UK. DSEI has carried out "hands on" programs for children in infant development, and later in language and reading skills. The organization pioneered fully inclusive education from 1988, a significant move for national and international bodies involving parents and professionals (Buckley & Bird, 2002; Buckley & Sacks, 2002).

On state-province, national, and international levels, major conferences and congresses of DSI, NDSC, and other Down syndrome organizations have become meeting places for parents to share ideas and concerns, along with opportunities for family support. The dynamic developed through such associations and agencies resulted in interaction with the United Nations and included DSI advocacy for recognition, such as the proclamation by the United Nations of "World Down Syndrome Day" (https://worlddownsyndromeday.org/united-nations-resolution-world-down-syndrome-day). At these international conferences and congresses, presented papers are often later published.

In addition to these conference-linked publications, parent groups have had incredible success in publishing easy-to-access guides on a host of topics. In the early 2000s, for example, the Down Syndrome Educational Trust commissioned 12 short books. Based on research and practice and replete with copious photographs illustrating the experiences and needs of adults with Down syndrome and their families, these books touched on topics including: an overview including quality of life; advocacy; spiritual well-being; information technology; drama and the arts; international and cultural aspects; recreation; transition to employment; families; the law; inclusive post-secondary (tertiary) education; and community and independent living. Many authors commented on the need to draw on research that included individuals with Down syndrome and with ID more generally. Other organizations, such as Down's Syndrome Scotland, have also published accessible guides (Watchman, 2003).

Throughout their existences, these parent advocacy organizations have included input from professionals and, increasingly, from individuals with Down syndrome themselves. Historically, regular contributors who related basic research to practice including Cliff Cunningham (1982, revised 2006), who helped parents respond to different or changed behavior in their children with Down syndrome. Similarly, Siegfried Pueschel (1988, 2006) worked with individuals with Down syndrome and their families on a number of medical and nonmedical topics. Such scientist-practitioner contributions were insightful and highly relevant to application across the lifespan of a person with the syndrome, covering such issues as mental health, medical issues and management, and behavioral and developmental issues, as well as the importance of sexuality and challenges of daily life.

To this day, however, the roles of professionals in these parent-centered organizations, and the role of self-advocates, continue to be addressed. For example, can professionals who did not have children with Down syndrome truly understand the needs of families with a child with the syndrome? What is or should be the appropriate role for self-advocates? Ultimately, who "speaks for" the population of individuals with Down syndrome—parents, professionals, self-advocates? More generally, individuals with Down syndrome are increasingly represented on the local and national boards of Down syndrome societies and speak at, or support the organization of, national and international assemblies. This positive outcome has led to greater involvement of people with the syndrome participating in a wide range of activities including paid employment, volunteering, co-researcher roles (Watchman, Mattheys, Doyle, Boustead & Rincones, 2020), speaking at conferences, and linking up together via conference venues and, more recently, the internet.

Concluding Thoughts

Focusing on the identification, causes, names, and early behavioral work on Down syndrome, this chapter highlights some major moments in a long history of advances. But beyond these advances, we also note that much remains to be done to help persons with Down syndrome and their families. Over the years, we have learned of the importance of collaboration among persons with Down syndrome, their parents, and professionals of varied backgrounds. Additionally, we have come to value inclusive bodies—both within the Down syndrome community and in persons with the syndrome participating in the wider community—which help encourage people to be heard and understood. Such inclusive efforts hold within them the ability to affect policy and services. Local efforts soon become represented globally, including associations in countries such as China and India, and individuals with Down syndrome themselves increasingly take part in their own organizational activities. Although many difficult issues remain, from even these few historical events we glimpse the prospects for a brighter future for persons with Down syndrome.

Acknowledgments

Thanks go the following colleagues:

Professor Emeritus Maire Percy for her comments on genetics of Down syndrome.

Mr. Ian Jones-Healey, archivist, Langdon Down Museum and Down's Syndrome Association, for information and useful discussions concerning Dr. Langdon Down and Normansfield.

Also to my wife, Patricia Mary Brown, BA, Cert. PSW, for past and present discussions and editorial comments (on this chapter).

References

Allen, G., Benda, C. E., Böök, J. A., Carter. C. O., Ford, C. E., Chu, C. H., Hanhart, G., . . . Yannet, H. (1961). Mongolism [Letter to the editor]. *The Lancet, 1*, 775. https://scholar.google.com/intl/us/scholar/citations.html

Baumeister, A. A. (1968). *Mental retardation*. London: University of London Press.

Bertoli, M., Biasini, G., Calignano, M. T., Celani, G., De Grossie, G., Digillio.M. C.,Fermariello, C. C., . . . Zuccalà, G. (2011). Needs and challenges of daily life for people with Down syndrome residing in the city of Rome, Italy. *Journal of Intellectual Disability Research, 55*(8), 801–820.

Bigby, C., Balandin, S., Fyffe, C., McCubbery, J., & Gordon, M. (2004). Retirement or just a change of pace: An Australian national survey of disability day services used by older people with disabilities. *Journal of Intellectual & Developmental Disability, 29*(3), 239–254. https://doi.org/10.1080/1366825041233 1285145

Bleyer, A. (1934). Indications that Mongoloid imbecility is a gametic mutation of degressive type. *American Journal of Diseases of Children, 47*(2), 342–348. https://doi.org/10.1001/archpedi.1934.01960090083006

Borthwick, C. (1996). Racism, IQ and Down's syndrome. *Disability & Society, 11*(3), 403–410.

Brinkworth, R. (1973). The unfinished child. Effects of early home training on the Mongol infant. Referenced In A. D. B. Clarke & A. M. Clarke (Eds.), *Mental retardation and behavioral research* (p. 823). Edinburgh and London: Churchill Livingstone.

Brockett, L.P.(1880). *In memory of Edouard Seguin, M.D: Being remarks made by some of his friends at the lay funeral service held October 31, 1880.* (1880). G. P. Putman and Sons. https://collections.nlm.nih.gov/bookviewer?PID=nlm:nlmuid-56220570R-bk

Brown, I., & Brown, R. I. (2003). *Quality of life and disability: An approach for community practitioners*. London: Jessica Kingsley Pubs.

Brown, R. I. (1976). *Psychology and education of slow learners*. Student Library of Education. London: Routledge and Kegan Paul.

Brown, R. I. (1994). Down syndrome and quality of life: Some challenges for future practice. *Down's Syndrome Research and Practice, 2*, (1), 19–30.

Brown, R. I. (1996). Partnership and marriage in Down syndrome. *Down syndrome Research and Practice, 4*(3), 96–99.

Brown, R., & Shearer, J. (1999). Challenges for inclusion within a quality of life model for the 21st century. *Australasian Journal of Special Education, 22*, 180–194.

Buckley, S., & Bird, G. (2002). Cognitive development and education: Perspectives on Down syndrome from a twenty-year research programme. In M. Cuskelly, A. Jobling, & S. Buckley (Eds.), *Down syndrome across the life span* (pp. 66–80). London: Whurr.

Buckley, S., & Sacks, B. (2002). An overview of the development of teenagers with Down syndrome (11-16 years). In S Buckley & G. Bird (Eds.), *Down syndrome issues and information.* Southsea, Hampshire, UK: Down syndrome Educational Trust.

Burack, J. A. (1990). Differentiating mental retardation: The two-group approach and beyond. In R. M. Hodapp, J. A. Burack, & E. Zigler (Eds.), *Issues in the developmental approach to mental retardation* (pp. 27–48). New York: Cambridge University Press.

Burgoyne, K., Baxter, R. & Buckley, S. (2014). Supporting the literacy skills of children with Down syndrome. In R. Faragher & B. Clarke (Eds.), *Educating learners with Down syndrome* (pp 195–220). Oxford: Routledge Education.

Cant, T. W., Gerrard, J. W., & Richards, B. W. (1953). A girl of mongoloid appearance and normal intelligence. *Journal of Mental Science, 99*(416), 560–563.

Capie, A., Contardi, A., & Doehring, D. (2006). Transition to employment. Adult Series: *Down Syndrome Issues and Information.* Southsea, Hampshire, UK: Down Syndrome Educational Trust.

Carr, J. (1975). *Young children with Down's syndrome: Their development, upbringing and effect on their families.* London: Butterworth.

Carr, J. (1995). *Down's syndrome: Children growing up.* Cambridge: Cambridge University Press.

Carr, J., & Collins, S. (2014). Ageing and dementia in a longitudinal study of a cohort with Down syndrome. *Journal of Applied Research in Intellectual Disabilities, 27*(6), 555–563.

Carter, K. C. (2002). Early conjectures that Down syndrome is caused by chromosomal nondisjunction. *Bulletin History of Medicine, 76*(3), 528–563.

Chicoine, B., McGuire, D., Hebein, S., & Gilly, D. (1994). Development of a clinic for adults with Down syndrome. *Mental Retardation, 32*(2), 100–106.

Clarke, A. M., & Clarke, A. D. B. (1958). *Mental deficiency: The changing outlook.* London: Methuen.

Cunningham, C. (1987). Early intervention in Down's syndrome. In G. Hosking and G. Murphy (Eds.) *Prevention of mental handicap: A world view.* Royal Society of Medicine Services International Congress and Symposium Series No. 112, published by Royal Society of Medicine Services Limited.

Cunningham, C. (1996). Families of children with Down syndrome. *Down Syndrome Research and Practice, 4*(3), 87–95.

Cunningham, C. (2006). *Down syndrome: An introduction for parents and teachers* (3rd ed.). London: New Horizons Series.

Dalton, A. J., & Wisniewski, H. M. (1990). Down's syndrome and the dementia of Alzheimer's disease. *International Review of Psychiatry, 2,* 41–50.

Davenport, C. B. (1932). Mendelism in man. *Proc 6th Intern Cong Genetics, 1,* 135–140.

Down, L. J. (1866). Observations on an ethnic classification of idiots. Clinical lecture reports. *London Hospital, 3,* 259–262.

Fanconi, G. (1939). Die Mutationstheorie des Mongolismus. *Schweizerische Medizinische Wochenschrift, 20,* 995–996.

Faragher, R., Broadbent, C., Brown, R. I., & Burgess, J. (2014). Applying the principles of quality of life to education. In J. Merrick (Ed.), *Public health yearbook, 2014* (pp. 131–148). Hauppauge, NY: Nova Science Publishers.

Faragher, R., & Clarke, B. (2014). Mathematical profile of the learner with Down syndrome. In R. Faragher & B. Clarke (Eds.), *Educating learners with Down*

Gautier, M., & Harper, P. S. (2009). Fiftieth anniversary of trisomy 21: Returning to a discovery. *Human Genetics, 126,* 317–324. https://doi.org/10.1007/s00439-009-0690-1

Gibson, D. (1978). *Down's syndrome: The psychology of mongolism.* London: Cambridge University Press.

Glover, G., Williams, R., Heslop, P., Oyinlola, J., & Grey, J. (2017). Mortality in people with intellectual disabilities in England. *Journal of Intellectual Disability Research, 61,* 62–74.

Gold, M. (1980). *Try another way: Training manual.* Research PrChampaign, Ill.

Gunzburg, H. C. (1974). Educational planning for the mentally handicapped. In A. M. Clarke & A. D. B. Clarke (Eds.), *Mental deficiency: The changing outlook* (pp. 628–652). London: Methuen.

Hassold, T. J., & Patterson, D. (Eds.). (1999). *Down syndrome: A promising future, together.* New York: Wiley.

Hayden, A. H., & Dimitriev, V. (1975). The multidisciplinary pre-school program for Down's syndrome children at the University of Washington model pre-school center. In B. Z. Friedlander, G. M. Sterrit, & G. E. Kirk (Eds.), *Exceptional infant: Assessment and intervention, 3,* 193–221. New York: Brunne/Mazel.

Hughson E. A., & Uditsky, B. (2007). *Inclusive post-secondary (tertiary) education for adults with Down syndrome and other developmental disabilities: A promising path to an inclusive lifestyle.* Down Syndrome Education. Down Syndrome Educational Trust.

Séguin, É. (1866). Idiocy: its diagnosis and treatment by the physiological method as cited in Kate Brousseau, *Mongolism: A study of the physical and Mental characteristics of Mongolism Inmbeciles.* London, 1928,1-2.

Jacobs, P. A., Baikie, A. G., Court Brown, W. M., & Strong, J. A. (1959). The somatic chromosomes in mongolism. *Lancet, 1*(7075), 710.

McCarthy, J. M. (1965). *Patterns of psycholinguistic development of mongoloid and non-mongoloid severely retarded children.* [Doctoral dissertation, University of Illinois at Urbana-Champaign]. ProQuest Dissertation & Theses Global. https://www.proquest.com/docview/302117479?pq-origsite=gscholar&fromopenview=true

Mitchell, D. (2017). *Diversities in education: Effective ways to reach all learners.* London: Routledge.

Moni, K. B., & Jobling, A. (2010). Reading-related literacy learning of young adults with Down syndrome: Findings from a three year teaching and research program. *International Journal of Disability, Development and Education, 48*(4), 377–394. https://doi.org/10.1080/10349120120094275

National Down Syndrome Society (NDSS). (2020). Health-care providers: Down Syndrome Specialty Clinics Database. Accessed on June 2, 2020, from https://www.ndss.org/resources/healthcare-providers/

Nirje, B. (1969). The normalisation principle and its human management implications. In R. B. Kugel & W. Wolfensberger (Eds.), *Changing patterns in residential services for the mentally retarded* (pp. 179–195). President's Committee on Mental Retardation.

O'Connor, N., & Hermelin, B. (1974). Specific deficits and coding strategies. In A. M. Clarke & A. D. B. Clarke (Eds.), *Mental deficiency: The changing outlook.* (pp. 330–349). London: Methuen.

Parmenter, T. R. (1976). The vocational development of the learning disabled. Implications for life-long learning. *Australian Journal of Mental Retardation, 4*(1), 8–14.

Penrose, L. S. (1939). Mental disease and crime: Outline of a comparative study of European statistics. *British Journal of Medical Psychology, 18*(1), 1–15. https://doi.org/10.1111%2Fj.2044-8341.1939.tb00704.x

Penrose, L. S. (1949a). *Biology of mental defect.* London: Sidgwick and Jackson Ltd.

Penrose, L. S. (1949b). The incidence of Mongolism in the general population. *Journal of Mental Science, 95,* 685–688.

Penrose, L. S., & Smith, G. F. (1966). *Down's anomaly.* London: J. and A. Churchill, Ltd.

Penwill, M. (1958). Speech disorders and therapy in mental deficiency. In A. M. Clarke & A. D. B. Clarke, *Mental deficiency: The changing outlook* (pp. 393–421). London: Methuen.

Pueschel, S. M. (2006). *Adults with Down syndrome.* Baltimore, MD: Paul H. Brookes.

Pueschel, S.M. (1988). *The young person with Down syndrome: Transition from adolescence to adulthood.* Baltimore, MD: Paul H. Brookes Publishing.

Southwick, W. E. (1939). Time and stage in development at which factors operate to produce Mongolism" *Amer. J. Dis. Child., 57,* 68–89.

Stratford, B. (1989). *Down syndrome: Past, present and future.* London and New York: Penguin Books.

Strippoli, P., Pelleri, M. C., Caracausi, M., Vitale, L., Piovesan, A., Locatelli, C., . . . Barisani, D. (2013). An integrated route to identifying new pathogenesis-based therapeutic approaches for trisomy 21 (Down syndrome) following the thought of Jérôme Lejeune. *Sci Postprint, 1*(1), e00010.

Tizard, J. (1964). *Community services for the mentally handicapped.* Oxford: Oxford University press.

Torr, J., Strydom, A., Patti, P., & Jokinen, N. (2010). Aging in Down syndrome: Morbidity and mortality. *Journal of Policy and Practice in Intellectual Disabilities, 7,* 70–81.

Tredgold, A. F. (1914) *Mental deficiency (Amentia).* London: Balliere, Tindall, & Cox.

Turpin, R., Caratzali, A., & Rogier, H. (1937). Étude étiologique de 104 cas de mongolisme et considérations sur la pathogénie de cette maladie (pp. 154–164). *1er Congrès Latin d'Eugénique: Rapport.*

UK Education Act. (1870). https://www.parliament.uk/about/living-heritage/transformingsociety/livinglearning/school/overview/1870educationact/

U.K. Mental Deficiency Acts of 1913. http://www.educationengland.org.uk/documents/acts/1913-mental-deficiency-act.html

Vardhan, G. (2011). Jean-Etienne Dominique Esquirol. *Archives of Mental Health, 12*(1), 37.

Waardenburg, P. J. (1932). *Das Menschliche Auge und seine Erbanlagen.* Martinus, Nijhoff, Den Haag.

Ward, O. (1999). John Langdon Down: The man and the message. *Down Syndrome Research and Practice, 6*(1), 19–24. https://doi.org/10.3104/perspectives.94

Watchman, K. (2003) *It's your move—the development of a guide for GP's in the diagnosis of dementia in people with Down's syndrome*. Edinburgh: Down's Syndrome Scotland.

Watchman, K., Mattheys, K., Doyle A., Boustead, L., & Rincones O. (2020). Revisiting photovoice: Perceptions of dementia among researchers with intellectual disability. *Qualitative Health Research* , *30*(7), 1019–1032. https://doi.org/10.1177%2F1049732319901127

Wishart, J. G. (1996). Avoidant learning styles and cognitive development in young children. In B. Stratford & P. Gunn (Eds.), *Approaches to Down syndrome*. London: Cassell.

Wolfensberger, W. (1970). The principle of normalization and its implications to psychiatric services. *American Journal of Psychiatry*, *127*(3), 291–297.

Wright, D. (2011). *Downs: The history of a disability*. Oxford: Oxford University Press.

CHAPTER

2 Developmental Traditions in the Study of Persons With Down Syndrome

Jacob A. Burack, Jessica Lai, Jillian Stewart, *and* Oriane Landry

Abstract

This chapter is focused on two lines of pioneering scholarship that were initiated more than a half century ago but continue to resonate in the contemporary study and understanding of the development of persons with Down syndrome. In one line, Janet Carr followed a cohort of persons with Down syndrome from infancy through well into adulthood and provided data about virtually every aspect of their lives, as well as the lives of their families. In a second line, Edward Zigler articulated a developmental approach to the study of persons with intellectual disability that was expanded by Dante Cicchetti and colleagues to also encompass persons with Down syndrome, and by extension persons with other specific physiological etiologies associated with intellectual disability. Both these lines of work contributed to the revised scholarly and lay narratives about persons with Down syndrome in which the emphasis is on the whole person and ways of being rather than on defects and differences.

Key Words: intellectual disability, Down syndrome, developmental approach, longitudinal study, Janet Carr, Edward Zigler, Dante Cicchetti

The study of the development of persons with Down syndrome emanates from two research lines that are clearly distinct despite the considerable overlap in their foci on the manifestation of the phenotype over time and how persons with this condition traverse the lifespan. One of these research lines was the remarkable longitudinal work by Janet Carr that began in 1963 and spanned more than a half century (Carr, 1970a, 1970b, 1975, 1988, 2000, 2003, 2005, 2008, 2012; Carr & Collins, 2014, 2018). Carr's exhaustive and comprehensive research program, which covered development across the cognitive, social, and emotional domains, as well as relationships with family members, was exclusively focused on persons with Down syndrome. In contrast, the second line of research emerged around the same time as part of a much broader nascent movement in the academic scholarship of developmental psychology to integrate classic developmental theory and methodology in the study of persons with atypical developmental histories due to any number or combination of physiological or experiential reasons. Some of the earliest foundational writings in this area of scholarship, known as developmental psychopathology, included a series of papers by Edward Zigler (1966, 1967, 1969), in which he introduced a developmental approach to the study of persons with intellectual disability. Within a decade, Dante Cicchetti and colleagues would expand that approach to include a focus on the social development of children with Down syndrome (for summaries, please see Cicchetti & Beeghly, 1990a; Cicchetti & Ganiban, 1990; Cicchetti & Pogge-Hesse, 1982). Much of that early work by Cicchetti, his colleagues, and a few other pioneers was reviewed and highlighted in Cicchetti and Beeghly's (1990b) landmark edited volume, *Children with Down syndrome: A Developmental Perspective*, the sole academic handbook on persons with Down syndrome based in a developmental framework prior to the publication of the present volume. As is evident in our volume, the study of the development of persons with Down syndrome has grown considerably in the interim three decades since the Cicchetti and Beeghly volume with regard to the numbers of researchers, related disciplines, methodologies, and domains of functioning that are examined.

In this chapter, we briefly review both the Carr and Zigler-Cicchetti lines of research to provide a backdrop against which to interpret the contributions to this volume and the contemporary research on the developmental study of persons with Down syndrome. In doing so, we note the common commitment to understanding the development of persons with Down syndrome despite the considerable differences in contextualization and methodological approaches between these two foundational lines of research.

Janet Carr's Longitudinal Research on Persons With Down Syndrome

In 1963, Carr, who was working as a clinical psychologist at the time, was invited to join a group that had initiated a longitudinal study intended to follow the early lives of a group of infants with Down syndrome born between December 1963 and November 1964 in three boroughs of London and the county of Surrey in the United Kingdom (Carr, 1970a; Murphy & Carr, 2020). Initially, the study involved the evaluation of the developmental trajectories of these infants during their first 4 years of life. However, coinciding with medical advances that allowed persons with Down syndrome to live well into their adult years, the study of long-term outcomes became possible. Inspired by this new opportunity, Carr extended and broadened the scope of the study of these infants to follow their development and relationships with their families throughout their prolonged lifespan. Her commitment to sustaining contact and good rapport with the participating families, largely by sending Christmas cards and by conducting most of the testing personally, was rewarded by the continuous enrollment of a remarkably substantial proportion of the participants for the next half century (Carr & Collins, 2018). Consequently, this landmark longitudinal study led to extraordinary amounts of information about various aspects of the unique development of persons with Down syndrome until the age of 50 years, including their biological, cognitive, and social growth; their relationships with their family members and other persons; involvement in various aspects of the society in which they lived; and the effects of aging and dementia.

At the study's onset, 54 infants with Down syndrome were enrolled, as was a comparison group of typically developing infants matched on age, sex, and socioeconomic factors. The participants with Down syndrome were assessed several times over their first 4 years of life, and again at 11, 16, 21, 30, 35, 40, 45, 47, and 50 years of age (Carr, 1970a, 1975, 1988, 2000, 2003, 2008, 2012; Carr & Collins, 2014, 2018). The typically developing participants were tested at the same age points as the participants with Down syndrome until 3 years of age, after which their testing ceased and information about them was provided solely by their mothers or primary caregivers. Carr also highlighted the role of environmental influences by providing comparisons of those who lived at home with their families and those who were raised in foster homes or institutions. For those who grew up at home, Carr also considered socioeconomic factors as reflected in the nature of the father's or male guardian's employment. In keeping with the emphasis on understanding the life experiences and the quality of life of persons with Down syndrome and their families, the mothers or primary caregivers of both the participants with Down syndrome and the typically developing participants were interviewed when the participants were 15 months old, 4 years old, and at all subsequent test ages, with the exceptions of 16 years old and after age 45 years for the typically developing participants (Carr, 1970b, 1988, 2005; Carr & Collins, 2018).

Over the participants' lifespan, Carr expanded and extended the repertoire of tests and measures to reflect the burgeoning salient issues of the particular age period from infancy through childhood, and from early adulthood to mid-life status. The initial testing with the participants with Down syndrome, from 6 weeks to 4 years of age, involved the administration of the Bayley Infant Scales (Bayley, 1969) to assess mental and motor development (Carr, 1975). At age 11 years, the Merrill-Palmer Scale (Stutsman, 1948) and the Reynell Language Scale (Reynell, 1969) were administered to assess cognitive development and language skills, respectively. After direct testing of the participants was suspended for a decade, it began again at age 21 years, with measures of many different aspects of cognitive, verbal, and academic skills (Carr, 1988). With the increase in life expectancy for persons with Down syndrome, batteries of tests used to assess memory and progression of dementia were added from age 30 years onward to better understand their cognitive progress or decline in adulthood (Carr, 2003; Carr & Collins, 2018). At 15 months, 4 years, and all subsequent time points with the exception of 16 years, measures of daily living skills of the participants and the health and well-being of the family members were also included using a guided interview schedule administered to the mothers or primary caregivers of the participants from both groups (Carr, 1970b, 1975, 1988; Carr & Collins, 2018). Thus, across the decades, Carr provided a broad swath of information across virtually all areas of functioning for persons with Down syndrome from infancy to 50 years of age.

Cognitive Development of Participants With Down Syndrome

With the early administration of the Bayley scales, cognitive development was the longest-standing focus of Carr's research. Several unique patterns of cognitive development were identified among the participants with Down syndrome. Consistent with prior evidence (Dameron, 1963; Dicks-Mireaux, 1966), the IQ scores of the children with Down syndrome declined over the first 4 years of life, from a mean IQ of 80 at 6 months of age to 45 at 4 years of age, indicating a deceleration of development rather than a loss of skills (Carr, 1975). Despite the continued decline in IQ from the outset of the study to age 11 years, an unexpected increase in average IQ was evident at age 21 years (Carr, 1988). Carr suggested that this increase was likely a function, at least to some degree, of the use of rather disparate tools to measure IQ at different ages. Whereas at 11 years IQ was measured with the Merrill-Palmer Scale (Stutsman, 1948), which includes verbal items, at 21 years and onward it was measured with the Leiter International Performance Scale (Leiter, 1980), which does not include verbal items. For those who were not affected by dementia, the mean IQ score of these participants remained stable throughout most of adulthood, with scores ranging in the mid-40s, until a significant decline at age 50 years (Carr, 2003, 2012; Carr & Collins, 2014, 2018).

Several of the other cognition-related patterns identified by Carr arose from her focus on understanding developmental outcomes in relation to various social determinants such as the setting in which the children were raised, including residential and socioeconomic status. At the time of the study, the prevailing preconception was that persons with Down syndrome who lived outside of their family homes were placed at a developmental disadvantage, as evidenced by lower IQ scores among those who were raised in institutions (Centerwall & Centerwall, 1960; Shipe & Shotwell, 1965). Consistent with this finding, the participants with Down syndrome at age 4 years who lived in institutions and foster homes scored lower on the IQ tests than the participants who were raised at home (Carr, 1975). Additionally, social class was associated with cognitive and academic outcomes, as the participants with Down syndrome from families designated as higher social class performed significantly better on language, arithmetic, and reading tests at ages 11 years and 21 years, with significant differences in performance on language tests continuing to be sustained through the ages of 30 years and 35 years (Carr, 1988, 2000, 2003).

Although examples of the relatively superior performance among the participants with Down syndrome who lived in their family homes and were raised in more favorable socioeconomic circumstances were observed over the years, the overall differences between the groups appeared to narrow and diminish as the cohort aged. For example, those who lived at home demonstrated significantly higher IQ scores at age 4 years (Carr, 1975), but this cognitive advantage was not maintained at the later test ages (Carr, 1988, 2000, 2003). With respect to social class, significant differences between the groups were only consistently seen for performance on language tests, but not for the other tests of academic skills (Carr, 1988, 2000, 2003). While the interpretation and analyses of these data may be limited by the small participant group and the gradual attrition of participants throughout the study, these findings, nonetheless, provided considerable insights regarding the role of environments on cognitive and educational outcomes at different points in the lifespan.

Carr also noted sex differences in patterns of cognitive development among the participants with Down syndrome over the course of her research. From as early as 6 weeks until 21 years of age, the female participants with Down syndrome exhibited significantly higher IQs as compared to their male peers (Carr, 1970a, 1975, 1988). Despite fluctuations in IQ scores over time, the scores of the females, in general, remained ever slightly higher than males across the 50 years of testing (Carr, 2000, 2003, 2012; Carr & Collins, 2014, 2018). Moreover, the relative strengths among the females also appeared to extend to other aspects of development. For example, in the case of language abilities, the advantage for the females was consistent over time, with statistically significant differences in scores of expressive language and comprehension at most test ages (Carr, 1988, 2000, 2003, 2012; Carr & Collins, 2014, 2018). Concordantly, the females also scored consistently higher on reading and arithmetic tests at age 21, 30, and 35 years, with the differences being statistically significant at the 21-year age point (Carr, 1988, 2000, 2003). Despite the female sex advantage in cognitive performance among the females for most of the span of the study, all of the participants diagnosed or suspected to be affected by dementia at 47 years of age were females, and four of the five participants diagnosed with dementia at 50 years of age were females.

Everyday Life of the Participants With Down Syndrome and Their Families

As further evidence of Carr's devotion to her participants with Down syndrome, she extended the focus to provide a more holistic perspective through the evaluation both of their adaptive functioning and daily lives broadly construed and of the quality of life and life experiences of their family members. With respect to the adaptive functioning of the participants with Down syndrome, the mother and caregiver reports pointed to considerable accomplishments in development throughout the lifespan, but also to some challenges. For example, the participants appeared to make steady progress in daily living skills, such as skills in feeding, bathing, dressing, and toileting throughout childhood to early adulthood; although less than half of the group were fully independent in all four areas of skills by the age of 21 years (Carr, 1988). This gradual positive trend of improvement in daily living skills was maintained until age 30 years and thereafter began to deteriorate until age 50 years (Carr, 2000, 2003, 2012; Carr & Collins, 2014, 2018). With regard to the daily lives of the participants with Down syndrome, Carr highlighted their limited autonomy and social lives as compared to the typically developing comparison group. At the 40-year age point of the study, Carr (2008) noted that many of the persons with Down syndrome were able to develop friendships over the course of their lives, but only a small subset reported having a best friend and less than a quarter reported having or having had a romantic relationship. Employment rates also followed similar trends as very few of the participants with Down syndrome were actively engaged in the workforce. At

40 years of age, none of the participants were employed full-time, and less than a quarter were employed part-time. The majority of the cohort from age 21 years onward were substantially restricted in their activities, such as being prohibited from staying at home alone for longer than an hour or wandering beyond the garden without supervision (Carr, 1988, 2008). Although the overall picture regarding the everyday life and social functioning of the participants with Down syndrome appeared to be less fulfilling when compared to their typically developing counterparts, Carr considered the achievements that were made throughout development as major accomplishments that should be welcomed and celebrated, as they pointed to both greater independence for the participants and a reduced responsibility for caregiving for their families and caretakers.

Despite the challenges experienced by the persons with Down syndrome, their family members appeared to experience relatively few adverse consequences, as reflected in Carr's study of the overall health and well-being of the mothers, siblings and, to a lesser extent, fathers. For example, when compared to the parents of the typically developing participants, the parents of the participants with Down syndrome reported comparable rates of marital discord and lower rates of divorce (Carr, 1988, 1995). The number of mothers who reported that their child with Down syndrome caused difficulties for their siblings declined with age. Although a small number of mothers considered having a child with Down syndrome to be troublesome for the siblings, the overall consensus was that the experience of having a child with Down syndrome at home was generally positive for the siblings (Carr, 1995, 2005). In addition, Carr (2005) noted that at the 30- and 35-year points of the study, the majority of the mothers of the participants with Down syndrome reported that they were in good health, had an adequate social life, and did not feel particularly burned out or depressed, although they also reported relatively poorer overall life satisfaction, saw less of their families, and had more restricted social lives and holidays than did the mothers of the typically developing participants. These differences between the two groups of mothers were minor and were not consistently observed at every time point. Further, any disparity in scores between the two groups could be partially attributed to the attrition of the more vulnerable and disadvantaged mothers of the typically developing participants (Carr, 2005). As a result, Carr emphasized that any deleterious effects of a child with Down syndrome were considerably less pronounced and devastating than had been portrayed in the common medical and societal narratives.

Carr's extraordinary half-century-long study resulted in a rich body of knowledge and a uniquely informed narrative about the development of persons with Down syndrome across virtually every aspect of their lives, including their cognitive, social, and emotional growth; their relationships with their family; and their functioning in the real world, as well as the challenges that they and their families faced at various life stages. This broad overview across 50 years of life continues to be essential to the scientific, professional, and societal understanding of persons with Down syndrome.

The Zigler-Cicchetti Developmental Approach

In contrast to Carr's exclusive focus on persons with Down syndrome, Zigler (1967, 1969) articulated a developmental approach to the study of persons with intellectual disability generally that was initially applied to persons with "familial" intellectual disability (i.e., those whose intellectual disability was considered to be due to the genetic transmission of lower levels of intelligence and impoverished environmental factors rather than to any identifiable physiological condition or syndrome). An expanded version of this developmental approach was subsequently applied by Cicchetti and colleagues (e.g., Cicchetti & Beeghly, 1990a; Cicchetti & Ganiban, 1990; Cicchetti & Pogge-Hesse, 1982) specifically to persons with Down syndrome, but with implications for the study of all persons with any type of physiological condition or syndrome associated with intellectual disability. Rather than segregating the study of persons with Down syndrome or other syndromes or conditions from mainstream developmental research, the challenge was to provide a framework in which these populations could be studied with rigor and precision within the context of universal developmental processes. This approach reflected a stark departure from, or even a rejection of, the prevailing notions of intellectual disability at the time, which were coined by Zigler and colleagues as "defect theories" as they were almost exclusively focused on identifying impairments in one or more specific cognitive processes or functions that differentiated persons with intellectual disability from everyone else (for a collection of papers regarding the developmental versus defect approaches to intellectual disability, please see Zigler & Balla, 1982).

Originally trained as a clinical psychologist, Zigler's career spanned more than a half-century as a researcher, policy maker, and advocate for children and their families from all sorts of backgrounds and with all sorts of levels of abilities. For example, early in his career, Zigler was tapped by President Lyndon B. Johnson to join the committee that founded the Head Start program, the seminal early intervention program oriented toward low-income children and their parents (mostly mothers) aimed at benefiting long-term academic outcomes. Throughout the rest of his life, Zigler would continue to work with and advocate for these children and their families, for children with histories of maltreatment, for children with intellectual disability, and for essentially all children whose development was at risk for any number of reasons. All this work was guided by the three premises that (a) developmental theory could and should be applied to all children; (b) developmental research must include consideration of the whole child, including the child's biological, cognitive, social, and emotional well-being, as well as relationships with family members and other persons and aspects of the society in which the child lives; and (c) the rigor of developmental research in all contexts and with all children must meet the highest scientific standards of the time (for reviews, see Burack, Evans et al., 2021b; Burack, Russo et al., 2021a). These integrative ideas were articulated in a series of papers in the mid- to late 1960s in which Zigler (e.g., 1966, 1967, 1969) formalized a developmental approach to intellectual disability that was based in universal developmental theory.

The essential quandary in this new approach to intellectual disability was: How could the developmental patterns, or structures, of populations with specific organic etiologies, such as Down syndrome, and their distinct profiles of strengths and weaknesses fit within the traditional notions and constraints of universal structures of development? This developmental question was the basis of Cicchetti's (1977) Ph.D. dissertation, *Affective Development in Down's Syndrome Infants: An Organizational Perspective,* and foundational to a series of empirical studies and conceptual papers and chapters. Along with his colleagues (e.g., Cicchetti & Serafica, 1981; Cicchetti & Sroufe, 1976, 1978), Cicchetti extended Zigler's developmental approach to the study of the social development of persons with Down syndrome. Unlike Zigler's emphasis on persons with familial intellectual disability, whose IQ could be thought to be the outcome of the genetic transmission of intelligence and environmental conditions and therefore within the normal distribution of intelligence, the study of persons with Down syndrome involved a population with a clear physiological basis and with obvious medical, physical, and behavioral characteristics that impacted IQ in ways not seen among the general population. This unique phenotype of Down syndrome presented a particularly daunting theoretical challenge to any developmental conceptualization.

The need to integrate a population-specific pattern of functioning within a traditional developmental perspective that was usually applied to typical developmental patterns led Cicchetti and colleagues to label their model as a "liberal" developmental approach. They tasked themselves with reconciling and making sense of the unique profile of persons with Down syndrome within the framework of universal developmental theories. These early articulations (Cicchetti & Beeghly, 1990a; Cicchetti & Pogge-Hesse, 1982) were highlighted in their contribution to Zigler and colleagues' early edited volumes on intellectual disability, *Mental Retardation: The Developmental-Difference Controversy* (Zigler & Balla, 1982), and the *Issues in the Developmental Approach to Mental Retardation* (Hodapp, Burack, & Zigler, 1990). Conversely, Hodapp and Zigler articulated the developmental foundation to the study of persons with intellectual disability as it could apply to persons with Down syndrome (Cicchetti and Beeghly, 1990b). Across these chapters, the prevailing theme was that the study of children with Down syndrome provided a compelling extension of developmental theory and principles that were previously only applied to the study of typically developing persons and by Zigler to persons with familial intellectual disability. As Cicchetti and Ganiban (1990) highlighted, the application of developmental theory and methodology is largely guided by Werner's (1957) universal organismic-developmental approach in which typical and atypical patterns of development are reconciled. Within this context, the study of persons with Down syndrome provided a particularly stringent test of the universality of developmental theory with the task of finding coherence among developmental patterns that appear to diverge so significantly from the typical structure of development (Wagner, Ganiban, & Cicchetti, 1990).

The state of the art of thinking about children with Down syndrome in 1990 included consideration of the whole child and a transactional conception of how children interact with their environments and how those in the environment respond to them. Biopsychosocial transactional models prompted the notion that what any child puts out into the world elicits responses that are driven by the unique circumstances of the responder, the context in which the interaction occurs, and the child themselves. The central themes of the volume revolved around the normalcy and uniqueness questions: Do children with Down syndrome differ from typically developing children, and if so do they differ in ways that are unique to Down syndrome (different from other children with intellectual disability), or is their difference merely a slowing down of the pace of skill acquisition? Consistent with the liberal developmental approach proposed by Cicchetti and colleagues, the specific emphasis was on the organization and coherence of development within or between specific domains of development. Reflecting the whole child approach, these types of developmental issues were addressed across a range of domains, including cognitive, social, emotional, linguistic, and familial, as well as various sub-domains within some of these broad topics.

Conclusions

As we conclude this chapter, we note that both Janet Carr and Edward Zigler passed away in the interim since this volume was initiated. Carr was originally slated to lead off this volume with a retrospective chapter in which she would review her life's work, but unfortunately that never came about. As a result, one of our goals in this chapter was to provide a glimpse into Carr's compelling legacy in the study and understanding of the development of persons with Down syndrome over their increasingly expanded lifespan. Her work was elegant, thorough, and visionary. Carr addressed the whole person with Down syndrome throughout the first 50 years of life as she included measures on cognitive, language, social, and emotional development, as well as on various aspects of parent well-being. This emphasis on the whole person was also central to Zigler's work with persons with intellectual disability more generally, as he highlighted the essential role of motivational-personality factors in development that both were affected by life experiences and affected every aspect of functioning and well-being. With this common theme, Carr and Zigler contributed to a changing narrative in which persons with Down syndrome and those with intellectual disability more generally were viewed with regard to their humanity and ways of being rather than with regard to deficits or limitations.

This type of reframing of attitudes was reflected in Cicchetti and colleagues' application of developmental theory to persons with Down syndrome. For example, in describing their rationale for applying a developmental approach to the study of persons with Down syndrome, Cicchetti and Pogge-Hesse (1982) rejected the deficit approach because it did not include consideration of the essential aspects of development that are common to all children—organization, integration, and adaptation. In stark contrast, they argued that "the important and challenging research questions concern the developmental process" (p. 279). This imperative was at the heart of the efforts to expand the developmental approach to entail the search for universal coherence even across patterns of development, such as seen among persons with Down syndrome that did not appear to conform to the norm (e.g., Cicchetti & Beeghly, 1990a; Cicchetti & Ganiban, 1990; Cicchetti & Serafica, 1981; Cicchetti & Sroufe, 1978). Thus,

> the goal of the work was not to study "does x have y" but rather "in what way does x use y" and does a particular mental structure interact with other mental structures in the same way in one. . . group as in another?
>
> *(Cicchetti & Pogge-Hess, 1982, p. 313)*

Cicchetti and Beeghly's (1990b) collection of chapters on the cutting-edge knowledge of specific areas and sub-areas of functioning among persons with Down syndrome, mostly infants and young children, was a first attempt to identify and delineate the ways that their development is organized. As evidenced in this volume, three decades later, this topic-focused approach continues to prevail in the study of persons with Down syndrome, as it does with other groups of persons with a specific type of intellectual disability or developmental condition (e.g., Burack et al., 2012).

The volume, like Ciccheti and Beeghly's (1990b), is organized around the study of clearly defined areas of functioning among persons with Down syndrome at specific mental and/or chronological ages, usually in relation to typically developing persons and sometimes in relation to groups of persons with other conditions associated with intellectual disability. As is the case generally with contemporary scientific work, the advantage of this approach is the advent of increasingly sophisticated, often technologically advanced, and rigorous methodologies that can contribute to similarly nuanced and fine-tuned conceptualizations or theories of functioning and abilities. However, this approach also comes with its limitation as it represents the type of fractionated science that dominates contemporary research and, in our case, leads to a limited understanding of the developmentally organized whole person. In keeping with both the Carr and Zigler/Cicchetti legacies, we tried to emulate the whole-person approach to understanding persons with Down syndrome by covering a wide range of topics in this volume, with leading scholars in the field contributing the relevant theory and empirical findings. However, as is the case with virtually all aspects of research, and especially research about specific populations, our current knowledge reflects a hit-or-miss type of understanding depending on the expertise and interest of the experimenter in relation to the specific ages or developmental levels of the participants who are available. Thus, rather than depicting some coherent picture or body of knowledge, this work reflects a mosaic approach in which pieces need to be fit together to provide some larger narrative about the development of persons with Down syndrome. This leads to a clearly more disjointed picture than provided by Janet Carr but also reflects the considerable advances over the past few decades in understanding the development of persons with Down syndrome across many different aspects of their lives.

References

Bayley, N. (1969). *Manual for the Bayley scales of infant development.* Psychological Corporation.

Burack, J. A., Russo, N., Flores, H., Iarocci, G., & Zigler, E. (2012). The more you know the less you know, but that's OK: Developments in the developmental approach to intellectual disability. In J. A. Burack, R. M. Hodapp, G. Iarocci & E. Zigler (Eds.), *The Oxford handbook of intellectual disability and development* (pp. 3–10). Oxford University Press.

Burack, J. A., Russo, N., Evans, D. W., Napoleon, J. S., Goldman, K., & Iarocci, G. (2021a). Developmental perspectives on the study of persons with intellectual disability. *Annual Review of Clinical Psychology, 17,* 339–363. https://doi.org/10.1146/annurev-clinpsy-081219-090532

Burack, J. A., Evans, D. W., Napoleon, J. S., Weva, V. K., Russo, N., & Iarocci, G. (2021b). The science of humanity and the humanity of science: Perspectives on Ed Zigler's contributions to developmental psychopathology and the study of all children. *Development and Psychopathology, 33,* 441–452. https://doi.org/10.1017/S0954579420002011

Carr, J. (1970a). Mental and motor development in young Mongol children. *Journal of Intellectual Disability Research, 14*(3), 205–220. https://doi.org/10.1111/j.1365-2788.1970.tb01116.x

Carr, J. (1970b). Mongolism: Telling the parents. *Developmental Medicine & Child Neurology, 12*(2), 213–221. https://doi.org/10.1111/j.1469-8749.1970.tb01892.x

Carr, J. (1975). *Young children with Down's syndrome: Their development, upbringing, and effect on their families.* Butterworth for the Institute for Research into Mental and Multiple Handicap.

Carr, J. (1988). Six weeks to twenty-one years old: A longitudinal study of children with Down's syndrome and their families. *Journal of Child Psychology and Psychiatry, 29*(4), 407–431. https://doi.org/10.1111/j.1469-7610.1988.tb00734.x

Carr, J. (1995). *Down's syndrome: Children growing up.* Cambridge University Press.

Carr, J. (2000). Intellectual and daily living skills of 30-year-olds with Down's syndrome: Continuation of a longitudinal study. *Journal of Applied Research in Intellectual Disabilities, 13*(1), 1–16. https://doi.org/10.1046/j.1468-3148.2000.00003.x

Carr, J. (2003). Patterns of ageing in 30–35-year-olds with Down's syndrome. *Journal of Applied Research in Intellectual Disabilities, 16*(1), 29–40. https://doi.org/10.1046/j.1468-3148.2003.00129.x

Carr, J. (2005). Families of 30–35-year olds with Down's syndrome. *Journal of Applied Research in Intellectual Disabilities, 18*(1), 75–84. https://doi.org/10.1111/j.1468-3148.2004.00226.x

Carr, J. (2008). The everyday life of adults with Down syndrome. *Journal of Applied Research in Intellectual Disabilities, 21*(5), 389–397. https://doi.org/10.1111/j.1468-3148.2007.00418.x

Carr, J. (2012). Six weeks to 45 years: A longitudinal study of a population with Down syndrome. *Journal of Applied Research in Intellectual Disabilities, 25*(5), 414–422. https://doi.org/10.1111/j.1468-3148.2011.00676.x

Carr, J., & Collins, S. (2014). Ageing and dementia in a longitudinal study of a cohort with Down syndrome. *Journal of Applied Research in Intellectual Disabilities, 27*(6), 555–563. https://doi.org/10.1111/jar.12093

Carr, J., & Collins, S. (2018). 50 years with Down syndrome: A longitudinal study. *Journal of Applied Research in Intellectual Disabilities, 31*(5), 743–750. https://doi.org/10.1111/jar.12438

Centerwall, S. A., & Centerwall, W. R. (1960). A study of children with Mongolism reared in the home compared to those reared away from the home. *Pediatrics, 25*(4), 678–685.

Cicchetti, D. (1977). *Affective development in Down's syndrome infants: An organizational perspective* (Publication No. 7809641) [Doctoral dissertation, University of Minnesota]. ProQuest Dissertations & Theses Global.

Cicchetti, D., & Beeghly, M. (1990a). An organizational approach to the study of Down syndrome: Contributions to an integrative theory of development. In D. Cicchetti, & M. Beeghly (Eds.), *Children with Down syndrome: A developmental perspective* (pp. 29–62). Cambridge University Press.

Cicchetti, D., & Beeghly, M. (Eds.). (1990b). *Children with Down syndrome: A developmental perspective.* Cambridge University Press.

Cicchetti, D., & Ganiban, J. (1990). The organization and coherence of developmental processes in infants and children with Down syndrome. In R. M. Hodapp, J. A. Burack & E. Zigler (Eds.), *Issues in the developmental approach to mental retardation* (pp. 169–225). Cambridge University Press.

Cicchetti, D., & Pogge-Hesse, P. (1982). Possible contributions of the study of organically retarded persons to developmental theory. In E. Zigler & D. Balla (Eds.), *Mental retardation: The developmental-difference controversy* (pp. 277–318). Lawrence Erlbaum Associates.

Cicchetti, D., & Serafica, F. C. (1981). The interplay among behavioral systems: Illustrations from the study of attachment, affiliation, and wariness in young Down's syndrome children. *Developmental Psychology, 17*(1), 36–49. https://doi.org/10.1037//0012-1649.17.1.36

Cicchetti, D., & Sroufe, L. A. (1976). The relationship between affective and cognitive development in Down's syndrome infants. *Child Development, 47*(4), 920–929. https://doi.org/10.1111/j.1467-8624.1976.tb02271.x

Cicchetti, D., & Sroufe, L. A. (1978). An organizational view of affect: Illustration from the study of Down's syndrome infants. In M. Lewis & L. Rosenblum (Eds.), *The development of affect* (pp. 309–350). Plenum Press.

Dameron, L. E. (1963). Development of intelligence of infants with Mongolism. *Child Development, 34*(3), 733–738. https://doi.org/10.2307/1126766

Dicks-Mireaux, M. J. (1966). Development of intelligence of children with Down's syndrome: Preliminary report. *Journal of Mental Deficiency Research, 10*(2), 89–93. https://doi.org/10.1111/j.1365-2788.1966.tb00176.x

Hodapp, R. M., Burack, J. A., & Zigler, E. (Eds.). (1990). *Issues in the developmental approach to mental retardation.* Cambridge University Press.

Leiter, R. G. (1980). *Leiter international performance scale: Instruction manual.* Stoelting.

Murphy, G., & Carr, S. (2020). Dr Janet Carr: Obituary. *Journal of Applied Research in Intellectual Disabilities, 33*, 1541–1543 https://doi.org/10.1111/jar.12766

Reynell, J. (1969). *Reynell developmental language scales.* National Foundation for Educational Research.

Shipe, D., & Shotwell, A. M. (1965). Effect of out-of-home care on Mongoloid children: A continuation study. *American Journal of Mental Deficiency, 69*(5), 649–652.

Stutsman, R. (1948). *Merrill-Palmer scale of mental tests.* Western Psychological Services.

Wagner, S., Ganiban, J., & Cicchetti, D. (1990). Attention, memory, and perception in infants with Down syndrome: A review and commentary. In D. Cicchetti & M. Beeghly (Eds.), *Children with Down syndrome: A developmental perspective* (pp. 147–179). Cambridge University Press.

Werner, H. (1957). The concept of development from a comparative and organismic point of view. In D. B. Harris (Ed.), *The concept of development* (pp. 125–148). University of Minnesota Press.

Zigler, E. (1966). Mental retardation: Current issues and approaches. In L. W. Hoffman & M. L. Hoffman (Eds.), *Review of child development research: Volume 2* (pp. 107–168). Russell Sage Foundation.

Zigler, E. (1967). Familial mental retardation: A continuing dilemma. *Science, 155*(3760), 292–298. https://doi.org/10.1126/science.155.3760.292

Zigler, E. (1969). Developmental versus difference theories of mental retardation and the problem of motivation. *American Journal of Mental Deficiency, 73*(4), 536–556.

Zigler, E., & Balla, D. (Eds.). (1982). *Mental retardation: The developmental-difference controversy.* Lawrence Erlbaum.

SECTION 2

Social Development and Family Relations

CHAPTER

3 Social-Emotional Competence in Down Syndrome

Amanda D. Nunnally *and* Connie L. Kasari

Abstract

This chapter aims to synthesize historical and contemporary literature to provide an overarching understanding of social-emotional competence in individuals with Down syndrome, where social-emotional competence refers to the skills necessary to allow for successful social relationships, as well as the ability to regulate the experience and expression of emotions. Using the framework of Rose-Krasnor's prism model, this chapter addresses each of the four components that underlie the development of social-emotional competence: self-regulation, social awareness, prosocial orientation, and social problem-solving. The development of each of these components is described for individuals with Down syndrome, and a description of the typical developmental trajectory is given for reference. The short-term and long-term implications of each component are also discussed, as they relate to the individual's overall social-emotional competence. This overview aims to highlight what is known regarding social-emotional competence in individuals with Down syndrome, as well as to identify areas in which knowledge is lacking.

Key Words: Down syndrome, social-emotional competence, self-regulation, social awareness, prosocial orientation, social problem-solving

Introduction

Individuals with Down syndrome (DS) have historically been regarded as having a relative strength in their social abilities and are commonly described as being very sociable, affectionate, happy, and skilled at understanding others (Gibbs & Thorpe, 1983). This perception led to the coining of the term "Down Syndrome Advantage" (Hodapp, Ly, Fidler, & Ricci, 2001), which refers to a phenomenon in which families of individuals with DS report less stress (Hodapp et al., 2001) and more positive benefits (Burke, Fisher, & Hodapp, 2012) than families of individuals with other developmental disabilities. Since this was a prevailing belief, researchers operated under the assumption that social-emotional development in children with DS mirrored the developmental trajectory of typically developing (TD) children. However, in recent years, both differences and similarities in social-emotional competence have been identified between individuals with DS and their TD counterparts. Further evidence suggests that individuals with DS may follow a different trajectory in the development of components necessary for social-emotional competence.

Broadly, the term "social-emotional competence" has been used to refer to the skills necessary to allow for successful social relationships, as well as the ability to regulate the experience and expression of emotions (Rose-Krasnor & Denham, 2009). Together, these skills create the foundation for successful social interactions, marked by sustained peer engagement and positive emotion expression (Rose-Krasnor & Denham, 2009). Social-emotional competence has implications beyond peer relationships, with developmentally appropriate social-emotional competence in TD preschoolers predicting more positive attitudes towards school, better school adjustment, and future academic achievement (Birch, Ladd, & Blecher-Sass, 1997; Ladd, Birch, & Buhs, 1999; Ladd, Kochenderfer, & Coleman, 1996).

Social-Emotional Competence

Social-emotional competence is a complex and multi-faceted construct, comprised of various skills and abilities that enable an individual to succeed at two fundamental developmental tasks: (a) Sustaining positive engagement with peers and (b) regulating emotional experience and expressiveness (Rose-Krasnor & Denham, 2009). In order to identify the various components that comprise social-emotional competence and to elucidate the theoretical relationships among them, Rose-Krasnor (Rose-Krasnor & Denham, 2009) provides a prism model of social-emotional competence. At the base level of the model, Rose-Krasnor identifies four components that serve as the building blocks for social-emotional competence: self-regulation, social awareness, prosocial orientation, and social problem-solving. Each of the four components subsumes several traits that will be explored and expounded upon in this chapter.

In the second tier of the theoretical model, Rose-Krasnor identifies success in attaining both intra- and interpersonal goals as necessary for successful social interactions and social development (Rose-Krasnor & Denham, 2009). The inclusion of both intra- and interpersonal goal attainment in the second tier of the model is based on the conclusion that each is representative of a different aspect of social-emotional development. The successful achievement of intrapersonal goals, or goals that are based on an individual's own needs and desires, is thought to be indicative of the development of autonomy and agentic development, whereas interpersonal goal attainment is indicative of social development (Rose-Krasnor & Denham, 2009). The combination of these two types of goal-oriented behaviors is thought to be necessary for overall social-emotional competence.

At the top tier of the prism model of social-emotional competence lies "effectiveness in interaction," which is thought to be a result of successful goal-oriented behavior that meets both short- and long-term developmental needs. In order to be effective in social interactions, an indicator of social-emotional competence, an individual must develop a strong foundation in a range of social and emotional skills. Furthermore, an individual must then be able to apply these abilities to organize and achieve both intra- and interpersonal goals. The culmination of these skills and abilities leads to effective social interactions and, as such, social-emotional competence.

Social-Emotional Competence in Children With Down Syndrome

Broadly, children with Down syndrome have been found to have a mixed profile of strengths and weaknesses in social-emotional competence. When compared to children with other types of intellectual and developmental disabilities, children with DS displayed better social adaptation and overall social outcomes once chronological age (CA) and IQ were taken into consideration (Cebula & Wishart, 2008; Wishart, Cebula, Willis, & Pitcairn, 2007). Relative weaknesses in the social-emotional profile of children with DS emerged when looking at more discrete skills such as social cognition, emotion recognition, emotion expressiveness, and emotion regulation (Abbeduto, Evans, & Dolan, 2001; Cebula, Wishart, Willis, & Pitcairn, 2017; Fidler, Barrett, & Most, 2005; Jahromi, Gulsrud, & Kasari, 2008; Kasari & Freeman, 2001; Kasari, Mundy, Yirmiya, & Sigman, 1990; Wishart & Pitcairn, 2000). Despite these weaknesses, children with DS also showed relative strengths in social motivation and emotion responsiveness when compared to children with other types of intellectual and developmental disabilities (Fidler, Most, Booth-LaForce, & Kelly, 2008; Kasari, Freeman, Mundy, & Sigman, 1995; Kasari, Freeman, & Bass, 2003). This combination of strengths and weaknesses makes for a very unique social-emotional profile for children with DS. A better understanding of this unique profile and the way in which it impacts the developmental trajectory of children with DS will contribute to a better understanding of how caregivers, teachers, and service providers can best facilitate optimal social-emotional development in this population.

In this review, we will describe the developmental trajectory of each individual component of social-emotional among children with DS, as outlined in the base level of Rose-Krasnor's prism theory of social-emotional competence. In order to contextualize the discussion of each component in DS, the reader will be oriented to the developmental trajectory and milestones in typical development. We will also discuss the implications of these components as relating to effectiveness in social interaction, the fundamental developmental task that is thought to represent the achievement of social-emotional competence.

Components of Social-Emotional Competence

According to Rose-Krasnor's (Rose-Krasnor & Denham, 2009) prism model of social-emotional competence, there are four base components that are foundational to achieving social-emotional competence: self-regulation, social awareness, prosocial orientation, and social problem-solving. In order to discuss the components that predicate the development of social-emotional competence, it is important to first address how children begin to experience their emotions, a process that has been referred to as emotion expression.

Emotion Expression

Emotion expression refers to the frequency, intensity, and duration of basic and complex emotions experienced by an individual (Denham, 2006). These affective expressions are foundational for effective social interactions, as they allow children to signal whether they need others to alter or persist with their goal-directed behavior (Campos, Mumme, Kermoian, & Campos, 1994). They also allow children to use emotional communication to nonverbally express their feelings toward certain social situations or events. Among TD preschoolers, a child's profile of emotion expressiveness is related to the child's perceived effectiveness in social interactions (Denham, 2006).

Beginning very early in life, TD infants are capable of expressing emotions. Researchers have reported evidence of infants expressing basic emotions such as happiness, sadness, and anger, although, at first, they may not be intentional or functional (Izard & Malatesta, 1987). Facial expressions are considered some of the earliest forms of nonverbal communication used by infants, and they play an important role in the socialization of children. When children display emotion expressions, whether they are negative or positive expressions, they elicit certain responses from their caretakers. These responses may include meeting the child's needs, which teaches the child an important lesson regarding eliciting assistance from their caretaker, or the labeling of emotions, which contributes to the child's socialization and understanding of their own emotions (Lewis & Michalson, 1983).

Early evidence indicated that children with DS had low postural tone, lessened intensity of affective expression, and greater variability in temperament (Bridges & Cicchetti, 1982; Cicchetti & Sroufe, 1978; Emde, Kligman, Reich, & Wade, 1978). Contradictory evidence has since emerged, suggesting that children with DS (MA = 26 months) display similar amounts of affect as MA-matched TD children (Kasari et al., 1990), although qualitative differences may be apparent. In a second study conducted by Kasari and colleagues (1990) with preschool-aged children with DS (MA = 26 months), researchers observed children's facial expressions as they interacted with an experimenter. The children with DS displayed similar amounts of affective expression as their TD MA-matched counterparts. Although the children with DS showed comparable frequency of emotion expressions as the MA-matched TD children, qualitative differences were seen in the way that the children expressed positive emotions. The children with DS displayed more slight smiles than the TD children and appeared to shift facial expressions more frequently than their TD counterparts, leading to less sustained emotional expressions. These findings seem to be consistent with evidence of lessened intensity of positive affect and more variability in temperament as reflected by the frequent shifts of affective states among children with DS (Emde et al., 1978, Bridges & Cicchetti, 1982).

Positive affect and indeed the sociability effect with DS children yield inconsistent findings across studies. Some researchers have found evidence of greater positive affect among children with DS (Capps, Kasari, Yirmiya, & Sigman, 1993; Kasari & Sigman,

1996), while others have found evidence of less positive affect than their TD peers (Bieberich & Morgan, 2004; Brooks-Gunn & Lewis, 1982). These conflicting findings may be due to differences in methodology, mainly in sample characteristics and measurement strategies (Sigman & Ruskin, 1999). This seems especially likely since different studies of emotion expression in children with DS tend to vary in the ages of the participants (Bieberich & Morgan, 2004; Brooks-Gunn & Lewis, 1982; Kasari & Sigman, 1996). When age is considered, the evidence appears to suggest that young children with DS appear to display positive affect as frequently as their TD peers, but that these displays tend to decrease as children age. In addition, children with DS have been reported to have increasingly negative affect as they grow older (Fidler et al., 2005). Together, these findings indicate that children with DS tend to express emotion comparably to TD children early in life, despite some qualitative differences in intensity and shifting of expression. Differences in emotion expression between children with DS and TD children seem to appear as the children approach middle and later childhood, which may be related to a slowing in development of cognitive abilities that children with DS experience during childhood.

Complex emotions, such as shame, guilt, and pride, begin to emerge in TD children between the ages of 1 and 2 years and continue to evolve and differentiate as children grow older (Lewis, 1993). The emergence of these complex emotions is preceded by the development of certain cognitive antecedents, such as the ability to recognize oneself as distinct from others and the ability to engage in perspective taking (Sigman & Ruskin, 1999).

As the emergence of complex emotion expression relies upon the development of socio-cognitive skills (Sigman & Ruskin, 1999) that may be impaired among children with DS (Abbeduto et al., 2001), the study of the manifestation of complex emotions is difficult in this population. In the only study on the expression of complex emotions among children with DS that was found in a search of studies on shame, guilt, or pride among children with DS, Hughes and Kasari (2000) asked children (MA = 40 months) with DS to complete a moderately challenging puzzle task in the presence of their mother. The children's interactions with their caregivers were analyzed for positive affect; social orientation, such as calling the adult's attention to the task; and task-related behaviors, such as verbal exclamations like "I did it!" Hughes and Kasari used these three types of behaviors as indicators of pride because young children typically show pride in their accomplishments by smiling and sharing their work with adults, as well as by making statements regarding their success. As compared to the group of MA-matched TD children, the behavior of the children with DS indicated pride, with greater social orientation and more task-related behaviors (Hughes & Kasari, 2000). Although this study offers some insight into the way pride may be expressed among this population, more research is needed on the manifestation of other complex emotions, such as guilt and shame, among children with DS.

Self-Regulation

Emotion regulation. The ability to monitor, evaluate, and modify emotional reactions is called emotion regulation (Thompson, 1994). A separate construct from emotion reactivity, or the experience of the emotion itself, emotion regulation is the process of regulating one's experience of a given emotion (Eisenberg & Spinrad, 2004). In typical development, children show evidence of emotion regulatory behavior as early as 5 months of age (Stifter & Braungart, 1995), as they display self-soothing behaviors or orientation to caregiver as a means of reducing emotional reactivity.

These regulatory strategies become more sophisticated with age, moving from physical self-soothing behaviors in the first year of life (Tronick, 1989) to include a new and more complex use of objects and interactions to regulate emotional states as the child develops (Diener & Mangelsdorf, 1999). By preschool age, children display cognitively sophisticated strategies, such as attentional shifting to active engagement, as a child may purposefully shift their attention to a new task in order to regulate their emotions (Morris et al., 2011). These changes are attributed to advances in cognitive, motor, and language development that occur over the first 5 years of life, enabling children to implement a broader range of emotion regulation strategies than in infancy.

The role of the caregiver is also essential to the process of children's regulation of their own emotions. For example, Field (1994) found that mothers regulate their infant's emotional states by providing appropriate stimulation, modulating the infant's arousal, and responding reciprocally to the infant's reactions, and Denham (1993) found that mothers responded emotionally to their children in systematic and temporally contingent ways, indicating that the pattern of coregulation continues with development. In addition to actively assisting children in the regulation of their emotions, the mere presence of a caregiver increases the likelihood that toddlers will engage in emotion regulatory behaviors (Grolnick, Bridges, & Connell, 1996).

By preschool years, the importance of children's emotion regulation capabilities in facilitating effective social interaction becomes increasingly apparent. Children with positive emotion regulation skills are perceived by teachers to be more successful in social interactions than children with poor emotion regulation capabilities (Denham, 2006). Additionally, children who experience difficulties with emotion regulation are more likely to report experiencing peer rejection (Hamre & Pianta, 2005; Ladd, Herald, & Kochel, 2006).

Emotion regulation in children with Down syndrome. Earlier discussion of emotion expression in children with DS revealed mixed reports of positive emotion expression in this population (Bieberich & Morgan, 2004; Brooks-Gunn & Lewis, 1982; Capps et al., 1993; Kasari & Sigman, 1996). It appears that while younger children with DS appear to exhibit similar levels of positive affect as their TD peers, they exhibit increasing levels of negative affect with age (Fidler et al., 2005). An understanding of emotion regulation capabilities in individuals with DS may yield a more complete understanding of why this increase may occur. In a study of negative emotion expression and emotion regulation during a task meant to elicit frustration, Jahromi et al. (2008) found that children with DS (MA = 49 months) expressed greater rates of negativity and frustration as compared to MA-matched TD children. In addition, while the TD children relied on goal-directed strategies to regulate their frustration, the children with DS tended to orient themselves toward the experimenter without seeking assistance. These findings suggest that children with DS may struggle with using goal-oriented emotion regulation strategies when confronted with a frustrating task, instead of opting to abandon the task and look to others for soothing. This finding is consistent with evidence that children with DS may be limited in their use of regulatory strategies to modulate the negative emotionality that is associated with behavioral control (McIntyre, Blacher, & Baker, 2006).

Some have speculated that children with DS may struggle with regulating negative emotions as a result of their decreased negative affect as infants. This theory posits that infants with decreased negative affect may have less exposure to caregiver coregulation as well as fewer opportunities to attempt to regulate their own emotions (Cicchetti, Ganiban, & Barnett, 1991; Stifter, Spinrad, & Braungart-Rieker, 1999), and as such would have fewer opportunities to develop emotion regulation skills. This pattern of low negative affect in early childhood begins to change in middle and late childhood, with findings that individuals with DS appear to display an increase in negative emotion expression as they age, likely related to a plateau in cognitive abilities that they experience during childhood (Fidler et al., 2005). This increase in negative affect corresponds with the emergence of a range of behavior problems such as noncompliance, stubbornness, disobedience, and inability to delay gratification (Coe et al., 1999; Cuskelly & Dadds, 1992; Cuskelly, Zhang, & Hayes, 2003; Dykens & Kasari, 1997; Fidler, Hepburn, & Rogers, 2006; Gath & Gumley, 1987; Kopp, 1982). A combination of increased negative emotionality and impaired emotion regulation capabilities may be responsible, in part, for the emergence of such behavioral problems in children with DS (Jahromi et al., 2008), indicating the important role that emotion regulation plays in the socioemotional development of individuals with DS.

Behavioral Regulation

Behavioral regulation refers to a range of skills that serve to support adaptive social and nonsocial responses (Calkins, 1994; Thompson, 1994), including complying with directives and delaying gratification (Kopp, 1982). The ability to effectively regulate behavior has been positively linked to the ability to sustain positive peer interactions in TD children (Mischel, Shoda, & Rodriguez, 1989; Spinrad et al., 2006). It is theorized that these positive outcomes occur as a result of the ability to inhibit inappropriate social responses and to foster appropriate social behaviors (Arsenio & Lemerise, 2004; Eisenberg et al., 1994; Eisenberg, Fabes, & Spinrad, 2006).

Compliance. Compliance, or the ability to observe societal standards of conduct and regulate one's behavior accordingly, is considered to be the earliest behavioral manifestation of a child's ability to regulate their own behavior (Kopp, 1982). Among TD children, the ability to comply with caregivers' requests by initiating, maintaining, or ceasing behavior emerges between 12 and 18 months (Kopp, 1982). By 24 months of age, TD children are able to begin to regulate their own behavior, even in the absence of external influence. Within the literature on the development of compliance, a distinction is made between two forms of compliance: committed compliance and situational compliance. When a child is wholeheartedly invested in a task given to them, following directives in a self-regulated manner without the need for external control, the child is said to exhibit committed compliance. Situational compliance, on the other hand, refers to instances in which the child is receptive to directives and completes the task given to them but needs external guidance in order to sustain compliance (Kochanska, Tjebkes, & Fortnan, 1998). Among TD children, committed compliance and situational compliance are negatively correlated and seem to have opposite developmental trajectories because committed compliance increases with age whereas situational compliance decreases with age (Crockenberg & Litman, 1990; Kochanska, Coy, & Murray, 2001; Kuczynski, Kochanska, Radke-Yarrow, & Girnius Brown, 1987).

Beyond being the earliest indicator of emerging behavior-regulation abilities, compliance has been found to be a hallmark of early childhood development, as it is predictive of both concurrent and future child outcomes. In a longitudinal study, children were assessed at 36 months and 54 months of age on measures of compliance and social efficacy (Ramani, Brownell, & Campbell, 2010). Results revealed that, at both time points, children who were more compliant with adults appeared to have more positive peer interactions and fewer negative peer interactions. These findings indicate a stable relationship between children's compliance behaviors and their efficacy in social interactions over time, a relationship that begins fairly early in life.

Compliance in children with Down syndrome. Landry, Garner, Pirie, and Swank (1994) sought to better understand compliance to maternal requests among children with DS across different social contexts. A group of children with DS and a group of MA-matched TD children (DS mean = 29.07 months; TD mean = 31.82 months) were asked to complete two tasks with their mothers. In the first task, the children were allowed 5 minutes to complete a difficult puzzle with their mothers. For the second task, the mothers were asked to engage their children in a 5-minute tea party and were given cookies, juice, and a tea set. The TD children were more compliant than the children with DS during the tea party task, but not during the puzzle task. The findings also revealed that the children's compliant behaviors were positively related to their expressive language abilities. The findings of this study also indicated that children with DS were more likely to respond to maternal directives with compliance than to suggestive requests on the tea task but not for the puzzle task. These findings indicate that the differences between the children with DS and the TD comparison group was associated with context, request strategies, and children's expressive language abilities.

In addition to behavioral observations, researchers have also relied on parent and teacher reports in order to better understand behavioral patterns in children with DS. Daunhauer and colleagues (2014) explored how the teachers of children with DS (n = 26, MA = 47.88 months) rated their students on measures related to school functioning using the School Function Assessment. Findings of this study revealed within-group strengths and challenges for the sample, as measured by the School Function Assessment, with relative strengths reported in the ability to complete physical tasks without assistance and relative challenges in social-cognitive tasks, such as compliance with adult directives.

Researchers have also relied on parent reports of their children's behavior regulation and effectiveness in social interaction. In a study comparing children with DS and TD children matched on CA (mean = 9.7 years), both parents and teachers reported the children with DS as exhibiting more noncompliant behaviors than their TD peers (Coe et al., 1999). A weakness of this study lies in the fact that MA-matched participants were not included for comparison, but the study nonetheless provides insight as far as the consistency of reporting between teachers and parents.

Delay of gratification. A foundational element of behavior regulation is the ability to delay gratification for the sake of future consequences. In a study conducted by Spinrad and colleagues (2006), measures of behavior regulation in TD children (CA = 73.58 months) were found to be predictive of children's popularity as measured by their teachers, and this relationship remained stable at a 2-year follow-up.

In a widely replicated study, Mischel, Ebbesen, and Raskoff Zeiss (1972) assessed behavior regulation using an experimental delay-of-gratification paradigm with TD preschoolers (age = 3–5 years), during which the participants were asked to sit at a table furnished with a bell and were shown reward objects that were previously determined to be desirable to the child. An experimenter then asked the child which of the two rewards was more favorable to them (e.g., one or two marshmallows). Once the child indicated their preference, the experimenter then explained to them the contingency. The experimenter was to leave the room for 15 minutes, and if the child waited for the experimenter to return, they were allowed to have the preferred reward (e.g., two marshmallows). Alternatively, the child could ring the bell in order to summon the experimenter, but subsequently they would only receive the less preferred reward (e.g., one marshmallow; Mischel et al., 1972; Mischel & Underwood, 1974). In a follow-up study, Shoda, Mischel, and Peake (1990) found that the children who were able to wait for the full

15-minute delay period as preschoolers were reported by their parents as being more socially competent as adolescents.

Casey et al. (2011) assessed the same group of individuals 40 years later on their ability to control impulses, as measured by subjects' behavioral responses to alluring and neutral stimuli, and found that the individuals who were less able to delay gratification as preschoolers showed more difficulty in suppressing responses to the alluring stimuli as adults. These findings suggest that the ability to delay gratification is a relatively stable individual characteristic across the lifespan in TD individuals and that it serves as an early indicator of social-emotional competence throughout childhood and adolescence.

Delay of gratification in children with Down syndrome. Given the established relationship between the ability to delay gratification and successful peer relationships in TD children, it is important to understand the relationship between these constructs among individuals with DS and whether the relationships differ from those seen in TD individuals. Kopp (1990) conducted a study in which children with DS (MA = 29 months) were compared to MA-matched TD children on their performance on two delay-of-gratification tasks. In the first task, the children sat across the table from an experimenter, with a bright red telephone between them. After showing the child the telephone, the experimenter explained that they must leave the room and asked the child not to touch the toy until they returned. On average, the TD children were able to delay their impulse to inspect the toy for a significantly longer amount of time than did the children with DS. In a second task, the children were seated across from an experimenter with three plastic cups on the table between them. Beneath one of the cups, the experimenter had hidden a raisin, and the children were asked to wait before looking for the raisin. Again, the children with DS waited less time than their TD counterparts to look for the raisin.

Cuskelly, Zhang, and Hayes (2003) examined delay of gratification in a MA-matched sample of TD children and children with DS, this time using a sample with a slightly older MA (DS mean = 56.2 months; TD mean = 54.8 months) and tasks which included both self-imposed and other-imposed delay of gratification. In the first other-imposed delay task, the children were seated at a table with their favorite food placed in front of them among other less tempting options. The mothers instructed their children not to eat the food until instructed to do so. In the second other-imposed delay task, the children were shown a gift-wrapped box and were told not to open it until the experimenter returned to the room. The groups differed when comparing waiting time for the gift task, but not for the tea task. The self-imposed delay task used in this study, modeled on the task used by Mischel and Underwood (1974), asked children to choose between a red fire engine with several intriguing features and a white jeep with no special features. Once making their choice, the children were told that the experimenter needed to leave the room, and that they must wait for the experimenter to return in order to play with their preferred toy. They were also given the alternative option that they could summon the experimenter back at any time by ringing a bell but, once they do, they would only be able to play with the less preferred toy. The children with DS waited significantly less time than the TD children before summoning the experimenter to return. Furthermore, only 20 percent of the children in the DS group waited for the experimenter to return, whereas 66 percent of the TD children were able to wait for the experimenter to return.

Similar results were found among a group of adolescents (n = 29) with DS (mean CA = 14.75 years; mean MA = 65.92 months) when asked to complete a delay of gratification task similar to Mischel et al.'s (1972) marshmallow task (Cuskelly & Stubbins, 2006). The participants were offered a choice of two small rewards and told that they could have the preferred reward if they could wait 15 minutes for the experimenter to return to the room, or they could summon the experimenter at any time and receive the lesser of the rewards. The participants completed the task twice, once during the initial visit to the laboratory and again upon their return. The sample of adolescents with DS displayed a range of abilities on the first iteration of the task, with 11of the 29 participants waiting the full 15 minutes for the reward and 12 of the 29 participants waiting less than 2 minutes, with the rest of the participants falling between. The mean waiting time was 332.38 seconds for the first administration of the task and 407.28 seconds for the second one. Waiting times for the two tasks were significantly correlated ($r = 0.61$, $p< 0.001$).

Altogether, the findings from these studies indicate that younger individuals with DS show greater difficulty in delaying gratification than older individuals with DS, and that TD individuals, both younger and older, were able to delay gratification for longer than individuals with DS. In addition, the findings suggest that the ability to delay gratification among children with DS may be contingent upon the situation, as evidenced by Cuskelly et al. (2003). The findings of these studies indicate a need to better understand how the ability to delay gratification develops over time for individuals with DS and what factors contribute to the within-group differences seen in this population.

Social Awareness

The second of the base components identified in Rose-Krasnor's prism model, social awareness, refers to "the abilities to identify and act upon one's awareness of the thoughts and feelings of others" (Rose-Krasnor & Denham, 2009, p.171). This type of social awareness is otherwise referred to in the literature as emotion knowledge, a multi-dimensional construct that encompasses emotion recognition and emotion situation knowledge (Basset, Denham, Mincic, & Graling, 2012).

Emotion knowledge. Emotion knowledge refers to the broader construct of emotion recognition and emotion situation knowledge (Bassett et al., 2012). While emotion recognition refers to the ability to identify and label other people's emotional states based on facial expression, emotion situation knowledge refers to the ability to understand how certain contexts and situations may elicit specific emotions (Fine, Izard, & Trentacosta,

2006; Morgan, Izard, & King, 2010). These two aspects of emotion knowledge do not appear to develop simultaneously in TD, as emotion recognition begins to emerge around the age of 3, and emotional situation knowledge begins to emerge at the end of preschool (Heinze, Miller, Seifer, Dickstein, & Locke, 2015; Bassett et al., 2012) and continues to develop through the course of childhood. Emotion knowledge plays a critical role in children's peer interactions by allowing children to identify and interpret other's cues, generating and evaluating possible responses, and enacting behaviors appropriately (Sette, Spinrad, & Baumgartner, 2016). Researchers have consistently reported the connection between emotion knowledge and children's effective social interactions. The findings from a meta-analysis indicated a relationship between successful social interaction and emotion knowledge across moderator subgroups, such as the age of the child and the respondent for the measure of social competence (Trentacosta & Fine, 2010). Significant relationships were found between emotion knowledge and both internalizing and externalizing behaviors in children. The magnitude of the relationship between emotion knowledge and internalizing behaviors was found to be nearly identical to the magnitude of the relationship between emotion knowledge and externalizing behaviors, both falling into the small-to-medium range as measured by established criteria regarding magnitude of effect sizes. These findings indicate that the development of emotion knowledge is inextricably related to maladaptive behaviors and the ability to engage in effective social interactions among TD developing children, regardless of the child's age or who reported the information. The established relationship between emotion knowledge and the ability to successfully navigate social interactions reveals a possible early target to help facilitate developmentally appropriate social-emotional development in both TD children and children with DS.

Emotion recognition. Emotion recognition refers to the ability to identify and label other people's emotional states based on facial expression. Among TD children, the ability to discriminate between static images of happiness and sadness has been identified in infants as young as 4 months old (Young-Browne, Rosenfeld, & Horowitz, 1977). This ability continues to develop as the child matures, and by the age of 4 years TD children are found to be adept at identifying and labeling basic emotions with almost perfect accuracy (Widen & Russel, 2003). The ability to identify and label more complex emotions, such as shame and guilt, emerge over the course of childhood (Durand, Gallay, Seigneuric, Rubichom, & Baudouin, 2007; Székely et al., 2011). Although children of 10 years appear to perform comparably to adults in their identification of emotion expression (Durand et al., 2007), they still seem to struggle with detecting more subtle emotion expressions (Thomas, De Bellis, Graham, & LaBar, 2007).

A central component of adaptive social functioning, good emotion-recognition capabilities among TD children have been associated with fewer internalizing and externalizing symptoms as well as better academic performance (Denham et al., 2003; Trentacosta

& Fine, 2010; Trentacosta, Izard, Mostow, & Fine, 2006). In addition, individuals with better developed emotion regulation capabilities are better at predicting and interpreting others' mental states and engaging in appropriate self-regulatory behaviors that allow for successful social interactions with others (Denham et al., 2003; Lemerise & Arsenio, 2000).

Emotion recognition in children with Down syndrome. The findings regarding emotion-recognition capabilities of young children with Down syndrome (DS) are mixed, with some evidence that emotion recognition is unaffected (Kasari et al, 2001) and other evidence that children with DS underperform on measures of emotion recognition as compared to CA-matched TD children as well as developmentally matched children with other developmental disorders (Kasari & Freeman, 2001). Difficulties appear to occur in the recognition of anger, fear, and sadness (Bouras, Turk, & Cornish, 1998; Kasari & Freeman, 2001), as children with DS (MA = 4.70 years), in comparison to MA-matched children with William's syndrome and MA-matched TD children, tend to identify negative expressions as positive ones (Porter, Coltheart, & Langdon, 2007). In addition to the recognition of negative emotions, the recognition of complex emotions such as surprise and fear may also be impaired among children with DS (Cebula et al., 2017; Wishart & Pitcairn, 2000). It has been speculated that these emotion-recognition deficits may result from a slowing in the development of emotion-recognition abilities that occur between the ages of 3 and 4 years (Kasari & Freeman, 2001). In a longitudinal study of the development of emotion recognition among TD children, children with DS, and children with non-specified intellectual disability (NSID) matched on developmental age (MA = 45 months at entry), Pochon and Declercq (2014) reported that the emotion-recognition abilities of TD children developed more rapidly over time than children in either the DS or NSID groups. This trend appears to hold with age, as adults with DS were found to perform worse on a task of negative emotion recognition but better on recognizing positive emotions as compared to TD children matched on receptive language abilities (Hippolyte, Barisnikov, Van der Linden, & Detraux, 2009).

In addition to longitudinally examining the development of emotion recognition in children with DS, Pochon and Declercq (2014) also endeavored to identify the underlying mechanism that is responsible for challenges in emotion recognition in children DS. One theory posits that the emotion-recognition tasks that are typically used to measure these abilities in children are not able to differentiate between difficulties that are attributable to challenges with using emotion labels or to difficulties in perceptual facial processing abilities (Lindquist & Gendron, 2013). In order to tease apart these constructs, Pochon and Declerq (2014) compared children with DS (MA = 45 months) with developmentally matched TD children and children with NSID. The children were asked to complete two tasks, one control task involving the identification of pictures of animals and an experimental task which involved the identification of photographs of faces displaying a range of facial expressions. In both tasks, the pictures that were presented to the participants were paired with a vocalization and the children were asked to identify the correct animal or person who made the vocalization. The findings indicated that the children with DS, but not children with NSID, underperformed as compared with their TD peers in the identification of facial expressions using emotion labels (Pochon & Declerq, 2014).

In a similar study of emotion recognition across contexts, Cebula et al. (2017) compared children with DS (MA = 4.27 years) with TD children and children with NSID matched for developmental on measures that differentially target emotion labeling and facial processing. Consistent with previous findings, they reported that the children with DS struggled in the identification of fear but successfully identified other basic emotions such as happiness and sadness. Additionally, they indicated that these difficulties in recognizing fear were not linguistic in nature, as the differences persisted in conditions in which emotion labels were not required for the task. Although findings between these two studies are consistent with findings of relative impairments in emotion labeling, Cebula and colleagues (2017) contradict Pochon and Declerq's (2014) assertion that children with DS underperformed as compared with their TD peers in the identification of facial expressions as a function of the use of emotion labels. Pochon and Declercq (2014) required their participants to match an emotion to a vocalization, whereas Cebula et al. (2017) only required their participants to match pictures of adults displaying the same facial expression. This leads to the conclusion that relative deficits in emotion labeling are not attributable to measurement differences.

In order to facilitate future intervention to support adaptive social functioning, we need to better understand the emotion-recognition profile that is unique to individuals with DS and the underlying processes that contribute to relative differences in the recognition of complex and negative emotions in comparison to MA-matched TD counterparts. Given that these differences appear to be a result not of measurement differences, but rather of an underlying difficulty in the recognition of certain emotions among individuals with Down syndrome, future work should be focused on identifying the underlying mechanism responsible for these emotion-recognition differences. This knowledge would contribute to the overall understanding of the construct in this population and would inform the development of targeted interventions in order to facilitate emotion-recognition development in individuals with DS.

Emotion situation knowledge. Emotion situation knowledge refers to the ability to understand how certain contexts and situations may elicit specific emotions (Fine et al., 2006; Heinze et al., 2015; Morgan, Izard, & King, 2010). This construct is set apart from emotion recognition in that it does not rely solely on the identification of facial expressions, but rather requires a more intricate understanding of the contexts which surround particular emotions. Emotion situation knowledge appears to be related to several child characteristics among TD children. For example, Heinze et al. (2015) found that emotion situation knowledge capabilities were positively related to age in a sample of TD Head Start preschoolers. They also reported that emotion situation knowledge was uniquely related to peers reporting whether they would like to play with the target child. Other factors that appear to contribute to emotion situation knowledge in TD children include the child's sex, with females exhibiting quicker development of emotion knowledge than males, and socio-economic status (SES), with indications that children from low-income families perform less well on measures of emotion knowledge (Denham et al., 2012).

Emotion situation knowledge is typically measured with tasks that rely upon vignettes, in which children are relayed an oral story and asked to identify the emotions that the central character may be experiencing (Garner & Waajid, 2008). A common criticism of such emotion situation knowledge measures is that the results may be confounded with receptive language abilities (Sette et al., 2016) among TD children, which could prove problematic when relying on such measures to determine emotion situation knowledge in populations that are known to exhibit receptive language deficits, such as persons with DS.

Emotion situation knowledge in children with Down syndrome. Among the studies on emotion situation knowledge among children with DS (Bouras et al., 1998; Kasari, Freeman, & Hughes, 2001), most involved tasks similar to the aforementioned vignette task based on children's receptive language abilities. In one example, Bouras et al. (1998) explored emotion knowledge in a sample of elementary-aged boys with fragile X syndrome (CA = 10.34 years; MA = 5.72 years) with comparison groups of children with DS matched on both CA and MA, and TD children matched on MA (CA = 10.82 years; MA = 5.11 years). The participants were presented with four drawings of a faceless figure in contexts which suggested one of four emotions: happiness, sadness, fear, or anger. Upon the presentation of each drawing, the participants were told a story regarding the context and what was happening to the figure in each picture. They were then presented with a set of four cards, each of which had a depiction of either a male or female face showing the distinctive features of each of the four emotions. The participants were asked to use the story to inform their choice in choosing the card with the facial expression that they would expect the faceless figure to be wearing in each of the four drawings. The children with DS (mean MA = 5.11 years) were significantly less successful than the MA-matched TD group (mean MA = 6.24 years) at pairing the correct facial expression with the appropriate vignette.

Kasari et al. (2001) also explored emotion knowledge in children with DS and a comparison group of TD children initially matched on a mean MA of 3 years, using a task commonly referred to as the "puppet interview" (Denham & Couchoud, 1990). In this task, a trained assessor acted out vignettes while narrating a story to the participants. During the narration, the assessor used appropriate facial expressions and tone of voice cues to accompany the story. Following the narration, the participants were asked to attach a schematic face representing an emotion expression to the doll, indicating that the puppet was experiencing the given emotion due to the context. At a MA of 3 years, the participants in both groups performed relatively poorly on the puppet interview task, with no significant differences detected between the two groups. At a later date, with both new participants and a subset of the original participants who had reached the MA of 4 years, the children with DS were significantly outperformed by the participants in the TD comparison group (mean MA = 4 years) as well as a comparison group comprised of children with intellectual disability (ID) of mixed etiology matched on MA (mean MA = 4 years). These findings led Kasari et al. (2001) to conclude that children with DS may experience a slowing in the development of emotion knowledge at or slightly before a MA of 4 years. In a third iteration of the puppet task, conducted at a 2-year follow-up, the authors' conclusions were supported by findings that the participants with DS did not display any significant increase in performance in comparison with the TD and ID groups. Along with the findings from Bouras et al. (1998), the evidence here suggests that children with DS experience difficulties when identifying emotion expressions using situational contexts, but the lag in their performance only becomes apparent at a MA of 3 years when they begin to underperform at situational emotion knowledge tasks in comparison to TD children matched on MA.

Measuring emotion knowledge in children with Down syndrome. Tasks traditionally used to assess emotion situation knowledge in children, both TD and with DS, rely heavily upon receptive linguistic comprehension (e.g., Bouras et al.,1998; Kasari & Freeman, 2001). That is, in order for children to perform well on the given tasks, they must have the requisite linguistic abilities to understand the context relayed orally by the assessor. The linguistic demands of these types of tasks are a common criticism of traditional emotion situation knowledge measures, since results may be confounded with receptive language abilities (Sette et al., 2016), even among TD children. This may prove even more problematic when assessing emotion situation knowledge in populations recognized to have poorer receptive linguistic comprehension skills, such as individuals with DS (Abbeduto, Warren, & Conners, 2007).

In order to address the possibility of measurement issues in assessing emotion knowledge in populations known to exhibit language impairments, Channell, Connors, and Barth (2014) developed the Emotion Judgement Test (EJT), which uses video clips in order to eliminate the challenge of language abilities. The EJT was initially used with children with DS (CA =11.44 years; MA = 4.66 years) and a comparison group of TD children matched on MA (mean = 4.65 years). The EJT consists of four short video clips starring a young male child as the protagonist. The video types varied only by emotion cue—face only, context only, face and context, and incongruent face and context. In the face-only type, the child's face was displayed making a neutral face which then forms into one of the three emotion expressions targeted by the task—happiness, sadness, or fear. In the context-only video, the child's face was obscured while the viewer observes the child engage in a situation that would commonly elicit a specific emotion (e.g., a balloon floating away is meant to elicit sadness). In the face and context video, the observer is exposed to both the situational context that elicits the emotional reaction as well as the child's contingent emotion expression. In the incongruent face and context video, the observer views the child engage in a situation and subsequently display an incongruous emotion expression. After showing the videos, an examiner asked the participant to indicate whether they thought the child was happy, sad, or scared. The examiner then provided the participants with three schematic faces indicating happiness, sadness, and fear, and asked the participant to point to the schematic that represented how the child felt.

The EJT, which was specifically designed to be used with persons with DS, differs from other emotion situation knowledge tasks in several ways. One, in order to compensate for attentional challenges often seen in this population, the task was intentionally designed to be brief and to allow for multiple trials per emotion. Two, no verbal language was used in the video clips, requiring participants to rely solely upon visual processing to understand the narrative depicted in the clip. Three, the decision to only include happiness, sadness, and fear in the task is based upon the approach-avoidance model by Lemerise and Arsenio (2000). Using this framework, happiness is considered a positive approach emotion, sadness a negative approach emotion, and fear a negative avoidance emotion. Fear was also chosen to be included based on the evidence that fear recognition may be uniquely impacted among persons with DS.

Using the EJT, Channell et al. (2014) found that children with DS and their TD MA-matched counterparts showed similar levels of emotion knowledge. They conducted a second study with the same group of participants in order to examine developmental trajectories of general emotion-recognition abilities in individuals with DS and TD individuals. A cross-sectional developmental trajectory approach was used, based on guidelines by Thomas et al. (2007). This method used the principles of analysis of covariance (ANCOVA) to examine group differences in both onset and gradient of developmental trajectory. The participants with DS and the TD participants showed similar rates of growth in emotion knowledge across MA, which was estimated using receptive language abilities. Channell et al. (2014) posited that these findings support the notion that emotion knowledge development is commensurate with receptive vocabulary in individuals with DS with a MA of 3 to 6 years.

These more recent findings might suggest that the emotion situation knowledge capabilities of persons with DS are commensurate with their MA, although delayed relative to their CA, thereby contradicting earlier evidence that children with DS are delayed in their emotion situation knowledge relative to both MA- and CA-matched TD children. If these differences can be attributed to differences in measurement, then comparisons in performance across different emotion situation tasks would be useful in discerning the underlying mechanism responsible for differences in emotion situation knowledge in children with DS. Alternatively, it is also plausible that these contradictory findings across measures point to an altogether artificial finding of challenges in emotion knowledge in DS. It is possible that the differences across measures may reflect weaknesses in areas related to emotion knowledge, rather than challenges in emotion knowledge abilities themselves. These questions offer potent areas for future exploration, in order to better understand whether a deficit in emotion knowledge truly exists in individuals with DS and, if so, what underlying mechanisms contribute to the manifestation of these deficits.

Prosocial Orientation

Prosocial orientation is identified by Rose-Krasnor as the third foundational component necessary to achieve social-emotional competence (Rose-Krasnor & Denham, 2009) and is defined as the tendency to voluntarily engage in behaviors intended to help or benefit others, such as empathic or emotion responsiveness (Eisenberg & Mussen, 1989; Ornaghi, Grazzani, Cherubin, Conte, & Piralli, 2015). The use of such prosocial behaviors in TD children appears to increase across early and middle childhood and is linked to the development of other abilities, including emotion regulation and language (Denham, 1993; Eisenberg et al., 1998, Eisenberg et al., 2006).

Emotion responsiveness. Emotion responsiveness, or empathic responsiveness, refers to the ability to deliver a congruent emotional response to another's emotions (Decety & Meyer, 2008). Although emotion responsiveness relies upon an individual's emotion knowledge, emotion knowledge capabilities do not guarantee successful emotion responsiveness. For example, among children with ASD who show relatively adequate emotion understanding abilities, performance on tests assessing emotion knowledge was not predictive of emotion responsiveness (Scheeren, de Rosnay, Koot, & Begeer, 2013).

Eisenberg (2000) suggests that empathic responses usually manifest as sympathy, personal distress, or some combination thereof. Sympathy is an emotional response stemming from the knowledge of another's emotional state and consists of feelings of concern and sorrow toward the other. Conversely, personal distress is a self-focused emotional reaction to the knowledge of the another's emotional state. Within this framework, emotion responsiveness can be both a self-directed response as well as an other-directed response. Emotion responsiveness can also be understood to encompass a third, more deliberate response: prosocial behavior, which refers to behaviors such as sharing, helping, comforting, and other positive social behaviors that are voluntary and intentional.

Prosocial behaviors emerge early in typically developing infants, with reports of infants under the age of 1 year appearing to comfort and respond empathically to their mothers when exhibiting distress (Zahn-Waxleret, Radkey-Yarrow, Wagner, & Chapman, 1992). These behaviors become more sophisticated with age, with toddlers between the ages of 1 and 2 years reported to engage in prosocial behaviors such as helping, comforting, and sharing (Rheingold, 1982). These studies have been replicated with findings that children between the ages of 18 and 24 months engage in helping behaviors, such as handing over missing objects in order to help someone complete a task (Warneken & Tomasello, 2006).

A wide range of quantitative and qualitative differences in prosocial behaviors are found among TD children (Zahn-Waxler et al., 1992). Findings from a series of studies by Eisenberg and colleagues (Eisenberg et al., 1990; Spinrad et al., 2006) indicated that children who exhibited physiological markers of sympathy, such as heart-rate deceleration and low skin conductance, were more likely to elect to engage in prosocial behaviors when given the opportunity to help others in distress. In contrast, children who responded to the distress of others with personal distress, indicated by high heart rate or skin conductance, were less likely to engage in prosocial behaviors (Fabes, Eisenberg, & Eisenbud, 1993; Miller, Eisenberg, Fabes, & Shell, 1996).

The ability to respond to another person's emotions, especially in a prosocial manner, has important implications for a child's future social-emotional competence. In a 7-year study conducted by Chen and colleagues (2002), data was initially collected from 235 children (MA = 12 years), then again 7 years later from a subset of the original participants (n = 123). Results of this study indicated that prosocial orientation at the age of 12 years was associated with social-emotional competence 7 years later, as measured through peer interactions. This association between prosocial orientation and social-emotional competence has been widely replicated by researchers using both longitudinal and cross-sectional designs (Denham et al., 2003; Kuppens, Grietans, Onghena, & Michiels, 2009; McAuliffe, Hubbard, & Romano, 2009).

Emotion responsiveness in Down syndrome. Few studies have explored prosocial behavior in individuals with DS, and none have explored the construct longitudinally. In the few studies conducted to date, findings have indicated that children with DS struggled with responding appropriately to the facial expressions of others. In a study of emotion responsiveness in children with DS, Knieps, Walden, and Baxter (1994) found that children with DS tended to display positive emotion expressions in response to their parents' fearful expressions during a social-referencing paradigm in which they were presented an ambiguous stimulus that was paired with either positive or fearful verbal and nonverbal communications from their parents. This finding is particularly relevant considering the possible difficulties in the recognition of fear in children with DS (Kasari et al., 2001). Using a similar paradigm in which the assessors reacted to an unfamiliar stimulus in the presence of their child with DS, Kasari et al. (1995) found slightly discrepant evidence, as the children with DS with a MA of 3.35 years exhibited more neutral and negative facial expressions, while the MA-matched TD children tended to react with expressions of interest. In addition, while the TD children tended to shift their gaze between the ambiguous stimulus and the assessor, the children with DS tended to focus their gaze mainly on the assessor. Kasari et al. suggested that since children with DS tended to attend to the assessor's face more than their TD MA-matched counterparts, they failed to pay the requisite attention to the stimulus in relation to the emotional message of the assessor, and as such reacted differently than their TD peers.

Although children with DS appear to struggle with detecting distress in facial expressions, they do not appear to display a lower frequency of prosocial behaviors in comparison to TD children. Kasari et al. (2003) compared performance on a response-to-distress task in which an assessor initiates a clean-up task and then feigns an injury and begins to cry among children with DS, TD children, and children with ID of mixed etiology, all matched on a MA of approximately 4 years. The children with DS showed little positive or negative expressed emotion, but oriented more toward the "injured" assessor. In addition, the children with DS engaged in significantly more prosocial behaviors toward the assessor than did the children in either of the comparison groups. These findings suggest that, while children with DS may struggle in social referencing tasks in which they are required to respond to another's facial expressions in an appropriate manner, they tend to provide more comfort-seeking and prosocial behaviors to those they perceive to be in distress as compared to TD children and children with NSID of a MA of 4 years.

Social Problem-Solving and Peer Interaction

The final basic component of Rose-Krasnor's (Rose-Krasnor & Denham, 2009) prism model of social-emotional competence is social problem solving, which is described as the process in which children process social information, determine effective ways to solve peer conflict, set social goals, and then follow through in performing the behaviors necessary to meet those goals (Crick & Dodge, 1996; Rose-Krasnor & Denham, 2009). Peer interactions begin to take place in toddlerhood and become increasingly important during the preschool years. Navigating the norms and expectations of the playground can prove challenging for many TD children and can be even more so for a child with a developmental or intellectual disability. Children with DS have long been described as affable and socially charming, and these findings have been echoed in much of the literature surrounding the topic (Fidler et al., 2006; Kasari et al., 2003). Increased eye gaze and other-directed vocalizations have been reported among children with DS, including increased positive facial expressions such as smiling and increased levels of joint attention as compared to TD toddlers and toddlers with ID of mixed etiology matched on a MA of 3 to 4 years (Fidler et al., 2005; Kasari et al., 1995). These skills have been found to be positively related to successful social interaction and peer involvement in TD children and children with other developmental disabilities (Denham et al., 2003; Freeman, Gulsrud, & Kasari, 2015). In a study comparing children with DS with MA-matched children with and without developmental disabilities, Fidler et al. (2006) found that toddlers with DS showed relative strength in socializing, namely in play and interpersonal relationships.

In collecting information regarding peer relationships among children with DS (CA = 5–12 years), Freeman and Kasari (2002) found that most of the children reported peer friendships that met criteria for true friendship, namely reciprocal nomination in the friendship dyad, convergence between the parent and child nomination, and at least 6 months of stable friendship within the dyad. In addition, Sigman & Ruskin (1999) reported that, in comparison to MA-matched children with ASD and unspecified developmental disabilities (Mean = 18 months), the children with DS showed similar levels of peer interaction as the children with unspecified developmental disabilities and higher levels than the children with ASD. Despite such findings that children with DS appear to form friendships and have successful peer interactions, they also seem to face unique hurdles when engaging socially with their peers. For instance, children with DS appear to experience difficulties with more complex social situations such as the unstructured play time that is common in preschool and school settings (Guralnick, Connor, & Johnson, 2011). Difficulties in navigating these more complicated social settings, such as those involving several people, may arise from challenges in planning and problem solving that have been identified in children with DS, as these skills underlie many social interactions (Næss, Nygaard, Ostad, Dolva, & Lyster, 2017). In such complex situations, the guidance of a TD peer may be helpful in facilitating higher levels of group play (Guralnick et al., 2011). The body of work exploring the nature of peer relationships in children with DS suggests that these children have the social capabilities necessary to engage with their peers, but they may not be as incorporated in group play as often as their TD peers (Næss et al., 2017). These positive peer interactions between children with DS and their peers have the potential to manifest themselves in selective friendships, with the correct level of support and guidance from more experienced peer mentors and the selection of activities that are better suited to the cognitive abilities of children with DS.

Næss et al. (2017) found that the children with DS were more likely than either MA- or CA- matched TD children to be identified as having social problems (Næss et al., 2017). The social problems include having fewer friends than those in either group and having more conduct problems than the children in the CA-matched group. These findings of fewer friends among the children with DS is discordant with Freeman and Kasari's (2002) findings that children with DS are comparable to TD children in the number of true friendships that they report (Freeman & Kasari, 2002). These discrepancies may be attributable to a difference in the ages in the groups, since Freeman and Kasari (2002) used a range of ages from 5–12 years, whereas Næss et al. (2017) only included 6-year-old children. The notion that age and social competence are related in DS individuals is supported by evidence that, unlike TD children whose social problems decrease as they grow older, children with DS appear to have display more externalizing problems as they age (Næss et al., 2017).

Conclusions

Researchers have been interested in exploring the social and emotional development of individuals with DS for decades. Although much of the literature regarding the social-emotional development of individuals with DS is dated, there has been a recent resurgence in the study of certain aspects of development such as emotion knowledge and social relationships. In addition, advances in the methodology with which these constructs are explored have been identified as an area of recent interest. This chapter has sought to synthesize both historical and contemporary research in order to develop an overarching vision of the field.

Individuals with DS exhibit a unique social-emotional profile characterized by both relative strengths and weaknesses. Relative strengths were revealed in social motivation and emotion responsiveness when compared to other children with intellectual and developmental disabilities (Cebula & Wishart, 2008; Wishart, 2007; Wishart, Cebula, Willis, & Pitcairn, 2007). Children with DS appear to enjoy true friendships with their peers and exhibit higher rates of prosocial behaviors, strengths that could be further fostered by caretakers and teachers. Weaknesses were identified among more discrete skills such as social cognition, emotion recognition, and emotion regulation (Abbeduto et al., 2001; Cebula et al., 2017; Fidler et al., 2005; Jahromi et al., 2008; Kasari et al., 1990; Kasari & Freeman, 2001; Wishart & Pitcairn, 2000), although contradictory findings raise questions as to the legitimacy of these findings. Recognition of this unique combination of strengths and weaknesses, which differentiates individuals with DS from other populations, may contribute to a better understanding of the unique developmental trajectory of social-emotional development in this population.

Given the recent resurgence of interest in the field, this chapter offers a foundational understanding of what is, and is not, known about social-emotional development in individuals with DS. Future research is encouraged in areas in which there have been mixed or contradictory findings, such as emotion recognition and emotion knowledge. This should include the development of measures that are validated for use in this particular population. Replication of previous studies using population-appropriate measures and adequate sample sizes would solidify understanding of the development of these skills among individuals with DS.

In addition to the implications for future research on the development of social-emotional competence in DS, this chapter offers salient targets for intervention in order to facilitate development in areas of relative weakness, such as emotion regulation and emotion knowledge. In order to best serve this population, targeted and tailored interventions should be developed, giving careful consideration to the relative social strengths seen in individuals with DS. By leveraging the social strengths of individuals with DS, interventions targeting components of social-emotional development in DS may prove to be more successful, thus facilitating optimal long-term outcomes.

Acknowledgments

This chapter was supported by grants from the Merck Foundation and Health Resources Services Administration, UA3MC11055.

References

Abbeduto, L., Evans, J., & Dolan, T. (2001). Theoretical perspectives on language and communication problems in mental retardation and developmental disabilities. *Mental Retardation and Developmental Disabilities Research Reviews, 7*(1), 45–55.

Abbeduto, L., Warren, S. F., & Conners, F. A. (2007). Language development in Down syndrome: From the prelinguistic period to the acquisition of literacy. *Mental Retardation and Developmental Disabilities Research Reviews, 13*(3), 247–261.

Arsenio, W. F., & Lemerise, E. A. (2004). Aggression and moral development: Integrating social information processing and moral domain models. *Child Development, 75*(4), 987–1002.

Bassett, H. H., Denham, S., Mincic, M., & Graling, K. (2012). The structure of preschoolers' emotion knowledge: Model equivalence and validity using a structural equation modeling approach. *Early Education & Development, 23*(3), 259–279.

Bieberich, A. A., & Morgan, S. B. (2004). Self-regulation and affective expression during play in children with autism or Down syndrome: A short-term longitudinal study. *Journal of Autism and Developmental Disorders, 34*(4), 439–448.

Birch, S. H., Ladd, G. W., & Blecher-Sass, H. (1997). The teacher-child relationship and children's early school adjustment: Good-byes can build trust. *Journal of School Psychology, 35*(1), 61–79.

Bouras, N., Turk, J., & Cornish, K. (1998). Face recognition and emotion perception in boys with fragile-X syndrome. *Journal of Intellectual Disability Research, 42*(6), 490–499.

Bridges, F. A., & Cicchetti, D. (1982). Mothers' ratings of the temperament characteristics of Down syndrome infants. *Developmental Psychology, 18*(2), 238.

Brooks-Gunn, J., & Lewis, M. (1982). Affective exchanges between normal and handicapped infants and their mothers. In T. Field & A. Fogel (Eds.), *Emotion and early interaction* (pp. 161–188). Hillsdale, NJ: Erlbaum.

Burke, M. M., Fisher, M. H., & Hodapp, R. M. (2012). Relations of parental perceptions to the behavioural characteristics of adolescents with Down syndrome. *Journal on Developmental Disabilities, 18*(2), 50.

Calkins, S. D. (1994). Origins and outcomes of individual differences in emotion regulation. *Monographs of the Society for Research in Child Development,* 59(2–3), 53–72.

Campos, J. J., Mumme, D., Kermoian, R., & Campos, R. G. (1994). A functionalist perspective on the nature of emotion. *Japanese Journal of Research on Emotions, 2*(1), 1–20.

Capps, L., Kasari, C., Yirmiya, N., & Sigman, M. (1993). Parental perception of emotional expressiveness in children with autism. *Journal of Consulting and Clinical Psychology, 61*(3), 475.

Casey, B. J., Somerville, L. H., Gotlib, I. H., Ayduk, O., Franklin, N. T., Askren, M. K., . . . Glover, G. (2011). Behavioral and neural correlates of delay of gratification 40 years later. *Proceedings of the National Academy of Sciences, 108*(36), 14998–15003.

Cebula, K. R., & Wishart, J. G. (2008). Social cognition in children with Down syndrome. *International Review of Research in Mental Retardation, 35*, 43–86.

Cebula, K. R., Wishart, J. G., Willis, D. S., & Pitcairn, T. K. (2017). Emotion recognition in children with Down syndrome: Influence of emotion label and expression intensity. *American Journal on Intellectual and Developmental Disabilities, 122*(2), 138–155.

Channell, M. M., Conners, F. A., & Barth, J. M. (2014). Emotion knowledge in children and adolescents with Down syndrome: A new methodological approach. *American Journal on Intellectual and Developmental Disabilities, 119*(5), 405–421.

Chen, X., Liu, M., Rubin, K. H., Cen, G. Z., Gao, X., & Li, D. (2002). Sociability and prosocial orientation as predictors of youth adjustment: A seven-year longitudinal study in a Chinese sample. *International Journal of Behavioral Development, 26*(2), 128–136.

Cicchetti, D., Ganiban, J., & Barrett, D. (1991). Contributions from the study of high-risk populations to understanding the development of emotion regulation. In J. Garber & K. A. Dodge (Eds.), *The Development of Emotion Regulation and Dysregulation* (pp. 15–48). New York: Cambridge University Press.

Cicchetti, D., & Sroufe, L. A. (1978). An organizational view of affect: Illustration from the study of Down's syndrome infants. In M. Lewis (Ed.), *The development of affect* (pp. 309–350). Boston, MA: Springer.

Coe, D. A., Matson, J. L., Russell, D. W., Slifer, K. J., Capone, G. T., Baglio, C., & Stallings, S. (1999). Behavior problems of children with Down syndrome and life events. *Journal of Autism and Developmental Disorders, 29*(2), 149–156.

Crick, N. R., & Dodge, K. A. (1996). Social information-processing mechanisms in reactive and proactive aggression. *Child Development, 67*(3), 993–1002.

Crockenberg, S., & Litman, C. (1990). Autonomy as competence in 2-year-olds: Maternal correlates of child defiance, compliance, and self-assertion. *Developmental Psychology, 26*(6), 961.

Cuskelly, M., & Dadds, M. (1992). Behavioural problems in children with Down's syndrome and their siblings. *Journal of Child Psychology and Psychiatry, 33*(4), 749–761.

Cuskelly, M., & Stubbins, P. (2006). Self-imposed delay of gratification in adolescents with Down syndrome. *Journal on Developmental Disabilities, 12*(1 Suppl 2), 19–28.

Cuskelly, M., Zhang, A., & Hayes, A. (2003). A mental age-matched comparison study of delay of gratification in children with Down syndrome. *International Journal of Disability, Development and Education, 50*(3), 239–251.

Daunhauer, L. A., Fidler, D. J., Hahn, L., Will, E., Lee, N. R., & Hepburn, S. (2014). Profiles of everyday executive functioning in young children with Down syndrome. *American Journal on Intellectual and Developmental Disabilities, 119*(4), 303–318.

Decety, J., & Meyer, M. (2008). From emotion resonance to empathic understanding: A social developmental neuroscience account. *Development and Psychopathology, 20*(4), 1053–1080.

Denham, S. A. (1993). Maternal emotional responsiveness and toddlers' social-emotional competence. *Journal of Child Psychology and Psychiatry, 34*(5), 715–728.

Denham, S. A. (2006). Social-emotional competence as support for school readiness: What is it and how do we assess it? *Early Education and Development, 17*(1), 57–89.

Denham, S. A., Bassett, H. H., Thayer, S. K., Mincic, M. S., Sirotkin, Y. S., & Zinsser, K. (2012). Observing preschoolers' social-emotional behavior: Structure, foundations, and prediction of early school success. *The Journal of Genetic Psychology, 173*(3), 246–278.

Denham, S. A., Blair, K. A., DeMulder, E., Levitas, J., Sawyer, K., Auerbach–Major, S., & Queenan, P. (2003). Preschool emotional competence: Pathway to social competence? *Child Development, 74*(1), 238–256.

Denham, S. A., & Couchoud, E. A. (1990). Young preschoolers' understanding of emotions. *Child Study Journal, 20*(3), 171–192.

Diener, M. L., & Mangelsdorf, S. C. (1999). Behavioral strategies for emotion regulation in toddlers: Associations with maternal involvement and emotional expressions. *Infant Behavior and Development, 22*(4), 569–583.

Durand, K., Gallay, M., Seigneuric, A., Robichon, F., & Baudouin, J. Y. (2007). The development of facial emotion recognition: The role of configural information. *Journal of Experimental Child Psychology, 97*(1), 14–27.

Dykens, E. M., & Kasari, C. (1997). Maladaptive behavior in children with Prader-Willi syndrome, Down syndrome, and nonspecific mental retardation. *American Journal on Mental Retardation, 102*(3), 228–237.

Eisenberg, N. (2000). Emotion, regulation, and moral development. *Annual Review of Psychology, 51*(1), 665–697.

Eisenberg, N., Fabes, R., Miller, P. A., Shell, R., Shea, C., & May-Plumlee, T. (1990). Preschoolers' vicarious emotional responding and their situational and dispositional prosocial behavior. *Merrill-Palmer Quarterly*, 36, 507–529.

Eisenberg, N., Fabes, R. A., Murphy, B., Karbon, M., Maszk, P., Smith, M., . . . Suh, K. (1994). The relations of emotionality and regulation to dispositional and situational empathy-related responding. *Journal of Personality and Social Psychology, 66*(4), 776.

Eisenberg, N., Fabes, R. A., Shepard, S. A., Murphy, B. C., Jones, S., & Guthrie, I. K. (1998). Contemporaneous and longitudinal prediction of children's sympathy from dispositional regulation and emotionality. *Developmental Psychology, 34*(5), 910.

Eisenberg, N., Fabes, R. A., & Spinrad, T. L. (2006). *Handbook of child psychology*. John Wiley & Sons.

Eisenberg, N., & Mussen, P. (1989). *The Roots of Prosocial Behavior in Children* (Cambridge Studies in Social and Emotional Development). Cambridge: Cambridge University Press. https://doi.org/10.1017/CBO9780511571121

Eisenberg, N., & Spinrad, T. L. (2004). Emotion-related regulation: Sharpening the definition. *Child Development, 75*(2), 334–339.

Elliott, S. N., & McKinnie, D. M. (1994). Relationships and differences among social skills, problem behaviors, and academic competence for mainstreamed learning-disabled and nonhandicapped students. *Canadian Journal of School Psychology, 10*(1), 1–14.

Emde, R. N., Kligman, D. H., Reich, J. H., & Wade, T. D. (1978). Emotional expression in infancy: I. Initial studies of social signaling and an emergent model. In M. Lewis & L. Rosenblum (Eds.), *The development of affect: The genesis of behavior* (Vol. 1). New York, NY: Plenum.

Fabes, R. A., Eisenberg, N., & Eisenbud, L. (1993). Behavioral and physiological correlates of children's reactions to others in distress. *Developmental Psychology, 29*(4), 655.

Fidler, D. J., Barrett, K. C., & Most, D. E. (2005). Age-related differences in smiling and personality in Down syndrome. *Journal of Developmental and Physical Disabilities, 17*(3), 263–280.

Fidler, D., Hepburn, S., & Rogers, S. (2006). Early learning and adaptive behaviour in toddlers with Down syndrome: Evidence for an emerging behavioural phenotype? *Down Syndrome Research and Practice, 9*(3), 37–44.

Fidler, D. J., Most, D. E., Booth-LaForce, C., & Kelly, J. F. (2008). Emerging social strengths in young children with Down syndrome. *Infants & Young Children, 21*(3), 207–220.

Field, T. (1994). The effects of mother's physical and emotional unavailability on emotion regulation. *Monographs of the Society for Research in Child Development, 59*(23), 208–227.

Fine, S. E., Izard, C. E., & Trentacosta, C. J. (2006). Emotion situation knowledge in elementary school: Models of longitudinal growth and preschool correlates. *Social Development, 15*(4), 730–751.

Freeman, S. F., Gulsrud, A., & Kasari, C. (2015). Brief report: Linking early joint attention and play abilities to later reports of friendships for children with ASD. *Journal of Autism and Developmental Disorders, 45*(7), 2259–2266.

Freeman, S. F., & Kasari, C. (2002). Characteristics and qualities of the play dates of children with Down syndrome: Emerging or true friendships? *American Journal on Mental Retardation, 107*(1), 16–31.

Garner, P. W., & Waajid, B. (2008). The associations of emotion knowledge and teacher–child relationships to preschool children's school-related developmental competence. *Journal of Applied Developmental Psychology, 29*(2), 89–100.

Gath, A., & Gumlev, D. (1987). Retarded children and their siblings. *Journal of Child Psychology and Psychiatry, 28*(5), 715–730.

Gibbs, M. V., & Thorpe, J. G. (1983). Personality stereotype of noninstitutionalized Down Syndrome children. *American Journal of Mental Deficiency, 87*, 601–605.

Grolnick, W. S., Bridges, L. J., & Connell, J. P. (1996). Emotion regulation in two-year-olds: Strategies and emotional expression in four contexts. *Child Development, 67*(3), 928–941.

Guralnick, M. J., Connor, R. T., & Johnson, L. C. (2011). Peer-related social competence of young children with Down syndrome. *American Journal of Intellectual and Developmental Disabilities, 116*(1), 48–64.

Hamre, B. K., & Pianta, R. C. (2005). Can instructional and emotional support in the first-grade classroom make a difference for children at risk of school failure? *Child development, 76*(5), 949–967.

Heinze, J. E., Miller, A. L., Seifer, R., Dickstein, S., & Locke, R. L. (2015). Emotion knowledge, loneliness, negative social experiences, and internalizing symptoms among low-income preschoolers. *Social Development, 24*(2), 240–265.

Hippolyte, L., Barisnikov, K., Van der Linden, M., & Detraux, J. J. (2009). From facial emotional recognition abilities to emotional attribution: A study in Down syndrome. *Research in Developmental Disabilities, 30*(5), 1007–1022.

Hodapp, R. M., Ly, T. M., Fidler, D. J., & Ricci, L. A. (2001). Less stress, more rewarding: Parenting children with Down syndrome. *Parenting: Science and Practice, 1*(4), 317–337.

Hughes, M., & Kasari, C. (2000). Caregiver–child interaction and the expression of pride in children with Down syndrome. *Education & Training in Mental Retardation & Developmental Disabilities, 35*(1), 67–77.

Izard, C. E., & Malatesta, C. Z. (1987). Perspectives on emotional development I: Differential emotions theory of early emotional development. In J. D. Osofsky (Ed.), *Wiley series on personality processes. Handbook of infant development* (pp. 494–554). Oxford, UK: John Wiley & Sons.

Jahromi, L. B., Gulsrud, A., & Kasari, C. (2008). Emotional competence in children with Down syndrome: Negativity and regulation. *American Journal on Mental Retardation, 113*(1), 32–43.

Kasari, C., & Freeman, S. F. (2001). Task-related social behavior in children with Down syndrome. *American Journal on Mental Retardation, 106*(3), 253–264.

Kasari, C., Freeman, S. F., & Bass, W. (2003). Empathy and response to distress in children with Down syndrome. *Journal of Child Psychology and Psychiatry, 44*(3), 424–431.

Kasari, C., Freeman, S. F., & Hughes, M. A. (2001). Emotion recognition by children with Down syndrome. *American Journal on Mental Retardation, 106*(1), 59–72.

Kasari, C., Freeman, S., Mundy, P., & Sigman, M. D. (1995). Attention regulation by children with Down syndrome: Coordinated joint attention and social referencing looks. *American Journal on Mental Retardation, 100*(2), 128–136.

Kasari, C., Mundy, P., Yirmiya, N., & Sigman, M. (1990). Affect and attention in children with Down syndrome. *American Journal on Mental Retardation, 95*(1), 55–67.

Kasari, C., & Sigman, M. (1996). Expression and understanding of emotion in atypical development: Autism and Down syndrome. In M. Lewis & M. W. Sullivan (Eds.), *Emotional development in atypical children* (pp. 109–130). Mahwah, NJ: Lawrence Erlbaum.

Knieps, L. J., Walden, T. A., & Baxter, A. (1994). Affective expressions of toddlers with and without Down syndrome in a social referencing context. *AJMR-American Journal on Mental Retardation, 99*(3), 301–312.

Kochanska, G., Coy, K. C., & Murray, K. T. (2001). The development of self-regulation in the first four years of life. *Child development, 72*(4), 1091–1111.

Kochanska, G., Tjebkes, J. L., & Fortnan, D. R. (1998). Children's emerging regulation of conduct: Restraint, compliance, and internalization from infancy to the second year. *Child development, 69*(5), 1378–1389.

Kopp, C. B. (1982). Antecedents of self-regulation: A developmental perspective. *Developmental Psychology, 18*(2), 199.

Kopp, C. B. 1990. The growth of self-monitoring among young children with Down syndrome. In Cicchetti, D., & Beeghly, M., (Eds.). *Children with Down Syndrome: A Developmental Perspective* (pp. 231–251). Cambridge: Cambridge University Press.

Kuczynski, L., Kochanska, G., Radke-Yarrow, M., & Girnius-Brown, O. (1987). A developmental interpretation of young children's noncompliance. *Developmental Psychology, 23*(6), 799.

Kuppens, S., Grietens, H., Onghena, P., & Michiels, D. (2009). Associations between parental control and children's overt and relational aggression. *British Journal of Developmental Psychology,* 27(3), 607–623. https://doi.org/10.1348/026151008X345591

Ladd, G. W., Birch, S. H., & Buhs, E. S. (1999). Children's social and scholastic lives in kindergarten: Related spheres of influence?. *Child Development, 70*(6), 1373–1400.

Ladd, G. W., Herald, S. L., & Kochel, K. P. (2006). School readiness: Are there social prerequisites? *Early education and development, 17*(1), 115–150.

Ladd, G. W., Kochenderfer, B. J., & Coleman, C. C. (1996). Friendship quality as a predictor of young children's early school adjustment. *Child Development, 67*(3), 1103–1118.

Landry, S. H., Garner, P. W., Pirie, D., & Swank, P. R. (1994). Effects of social context and mothers' requesting strategies on Down's syndrome children's social responsiveness. *Developmental Psychology, 30*(2), 293.

Lemerise, E. A., & Arsenio, W. F. (2000). An integrated model of emotion processes and cognition in social information processing. *Child Development, 71*(1), 107–118.

Lewis, M. D. (1993). Emotion-cognition interactions in early infant development. *Cognition and Emotion, 7*(2), 145–170.

Lewis, M., & Michalson, L. (1983). The socialization of emotion. In M. Lewis & L. Michalson (Eds.), *Children's Emotions and Moods: Developmental Theory and Measurement* (pp. 157–230). Boston, MA: Springer.

Lindquist, K. A., & Gendron, M. (2013). What's in a word? Language constructs emotion perception. *Emotion Review, 5*(1), 66–71.

McAuliffe, M. D., Hubbard, J. A., & Romano, L. J. (2009). The role of teacher cognition and behavior in children's peer relations. *Journal of Abnormal Child Psychology, 37*(5), 665–677.

McIntyre, L. L., Blacher, J., & Baker, B. L. (2006). The transition to school: Adaptation in young children with and without intellectual disability. *Journal of Intellectual Disability Research, 50*(5), 349–361.

Miller, P. A., Eisenberg, N., Fabes, R. A., & Shell, R. (1996). Relations of moral reasoning and vicarious emotion to young children's prosocial behavior toward peers and adults. *Developmental psychology, 32*(2), 210.

Mischel, W., Ebbesen, E. B., & Raskoff Zeiss, A. (1972). Cognitive and attentional mechanisms in delay of gratification. *Journal of personality and social psychology, 21*(2), 204.

Mischel, W., & Underwood, B. (1974). Instrumental ideation in delay of gratification. *Child development, 45*(4), 1083–1088.

Mischel, W., Shoda, Y., & Rodriguez, M. I. (1989). Delay of gratification in children. *Science, 244*(4907), 933–938.

Morgan, J. K., Izard, C. E., & King, K. A. (2010). Construct validity of the Emotion Matching Task: Preliminary evidence for convergent and criterion validity of a new emotion knowledge measure for young children. *Social Development, 19*(1), 52–70.

Morris, A. S., Silk, J. S., Morris, M. D., Steinberg, L., Aucoin, K. J., & Keyes, A. W. (2011). The influence of mother–child emotion regulation strategies on children's expression of anger and sadness. *Developmental Psychology, 47*(1), 213.

Næss, K. B., Nygaard, E., Ostad, J., Dolva, A. S., & Lyster, S. A. H. (2017). The profile of social functioning in children with Down syndrome. *Disability and Rehabilitation, 39*, 1320–1331. https://doi.org/10.1080/09638288.2016.1194901

Ornaghi, V., Grazzani, I., Cherubin, E., Conte, E., & Piralli, F. (2015). "Let's talk about emotions!" The effect of conversational training on preschoolers' emotion comprehension and prosocial orientation. *Social Development, 24*(1), 166–183.

Pochon, R., & Declercq, C. (2014). Emotional lexicon understanding and emotion recognition: A longitudinal study in children with Down syndrome. *Journal of Developmental and Physical Disabilities, 26*(5), 549–563.

Porter, M. A., Coltheart, M., & Langdon, R. (2007). The neuropsychological basis of hypersociability in Williams and Down syndrome. *Neuropsychologia, 45*(12), 2839–2849.

Ramani, G. B., Brownell, C. A., & Campbell, S. B. (2010). Positive and negative peer interaction in 3-and 4-year-olds in relation to regulation and dysregulation. *The Journal of genetic psychology, 171*(3), 218–250.

Rheingold, H. L. (1982). Little children's participation in the work of adults, a nascent prosocial behavior. *Child Development, 53*, 114–125.

Rose-Krasnor, L., & Denham, S. (2009). Social-emotional competence in early childhood. In K. H. Rubin, W. M. Bukowski, & B. Laursen (Eds.), *Social, Emotional, and Personality Development in Context. Handbook of Peer Interactions, Relationships, and Groups* (pp. 162–179). New York, NY: The Guilford Press.

Scheeren, A. M., de Rosnay, M., Koot, H. M., & Begeer, S. (2013). Rethinking theory of mind in high-functioning autism spectrum disorder. *Journal of Child Psychology and Psychiatry, 54*(6), 628–635.

Sette, S., Spinrad, T. L., & Baumgartner, E. (2016). The relations of preschool children's emotion knowledge and socially appropriate behaviors to peer likability. *International Journal of Behavioral Development, 41*(4), 532–541. https://doi.org/10.1177/0165025416645667

Shoda, Y., Mischel, W., & Peake, P. K. (1990). Predicting adolescent cognitive and self-regulatory competencies from preschool delay of gratification: Identifying diagnostic conditions. *Developmental psychology, 26*(6), 978.

Sigman, M., & Ruskin, E. (1999). Continuity and change in the social competence of children with autism, Down syndrome, and developmental delays. *Monographs of the Society for Research in Child Development, 64*(1), 1–114. https://doi.org/10.1111/1540-5834.00002

Spinrad, T. L., Eisenberg, N., Cumberland, A., Fabes, R. A., Valiente, C., Shepard, S. A., . . . Guthrie, I. K. (2006). Relation of emotion-related regulation to children's social competence: A longitudinal study. *Emotion, 6*(3), 498.

Stifter, C. A., & Braungart, J. M. (1995). The regulation of negative reactivity in infancy: Function and development. *Developmental Psychology, 31*(3), 448.

Stifter, C. A., Spinrad, T., & Braungart-Rieker, J. (1999). Toward a developmental model of child compliance: The role of emotion regulation in infancy. *Child Development, 70*(1), 21–32.

Székely, E., Tiemeier, H., Arends, L. R., Jaddoe, V. W., Hofman, A., Verhulst, F. C., & Herba, C. M. (2011). Recognition of facial expressions of emotions by 3-year-olds. *Emotion, 11*(2), 425.

Thomas, L. A., De Bellis, M. D., Graham, R., & LaBar, K. S. (2007). Development of emotional facial recognition in late childhood and adolescence. *Developmental Science, 10*(5), 547–558.

Thompson, R. A. (1994). Emotion regulation: A theme in search of definition. *Monographs of the Society for Research in Child Development, 59*(2–3), 25–52.

Trentacosta, C. J., & Fine, S. E. (2010). Emotion knowledge, social competence, and behavior problems in childhood and adolescence: A meta-analytic review. *Social Development, 19*(1), 1–29.

Trentacosta, C. J., Izard, C. E., Mostow, A. J., & Fine, S. E. (2006). Children's emotional competence and attentional competence in early elementary school. *School Psychology Quarterly, 21*(2), 148.

Tronick, E. Z. (1989). Emotions and emotional communication in infants. *American Psychologist, 44*(2), 112.

Warneken, F., & Tomasello, M. (2006). Altruistic helping in human infants and young chimpanzees. *Science, 311*(5765), 1301–1303.

Widen, S. C., & Russell, J. A. (2003). A closer look at preschoolers' freely produced labels for facial expressions. *Developmental Psychology, 39*(1), 114.

Wishart, J. G. (2007). Socio-cognitive understanding: A strength or weakness in Down's syndrome? *Journal of Intellectual Disability Research, 51*(12), 996–1005.

Wishart, J. G., Cebula, K. R., Willis, D. S., & Pitcairn, T. K. (2007). Understanding of facial expressions of emotion by children with intellectual disabilities of differing aetiology. *Journal of Intellectual Disability Research, 51*(7), 551–563.

Wishart, J. G., & Pitcairn, T. K. (2000). Recognition of identity and expression in faces by children with Down syndrome. *American Journal on Mental Retardation, 105*(6), 466–479.

Young-Browne, G., Rosenfeld, H. M., & Horowitz, F. D. (1977). Infant discrimination of facial expressions. *Child Development, 48*(2), 555–562.

Zahn-Waxler, C., Radke-Yarrow, M., Wagner, E., & Chapman, M. (1992). Development of concern for others. *Developmental Psychology, 28*(1), 126.

CHAPTER

4 Young Children With Down Syndrome: Mother–Child Dyadic Relationships

Penny Hauser-Cram, Ashley C. Woodman, *and* Linda Gilmore

Abstract

This chapter is focused on the mother-child dyadic relationship in families where a young child has Down syndrome. Because mothers enter into a relationship with a child within a particular context, a sociocultural perspective on parenting a child with Down syndrome promotes a deeper understanding of interaction in the mother-child dyad. Both the role of the family system, including positive parenting, and the contributions of the child's attributes, especially temperament, are considered. Specific literature on the mother-child dyad is discussed, including maternal language input, the role of maternal directives during structured and unstructured tasks, and studies on autonomy-supportive parenting. Suggestions for future research include developing studies that focus on maternal strengths as well as conducting investigations that recognize the importance of the sociocultural context in which mother-child dyadic relationships are developed.

Key Words: mother-child relationship, Down syndrome, temperament, positive parenting, autonomy, directives, stigma

Young Children With Down Syndrome: Mother-Child Dyadic Relationships

From the perspective of the bioecological model, proximal processes operate as the engines of development (Bronfenbrenner & Evans, 2000; Bronfenrenner & Morris, 1998). Such processes encompass increasingly complex reciprocal interactions that occur on a regular basis over an extended period of time. The interaction that occurs within the mother-child relationship is a prime example of such processes that serve to contribute centrally to a child's development. In this chapter, we consider the mother-child dyadic relationship in families in which the child has Down syndrome. We begin with a brief discussion of the role of the sociocultural perspective on disability, as this view permeates the various ecological niches of the family. Next, we turn to the importance of family dynamics in fostering mother-child interaction. Given increasing evidence of the detrimental role of high levels of stress in families (Shonkoff et al., 2012), we consider the various components of stress experienced by mothers in families in which a child has Down syndrome. Because children elicit reactions in the dyadic relationship, we review the literature on temperament in children with Down syndrome and examine how children's dispositions and behaviors contribute to dyadic interactions. Next, we analyze the empirical literature on mother-child interaction in dyads in which a child has Down syndrome and discuss the various interpretations of the findings. In that section, we include a discussion about the research on maternal verbal input to a child with Down syndrome as well as on maternal-child interactions during unstructured situations, such as play, and structured situations, such as teaching tasks. In the final section, we discuss the areas ripe for future scholarship, including the need for increased focus on dimensions of positive parenting.

Sociocultural Perspectives on Disability

Parenting a child with Down syndrome was at one time considered fraught with psychological difficulties, including parental mourning and prolonged sadness (see, for example, Solnit & Stark, 1961). Despite a research emphasis on the positive ways in which a child with disabilities may contribute to the family (e.g., Goddard, Lehr, & Lapadat, 2000; Hastings, Beck, & Hill, 2005), much attention continues to be paid to the multiple challenges of parenting a child with Down syndrome. Some of those challenges relate to the child's health and developmental needs, whereas others emerge from sociocultural perspectives on disability, including the stigma associated with disability (Lalvani, 2011).

Sociocultural views of disability are central to the perspectives of mothers as they parent a child with Down syndrome. The results of several analyses in which the perceptions of parents of children with Down syndrome and other developmental disabilities in Anglo and Latino families living in the United States have been compared indicate that Latino parents report a more positive impact of raising a child with Down syndrome (Blacher, Baker, & Berkovits, 2013). In a study by Skinner, Correa, Skinner, and Bailey (2001), a high proportion of Latino parents reported that they viewed their child as a blessing from God and a sign of their worthiness as parents. This suggests a positive view of both their child and themselves as capable parents.

The findings from studies conducted in a range of cultures indicate that parents frequently view their child with Down syndrome as a gift determined by supernatural powers. For example, in a study of health professionals, researchers, and parents of children with Down syndrome in Pakistan, many parents acknowledged that the birth of a child with Down syndrome was due to the "will of Allah." Some believed that they had been "chosen" to be the child's parent, while others considered that having a child with Down syndrome was a symbol of good luck (Bryant, Ahmed, Ahmed, Jafri, & Raashid, 2011). A view of the child with intellectual disabilities as a gift was also endorsed in a study of South Asian Indian immigrants who were members of a Hindu temple in the United States (Gabel, 2004). The mothers reported that members of their families, including themselves, were given the gift of this child to repair sins of previous lives. As a result, they considered it important to "suffer through" without complaint because the child was potentially teaching them lessons. Cheng and Tang (1995) described a somewhat similar response by parents of Chinese children with disabilities living in China: their approaches included coping strategies of forbearance, coupled with prayers to ancestors and bids to supernatural powers. In a review of studies on families with a child with Down syndrome in East Asian countries, Choi and Van Riper (2017) emphasized the importance of Confucian values to maintaining family harmony. Such values, largely defined by age and gender, require a balancing of needs of various family members. Choi and Van Riper found that parenting demands differed from those emphasized in Western cultures. For example, parents of children with Down syndrome in Western countries often focus on their children's problem behaviors, whereas parents in East Asian countries emphasize the daily caretaking demands and the challenges due to the stigma experienced by the family (Choi & Van Riper, 2017).

Stigma related to children with intellectual disabilities, such as those with Down syndrome, is a theme of several investigations. For example, in studies conducted in Pakistan, mothers of children with intellectual disabilities discussed the way in which the experiences of stigma prevented them from fully participating in community activities (Mirza, Tareen, Davidson, & Rahman, 2009). These mothers also expressed their experience of "otherness" as parents and endorsed feelings of alienation from other families in their community (Ali & Rafique, 2015). In China, the shame associated with having a child with an intellectual disability and the consequent fear of discrimination may lead many families to keep their child a secret and to avoid seeking help outside the family (Su, Cuskelly, Gilmore, & Sullivan, 2018; Wong et al., 2004). As these various inquiries indicate, mothers in all cultures enter into interactions with their child infused with sociocultural perspectives on the meaning of intellectual disability and the role of mothers in parenting children.

Lalvani (2011) indicated that mothers of young children with Down syndrome in North America encounter two cultural narratives: that of idealized motherhood and that of the sociocultural meaning of disability. Within these narratives, mothers of children with Down syndrome may be viewed as having "diminished parenthood" (Landsman, 2005) or, alternatively, as being "special" or "chosen" (Lalvani, 2008). These discrepant narratives have long histories across many cultural groups (O'Hara & Bouras, 2007). Both perspectives reveal the sociocultural stigma associated with having a child with a condition such as Down syndrome.

In families in which a child has Down syndrome, even the medical diagnosis itself can be stigmatizing, as it might imply an assignment of culpability based on genetic variation (Davis & Manago, 2016). Moreover, mothers of children with Down syndrome in Western countries often report that the stigma they experience to some extent has emerged from the medical community itself because health care providers often present a child's diagnosis as a "tragedy" or a "burden" (Lalvani, 2011). Some claim that the medicalization of the disability, which may include the discussion of medical procedures such as those for heart defects common among children with Down syndrome, can neglect the focus on the whole child. Such focus on the medical needs of a child may fortify rather than lessen the moral stigma experienced by mothers of a child with a disability (Davis & Manago, 2016). In a quantitative and qualitative study of 81 mothers of children with disabilities in the United States, Green (2003) found that maternal reports of both stigma and objective burden of parenting predicted mothers' reports of subjective burden and distress. Based on Goffman's (1963) classic theoretical work on stigma, which suggests that stigma can extend to others with whom an individual associates, Green proposed that many mothers of children with disabilities experience both stigma and "courtesy stigma," a devaluing through association. According to this view, societal stigma both devalues individuals with disabilities and those who provide care, nurturing, and support to them.

Sauer and Lalvani (2017) proposed that rather than focusing primarily on the individual parent, disability studies provide an examination of the sociopolitical and institutional climates that promote stigmatized views of disability. Most researchers of mother-child interaction in dyads in which a young child has Down syndrome focus on the proximal system of the family and do not fully discuss the larger sociocultural context in which such family dynamics occur (Hauser-Cram, Howell-Moneta, & Young, 2012). Nevertheless, in considering the literature on the mother-child dyad, the importance of the sociocultural ecosystem must be considered for it is embedded in the questions posed by researchers and, as such, guides views of appropriate and inappropriate interactions between the children and their mothers.

The Family System and Parenting Stress

The family system provides the most proximal setting for the young child. In line with the sociocultural view that parenting a child with a disability is often associated with rewards and satisfactions (Goddard et al., 2000; Hastings et al., 2005), a comprehensive view of family experiences also includes the unique challenges posed by the demands of parenting. Some of those challenges result in parenting stress, and as a result much research has been devoted to understanding such stress in parents (primarily mothers) of children with Down syndrome. Most evidence indicates that, as a group, mothers of children with Down syndrome exhibit higher levels of stress during their child's early years than do mothers of typically developing children (Hamlyn-Wright, Draghi-Lorenz, & Ellis, 2007; Nes et al., 2014; Roach, Orsmond, & Barratt, 1999). Moreover, stress levels tend to increase for those mothers over the early to middle childhood period (Hauser-Cram, Warfield, Shonkoff, & Krauss, 2001) and are associated with increases in children's externalizing problem behaviors (Eisenhower, Baker, & Blacher, 2005).

Although stress levels among parents of children with Down syndrome tend to be higher than parents of children with typical development, they also tend to be lower than those reported by parents of children with other developmental disabilities. When considering parents of children across a range of disabilities, researchers have proposed a "Down syndrome advantage" for parents, especially mothers. This proposal, based largely on studies of parents of young children with Down syndrome in comparison to those of children with other developmental disabilities, was first described by Hodapp, Ricci, Ly, and Fidler (2003). They suggested that children with Down syndrome are easier to parent than children with other types of developmental disabilities because of their particular temperament and behavioral characteristics. The Down syndrome advantage appears to extend also to adolescence and young adulthood. Lower levels of stress are reported by both mothers (Abbeduto et al., 2004) and fathers (Hartley, Seltzer, Head, & Abbeduto, 2012) of adolescents and young adults with Down syndrome compared to parents of those with fragile X and autism. Hodapp et al. (2003) suggested that the advantages were likely due to lower levels of challenging behavior among individuals with Down syndrome. Other researchers have pointed to the importance of considering confounding variables, such as parental socioeconomic status and parental age, that may contribute to such findings (e.g., Glidden, Grein, & Ludwig, 2014). In a longitudinal study of parenting stress trajectories, Most, Fidler, Booth-Laforce, and Kelly (2006) reported that the stress levels of mothers of young children with Down syndrome, in comparison to a group of young children with mixed etiologies, were lower when the children were 15 months of age, a finding that supports the "advantage." However, they found that the stress levels increased by the time the children were 45 months of age, at which point the stress levels in the two groups were similar. They suggested that as children grew older their cognitive delays, language delays, and problem behaviors became more apparent and likely contributed to the relatively higher parenting stress levels reported during the preschool, in comparison to the toddler, ages. Nevertheless, the discussion around the "Down syndrome advantage" centers on questions about whether children with Down syndrome have temperaments and related dispositional qualities that make them generally easier to parent than children with other disabilities.

The Role of Child Temperament

Temperament, defined as constitutionally based individual differences in reactivity and self-regulation, influenced by genetic inheritance, maturation, and experience (Rothbart, 1981; Rothbart & Derryberry, 1981), can be observed in an individual's emotional, attentional, and motor activity. Several key questions arise when considering the use of traditional measures of temperament in children with disabilities. As most measures of temperament are standardized for specific age groups, should children with disabilities be compared to their same-age peers, or to peers of the same developmental age? Do behavioral indicators of temperament have the same meaning for children with disabilities? For example, high intensity of mood is considered a sign of a difficult temperament, yet Goldberg and Marcovitch (1989) argued that extremely low intensity of emotional expression may be problematic for parents of children with disabilities. Are behavioral indices of temperament more difficult to ascertain in children with disabilities?

In an initial study of child temperament, Nygaard, Smith, and Torgersen (2002) evaluated the validity and reliability of the Children's Behavior Questionnaire (CBQ; Ahadi,

Rothbart, & Ye, 1993) among children with Down syndrome, children born prematurely, and children with typical developmental histories in Norway, China, and the United States. In line with previous research with this measure, a principal component analysis yielded three factors for all the groups of children: surgency/positive affect, negative emotionality, and effortful control. However, discrepancies in the factor structure were found across the groups. For example, the surgency factor, consisting of positive affect, high intensity, showing pleasure and little shyness, was more influenced by emotional processes (discomfort, fear, smiling, and laughing) and less influenced by effortful control (approach, attentional shifting) for the children with Down syndrome as compared to the children born prematurely and the children with typical developmental histories. The expression of happiness was less associated with effortful control in the children with Down syndrome as compared to those in the other groups. The mean internal consistency across subscales was also relatively lower for the children with Down syndrome. These findings highlight the need for further research on the validity and reliability of measures of temperament for children with Down syndrome.

Temperament in Children With Down Syndrome

Interest in the temperamental profiles of children with Down syndrome began in the 1980s (for reviews, see Beeghly, 1998; Goldberg & Marcovitch, 1989). Since then, most studies have focused on comparing mean level differences for children with and without Down syndrome. Several of the early researchers were specifically motivated to challenge the prevailing stereotype that children with Down syndrome were temperamentally "easy." For example, Bridges and Cicchetti (1982) questioned the dominant view of infants with Down syndrome as "placid, humorous, cheerful, friendly, easy children" (p. 238). Whereas children with Down syndrome had been assumed to represent a uniform, homogenous group with respect to personality characteristics, Bridges and Cicchetti (1982) found a wide range of temperamental variation among children with Down syndrome in line with similar research on typical development at the time (Baron, 1972; Gunn & Berry, 1985).

For decades, researchers have failed to find evidence for a personality stereotype of individuals with Down syndrome as more pleasant, more affectionate, and more behaviorally passive (Fidler, 2006). However, this perception seems to persist. In an Australian sample of 1,228 members of the general community, Gilmore (2006) identified a common stereotype of individuals with Down syndrome as being affectionate, loving, and happy. These positive perceptions mirrored the findings of an earlier community study of 2,591 Australians that included 538 experienced teachers (Gilmore, Campbell, & Cuskelly, 2003). High proportions (70 to 85 percent) of participants in both groups believed that children with Down syndrome are more affectionate, friendlier, and happier than other children. Parents may also endorse this stereotype. In her classic longitudinal study of children with Down syndrome, Carr (1995) indicated that a large percentage of mothers described their children as "cheerful," "generous," and "fun." Similarly, several investigators have indicated that children with Down syndrome may have easier temperamental dispositions compared to children with other intellectual and developmental disabilities (Ganiban, Wagner, & Cicchetti, 1990; Kasari & Sigman, 1996; Shonkoff, Hauser-Cram, Krauss, & Upshur, 1992; Stoneman, 2007; Stores, Stores, Fellows, & Buckley, 1998), although, as stated by Nygaard et al. (2002), "the problem with this literature is that for each paper reporting a difference, there exists another study reporting failure to replicate" (p. 62). Several factors complicate the ability to abstract patterns from the literature on group comparisons. First, researchers use different methods (e.g., observation vs. questionnaire) and different instruments, and there is little consistency across these methods regarding the dimensions being measured. Second, the demographics of the samples may differ considerably with respect to age, gender, birth weight, racial/ethnic background, culture, and socioeconomic status, and such demographic features may relate to ratings of temperament. Third, much of the research on temperament in children with Down syndrome is limited by small sample sizes. Variation in research methodology and populations studied will eventually yield a more robust picture of temperament in children with Down syndrome, but the number of studies on this topic is fairly limited to date.

Most comparative studies are inconclusive, but differences in persistence between children with Down syndrome and children with typical development have often been reported (Bridges & Cicchetti, 1982; Green, Dennis, & Bennets, 1989; Gunn & Berry, 1985; Gunn & Cuskelly, 1991; Marcovitch, Goldberg, MacGregor, & Lojkasek, 1986; Pueschel & Myers, 1994; Ratekin, 1996). Children with Down syndrome are generally perceived to be less persistent than their peers. Motivation to persist with challenges has been identified as an area of particular difficulty for children with Down syndrome (Ruskin, Mundy, Kasari, & Sigman, 1994; Wishart, 1991, 1993), although this is not a consistent finding. Some researchers have found no differences between children with Down syndrome and typically developing children of the same mental age, although parent reports of their children's persistence tend to be less positive (Gilmore & Cuskelly, 2011; Gilmore, Cuskelly, & Hayes, 2003; Glenn, Dayus, Cunningham, & Horgan, 2001). The inconsistent findings may be related to different methodological approaches, especially when persistence is measured during structured tasks versus free play. Without structure, children with Down syndrome may have more difficulty sustaining their effort.

Although parent reports may be more valid as they are based on observations of their child across many times and settings, parents' perceptions may be based on comparisons of their child with same-age peers, rather than those of the same mental age—a comparison that is more common in laboratory studies of persistence (Gilmore & Cuskelly, 2011). Thus, the low persistence may be an inherent characteristic of children with Down syndrome, an acquired pattern of behavior due to a history of frustrating experiences, or a phenomenon that is associated with other core features of Down syndrome. Fidler (2006) argued that a personality profile characterized by low persistence may emerge as a secondary phenotype in individuals with Down syndrome. She suggested that poorer persistence in young children with Down syndrome could be the indirect result of emerging difficulties with instrumental and strategic thinking. Thus, toddlers with Down syndrome may abandon challenging situations because they are not able to generate new, more viable strategies to complete the task.

Positive-Parenting Dynamics

Perceived difficulties with persistence and other problem behaviors may challenge parents of children with Down syndrome to a greater extent than parents of children with typical development, and some of those challenges likely emerge in parenting dynamics, especially in mother-child interactions. This is why parenting stress is one of the most frequently studied responses in mothers of children with Down syndrome. High levels of stress can lead to disruptive parenting, but protective factors in the family, community, and culture can moderate parenting stress, leading to positive-parenting practices (Masarik & Conger, 2017). Investigations of positive-parenting behaviors delineate critical aspects of family dynamics. Parents who demonstrate positive parenting are warm in their interactions with a child, sensitive to their child's needs and signals, affectionate, supportive, and predictable (Barber, Stolz, Olsen, Collins, & Burchinal, 2005). Positive parenting is associated with secure attachment across cultures (van IJzendoorn & Sagi-Schwartz, 2008), and with more advantageous child cognitive and social outcomes, including effective emotion regulation (Mesman, van IJzendoorn, & Bakermans-Kranenburg, 2012).

Maternal sensitivity is a key dimension of positive parenting. Conceptual definitions vary, but maternal sensitivity generally involves maternal displays of warmth and affiliation in responding contingently to a child and providing a child with social-emotional support (Landry, Smith, & Swank, 2006). The importance of sensitive maternal responsiveness is central to several theoretical perspectives including attachment theory (Ainsworth, Blehar, Waters, & Wall, 1978), socialization theory (Grusec, Goodnow, & Kuczynski, 2000), and sociocultural theory (Rogoff & Morelli, 1989). Substantial research on typically developing children points to the importance of maternal sensitivity during the early childhood years in enhancing children's emotional control of behavior (Deater-Deckard, Ivy, & Petrill, 2006; Ispa, Su-Russell, Palermo, & Carlo, 2017; Spinrad et al., 2012). Through sensitive parenting, mothers model positive interaction styles for children (Darling & Steinberg, 1993). Sensitive parenting also fosters feelings of self-control and self-efficacy in children (Bornstein & Tamis-LeMonda, 1989; Mintz, Hamre, & Hatfield, 2011). Mothers who show sensitivity in their interactions with their young children have children who display more positive self-regulatory behaviors (Eisenberg, Spinrad, & Smith, 2004) and exhibit fewer behavior problems (Dodge & Pettit, 2003).

In one study of positive parenting in dyads in which a child has a disability, Niccols and Feldman (2006) examined the interactions of mothers with 2-year-olds with developmental delays and found those children whose mothers demonstrated higher levels of sensitivity had lower levels of behavior problems both concurrently and a year later. In a follow-up study of children aged 2 and 3 years with Down syndrome specifically, Niccols, Milligan, Chisholm, and Atkinson (2011) analyzed the relation between maternal sensitivity in interactions with children and children's aggressive behaviors 2 years later. The mothers who displayed higher levels of maternal sensitivity had children with Down syndrome who later displayed lower levels of externalizing behavior problems.

Some researchers have suggested that parents of children with disabilities display lower levels of positive parenting than parents of children without disabilities. For example, Blacher, Baker, and Kaladjian (2013) conducted a comprehensive longitudinal comparison of maternal behaviors with preschool-aged children (at ages 3, 4, and 5 years) with a disability (Down syndrome, autism spectrum disorders, cerebral palsy, undifferentiated delay) in relation to the behaviors of mothers of typically developing children in both unstructured and structured settings. The unstructured tasks included free play, whereas the structured tasks involved clean-up and problem-solving activities; these task categories differed by the demands placed on the mother and child. Blacher et al. defined positive parenting as demonstrating positive affect, sensitivity, stimulation of cognition, and low detachment during interactions and negative parenting as engaging in intrusive behaviors and negative affect. They found that the parents of both the typically developing children and the children with disabilities demonstrated more positive parenting in the unstructured or free-play activity in which few task demands were present. In unstructured activities, mothers of children with Down syndrome demonstrated more positive parenting than those of children in all other groups. Over the preschool year, the mothers of the children with Down syndrome demonstrated a noticeable increase in positive parenting during structured tasks, although they also demonstrated high levels of negative parenting, resulting from high levels of intrusion. Blacher et al. suggested that the mothers of the children with Down syndrome may have learned certain behavioral techniques that range from overtly intrusive to appropriately directive. As we discuss in a later section, the issue of whether maternal directives with children with Down syndrome are a beneficial or intrusive part of interacting has been a theme in much research on mothers of children with Down syndrome.

In a meta-analysis of 14 studies of parenting children with disabilities, Dyches, Smith, Korth, Roper, and Mandleco (2012) considered various dimensions of positive parenting, such as maternal sensitivity, joint attention, engagement in play, maternal responsiveness, praise, turn-taking control, and avoidance of intrusive interactions. They found that such parenting had a moderate relation to child outcomes, including children's level of play, social behaviors, and adaptive behaviors. The impact of positive parenting on child outcomes did not differ by type of disability. Specifically, children with Down syndrome were found to benefit from positive-parenting approaches to the same extent as their peers with other developmental disabilities. This suggests that, similar to typically developing children and children with other disabilities, positive parenting is valuable for children with Down syndrome.

Mother-Child Interactions in Dyads Where a Child Has Down Syndrome

Mothers interact with their young children in multiple settings and contribute many elements to their children's experiences. In this section, we consider the research on two types of mother-child interactions. First, we focus on maternal language input because it serves an increasingly important aspect of mother-child interactions during the early childhood years. Next, we consider mother-child interaction during play as well as in structured activities.

Maternal Language Input

Children with Down syndrome tend to have several syndrome-specific features of language difficulties, especially related to expressive syntax language processes that are highly dependent on phonological short-term memory (Abbeduto et al., Chapter 18, this volume; Abbeduto, Warren, & Conners, 2007). Studies on maternal input to children with Down syndrome have largely been focused on the structural features of maternal language, such as mean length of utterance (MLU) and aspects of syntactic complexity (Venuti, de Falco, Esposito, Zaninelli, & Bornstein, 2012). In general, the findings from such studies indicate that the structural aspects of maternal language input relate to children's comprehension, rather than to production levels (Chapman & Raining Bird, 2012).

As emphasized by D'Souza, D'Souza, and Karmiloff-Smith (2017), language development is an experience-dependent process. Neural connectivity and circuitry related to language processing change as a function of language input. Therefore, the variation and level of complexity of language input provided by a mother (and presumably by others who interact with a child) lead to the child's developing lexical skills. In one small but instructive study, mothers of children with Down syndrome were found to use precise names when talking to their children, whereas mothers of typically developing children used more general categories (Cardoso-Martins & Mervis, 1985). As D'Souza et al. indicated, parents may employ such precise naming based on their assessments of what a child can learn, but such restrictive labeling may also prevent children from readily developing category discrimination. Additional evidence of the use of specific lexical strategies was reported by Zampini, Fasolo, and D'Odorico (2012) in a comparison study of maternal linguistic input to 24-month-old children with and without Down syndrome. The mothers of the children with Down syndrome used simpler linguistic strategies than mothers of typically developing children, as they produced simpler vocabulary and used more routines and onomatopoeic words when addressing their children. These findings led Zampini et al. to speculate that mothers of children with Down syndrome provide input that is not sufficiently complex given their child's level of understanding.

Although mothers of children with Down syndrome may provide verbal input that is less complex than that used by other mothers, they tend to complement their communication with gestures to a greater extent than other mothers. Iverson, Longobardi, Spampinato, and Caselli (2006) reported that mothers of 4-year-old children with Down syndrome produced more deictic gestures than did mothers of typically developing children of the same age. Iverson et al. proposed that the use of such gestures may assist in joint attention between a mother and child. Despite their high degree of social interest, young children with Down syndrome often have difficulty in acquiring important components of joint attention (Abbeduto et al., 2007), and their mothers' use of gestures may assist them in this interactive process.

Mothers of children with Down syndrome appear to use additional strategies, such as employing high levels of affect when interacting with their child. In a study on maternal functional speech to children with Down syndrome, autism spectrum disorder, and typically developing children, Venuti et al. (2012) considered maternal use of information-salient speech and affect-salient speech to children with developmental ages around two years. They found that the mothers in all the groups used more information-salient than affect-salient speech, but that the mothers of children with Down syndrome in particular used more affect-salient speech as compared to the mothers of the typically developing children. They speculated that the high level of affect displayed by the mothers could be related to the Down syndrome phenotype, reasoning that the facial features of children with Down syndrome often resemble those of younger children, evoking high levels of affective responses from their mothers. Parenting styles typically used with very young children were also reported in a study by Fidler (2003) of parental vocalizations to children with Down syndrome. She indicated that parents of children with Down syndrome raised the pitch of their voice and used wider pitch variance than the parents of comparison children with other etiologies. Such high pitch and large pitch variation is typical of parents in their interactions with very young children. Questions remain about whether such maternal verbal input is overly simplistic or appropriate to the child's level of maturity. Further consideration of maternal-child interactions in the context of the language development of individuals with Down syndrome can be found in Chapter 18 (Abbeduto) of this volume.

Mother-Child Interactions

Similar questions emerge about the role of maternal interactions in the analyses of research on the mother-child dyad during structured situations, such as teaching, and during unstructured situations, such as play. Although this body of research is often focused on maternal input, the child's contributions, not just status, are critical to consider as well. For example, Mitchell, Hauser-Cram, and Crossman (2015) found that both mothers and young children with Down syndrome (age 3 years) displayed more contingent behaviors toward each other than did the members of mother-dyads in which a child had other types of developmental etiologies. These results were maintained when confounding variables, such as maternal levels of education and social support, were controlled. Such findings emphasize the value of considering bidirectional responsivity between mother and child in studying such interactions.

The importance of this fluid exchange between mothers and children with Down syndrome is central to the study of mother-child dyads. Many early studies on maternal interaction with children with Down syndrome indicated that mothers tend to use more directives in such transactions (Marfo, 1990). In an analysis of such studies, Marfo (1990) emphasized that negative connotations emerge from the attributions of over-zealous control by mothers of children with Down syndrome. A question emerges, however, as to whether such directives serve intrusive functions or act as reparative and facilitative functions. The differences observed in maternal behavior may reflect appropriate adaptations by mothers of children with Down syndrome. Such adaptations may be necessary because young children with Down syndrome tend to demonstrate decreased emotionality and responsiveness to their environment (Jahromi, Gulsrud, & Kasari, 2008), difficulties with sustained attention (Edvardson et al, 2014), and challenges with appropriate use of social skills when presented with learning tasks (Wishart, Willis, Cebula, & Pitcairn, 2007). In one study, Gilmore, Cuskelly, Jobling, and Hayes (2009) found that maternal directiveness and autonomy support of children with Down syndrome were related to the children's behaviors, specifically their task persistence, whereas no such relationships were evident in the typically developing dyads. The direction of effect was uncertain, but mothers of children with Down syndrome may be more likely to act in ways that respond to their child's task behaviors. Another possibility is that maternal behaviors, especially directiveness and autonomy support, may have more impact for children with Down syndrome than for typically developing children.

The results of many, but not all, studies suggest that mothers of young children with Down syndrome use more directives, but are concomitantly more supportive during play than mothers of typically developing children of similar chronological and mental ages (Roach, Barratt, Miller, & Leavitt, 1998). However, some researchers have found that mothers of children with Down syndrome do not differ from other mothers in their use of directives in some contexts (Gilmore & Cuskelly, 2009). For example, Hughes and Kasari (2000) found that although mothers of children with Down syndrome, in comparison to mothers of typically developing children, were more directive in play-based situations, they did not differ when engaged in joint problem-solving tasks. Reconciling discrepant findings about maternal directiveness across studies is challenging because of the differing operational definitions and methodologies that have been employed. Children's ages and the contexts in which observations are made (e.g., free play versus structured tasks) need to be considered too. The overall affective quality of the interaction is an additional important dimension. For example, Venuti, de Falco, Giusti, and Bornstein (2008) reported that children with Down syndrome display more sophisticated behaviors within interactions that have high levels of affective quality. Therefore, a combination of directives and supportive structures observed in positive parenting may be optimally functional for children with Down syndrome.

Mothers of children with Down syndrome may be more likely than other mothers to adopt teaching strategies in their interactions with their young child. For example,

Pino (2000) compared observations of eight mothers of preschool children with Down syndrome to those of eight mothers of children developing typically in two types of activities: meal time (considered a structured activity) and unstructured play. The two groups were similar in relation to level of receptive language development and maternal levels of education. The mothers of the children with Down syndrome did not differ from the other mothers in the use of strategies to manage their child's behavior, but demonstrated more strategies, such as explaining, demonstrating, labeling, and questioning, indicative of a teaching role. Pino proposed that these differences might be attributed to the parent training received by the mothers of children with Down syndrome, although no direct evidence on this point was available.

Autonomy-Supportive Parenting

Early intervention programs often encourage parents to provide high levels of scaffolding, continual encouragement and stimulation, and prompt acknowledgement of child performance using praise and rewards. Such responses, while potentially being effective in the short-term, may lead to dependence on external sources of structure and motivation. Researchers of typically developing children have demonstrated the critical importance of encouraging a child's autonomy (van der Kaap-Deeder, Vansteenkiste, Soenens, & Mabbe, 2017). Supporting autonomy means giving children opportunities to make their own choices and to solve problems with sensitive and developmentally appropriate support, and without unnecessary interference, from parents (Evans & Boucher, 2015; Gilmore & Cuskelly, 2014). A crucial element of autonomy-supportive parenting is adult awareness of, and attunement to, a child's needs and abilities. As will be discussed later, due to factors such as parents' goals or difficulty in reading the child's intentions, attunement may be more difficult when the child has a developmental disability such as Down syndrome. For example, van der Kaap-Deeder et al. (2017) pointed out that autonomy-suppressing or autonomy-thwarting environments are likely to "minimize, ignore or deny the child's perspective" (p. 238), although low levels of support for autonomy are not necessarily accompanied by high levels of control and intrusive directiveness.

With typically developing children, maternal support for autonomy has been shown to be important for the development of children's self-regulation (Brenning, Soenens, Van Petegem, & Vansteenkiste, 2015), social-emotional functioning (Matte-Gagné, Harvey, Stack, & Serbin, 2015), and competence (Bindman, Pomerantz, & Roisman, 2015; Joussemet, Koestner, Lekes, & Landry, 2005). Autonomy support may have even greater benefits for children with Down syndrome. For example, as mentioned earlier, Gilmore et al. (2009) reported higher levels of persistence by children with Down syndrome whose mothers displayed more autonomy-supportive behaviors, whereas there was no association for typically developing children. Although parents are more likely to respond with greater direction when they perceive their child needs assistance to stay on task, direction can be provided sensitively in ways that are also supportive of a child's autonomy.

For instance, gentle encouragement includes prompting and giving suggestions, whereas insensitive, intrusive directiveness involves taking over or not allowing the child to make independent attempts prior to intervening.

Even when parents recognize the value of supporting their child's autonomy, many personal, contextual, and situational factors can constrain their capacity to do so (Mageau, Bureau, Ranger, Allen, & Soenens, 2016). The goals that parents have for their child may influence the extent to which autonomy is a priority for them. For example, Mageau et al. (2016) found that parents who reported endorsing mastery rather than performance goals for their typically developing children were more likely to behave in ways that their sons or daughters perceived as autonomy-supportive. Parents of children with Down syndrome may also be more likely to encourage a child's autonomy if their focus is on the development of competence rather than on comparisons with peers. Child characteristics, too, are likely to have an effect on the extent to which parents are supportive of autonomy. Waiting for signs that a child requires assistance before intervening is an important autonomy-supportive strategy (Grolnick, Gurland, DeCourcey, & Jacob, 2002), but children with Down syndrome may not communicate their needs effectively or parents may miss subtle cues (Gilmore, Ryan, Cuskelly, & Gavidia-Payne, 2016). Similarly, difficulties with motor skills and sensory issues will mean that children with Down syndrome require more direction and assistance.

Supporting autonomy in sensitive, developmentally appropriate ways takes considerable time and effort on the part of the parent. As in families of typically developing children (Grolnick, Price, Beiswenger, & Sauck, 2007), there are times when parents of children with Down syndrome decide it is quicker and easier to respond in a directive fashion and to take control of a situation, either due to competing demands or because of safety concerns (Gilmore et al., 2016). In assessing the findings of research that involves observations from a single session in one context, it is difficult to know whether the snapshot of mother-child behavior reflects typical behavior. Parents of a child with Down syndrome may be particularly sensitive to being observed, either because they are trying to behave in ways that they believe to be optimal or because they wish their child to perform well. For example, in their observational study of mothers of young children with Down syndrome, Gilmore et al. (2016) speculated that anxiety about being observed, and potentially judged, may have triggered atypical behaviors for some of the mothers. In addition, compared with free-play situations, structured settings that require the child, or the parent-child dyad, to complete a specified task may elicit more directive parent behaviors.

Implications and Future Research Directions

Mothers interact with young children in the context of the family as well as within the broader socioecological cultural context. In families with a young child with Down syndrome, research has been focused on maternal interactions, often to the exclusion of considering the interactions of other family members, such as fathers and siblings and the family system more generally. As a result, the literature on parent-child studies in dyads where a child has Down syndrome has largely focused on maternal behaviors, with much attention on maternal directives. As a whole, this line of research has touched on critical questions, such as identifying supportive versus interfering directives (Green, Caplan, & Baker, 2014), but further differentiation is needed. Moreover, research on the ways in which children themselves elicit responses from mothers would contribute to a fuller understanding of such interactions. Since some investigators indicate that children with Down syndrome struggle with persistence on challenging tasks (Fidler, 2006), directives, at least those in the form of re-directing attention and scaffolding children's behaviors, may be beneficial to children during task-oriented endeavors. Distinguishing such situations from those of unstructured play, where mothers tend to show greater affection and less directiveness (Blacher, Baker, & Kaladjian, 2013), is also central to further study of the mother-child dyad.

Broader issues emerge, however, when assessing the bulk of the research literature on mother-child interactions. Most of the research emanates from Western cultures. Mothers of children with Down syndrome in many Western cultures tend to be involved in early intervention and related programs from the time a child is very young. As has been suggested by some researchers, these mothers may be especially sensitive to suggestions provided by service providers that encourage maternal directiveness as a way to support their children's activities because children with Down syndrome tend to enter such programs at a very young age (Blacher, Baker, & Kaladjian, 2013; Pino, 2000). Additionally, most studies involve observations of mothers and children and—as with any observational study—mothers may react differently in situations where they are knowingly observed. This may be especially true in dyads where a child has Down syndrome because mothers may tend to focus on their child's success with tasks (Gilmore et al., 2016). Future studies on children's processes and parental meanings ascribed to those processes during challenging task situations would provide valuable information to researchers, service providers, and mothers themselves.

An overarching question emanating from this research is why so many studies on mothers' interactions with their child with Down syndrome are focused on maternal inadequacies rather than maternal strengths. Admittedly, such investigations may yield valuable recommendations for intervention programs, but this focus, to the exclusion of investigating the full array of maternal behaviors, may also augment the stigmatizing effects that parents experience when they have a child with Down syndrome (Sauer & Lalvani, 2017). Mothers may be led to believe that they are insufficient teachers of their children. Studies of positive-parenting behaviors (Dyches et al., 2012) and of the ways in which mothers of children with Down syndrome support children's autonomy (Gilmore at al., 2016) are emerging but are still few in number. Such studies may stimulate an expanded focus on various features of the mother-child dyad by considering additional maternal behaviors that are beneficial to children's development. Future research aimed at investigating aspects of positive parenting in families where a child has Down syndrome would add valuable insight into the full range of maternal experiences and interactions that support the overall development of children.

References

Abbeduto, L., Seltzer, M. M., Shattuck, P., Krauss, M. W., Orsmond, G., & Murphy, M. M. (2004). Psychological well-being and coping in mothers of youths with autism, Down Syndrome or Fragile X syndrome. *American Journal on Mental Retardation, 109*, 237–254.

Abbeduto, L., Warren, S. F., & Conners, F. A. (2007). Language development in Down syndrome: From the prelinguistic period to the acquisition of literacy. *Mental Retardation and Developmental Disabilities Research Reviews, 13*(3), 247–261. doi:10.1002/mrdd.20158

Ahadi, S. A., Rothbart, M. K., & Ye, R. (1993). Children's temperament in the US and China: Similarities and differences. *European Journal of Personality, 7*(5), 359–377. doi:10.1002/per.2410070506

Ainsworth, M. D. S., Blehar, M. C., Waters, E., & Wall, S. (1978). *Patterns of attachment: A psychological study of the strange situation*. Oxford: Erlbaum.

Ali, R., & Rafique, S. (2015). The challenges of disability in Pakistan: Listening to the voices of mothers. *European Scientific Journal, 11*(32), 364–375.

Barber, B. K., Stolz, H. E., Olsen, J. A., Collins, A., & Burchinal, M. (2005). Parental support, psychological control, and behavioral control: Assessing relevance across time, culture, and method. *Monographs of the Society for Research in Child Development, 70*(4), vii, 125–137. doi:10.1111/j.1540–5834.2005.00365.x

Baron, J. (1972). Temperament profile of children with Down's syndrome. *Developmental Medicine & Child Neurology, 14*, 640–643. doi:10.1111/j.1469–8749.1972.tb02646.x

Beeghly, M. (1998). Temperament in children with Down syndrome. In J. A. Rondal, J. Perara, & L. Nadel (Eds.), *What do we know about Down syndrome: A review of current knowledge* (pp. 111–123). London: C. Whurr.

Bindman, S. W., Pomerantz, E. M., & Roisman, G. I. (2015). Do children's executive functions account for associations between early autonomy-supportive parenting and achievement through high school? *Journal of Educational Psychology, 107*, 756–770. doi:10.1037/edu0000017

Blacher, J., Baker, B. L., & Berkovits, L. D. (2013). Family perspectives on child intellectual disability: Views from the sunny side of the street. In M. L. Wehmeyer (Ed.), *The Oxford handbook of positive psychology and disability* (pp. 166–181). New York: Oxford University Press.

Blacher, J., Baker, B. L., & Kaladjian, A. (2013). Syndrome specificity and mother-child interactions: Examining positive and negative parenting across contexts and time. *Journal of Autism and Developmental Disorders, 43*(4), 761–774. doi:10.1007/s10803-012-1605-x

Bornstein, M. H., & Tamis-LeMonda, C. (1989). Maternal responsiveness and cognitive development in children. *New Directions for Child Development, 43*, 49–61. doi:10.1002/cd.23219894306

Brenning, K., Soenens, B., Van Petegem, S., & Vansteenkiste, M. (2015). Perceived maternal autonomy support and early adolescent emotion regulation: A longitudinal study. *Social Development, 24*, 561–578. doi:10.1111/sode.12107

Bridges, F. A., & Cicchetti, D. (1982). Mothers' ratings of the temperament characteristics of Down syndrome infants. *Developmental Psychology, 18*(2), 238–244. doi:10.1037/0012-1649.18.2.238

Bronfenbrenner, U., & Evans, G. W. (2000). Developmental science in the 21st century: Emerging questions, theoretical models, research designs and empirical findings. *Social Development, 9*(1), 115–125. doi:10.1111/1467-9507.00114

Bronfenbrenner, U., & Morris, P. A. (1998). The ecology of developmental processes. In W. Damon & R. M. Lerner (Eds.), *Handbook of child psychology: Theoretical models of human development* (5th ed., Vol. 1, pp. 993–1028). New York: Wiley.

Bryant, L. D., Ahmed, S., Ahmed, M., Jafri, H., & Raashid, Y. (2011). "All is done by Allah": Understandings of Down syndrome and prenatal testing in Pakistan. *Social Science & Medicine, 72*(8), 1393–1399. doi:10.1016/j.socscimed.2011.02.036 02791

Cardoso-Martins, C., & Mervis, C. B. (1985). Maternal speech to prelinguistic children with Down syndrome. *American Journal of Mental Deficiency, 89*(5), 451–458.

Carr, J. H. (1995). *Down's syndrome: Children growing up*. New York: Cambridge University Press.

Chapman, R. S., & Raining Bird, E. K. (2012). Language development in childhood, adolescence, and young adulthood in persons with Down syndrome. In J. A. Burack, R. M. Hodapp, G. Iarocci, & E. Zigler (Eds.), *The Oxford handbook of intellectual disability and development* (pp. 167–183). New York: Oxford University Press.

Cheng, P., & Tang, C. S. (1995). Coping and psychological distress of Chinese parents of children with Down syndrome. *Mental Retardation, 33*(1), 10–20.

Choi, H., & Van Riper, M. (2017). Adaptation in families of children with Down syndrome in East Asian countries: An integrative review. *Journal of Advanced Nursing, 73*(8), 1792–1806. doi:10.1111/jan.13235

Darling, N., & Steinberg, L. (1993). Parenting style as context: An integrative model. *Psychological Bulletin, 113*(3), 487–496. doi:10.1037/0033-2909.113.3.487

Davis, J. L., & Manago, B. (2016). Motherhood and associative moral stigma: The moral double bind. *Stigma and Health, 1*(2), 72–86. doi:10.1037/sah0000019

Deater-Deckard, K., Ivy, L., & Petrill, S. A. (2006). Maternal warmth moderates the link between physical punishment and child externalizing problems: A parent-offspring behavior genetic analysis. *Parenting: Science and Practice, 6*(1), 59–78. doi:10.1207/s15327922par0601_3

Dodge, K. A., & Pettit, G. S. (2003). A biopsychosocial model of the development of chronic conduct problems in adolescence. *Developmental Psychology, 39*(2), 349–371. doi:10.1037/0012-1649.39.2.349

D'Souza, D., D'Souza, H., & Karmiloff-Smith, A. (2017). Precursors to language development in typically and atypically developing infants and toddlers: The importance of embracing complexity. *Journal of Child Language, 44*(3), 591–627. doi:10.1017/S030500091700006X

Dyches, T. T., Smith, T. B., Korth, B. B., Roper, S. O., & Mandleco, B. (2012). Positive parenting of children with developmental disabilities: A meta-analysis. *Research in Developmental Disabilities, 33*(6), 2213–2220. doi:10.1016/j.ridd.2012.06.015

Edvardson, S., Msallam, N., Hertz, P., Malkiel, S., Wexler, I. D., & Tenenbaum, A. (2014). Attention deficit hyperactivity disorders symptomatology among individuals with Down syndrome. *Journal of Policy and Practice in Intellectual Disabilities, 11*(1), 58–61. doi:10.1111/jppi.12069

Eisenberg, N., Spinrad, T. L., & Smith, C. L. (2004). Emotion-related regulation: Its conceptualization, relations to social functioning, and socialization. In P. Philippot & R. S. Feldman (Eds.), *The regulation of emotion* (pp. 277–306). Mahwah, NJ: Erlbaum.

Eisenhower, A. S., Baker, B. L., & Blacher, J. (2005). Preschool children with intellectual disability: Syndrome specificity, behaviour problems, and maternal well-being. *Journal of Intellectual Disability Research, 49*(9), 657–671. doi:10.1111/j.1365.

Evans, M., & Boucher, A. R. (2015). Optimizing the power of choice: Supporting student autonomy to foster motivation and engagement in learning. *Mind, Brain, and Education, 9*, 87–91. doi:10.1111/mbe/12073

Fidler, D. J. (2003). Parental vocalizations and perceived immaturity in Down syndrome. *American Journal on Mental Retardation, 108*(6), 425–434. doi:10.1352/0895-8017(2003)108<425:PVAPII>2.0

Fidler, D. J. (2006). The emergence of a syndrome-specific personality profile in young children with Down syndrome. *Down Syndrome: Research & Practice, 10*(2), 53–60. doi:10.3104/reprints.305

Gabel, S. (2004). South Asian Indian cultural orientations toward mental retardation. *Mental Retardation, 42*(1), 12–25. doi:10.1352/0047-6765

Ganiban, J. M., Wagner, S., & Cicchetti, D. (1990). Temperament and Down syndrome. In D. Cicchetti & M. Beeghly (Eds.), *Children with Down syndrome: A developmental perspective* (pp. 63–100). New York: Cambridge University Press.

Gilmore, L. (2006). Perceptions of Down syndrome in the Australian community. *Journal on Developmental Disabilities, 12*, 59–70.

Gilmore, L., Campbell, J., & Cuskelly, M. (2003). Developmental expectations, personality stereotypes, and attitudes towards inclusive education: Community and teacher views of Down syndrome. *International Journal of Disability, Development and Education, 50*, 65–76. doi:10.1080/1034912032000053340

Gilmore, L., & Cuskelly, M. (2009). A longitudinal study of motivation and competence in children with Down syndrome: Early childhood to early adolescence. *Journal of Intellectual Disability Research, 53*(5), 484–492. doi:10.1111/j.1365–2788.2009.01166.x

Gilmore, L., & Cuskelly, M. (2011). Observational assessment and maternal reports of motivation in children and adolescents with Down syndrome. *American Journal on Intellectual and Developmental Disabilities, 116*(2), 153–164. doi:10.1352/1944-7558-116.2.153

Gilmore, L., & Cuskelly, M. (2014). Mastery motivation in children with Down syndrome: Promoting and sustaining interest in learning. In R. Faragher & B. Clarke (Eds.), *Educating learners with Down syndrome: Research, theory, and practice with children and adolescents* (pp. 60–82). London: Routledge.

Gilmore, L., Cuskelly, M., & Hayes, A. (2003). A comparative study of mastery motivation in young children with Down's syndrome: Similar outcomes, different processes? *Journal of Intellectual Disability Research, 47*(3), 181–190. doi:10.1046/j.1365–2788.2003.00460.x

Gilmore, L., Cuskelly, M., Jobling, A., & Hayes, A. (2009). Maternal support for autonomy: Relationships with persistence for children with Down syndrome and typically developing children. *Research in Developmental Disabilities, 30*, 1023–1033. doi:10.1016/j.ridd.2009.02.005

Gilmore, L., Ryan, B., Cuskelly, M., & Gavidia-Payne, S. (2016). Understanding maternal support for autonomy in young children with Down syndrome. *Journal of Policy and Practice in Intellectual Disabilities, 13*, 92–101. doi:10.1111/jppi.12163

Glenn, S., Dayus, B., Cunningham, C., & Horgan, M. (2001). Mastery motivation in children with Down syndrome. *Down Syndrome: Research & Practice, 7*(2), 52–59. doi:10.3104/reports.114

Glidden, L. M., Grein, K. A., & Ludwig, J. A. (2014). The Down syndrome advantage: It depends on what and when you measure. *American Journal on Intellectual and Developmental Disabilities, 119*(5), 389–404. doi:10.1352/1944-7558-119.5.389

Goddard, J. A., Lehr, R., & Lapadat, J. C. (2000). Parents of children with disabilities: Telling a different story. *Canadian Journal of Counselling, 34*(4), 273–289.

Goffman, E. (1963). *Stigma: Notes on the management of a spoiled identity*. Englewood Cliffs, NJ: Prentice-Hall.

Goldberg, S., & Marcovitch, S. (1989). Temperament in developmentally disabled children. In G. A. Kohnstamm, J. E. Bates, & M. K. Rothbart (Eds.), *Temperament in childhood* (pp. 387–403). New York: Wiley.

Green, S. E. (2003). "What do you mean 'what's wrong with her?'": Stigma and the lives of families of children with disabilities. *Social Science & Medicine, 57*(8), 1361–1374. doi:10.1016/S0277-9536(02)00511-7

Green, S., Caplan, B., & Baker, B. (2014). Maternal supportive and interfering control as predictors of adaptive and social development in children with and without developmental delays. *Journal of Intellectual Disability Research, 58*, 691–703.

Green, J. M., Dennis, J., & Bennets, L. A. (1989). Attention disorder in a group of young Down's syndrome children. *Journal of Mental Deficiency Research, 33*(2), 105–122.

Grolnick, W. S., Gurland, S. T., DeCourcey, W., & Jacob, K. (2002). Antecedents and consequences of mother's autonomy support: An experimental investigation. *Developmental Psychology, 38*, 143–155. doi:10.1037/0012-1649.38.1.143

Grolnick, W. S., Price, C. E., Beiswenger, K. L., & Sauck, C. C. (2007). Evaluative pressure in mothers: Effects of situation, maternal and child characteristics on autonomy supportive versus controlling behavior. *Developmental Psychology, 43*, 991–1002. doi:10.1037/0012-1649.43.4.991

Grusec, J. E., Goodnow, J. J., & Kuczynski, L. (2000). New directions in analyses of parenting contributions to children's acquisition of values. *Child Development, 71*(1), 205–211. doi:10.1111/1467-8624.00135

Gunn, P., & Berry, P. (1985). Down's syndrome temperament and maternal response to descriptions of child behavior. *Developmental Psychology, 21*(5), 842–847. doi:10.1037/0012-1649.21.5.842

Gunn, P., & Cuskelly, M. (1991). Down syndrome temperament: The stereotype at middle childhood and adolescence. *International Journal of Disability, Development and Education, 38*(1), 59–70. doi:10.1080/0156655910380106

Hamlyn-Wright, S., Draghi-Lorenz, R., & Ellis, J. (2007). Locus of control fails to mediate between stress and anxiety and depression in parents of children with a developmental disorder. *Autism, 11*(6), 489–501. doi:10.1177/1362361307083258

Hartley, S. L., Seltzer, M. M., Head, L., & Abbeduto, L. (2012). Psychological well-being in fathers of adolescents and young adults with Down syndrome, Fragile X syndrome and autism. *Family Relations, 61*, 327–342. doi:10.1111/j.1741–3729.2011.00693.x

Hastings, R. P., Beck, A., & Hill, C. (2005). Positive contributions made by children with an intellectual disability in the family: Mothers' and fathers' perceptions. *Journal of Intellectual Disabilities, 9*(2), 155–165. doi:10.1177/1744629505053930

Hauser-Cram, P., Howell-Moneta, A., & Young, J. M. (2012). Dyadic interaction between mothers and children with Down syndrome or Williams syndrome: Empirical evidence and emerging agendas. In J. A. Burack, R. M. Hodapp, G. Iarocci, & E. Zigler (Eds.), *The Oxford handbook of intellectual disability and development* (pp. 318–333). New York: Oxford University Press.

Hauser-Cram, P., Warfield, M. E., Shonkoff, J. P., & Krauss, M. W. (2001). Children with disabilities: A longitudinal study of child development and parent well-being. *Monographs of the Society for Research in Child Development, 66*(3), 1–131. doi:10.1111/1540-5834.00151

Hodapp R. M., Ricci L. A., Ly T. M., & Fidler D. J. (2003) The effects of the child with Down syndrome on maternal stress. *British Journal of Developmental Psychology, 21*(1), 137–151.doi:10.1348/026151003321164672

Hughes, M., & Kasari, C. (2000). Caregiver–child interaction and the expression of pride in children with Down syndrome. *Education & Training in Mental Retardation & Developmental Disabilities, 35*(1), 67–77.

Ispa, J. M., Su-Russell, C., Palermo, F., & Carlo, G. (2017). The interplay of maternal sensitivity and toddler engagement of mother in predicting self-regulation. *Developmental Psychology, 53*(3), 425–435. doi:10.1037/dev0000267

Iverson, J. M., Longobardi, E., Spampinato, K., & Caselli, M. C. (2006). Gesture and speech in maternal input to children with Down's syndrome. *International Journal of Language & Communication Disorders, 41*(3), 235–251. doi:10.1080/13682820500312151

Jahromi, L. B., Gulsrud, A., & Kasari, C. (2008). Emotional competence in children with Down syndrome: Negativity and regulation. *American Journal on Mental Retardation, 113*(1), 32–43. doi:10.1352/0895-8017(2008)113[32:ECICWD]2.0.CO;2

Joussemet, M., Koestner, R., Lekes, N., & Landry, R. (2005). A longitudinal study of the relations of maternal autonomy support to children's adjustment and achievement in school. *Journal of Personality, 73*, 1215–1236. doi:10.1111/j.1467–6494.2005.00347.x

Kasari, C., & Sigman, M. (1996). Expression and understanding of emotion in atypical development: Autism and Down syndrome. In M. Lewis & M. W. Sullivan (Eds.), *Emotional development in atypical children* (pp. 109–130). Hillsdale, NJ: Erlbaum.

Lalvani, P. (2008). Mothers of children with Down syndrome: Constructing the sociocultural meaning of disability. *Intellectual and Developmental Disabilities, 46*(6), 436–445. doi:10.1352/2008.46:436–445

Lalvani, P. (2011). Constructing the (m)other: Dominant and contested narratives on mothering a child with down syndrome. *Narrative Inquiry, 21*(2), 276–293. doi:10.1075/ni.21.2.06lal

Landsman, G. (2005). Mothers and models of disability. *Journal of Medical Humanities, 26*(2–3), 121–139. doi:10.1007/s10912-005-2914-2

Landry, S. H., Smith, K. E., & Swank, P. R. (2006). Responsive parenting: Establishing early foundations for social, communication, and independent problem-solving skills. *Developmental Psychology, 42*(4), 627–642. doi:10.1037/0012-1649.42.4.627

Mageau, G. A., Bureau, J. S., Ranger, F., Allen, M., & Soenens, B. (2016). The role of parental achievement goals in predicting autonomy-supportive and controlling parenting. *Journal of Child and Family Studies, 25*(5), 1702–1711. doi:10.1007/s10826-015-0341-1

Marcovitch, S., Goldberg, S., MacGregor, D. L., & Lojkasek, M. (1986). Patterns of temperament variation in three groups of developmentally delayed preschool children: Mother and father ratings. *Journal of Developmental and Behavioral Pediatrics, 7*(4), 247–252. doi:10.1097/00004703-198608000-00006

Marfo, K. (1990). Maternal directiveness in interactions with mentally handicapped children: An analytical commentary. *Child Psychology & Psychiatry & Allied Disciplines, 31*(4), 531–549. doi:10.1111/j.1469–7610.1990.tb00796.x

Masarik, A. S., & Conger, R. D. (2017). Stress and child development: A review of the family stress model. *Current Opinion in Psychology, 13*, 85–90. doi:10.1016/j.copsyc.2016.05.008

Matte-Gagné, C., Harvey, B., Stack, D. M., & Serbin, L. A. (2015). Contextual specificity in the relationship between maternal autonomy support and children's socio-emotional development: A longitudinal study from preschool to preadolescence. *Journal of Youth and Adolescence, 44*, 1528–1541. doi:10.1007/s10964-014-0247-z

Mesman, J., van IJzendoorn, M. H., & Bakermans-Kranenburg, M. J. (2012). Unequal in opportunity, equal in process: Parental sensitivity promotes positive child development in ethnic minority families. *Child Development Perspectives, 6*(3), 239–250. doi:10.1111/j.1750–8606.2011.00223.x

Mintz, T. M., Hamre, B. K., & Hatfield, B. E. (2011). The role of effortful control in mediating the association between maternal sensitivity and children's social and relational competence and problems in first grade. *Early Education and Development, 22*(3), 360–387. doi:10.1080/10409289.2011.569317

Mirza, I., Tareen, A., Davidson, L. L., & Rahman, A. (2009). Community management of intellectual disabilities in Pakistan: A mixed methods study. *Journal of Intellectual Disability Research, 53*(6), 559–570. doi:10.1111/j.1365–2788.2009.01176

Mitchell, D. B., Hauser-Cram, P., & Crossman, M. K. (2015). Relationship dimensions of the "Down syndrome advantage." *Journal of Intellectual Disability Research, 59*(6), 506–518. doi:10.1111/jir.12153

Most, D. E., Fidler, D. J., Booth-Laforce, C., & Kelly, J. (2006). Stress trajectories in mothers of young children with Down syndrome. *Journal of Intellectual Disability Research, 51*(9), 501–514. doi:10.1111/j.1365–2788.2006.00796.x

Nes, R. B., Røysamb, E., Hauge, L. J., Kornstad, T., Landolt, M. A., Irgens, L. M., . . . Vollrath, M. E. (2014). Adaptation to the birth of a child with a congenital anomaly: A prospective longitudinal study of maternal well-being and psychological distress. *Developmental Psychology, 50*(6), 1827–1839. doi:10.1037/a0035996

Niccols, A., & Feldman, M. (2006). Maternal sensitivity and behaviour problems in young children with developmental delay. *Infant and Child Development, 15*(5), 543–554. doi:10.1002/icd.468

Niccols, A., Milligan, K., Chisholm, V., & Atkinson, L. (2011). Maternal sensitivity and overt aggression in young children with Down syndrome. *Brain and Cognition, 77*(2), 153–158. doi:10.1016/j.bandc.2011.06.007

Nygaard, E., Smith, L., & Torgersen, A. M. (2002). Temperament in children with Down syndrome and in prematurely born children. *Scandinavian Journal of Psychology, 43*(1), 61–71. doi:10.1111/1467-9450.00269

O'Hara, J., & Bouras, N. (2007). Intellectual disabilities across cultures. In D. Bhugra & K. Bhui (Eds). *Textbook of cultural psychiatry* (pp. 461–483). Cambridge UK: Cambridge University Press.

Pino, O. (2000). The effect of context on mother's interaction style with Down's syndrome and typically developing children. *Research in Developmental Disabilities, 21*(5), 329–346. doi:10.1016/S0891-4222(00)00046-9

Pueschel, S. M., & Myers, B. A. (1994). Environmental and temperament assessments of children with Down's syndrome. *Journal of Intellectual Disability Research, 38*(2), 195–202. doi:10.1111/j.1365–2788.1994.tb00374.x

Ratekin, C. (1996). Temperament in children with Down syndrome. *Developmental Disabilities Bulletin, 24*(1), 18–32.

Roach, M. A., Barratt, M. S., Miller, J. F., & Leavitt, L. A. (1998). The structure of mother-child play: Young children with Down syndrome and typically developing children. *Developmental Psychology, 34*(1), 77–87. doi:10.1037/0012-1649.34.1.77

Roach, M. A., Orsmond, G. I., & Barratt, M. S. (1999). Mothers and fathers of children with Down syndrome: Parental stress and involvement in childcare. *American Journal on Mental Retardation, 104*(5), 422–436.

Rogoff, B., & Morelli, G. (1989). Perspectives on children's development from cultural psychology. *American Psychologist, 44*(2), 343–348. doi:10.1037/0003-066X.44.2.343

Rothbart, M. K. (1981). Measurement of temperament in infancy. *Child Development, 52*(2), 569–578. doi:10.2307/1129176

Rothbart, M. K., & Derryberry, D. (1981). Development of individual differences in temperament. In M. E. Lamb & A. L. Brown (Eds.), *Advances in developmental psychology* (vol. 1, pp. 37–86). Hillsdale, NJ: Erlbaum.

Ruskin, E. M., Mundy, P., Kasari, C., & Sigman, M. (1994). Object mastery motivation of children with Down syndrome. *American Journal on Mental Retardation, 98*(4), 499–509.

Sauer, J. S., & Lalvani, P. (2017). From advocacy to activism: Families, communities, and collective change. *Journal of Policy and Practice in Intellectual Disabilities, 14*(1), 51–58. doi:10.1111/jppi.12219

Shonkoff, J. P., Garner, A. S., Siegel, B. S., Dobbins, M. I., Earls, M. F., McGuinn, L., . . . Wood, D. L. (2012). The lifelong effects of early childhood adversity and toxic stress. *Pediatrics, 129*(1), e232–e246. doi:10.1542/peds.2011–2663

Shonkoff, J. P., Hauser-Cram, P., Krauss, M. W., & Upshur, C. C. (1992). Development of infants with disabilities and their families: Implications for theory and service delivery. *Monographs of the Society for Research in Child Development, 57*(6), v–153.

Skinner, D. G., Correa, V., Skinner, M., & Bailey, D. B., Jr. (2001). Role of religion in the lives of Latino families of young children with developmental delays. *American Journal on Mental Retardation, 106*(4), 297–313.

Solnit, A. J., & Stark, M. H. (1961). Mourning and the birth of a defective child. *The Psychoanalytic Study of the Child, 16*(1), 523–537.

Spinrad, T. L., Eisenberg, N., Silva, K. M., Eggum, N. D., Reiser, M., Edwards, A., . . . Gaertner, B. M. (2012). Longitudinal relations among maternal behaviors, effortful control and young children's committed compliance. *Developmental Psychology, 48*(2), 552–566. doi:10.1037/a0025898

Stores, R., Stores, G., Fellows, B., & Buckley, S. (1998). Daytime behavior problems and maternal stress in children with Down's syndrome, their siblings, and non-intellectually disabled and other intellectually disabled peers. *Journal of Intellectual Disability Research, 42*, 228–237. doi:10.1046/j.1365–2788.1998.00123.x

Stoneman, Z. (2007). Examining the Down syndrome advantage: Mothers and fathers of young children with disabilities. *Journal of Intellectual Disability Research, 51*(12), 1006–1017. doi:10.1111/j.1365–2788.2007.01012.x

Su, H., Cuskelly, M., Gilmore, L., & Sullivan, K. (2018). Perceptions of support in Chinese mothers of a child with intellectual disability. *Journal of Developmental and Physical Disabilities, 30*, 509–525. doi:10.1007/s10882-018-9599-8

van der Kaap-Deeder, J., Vansteenkiste, M., Soenens, B., & Mabbe, E. (2017). Children's daily well-being: The role of mothers', teachers', and siblings' autonomy support and psychological control. *Developmental Psychology, 53*, 237–251. doi:10.1037/dev0000218

van IJzendoorn, M. H., & Sagi-Schwartz, A. (2008). Cross-cultural patterns of attachment: Universal and contextual dimensions. In J. Cassidy & P. R. Shaver (Eds.), *Handbook of attachment: Theory, research, and clinical applications* (2nd ed., pp. 880–905). New York: Guilford Press.

Venuti, P., De Falco, S., Esposito, G., Zaninelli, M., & Bornstein, M. H. (2012). Maternal functional speech to children: A comparison of autism spectrum disorder, Down syndrome, and typical development. *Research in Developmental Disabilities, 33*(2), 506–517. doi:10.1016/j.ridd.2011.10.018

Venuti, P., De Falco, S., Giusti, Z., & Bornstein, M. H. (2008). Play and emotional availability in young children with Down syndrome. *Infant Mental Health Journal, 29*(2), 133–152. doi:10.1002/imhj.20168

Wishart, J. G. (1991). Taking the initiative in learning: A developmental investigation of infants with Down syndrome. *International Journal of Disability, Development and Education, 38*(1), 27–44. doi:10.1080/0156655910380104

Wishart, J. G. (1993). The development of learning difficulties in children with Down's syndrome. *Journal of Intellectual Disability Research, 37*(4), 389–403. doi:10.1111/j.1365–2788.1993.tb00882.x

Wishart, J. G., Willis, D. S., Cebula, K. R., & Pitcairn, T. K. (2007). Collaborative learning: Comparison of outcomes for typically developing children and children with intellectual disabilities. *American Journal on Mental Retardation, 112*(5), 361–374. doi:10.1352/0895-8017.

Wong, S. Y., Wong, T. K. S., Martinson, I., Lai, A. C., Chen, W. J., & He, Y. S. (2004). Needs of Chinese parents of children with developmental disability. *Journal of Learning Disabilities, 8*(2), 141–158. doi:10.1177/1469004704042703

Zampini, L., Fasolo, M., & D'Odorico, L. (2012). Characteristics of maternal input to children with Down syndrome: A comparison with vocabulary size and chronological age-matched groups. *First Language, 32*(3), 324–342.

CHAPTER 5

Parenting the Child With Down Syndrome: Understanding—But Going Beyond—The "Down Syndrome Advantage"

Robert M. Hodapp *and* Ellen G. Casale

Abstract

Compared to parents of children with other types of intellectual disabilities, parents of children with Down syndrome experience less stress and more rewards, although this "Down syndrome advantage" mostly occurs compared to parents of children with autism and before groups are equated. Behaviorally, children with Down syndrome display more sociable interactional styles and baby-faced facial features, along with fewer instances of severe behavior problems. Demographically, parents of children with (versus without) Down syndrome average 5 years older when giving birth; parents are more often well educated, married, of higher socioeconomic status, and they likely provide these children greater financial and cultural resources. In most industrialized societies, rates of Down syndrome seem steady, with easily available, noninvasive prenatal testing counteracted by increasing numbers of women giving birth at older ages. Parenting children with Down syndrome relates to characteristics of children, their parents, and society, all of which intersect in important, underexplored ways.

Key Words: Down syndrome advantage, demographics, advanced maternal age, sociability, baby face, prenatal testing

With a research history from Britain's Victorian age until today, one would think that we know most everything there is to know about persons with Down syndrome. From Down's descriptions in the 1860s (c.f., Dunn, 1991), to Penrose's studies in the mid-20th century (Penrose, 1949; Penrose & Smith, 1966), to Gibson's (1978) behavioral review, and the more modern studies of the past 40 years, we as a field have learned much about Down syndrome. As chapters in this volume attest, we know a fair amount about the genetics, language, memory, health, and life-span development of individuals with Down syndrome. Yet despite the 150-year research history of Down syndrome, our knowledge might be considered wide but shallow. Using PsycINFO as the primary source, published research studies involving persons with Down syndrome rose from 607 during the 1980s to 1,140 during the 1990s (Dykens & Hodapp, 2001), with the last full decade (from 2000 to 2009) weighing in at 1,257 published studies. Though impressive, these numbers hide the fact that many studies used persons with Down syndrome as the comparison or contrast group, with the main focus on children or adults with autism, Williams syndrome, or some other condition. For this reason, many aspects of Down syndrome, though generally understood, lack more in-depth information.

Even more than our lack of detailed knowledge about the children themselves, we know little about their families. Again, several classic projects have been undertaken, notably those that longitudinally followed large cohorts of offspring with the syndrome in several areas of Britain (Carr, 1995, 2012; Cunningham, 1996, 2006). In other respects, however, our knowledge remains spotty, with more studies of families of children with different conditions lumped together rather than of families of children with Down syndrome per se.

In considering this state of affairs, one must question whether families of children with Down syndrome are, indeed, different from families of children with other forms of intellectual disability (ID). As we note below, our answer (detailed below) is a qualified yes, in that there may be a "Down syndrome advantage" for these families. But even if such families are coping better, one must still ask why. What is it about children with Down syndrome, or their families, or society at large that may lead these families to "do better" than families of children with other conditions?

In this chapter, we explore whether a so-called "Down syndrome advantage" exists and, if so, why. In doing so, we separate various outcomes, various people who might experience such an advantage, and various characteristics—of the child, parents-family, and society—that might predispose these families to do better. We then attempt to go beyond whether a Down syndrome advantage is evident to consider influences on parenting any child, whether it be one who is developing typically, has disability conditions more generally, or has Down syndrome.

The Down Syndrome Advantage: Definition and Current Status

Over the past several decades, researchers have noted that there may be an advantage for families of children with Down syndrome. We present below the definition and salient issues, as well as a review of the many studies of this issue.

The Down syndrome advantage has been described as follows: "compared to other children with disabilities, children with Down syndrome may help their parents to experience both less stress and more reward" (Hodapp, Ly, Fidler, & Ricci, 2001, p. 318). Another set of authors states: "Mothers of adults with Down syndrome experienced significantly less stress and less burden associated with caregiving than did the mothers of adults whose retardation was due to other factors, even after background factors such as maternal age and family size were controlled for" (Seltzer & Ryff, 1994, p. 22).

From these quotations, one can anticipate the main issues involved in studies of the Down syndrome advantage. Such concerns include:

(1) **Which outcomes are being examined?** From these quotes alone, we see mention of stress, rewards, and burden. In other studies, researchers examine aspects of parental stress—for example, parental pessimism or the child's demandingness—and related constructs such as parental well-being or depression. Beyond parents, sibling relationships (Hodapp & Urbano, 2007) and family's support from friends or community groups (Erikson & Upshure, 1989) have been studied. Recent researchers have begun examining specific aspects of the Down syndrome advantage as it relates to these outcomes.

(2) **What age(s) are the offspring?** Whereas Seltzer and colleagues (1994) focused on families of adults with Down syndrome, other researchers (e.g., Erikson & Upshure, 1989) examined families from early childhood on. Some have argued that a Down syndrome advantage may be age-specific, such that these families cope better when their children are at certain ages, less so at others (Glidden, Grein, & Ludwig, 2014). In this chapter, we limit ourselves to the childhood years, but even across those years the existence and/or strength of any advantage needs to be considered.

(3) **What is the nature of the comparison or contrast groups?** In most description statements, the hypothesized Down syndrome advantage is considered to be for families of children with Down syndrome relative to families of children with other types of conditions, with some comparisons also made to families of same-aged typically developing children (Roach, Orsmond, & Barrett, 1999). In particular, Stoneman (2007) argued that the Down syndrome advantage may instead be an "autism disadvantage," as many studies of the Down syndrome advantage entail comparisons of maternal stress levels when parenting children with Down syndrome versus parenting children with autism. More generally, levels of maternal stress seem higher for mothers of children with autism versus those with other conditions (Hayes & Watson, 2012).

(4) **Are critical background variables controlled for?** Of all background variables, researchers have been mostly interested in the mother's age at the birth of the child with Down syndrome. Although examined later, two issues arise. One, mothers of children with Down syndrome remain older than mothers of children with ID more generally (Hodapp, Burke, Finley, & Urbano, 2016). Although some researchers match or co-vary on maternal age, not all do so; on some occasions, once maternal age is co-varied, group differences in maternal stress are no longer apparent (e.g., Cahill & Glidden, 1996). Such discussions all relate to making an appropriate comparison, comparing groups who do not have pre-existing differences that might account for any differences in the outcomes that might appear.

But we also need to consider the correlates of maternal age. In most industrialized countries, mothers give birth to children with Down syndrome at median ages of about 32 years (Hodapp et al., 2016). What implications arise from giving birth to children with Down syndrome at maternal birth ages that, compared to typically developing children or to children with other conditions, are generally 5 or more years older? Although we examine this issue later, suffice for now to note that, by having disproportionate percentages of older mothers in the Down syndrome (vs. non-Down syndrome) group, we must consider both methodological and conceptual issues.

Studies of Parents

To synthesize research for and against the Down syndrome advantage, we searched psychology and educational databases for peer-reviewed articles on this issue. Limiting our search to parents of children with Down syndrome, we included the terms "Down syndrome," "mothers," "parental characteristics," and all related terms. Very few researchers were able to gather information from both the mothers and fathers, so studies with just mothers or both parents were included. We also performed both backward and forward searches, identifying relevant studies from the reference lists of already-chosen studies (i.e., "backward") and, via several databases, any studies that cited already-identified studies (i.e., "forward"). From these many studies, we chose only those with comparisons of parents-families of children with Down syndrome to other conditions and/or to groups of typically developing children.

The 36 studies that we could identify that were focused on the Down syndrome advantage are presented in Table 5.1. As shown in the table, 13 are focused on parents of children whose average age was below age 5 years; 12 of children 5–12 years; five of offspring 12-18 years; and six who were above 18 years. In each case, we organized by average age, acknowledging that certain participants might be younger or older than the stated ages. Columns indicate the study's authors and year, the number of participants in the Down syndrome group, the type and participant number of the comparison group, their age range or mean age, parent measures, whether a Down syndrome advantage was evident prior to any control-covariance procedures, which variable(s) were controlled-covaried, and, on the right-most column, whether a Down syndrome advantage continued to be evident once researchers performed control-covariance procedures.

As seen in the table, before controlling for any variables, virtually all studies include evidence of a Down syndrome advantage. This advantage appears in studies of parents of children across age ranges, parents of children with Down syndrome compared to those of children with different conditions, and parents measured on diverse outcome measures. In this initial, more global sense, then, an advantage does appear evident for parents of children with Down syndrome.

In delving more deeply, however, we need to consider the effects of a priori differences between the groups. Of the studies reviewed in Table 5.1, only 15 featured analyses that controlled for confounding variables, which ranged across maternal-related characteristics

Table 5.1. Literature Review of Comparative Studies of Down Syndrome across Measures of Parental Characteristics

	Sample Size						
(Author, Year)	DS (*N*)	Comparison Group (*N*)	Age range or Mean age	Parent Measures **Bolded measures** = DS Advantage Identified* = DS Advantage remained after control procedures	DS Adv.	Control Variables or Covariates	Still Exists?
Early Life (Birth – 5 years)							
Shonkoff et al., 1992	54	MI (77) DD (59)	$\bar{x}_{DS}$ = 3.4 mo. $\bar{x}_{MotorImp}$ = 11.5 mo. $\bar{x}_{DD}$ = 16 mo.	Child Improvement Locus of Control Scales; Family Adaptability and Cohesion Evaluation Scales; Nursing Child Assessment Teaching Scale; **Home Observation for Measurement of the Environment; Parent Stress Index**			
Atkinson et al., 1995	56		$\bar{x}_{DS}$ = 19.00 mo.	Approach–Avoidance Scale	Inconclusive		
Crawley & Spiker, 1983	18		$\bar{x}_{DS}$ = 2y	Bayley Mental Scale; **Created Measures for Mother-Child Interactions**; Maternal Characteristics			
Cahill & Glidden, 1996 *	34	Unmatched Mixed (74) Matched Mixed (34)	$\bar{x}_{DS}$ =28.71 mo. $\bar{x}_{UM}$ =33.6 mo. $\bar{x}_{M}$ =26.42 mo.	**Questionnaire on Resources and Stress;** Locke-Wallace Marital Adjustment Test; Family Strengths Scale; Beck Depression Inventory; Nelson Parental Satisfaction with Child Scale		When matched for: Child level of functioning, child age, marital status, family income	X

Mitchell et al., 2015	43	DD (54)	Longitudinal Study at age 3y	**Nursing Child Assessment Teaching Scale;** Parenting Stress Index; **Family Social Support Scale; Child Behavior Checklist;** Vineland		Mother and child characteristics	
						Maternal age and adaptive skills	X
Roach et al., 1999	41	TDC (53) SES Matched	< 5y	**Caregiving Difficulties**Parenting Stress Index Daily Caregiving		Chronological age and # of siblings	X
Fidler et al., 2006	24	DD (33)	< 5y old	**Infant Temperament Questionnaire-Revised; Child Behavior Checklist** (varied between 2nd and last time sampling)			
Hanson & Hanline, 1990	14	HI (9) NI (12)	$\bar{x}_{GrpTime1}$= 20.3 mo. $\bar{x}_{GrpTime2}$= 34.8 mo. $\bar{x}_{GrpTime3}$= 51 mo.	(Longitudinal 12–30 mo., 3y, 4y)**Parenting Stress Index**; Inventory of Parent Experiences			
Blacher et al., 2013	10	ASD (12) CP (9) DD (37) TDC (15)	30–90 mo.	(Longitudinal at 3, 4, 5y) **Mother-child observations for Interactions** *; Child Behavior Checklist; **Parent-Child Interaction Rating System**		Mother's education; child behavior problems	
Smith et al., 2014	29	DD (82)	28.66–31.28 mo.	**Parenting Stress Index***; **Parent Perceptions of Language** *; Sequences Inventory Communication Development – Revised; Vineland Adaptive Behavior Scales		Parent age; maternal age; adaptive behavior	

(*continued*)

Table 5.1. *Continued*

	Sample Size						
(Author, Year)	DS (*N*)	Comparison Group (*N*)	Age range or Mean age	Parent Measures **Bolded measures** = DS Advantage Identified* = DS Advantage remained after control procedures	DS Adv.	Control Variables or Covariates	Still Exists?
Eisenhower et al., 2005	12	DD (43) AUT (14) CP (10) TDC (136)	$\bar{x}_{DS}$ = 34.7 mo. $\bar{x}_{DD}$ = 36.0 mo. $\bar{x}_{TDC}$ = 35 mo. $\bar{x}_{AUT}$ = 36.5 mo. $\bar{x}_{CP}$ = 34.7 mo.	**Child Behavior Checklist** *(Increased in aggression from age 3 to 5)*; **Family Impact Questionnaire; Center for Epidemiological Studies Depression Scale**			
Duis et al., 1997	17	HI (16) 2 parent DD (19) Single Parent TDC (29) 2 parent TDC (35)	$\bar{x}_{Control}$ =4.1 $\bar{x}_{HI}$ =4.9 $\bar{x}_{DS}$ = 3.5 $\bar{x}_{DD}$ = 5.3 $\bar{x}_{SingleTDC}$ = 5.2	**Parenting stress index*** *(over other disabilities)*; Family Support Scale; Family Resource Scale; Family Adaptability and Cohesion Scales III Sibling; Behavior Rating Scale		Parent- and child-related stress across two-parent, single-parent TDC and disabilities groups	
Dabrowska &Pisula, 2010	51	AUT (51) TDC (57)	$\bar{x}_{DS}$ =4.3 $\bar{x}_{AUT}$ =4.8 $\bar{x}_{TDC}$ = 4.9	**Questionnaire of Resources and Stress for Families with Chronologically Ill or Handicapped Members;** Coping Inventory for Stressful Situations		Level of education, income, no. of children, task-oriented coping, emotion-oriented coping, avoidance-oriented coping	?
Early Childhood (5–11 years)							
Fidler, Hodapp, & Dykens, 2000	20	WS (20) SMS (20)	$\bar{x}_{DS}$ = 5.78 $\bar{x}_{WS}$ =6.13 $\bar{x}_{SMS}$= 5.61	**Questionnaire on Resources and Stress; Child Behavior Checklist**		Family income (covariate)	
Cuskelly et al., 1998	45	TDC (88)	4.6–7.6y & 12.6–15.6y	**Child Behavior Checklist;** Stress			

Stoneman, 2007	29	Mixed (32)	2.0–6.8y	**Center for epidemiologic Studies Depression Scale; Questionnaire on Resources and Stress**Family Support Scale; Parental Attitudes towards Childrearing Questionnaire; Temperament Assessment Battery; **Observed Maternal Warmth**		Income	X
Olsson & Hwang, 2003	51	ID (107) AUT (68) TDC (234)	$\bar{x}_{DS}$ = 5.3 $\bar{x}_{ID}$ =8.4 $\bar{x}_{AUT}$ = 9.8 $\bar{x}_{TDC}$= 8.2	**Hollingshead Four Factor Index of Social Position;** Created Survey: Family Composition, Professional Contact, Division of household chores, Parental work situation, Recreation and Vacation, **Positive Aspects**			
Holroyd & MacArthur, 1976	22DS$_1$ (4) DS$_2$ (9) DS$_3$ (9)	AUT$_1$ (4) AUT$_2$ (5) AUT$_3$ (13) Clinic$_1$(9) Clinic$_2$(11) Clinic$_3$ (12)	Group$_1$= 3–5y Group$_2$= 6–8y Group$_3$= 9–12y	**Questionnaire on Resources and Stress**Hollingshead Four Factor Index of Social Position			
Kasari & Sigman, 1997	13	ID (13) AUT (28) TDC (28)	8.26–11.61	Autism Behavior Checklist; **Behavior Style Questionnaire; Parenting Stress Index**; Parent-Child engagement			
Saunders & Morgan, 1997	18	AUT (18)TDC (18)	7–11y	Hollingshead 4-Factor analysis; **Questionnaire of Resources and Stress; Family Environment Scale**			

(*continued*)

Table 5.1. *Continued*

	Sample Size						
(Author, Year)	DS (*N*)	Comparison Group (*N*)	Age range or Mean age	Parent Measures **Bolded measures** = DS Advantage Identified* = DS Advantage remained after control procedures	DS Adv.	Control Variables or Covariates	Still Exists?
Griffith et al., 2010	19	AUT (19) Mixed (19)	$\bar{x}_{DS}$= 10.16 (3.86) $\bar{x}_{AUT}$= 9.98 (4.04) $\bar{x}_{Mixed}$ = 9.84 (4.18)	**Vineland Adaptive Behavior; Behavior Problems Inventory; Reiss Scales for Children's Dual Diagnosis; Nisonger Child Behavior Rating Form;** Questionnaire on Resources and Stress; **Kansas Inventory of Parental Perceptions;** Hospital Anxiety and Depression Scales; Family Satisfaction Scale; Satisfaction with Life Scale; Golombok Rust Inventory of Marital State			
Hodapp et al., 2003	27	Mixed (15)	$\bar{x}_{DS}$= 7.74 $\bar{x}_{Mixed}$=8.14	**Parenting Stress Index; Personality Rating Questionnaire;** Child Behavior ChecklistVineland Adaptive Behavior Scales			
Siklos & Kerns, 2006	32	ASD (56)	$\bar{x}_{DS}$= 11.08 $\bar{x}_{AUT}$= 7.98	**Family Needs Questionnaire;** Child Characteristics Questionnaire (created)			
Dumas et al., 1991	30	AUT (30) BD (30) TDC (60)		Parenting Stress Index; Eyberg Child Behavior Inventory; **Beck Depression Inventory**			

Noh et al., 1989	31	AUT (31) CD (35) TDC—matched (62)	$\bar{x}_{DS}$ = 9.11 $\bar{x}_{AUT}$= 9.34 $\bar{x}_{CD'}$= 6.43 $\bar{x}_{TDC}$ = 7.62	**Parenting Stress Index**		Child birth order, No. of Children, Income, Marital status, Mom's age, education and fathers age and education	?
Young Adult (12–18 years)							
Lanfranchi & Vianello, 2012	31	WS (40) FXS (42) PWS (31)	$\bar{x}_{DS}$=4.97 $\bar{x}_{WS}$=13.65 $\bar{x}_{FXS}$=13.50 $\bar{x}_{PWS}$=16.19	**Questionnaire of Resources and Stress; Parental Locus of Control Scale; Family Adaptability and Cohesion Scales III**			
Abbeduto et al., 2004	39	FXS (22) ASD (174)	$\bar{x}$ =16	**Center for Epidemiologic Studies Depression Scale; Questionnaire on Resources and Stress; Positive Affect Index;** Multidimensional Coping Inventory		Family income, maternal education, No. of children w/disability, Child gender, child age	X
Burke et al., 2012	42		$\bar{x}$ =15.12	Child Behavior Checklist; Reiss Profiles of Fundamental Goals and Motivational Sensitivities; **Beck Depression Inventory; Positive Perceptions in Families Questionnaire; Kansas Inventory of Parental Perceptions**; Positive Contributions Section; **COPE Questionnaire;** Transition Daily Rewards and Worries Questionnaire			
Lewis et al., 2006	19	FXS (19) FXS+AUT (9)	$\bar{x}_{DS}$=16.04 $\bar{x}_{FXS}$=15.83 $\bar{x}_{FXS+AUT}$=16.38	Positive Affective Index; **Subscales of Family Environment Scale; QRS Pessimism subscale**			

(*continued*)

Table 5.1. *Continued*

	Sample Size						
(Author, Year)	DS (*N*)	Comparison Group (*N*)	Age range or Mean age	Parent Measures **Bolded measures** = DS Advantage Identified* = DS Advantage remained after control procedures	DS Adv.	Control Variables or Covariates	Still Exists?
Corrice & Glidden, 2009^	56	DD (64)	$\bar{x}_{DS}$=16.70	Beck Depression Inventory; Questionnaire on Resources and Stress; **Subjective Well-being, child-related; Transition Daily Rewards and Worries Questionnaire**		Maternal age covariate, maternal and child age covariates	X
Adulthood (> 18 years)							
Glidden, Grein & Ludwig, 2014^	40	Mixed (45)	$\bar{x}_{DS}$=24.79 $\bar{x}_{DD}$=26.98	**Rearing impact; Subjective Well-Being (child);** Depression (DEP5)**; Transition Daily Rewards and Worries;** Adaptive Behavior Scale; NEO 5 Factor Personality Inventory		Maternal age, Child age, ABS Personal Self-Sufficiency	X
Seltzer, Krauss, & Tsunematsu, 1993	160	ID (253)	$\bar{x}$ =35.55	**Family Environment Scale; Questionnaire on Resources and Stress**		Maternal age, child age, family size	
Hamlyn-Wright, Draghi-Lorenz, & Ellis, 2007	223	AUT (265)TDC(131)	$\bar{x}_{DS}$=12.35 $\bar{x}_{AUT}$=13.51 $\bar{x}_{TDC}$=12.35	**Locus of Control Scale; Hospital Anxiety and Depression Scale; Created Stress measure**			

Blacher & McIntyre, 2006	59Anglo (23) Latino (36)	(Anglo; Latino)AUT (12; 11) CP (52;35) Mixed ID (63;50)	$\bar{x}_{Anglo}$=20.4 (2.3) $\bar{x}_{Latino}$=20.2 (2.8)	**SIB—R***; **Reiss Screen for Maladaptive Behavior*Family Impact Questionnaire***; Center for Epidemiologic Studies—Depression; Philadelphia Geriatric Center Morale Scale		Behavior Problems	
Holmes & Carr, 1991	20	AUT (19)	$\bar{x}_{DS}$ = 28 $\bar{x}_{AUT}$ = 24	**Handicaps, Behaviour and Skills Schedule; Vineland Social Maturity Scale;** Leiter International Performance Scale; Coping Schedule (created measure)			
Meta-Analyses							
Hayes & Watson, 2012		AUT		**Parenting Stress Index; Questionnaire on Resources and Stress**			

Note: Studies identified with an asterisk (*) utilize the same sample. Studies using the same population or data set are marked with a karat (^). A capital X (X) indicates that the Down syndrome advantage disappeared after controlling for identified variables. A question mark (?) indicates that the outcomes measured after considering covariates or control did not include the measures in which a Down syndrome advantage was indicated. Abbreviations included: motor impairment (MI); Down syndrome (DS); autism (AUT) or autism spectrum disorders (ASD); Fragile X syndrome (FXS); typically developing children (TDC); intellectual disability (ID); cerebral palsy (CP); developmental delay (DD); behavior disorder (BD); conduct disorder (CD); Prader-Willi syndrome (PWS); Smith-Magenis syndrome (SMS); Williams syndrome (WS); hearing impairment (HI); neurological impairment (NI) (e.g., age, education, SES, level of education, income), child characteristics (e.g., behavior, gender, age) and family characteristics (e.g., number of children with a condition, number of offspring). After controlling for one or more of these variables, evidence for the Down syndrome advantage remained in 7 of the 15 studies. Three issues seemed most important: (a) comparison group, (b) age of the child, and (c) measures.

Different comparison groups. Across the studies shown in Table 5.1, thirteen different conditions were used for comparison. The most common, representing nearly half of all studies, was autism (also noted as autism spectrum disorders). Of the 16 studies using individuals with autism as the comparison group, almost all showed an advantage for parents of children with Down syndrome. Compared to parents of children with autism, then, parents of children with Down syndrome showed advantages on measures of mother-child interactions (Blacher, Baker, & Kaladjian, 2013), maternal stress (Dabrowska & Pisula, 2010; Eisenhower, Baker, & Blacher, 2005; Holroyd & McArthur, 1976; Olsson & Hwang, 2003), maternal depression (Eisenhower et al., 2005; Griffith, Hastings, Nash, & Hill, 2010), family resources (Dabrowska & Pisula, 2010; Siklos & Kerns, 2006), and child behaviors (Griffith et al., 2010). In one study, the two groups no longer differed when controlling for family income, maternal age, number of children with a condition, and child gender and age (Abbeduto et al., 2004). Taken together, however, these 16 studies support Stoneman's (2007) argument that the Down syndrome advantage may, as well, be considered as an "autism disadvantage."

The picture seems less clear-cut when comparisons are made to parents of children with developmental disabilities or disabilities of mixed etiology. Fourteen studies with these comparison groups are reported in Table 5.1. These studies featured a wide range of outcome measures concerning parents, parent-child interactions, and parental perceptions of their child. Parent measures included stress (Duis, Summers, & Summers, 1997; Hodapp, Ricci, Ly, & Fidler, 2003; Mitchell, Hauser-Cram, & Crossman, 2015; Smith, Romski, Sevcik, Adamson, & Barker, 2014), depression (Stoneman, 2007), warmth (Stoneman, 2007), social support (Mitchell et al., 2015), and rewards and well-being (Corrice & Glidden, 2009). In addition to studies of parental interactive behaviors with their child (Blacher et al., 2003; Mitchell et al., 2015; Shonkoff, Hauser-Cram, Krauss, & Upshur, 1992), several studies also included parental perceptions of their child's problem behaviors (Fidler, Most, Booth-LaForce, & Kelly, 2006), and of language difficulties (Smith et al., 2014). Considered before any covariance procedures, most involved an advantage for the parents of children with Down syndrome. Whether these parents remain advantaged when confounding variables are controlled is more difficult to discern. Specifically, only six of these 14 studies controlled for family income and/or maternal age. Once these preexisting group differences were controlled for, the advantage for the Down syndrome group remained in three (of six) studies. Thus, strong conclusions cannot be made either way, at least with respect to comparing parents of children with Down syndrome versus those of children with developmental disabilities or mixed causes of intellectual disabilities.

Contrasts between parents of children with Down syndrome to parents of same-aged children who were typically developing are also instructive. In many of these studies, similar—and even better—outcomes were reported among parents in the Down syndrome group. For instance, mothers of children with Down syndrome reported similar numbers of family problems, similar positive ratings of behavior, and similar parent perceptions (Blacher et al., 2013; Cuskelly, Chant, & Hayes, 1998; Dumas, Wolf, Fisman, & Culligan, 1991; Noh, Dumas, Wolf, & Fisman, 1989; Roach et al., 1999). In two studies, mothers of young children with Down syndrome reported fewer behaviors on the Child Behavior Checklist (Cuskelly et al., 1998; Eisenhower et al., 2005). Parents of children with Down syndrome also rated lower child-related stress than single parents of typically developing children (Duis et al., 1997). However, other studies of mothers of children with Down syndrome include reports of higher levels of stress and depression when compared to mothers of typically developing children (Dabrowska & Pisula, 2010; Noh et al., 1989; Roach et al., 1999).

Different ages of the child. Whether a Down syndrome advantage is evident across the childhood years is also difficult to answer. As shown in Table 5.1, more than half of all studies included parents of children younger than age 12; from these studies, a Down syndrome advantage did seem evident for these parents. Specifically, 84 percent (21 of 25) of these studies revealed some level of a Down syndrome advantage. In contrast, only five studies involved offspring in the young adult range (12–18 years old), with 60 percent of these studies (3 of 5) supporting a Down syndrome advantage. To complicate matters, two of the studies in which the advantage in the young adult and adult years was discounted involved the same pool of participants (Corrice & Glidden, 2009; Glidden et al., 2014). In addition, evidence from several longitudinal studies indicated that the advantage disappears at different points in time, at least with respect to the parent's perceptions of their child's maladaptive behaviors (Fidler et al., 2006; Glidden et al., 2014). More research seems needed, especially longitudinal studies during the later childhood years.

Differing outcome measures. When asking about the Down syndrome advantage, one must also consider outcome measures. Most definitely, the Down syndrome advantage continues to be evident when comparing parents of children with Down syndrome and parents of children with autism on measures of stress and family resources. This conclusion can be seen both in a recent meta-analysis and in Table 5.1. Hayes and Watson (2012) conducted a meta-analysis across studies on the outcomes of families of children with autism on the Parenting Stress Index (PSI; Abidin, 1983) and the Questionnaire of Resources and Stress (QRS; Holroyd, 1987). Of the studies which included parents of children with Down syndrome in the meta-analysis, there was a significant effect in favor of the Down syndrome advantage as compared to the responses of parents of children with autism across these two measures.

Although the PSI and QRS were the most commonly used measures across studies, many researchers also used other measures and outcomes. Table 5.1 includes well over 20 different parent-reported outcome measures. Though some are repeated across studies, the types of outcomes which were found to be significant are noteworthy. Using similar measures, researchers found that the Down syndrome advantage is evident with (parent-reported) child-related measures such as the child-related stress on the PSI (Griffith et al., 2010), subjective well-being related to the child (Corrice & Glidden, 2009; Glidden et al., 2014), and parent-reported measures of child characteristics (Burke, Fisher, & Hodapp, 2012; Duis et al., 1997; Fidler et al., 2006; Griffith et al., 2010; Mitchell et al., 2015; Olsson & Hwang, 2003; Smith et al., 2014). Some studies also indicated a Down syndrome advantage when observing interactions between mothers and their children with Down syndrome during early childhood (Blacher et al., 2013; Crawley & Spiker, 1983; Mitchell et al., 2015; Shonkoff et al., 1992).

In summarizing these many studies, simple conclusions seem difficult to make because of differences in comparison groups, ages of children, and outcome measures. Still, at present, parents of children with Down syndrome appear to show better outcomes, especially compared to parents of children with autism and before researchers perform co-variance or other procedures to account for pre-existing group differences. More studies are obviously needed, and we now consider aspects of children themselves, their parents, and societal issues that might relate to the Down syndrome advantage and parenting more generally.

What Might Account for the Down Syndrome Advantage?

Although research may not be sufficiently advanced to answer this question, we provide tentative answers by identifying possible child, mother-family, and societal factors.

Aspects of the Child With Down Syndrome

Orientation toward others and personality. From Langdon Down on, individuals who interact with children with Down syndrome have noted the degree to which most individuals are oriented to other people. Such an outer-directed style, which has been described as the "Down syndrome personality," has also been criticized as being overly stereotypical (Enea-Drapeau, Carlier, & Huguet, 2012; Wishart & Johnston, 1990) and does not apply to all children with Down syndrome. Still, on average, infants and toddlers with Down syndrome seem more interested in looking to others as opposed to objects (Berger & Cunningham, 1981). Similarly, when faced with performing a difficult cognitive task, toddlers and older children with Down syndrome often engage in "party tricks" (Pitcairn & Wishart, 1994), or sets of social behaviors toward others that allow them to avoid performing the task itself (also, Fidler, Most, Booth-LaForce, & Kelly, 1997; Kasari & Freeman, 2001). In this sense, most children with Down syndrome appear to others to be sociable and outgoing.

At the same time, however, such strengths in sociability may be mostly limited to the lowest levels of social behavior, including such behaviors as looking to others and smiling. Cebula, Moore, and Wishart (2010) refer to such social—but lower-level—achievements as "social-perceptual abilities," differentiating these from higher-level social-cognitive abilities. On such higher-level social-cognitive tasks as theory of mind and emotion recognition, children with Down syndrome showed marked deficits compared to mental aged-matched typical children. As Cebula et al. (2010) illustrate, this social profile—with etiology-related strengths in social-perceptual abilities but weaknesses in social-cognitive abilities—then relates to later cognitive, social, and linguistic achievements of the children themselves, as well as to specific changes in the interactive behaviors of their parents, siblings, and peers.

Behavior problems. Children with Down syndrome generally show lower prevalence rates of severe psychopathology relative to other conditions. Although estimates vary, approximately 20 percent of children with Down syndrome appear to show high levels of maladaptive behavior/psychopathology as compared to 35–40 percent of other groups with intellectual disability or with such specific genetic disorders as Prader-Willi syndrome (Dykens & Kasari, 1997; Foley et al., 2016). However, approximately 5–10 percent of children with Down syndrome do show autism (DiGuiseppi et al., 2010), some show schizophrenia and other types of severe psychopathology (Dykens, et al., 2015; Foley et al. 2014), and, more generally, children with Down syndrome show higher levels of psychopathology when compared to typically developing children of the same age or cognitive levels (Dykens, 2007). Children with Down syndrome also frequently display stubbornness, speech problems, inattention, and hyperactivity (Dykens & Kasari, 1997; Stores, Stores, Fellows, & Buckley, 1998). Still, compared to others with intellectual disability (or even to children with several genetic conditions), "children with Down syndrome generally show lower rates of significant behavioral or emotional problems" (Dykens, 2007, p. 273).

Physical appearance. How others react to any person is, to some extent, influenced by how one looks. Although obvious, the influences of physical appearance have recently been considered by those interested in evolutionary psychology, the theory that specific human characteristics have helped our species to thrive over millennia (Bjorklund, 1997, 2018). One such characteristic involves neoteny, the way in which human infants have evolved a host of physical and behavioral characteristics to elicit nurturant behaviors from others. This nurturing from caregivers is partly elicited from infants' physical appearance—from faces that are rounder and that feature large, round eyes; a small chin; high cheekbones; and thick and pudgy lips (Bjorklund, 2018). Using this insight, Zebrowitz (1997) highlighted that humans perceive faces that are more "baby-like" as more naïve and as needing warm, protective responses (Hugenberg & Wilson, 2013; Zebrowitz & Montepare, 1992).

Children with Down syndrome also show more baby-like faces. Allanson, O'Hara, Farkas, and Nair (1993) found that, compared to the faces of same-aged typical children and of children with intellectual disability more generally, children with Down syndrome, on average, have more baby-like faces. Compared to those of typically developing children, such faces also elicited feelings of nurturance from adult raters (Fidler & Hodapp, 1999). Even within same-aged children with Down syndrome, those with more baby-like facial features elicited more nurturant reactions from raters. Although Down-syndrome facial features may mislead others' judgments of intelligence (Enea-Drapeau, Huguet, & Carlier, 2014), more infantile faces do elicit nurturant behaviors from others (Hugenberg & Wilson, 2013); this reaction from others also operates toward children with Down syndrome.

Aspects of Down Syndrome's "Associated" Characteristics

We noted that mothers were, on average, older when they gave birth to their children with Down syndrome, with evidence on this issue from the United States, Great Britain, and Australia (Hodapp et al., 2016). Across these three countries, the median age at which mothers give birth to the child with Down syndrome is 32 years, compared to 26–27 years for non-Down syndrome births. Roughly 10–12 percent of mothers are 40 years old or older when giving birth to their child with Down syndrome, as compared to 1–2 percent of mothers of newborns who do not have Down syndrome (Hodapp, Burke, & Urbano, 2012; Hodapp et al., 2016).

Although the presence of so-called "advanced maternal age" in Down syndrome has been noted for almost a century (Brousseau, 1928; Penrose, 1933), the wider implications of a mother's age have received less attention. However, as the demographers McLanahan and Jacobsen (2015) point out for the larger population, maternal age is tied to a host of other maternal, paternal, and familial characteristics. Thus, increasingly until mothers are in their early to mid-30s, those mothers who are older are also more likely to have had more years of formal education. In addition, older mothers are more likely to be married and to not get divorced. Due to assortative mating (i.e., individuals marrying spouses much like themselves), these fathers are themselves more likely to be older and to have higher levels of education. Also compared to other fathers in the general population, these older, more educated fathers are more often actively involved in their children's lives.

Many of these connections have yet to be formally examined among families of children with Down syndrome, although identical findings have been noted for these families on the few variables that have been examined. For example, in comparing mothers who gave birth to their child with Down syndrome below versus above 23 years of age, Hodapp and Urbano (2008) found higher percentages of younger (versus older) mothers had not graduated from high school when they gave birth, were unmarried, and were from neighborhoods that had a lower median socioeconomic status (SES). While preliminary, the demographic correlates of younger maternal age seem to hold as well for families of children with Down syndrome.

In the larger, non-Down syndrome population, maternal age also relates to a variety of parental practices and cultural benefits. Though harder to define, such practices and benefits involve experiences that more educated, middle-class parents routinely provide for their children. Compared to children of less-educated parents, such children are more likely to have parents who spend money on, play with, and read to them, as well as families who go to bookstores, movies, museums, zoos, and sporting events (McLanahan,

2004). Over the past few decades, the amount of such "cultural capital" has increased greatly for children of highly educated parents, even as it has remained the same or only slightly increased for children whose parents have less formal education (McLanahan & Jacobsen, 2015).

Among typical children whose mothers give birth at different ages, one also sees differing levels of certain behaviors, at least up through when mothers are in their late 20s (i.e., they do not continue increasing with maternal birth age for mothers giving birth in their 30s or 40s). More precisely, certain aspects of social support and of parental practices change with increased maternal age, whereas others do not. In a study of over 300 mothers of 5-month-old infants, Bornstein, Putnick, Suwalsky, and Gini (2006) noted that "in-home support" (defined as help from the father, books, and other written materials) increased with maternal birth age up through 29 years (but not beyond). Similarly, older mothers (at least until the mid- to late 20s) also provided higher frequencies and durations of input language to their infants, as well as increased amounts of maternal sensitivity and structuring during interactions. In contrast, other social support and parenting practice variables did not differ for older versus younger mothers. The age at which a mother gives birth thus relates to many—not all—supports and behaviors, at least through the late 20s. Currently, these relations to birth age among mothers of children with Down syndrome have not been examined.

Aspects of Culture

We here briefly discuss the prevalence of Down syndrome and the population of parents of these children, as well as the effects of cultural knowledge of the syndrome and parent groups.

Changing prevalence of Down syndrome? Seemingly every few months, news reports highlight yet another easy, quick, and (increasingly) noninvasive prenatal test for Down syndrome. At various points, such professional groups as the American College of Obstetricians and Gynecologists (2007) have even proposed that prenatal screening for Down syndrome should be universally provided to all pregnant women. As might be imagined, the Down syndrome community—consisting of self-advocates, parents, siblings, researchers, teachers, and clinicians—has decried the call for universal screening (e.g., Will, 2007). They have pointed out how new prenatal testing techniques are often not nearly as noninvasive as advertised; that such tests are not always reliable (and that false-positive results lead prospective parents to anxiety); and that children and adults with Down syndrome increasingly experience lives that are longer, less often medically compromised, and feature more activities and integration in the wider community (Buckley & Buckley, 2008). Parents have even wondered whether they will be the last generation to have children with Down syndrome (Rasmussen, Whitehead, Cottier, & Frias, 2008) and studies have appeared with titles such as "Is Down Syndrome a Disappearing Birth Defect?" (Collins et al., 2008).

In contrast, increasing numbers of women in the general population are waiting to have their children, usually to embark on post-college careers or education. As a result, increasing numbers of births are by older mothers. Indeed, in certain U.S. states with high levels of education, the median maternal age at birth now exceeds 30 years (e.g., Massachusetts Department of Public Health, 2014). For the US as a whole, the mean age at mother's first birth has risen dramatically, from 21.4 years in 1970, to 24.9 years in 2000, and to 26.3 years in 2014 (Mathews & Hamilton, 2002, 2016). The percentage of births to women 35 years or older has also risen, from 7.4 percent in 2000 to 9.1 percent in 2014 (Mathews & Hamilton, 2016). Given this change over the years, there should be increasing—not decreasing—numbers of newborns with Down syndrome.

With two contrasting forces operating, the numbers of newborns with Down syndrome appear to be either steady or rising slightly. This number, which in the US equals about 5,300 to 6,000 births per year, seems to have been reasonably steady over the years. In a study of "active registries" of all births across ten U.S. regions, the numbers of Down syndrome births were even found to increase over the years 1979 to 2003 (Shin et al., 2009). Taken together, the various factors—more widespread prenatal testing along with larger numbers of older mothers—may be partially cancelling each other out. Thus, while the numbers of Down syndrome births are fewer than predicted given the numbers of older mothers, the actual numbers of Down syndrome births do not seem to be declining from one year to the next.

Less often considered is that mothers of newborns with Down syndrome might be changing in other ways. Given that, in most industrialized countries, prenatal testing is offered to all pregnant women aged 35 and above, older mothers of newborns with Down syndrome may be either explicitly choosing not to receive such testing or, upon learning that the fetus has Down syndrome, actively choosing to carry their fetus to term. If so, we may be seeing increasing numbers of parents who explicitly choose to have and raise these children. This possibility (though not formally examined) conforms to the growing interest in adopting children with the syndrome, as attested to by various websites and by such organizations as the National Down Syndrome Adoption Network (NDSAN; see https://www.ndsan.org).

A changing population of parents? A second cultural influence involves parent groups. Present for families of children with many disorders, parent groups are organizations originated and directed primarily by parents, but which also include clinicians, teachers, and researchers. Such organizations usually are national in scope, with state and local chapters. On a national level, groups provide their members information via the web, booklets, and newsletters; organize yearly (often summer) conferences attended by hundreds of individuals of all ages, as well as by parents, siblings, researchers, group home workers, teachers, and clinicians; and advocate locally and nationally for greater services and for more research in the condition. Local chapters hold monthly meetings and fundraisers, organize camps and events for children with the condition, advocate for appropriate educational and other placements for individual children, sponsor monthly or quarterly sibling groups; and lobby state legislatures.

Given these services and supports, parent groups constitute an important presence in the lives of many families of children with various disability conditions. Though vastly understudied, these groups seem to have many beneficial effects (Shilling, et al., 2013). One, parents describe a shared social identity which fosters a sense of belonging, support, and empowerment. Two, parent groups allow members to learn from the experience of others. As one parent noted, "When you have a child with special needs, you don't know the best services, the best care, etc. You get that information from the group" (Solomon, Pistrang, & Barker, 2001, p. 121). Three, groups provide parents the opportunity for personal growth; parents report that, from participating in the group, they felt more confident when dealing with other people and they became more "assertive, 'tougher,' and felt less intimidated, inhibited, embarrassed, awkward, and shy" (Solomon et al., 2001, p. 124). Four, over time, parents appreciate the value of providing support to other parents. In interacting with another parent, then, "I felt that perhaps my hope too, was that maybe I could be of help to them; not always just for my support" (Ainbinder et al., 1998, p. 104). Granted, such groups help parents of children with many conditions, although in many countries the parent-support groups for parents of children with Down syndrome seem especially active and prominent.

Considered together, then, diverse factors may contribute to the Down syndrome advantage. Such potential correlates include aspects of the child, of parental age and other associated characteristics, and of the wider culture. We now detail future directions in the study of parents and families of children with Down syndrome.

Future Directions

Although many aspects of parenting children with Down syndrome remain either partially or totally unexplored, we highlight three main issues.

Parenting Children of Different Ages

As any parent knows, parenting differs for children of different ages and oftentimes requires different sets of parenting skills and behaviors. For this reason, most life-span family models differentiate parenting infants and young children from parenting teens (Carter & McGoldrick, 1980; Channell & Loveall, 2018; Martin, 2018). But when considering parenting children with Down syndrome, most studies focus on a single age-group, most often younger children (see Table 5.1). For the most part, studies ignore the idea of age-related changes or of parenting older children.

As the disability world increasingly appreciates teens and young adults, however, we appreciate as well that these issues also have a parent-family component. Specifically, in Down syndrome, many children may undergo a slight change in personality and increase in maladaptive behavior that influences parent–offspring relations during the later teen and early adult years (Dykens, 2007). Although not present for all children, many teens and young adults with Down syndrome may become more withdrawn and less outwardly social toward others (Dykens, Shah, Sagun, Beck, & King, 2002; Foley et al., 2016). In these later-teen years, parents generally experience lesser degrees of help from parent groups and service systems more generally. The teen and early adult years may also be the time when offspring with Down syndrome most require environmental stimulation-interactions to keep and increase earlier cognitive-adaptive gains (Foley et al., 2014; Shepperdson, 1995).

Partially or Totally Unexamined Issues

As we note above, basic parenting issues often remain unexamined in Down syndrome, especially the ties of demographics to parenting behaviors. Thus, whereas we have preliminary evidence that mothers (and fathers) of children with Down syndrome are, compared to the general population, older, better educated, and more likely to be married (Hodapp & Urbano, 2008), we do not know whether other ties also hold. As in the general population, are mothers who are older (versus younger) when they give birth to their child with Down syndrome also more likely to be married to more active fathers and to have families that provide the child more resources? Similarly, do parents who are older and more educated also act differently toward their offspring with Down syndrome than do younger parents? Although such ties appear among typically developing infants and their parents, we do not yet know whether such connections hold for parents and their children with Down syndrome.

Even more importantly, few studies are focused on many societal issues. What, exactly, is the role of prenatal testing for parents of children with Down syndrome in modern-day industrial societies? Are these parents explicitly choosing to have and raise their children with Down syndrome? If so, how do today's parents compare to parents of earlier generations? Are differences between older and younger parents of typically developing children operating the same way when parents in the Down syndrome group are both older chronologically *and* have chosen to parent their offspring with Down syndrome? Answers to these questions will allow us to update our knowledge about the status and needs of children with Down syndrome and their families as we progress into the 21st century.

Connections to Parenting Specific to Down syndrome

A final issue concerns connections. In the parenting literature in disabilities, certain connections exist between the child's behavior and parental coping, but these are mostly explored in relation to children with intellectual disability more generally. Most notably, there seems a connection between greater levels of child behavior problems and increased maternal stress. This connection has now been noted among groups with intellectual disability more generally (Eisenhower et al., 2005), for children with several different genetic conditions (e.g., Prader-Willi Syndrome; Hodapp, Dykens, & Masino, 1997), and for children with Down syndrome (Mitchell et al., 2015).

In the case of Down syndrome, however, additional etiology-related characteristics may also tie to parent or family functioning. We now know, for instance, that many children with the syndrome experience sleep problems, which may in turn tie to increased language problems (Edgin et al., 2015). Similarly, the congenital heart defects experienced by roughly half of all newborns with Down syndrome (Roizen, 2010) may relate as well to infant receptive and expressive language scores (Alsaied et al., 2016). In short, researchers are beginning to connect common physical-medical characteristics with specific behavioral sequelae. Those studying Down syndrome need to tie these physical, health, and behavioral characteristics to parent and family outcomes. Consider even the basic, bedrock issue of infant health. From large-scale studies of hospitalization and other health records, somewhere between one half to two thirds of all newborns with Down syndrome experience nonbirth hospitalizations over the first year of life (Dawson et al., 2014; So, Urbano, & Hodapp, 2007). Given that, for any family, the hospitalization of a young child is an incredibly stressful event, how do such hospitalizations affect parents, siblings, and the family as a whole? In short, we need to understand how parents are influenced by specific, commonly occurring child characteristics (e.g., health problems) and behaviors (e.g., maladaptive behaviors). Conversely, we need as well to understand the degree to which parents—especially those who may be more or less educated and/or able to provide resources to their children—influence their children with Down syndrome.

Conclusion: Going Beyond the Down Syndrome Advantage

Considering its 150 years of existence as a recognized syndrome, Down syndrome remains, relative to other, more recently discovered conditions, an under-researched condition that features areas of great knowledge and of little knowledge. As illustrated by the contributions to this volume, we have learned a great deal about certain areas of behavioral functioning, as well as specifics of the many medical and physical issues that these children face. Increasingly, researchers are tying this knowledge to these children's development, such that we can determine both how such profiles develop over age and the effects of particular cognitive-linguistic-adaptive strengths and weaknesses on functioning in other domains.

At the same time, however, we remain less knowledgeable about many aspects of the functioning of these children's parents and families. Mothers, fathers, and the families of these children, in particular, have only now begun to receive research attention. And, while we do know at least some about functioning in these families—witness Table 5.1's many studies of the Down syndrome advantage—we also continue to have major gaps in our knowledge. As noted above, we currently know little about the effects of maternal age on maternal (and paternal) behaviors, on how different types or amounts of parental behaviors affect children, and on how current generations of parents of children with Down syndrome may be more explicitly choosing these children.

Beyond calling for additional and more sophisticated studies, then, our call is for studies on new, heretofore unexplored issues and on those that tie together different aspects of Down syndrome. New issues include many aspects of parenting behaviors and of the effects of cultural changes on parents and families (e.g., prenatal testing, more integrated classroom placements). Connections include considerations of how these children's health problems influence their cognitive, linguistic, and adaptive functioning, but also on the perceptions, coping, and parenting behaviors of parents themselves. For a disorder first described in the 1860s, it is time to work towards more sophisticated, deeper understandings of children, parents, and families of children with Down syndrome.

References

References marked with an asterisk indicate studies included in Table 5.1's literature review.

*Abbeduto, L., Seltzer, M. M., Shattuck, P., Krauss, M. W., Orsmond, G., & Murphy, M. M. (2004). Psychological well-being and coping in mothers of youths with autism, Down syndrome, or Fragile X syndrome. *American Journal on Mental Retardation, 109*(3), 237–254. doi:10.1352/0895-8017(2004)109<237:PWACIM>2.0.CO;2

Abidin, R. R. (1983). *Parenting Stress Index.* Charlottesville, VA: Pediatric Psychology Press.

Ainbinder, J. G., Blanchard, L. W., Singer, G. H. S., Sullivan, M. E., Powers, L. K., Marquis, J. G., . . . Consortium to Evaluate Parent to Parent. (1998). A qualitative study of parent to parent support for parents of children with special needs. *Journal of Pediatric Psychology, 23,* 99–109.

Allanson, J. E., O'Hara, P., Farkas, G., & Nair, R. C. (1993). Anthropometric craniofacial pattern profiles in Down syndrome. *American Journal of Medical Genetics, 47,* 748–752.

American College of Obstetricians and Gynecologists Committee on Practice Bulletins. (2007). Screening for fetal chromosomal abnormalities. ACOG Practice Bulletin No. 77. *Obstetrics and Gynecology, 109,* 217–227.

Alsaied, T., Marino, B. S., Esbensen, A. J., Anixt, J. S., Epstein, J. N., & Cnota, J. F. (2016). Does congenital heart disease affect neurodevelopmental outcomes in Down syndrome? *Congenital Heart Disease, 11,* 26–33.

*Atkinson, L., Scott, B., Chisholm, V., Blackwell, J., Dickens, S., Tam, F., & Goldberg, S. (1995). Cognitive coping, affective distress, and maternal sensitivity: Mothers of children with Down syndrome. *Developmental Psychology, 31*(4), 668–676.

Berger, J., & Cunningham, C. C. (1981). Development of eye contact between mothers and normal versus Down syndrome infants. *Developmental Psychology, 17,* 678–689.

*Blacher, J., & McIntyre, L. L. (2006). Syndrome specificity and behavioural disorders in young adults with intellectual disability: Cultural differences in family impact. *Journal of Intellectual Disability Research, 50*(3), 184–198. doi:10.1111/j.1365–2788.2005.00768.x

*Blacher, J., Baker, B. L., & Kaladjian, A. (2013). Syndrome specificity and mother-child interactions: Examining positive and negative parenting across contexts and time. *Journal of Autism and Developmental Disorders, 43,* 761–774.

Bjorklund, D. F. (1997). The uses of immaturity in human development. *Psychological Bulletin, 122,* 153–169.

Bjorklund, D. F. (2018). How children invented humanity. *Child Development, 89,* 1462–1466.

Bornstein, M. H., Putnick, D. L., Suwalsky, J. T. D., & Gini, M. (2006). Maternal chronological age, prenatal and perinatal history, social support, and parenting of infants. *Child Development, 77,* 875–892.

Brousseau, K. (1928). *Mongolism.* London: Lippincott, Williams, & Wilkins.

Buckley, F., & Buckley, S. (2008). Wrongful deaths and rightful lives: Screening for Down syndrome. *Down Syndrome Research and Practice, 12*(2), 79–86.

*Burke, M. M., Fisher, M. H., & Hodapp, R. M. (2012). Relations of parental perceptions to the behavioural characteristics of adolescents with Down syndrome. *Journal on Developmental Disabilities, 18*(2), 50–58.

*Cahill, B. M., & Glidden, L. M. (1996). Influence of child diagnosis on family and parental functioning: Down syndrome versus other disabilities. *American Journal on Mental Retardation, 101*, 149–160.

Carr, J. (1995). *Down syndrome: Children growing up*. Cambridge, UK: Cambridge University Press.

Carr, J. (2012). Six weeks to 45 years: A longitudinal study of a population with Down syndrome. *Journal of Applied Research in Intellectual Disabilities, 25*, 414–422.

Carter, A. E., & McGoldrick, M. (Eds.). (1980). *The family life-cycle: A framework for family therapy*. New York, NY: Gardner Press.

Cebula, K. R., Moore, D. G., & Wishart, J. G. (2010). Social cognition in children with Down's syndrome: Challenges to research and theory building. *Journal of Intellectual Disability Research, 54*, 113–134.

Channell, M. M., & Loveall, S. J. (2018). Post-high school transition for individuals with Down syndrome. *International Review of Research in Developmental Disabilities, 54*, 105–136.

Collins, V. R., Muggli, E. E., Riley, M., Dip, G., Palma, S., & Halliday, J. L., (2008). Is Down syndrome a disappearing birth defect? *Journal of Pediatrics, 152*, 20–24.

*Corrice, A. M., & Glidden, L. M. (2009). The Down syndrome advantage: Fact or fiction? *American Journal on Intellectual and Developmental Disabilities, 114*, 254–268.

*Crawley, S. B., & Spiker, D. (1983). Mother–child interactions involving two-year-olds with Down syndrome: A look at individual differences. *Child Development, 54*(5), 1312–1323. doi:10.2307/1129684

Cunningham, C. C. (1996). Families of children with Down syndrome. *Down Syndrome Research and Practice, 4*(3), 87–95.

Cunningham, C. C. (2006). *Down syndrome: An introduction for parents and carers* (3rd ed.). London: Souvenir Press.

*Cuskelly, M., Chant, D., & Hayes, A. (1998). Behaviour problems in the siblings of children with Down syndrome: Associations with family responsibilities and parental stress. *International Journal of Disability, Development and Education, 45*(3), 295–311. doi:10.1080/1034912980450305

*Dabrowska, A., & Pisula, E. (2010). Parenting stress and coping styles in mothers and fathers of pre-school children with autism and Down syndrome. *Journal of Intellectual Disability Research, 54*(3), 266–280. doi:10.1111/j.1365–2788.2010.01258.x

Dawson, A. L., Cassell, C. H., Oster, M. E., Olney, R. S., Tanner, J. P., Kirby, R. S., . . . Grosse, S. D. (2014). Hospitalizations and associated costs in a population-based study of children with Down syndrome born in Florida. *Birth Defects Research Part A—Clinical and Molecular Teratology, 100*, 826–836. doi:10.1002/bdra.23295

DiGuiseppi, C., Hepburn, S., Davis, J. M., Fidler, D. J., Hartway, S., Lee, N. R., . . . Robinson, C. (2010). Screening for Autism Spectrum Disorders in children with Down syndrome: Population prevalence and screening test characteristics. *Journal of Developmental and Behavioral Pediatrics, 31*, 181–191.

*Duis, S. S., Summers, M., & Summers, C. R. (1997). Parent versus child stress in diverse family types: An ecological approach. *Topics in Early Childhood Special Education, 17*(1), 53–73. doi:10.1177/027112149701700107

Dunn, P. M. (1991). Dr. Langdon Down (1828–1896) and "mongolism." *Archives of Diseases of Childhood, 66*, 827–828.

*Dumas, J. E., Wolf, L. C., Fisman, S. N., & Culligan, A. (1991). Parenting stress, child behavior problems, and dysphoria in parents of children with autism, Down syndrome, behavior disorders, and normal development. *Exceptionality, 2*(2), 97–110. doi:10.1080/09362839109524770

Dykens, E. M. (2007). Psychiatric and behavioral disorders in persons with Down syndrome. *Mental Retardation and Developmental Disabilities Research Reviews, 13*, 272–278.

Dykens, E. M., & Hodapp, R. M. (2001). Research in mental retardation: Toward an etiologic approach. *Journal of Child Psychology and Psychiatry, 42*, 49–71.

Dykens, E. M., & Kasari, C. (1997). Maladaptive behaviour in children with Prader-Willi syndrome, Down syndrome, and non-specific mental retardation. *American Journal on Mental Retardation, 102*, 228–237.

Dykens, E. M., Shah, B., Davis, B., Baker, C., Fife, C., & Fitzpatrick, J. (2015). Psychiatric disorders in adolescents and young adults with Down syndrome and other intellectual disabilities. *Journal of Neurodevelopmental Disorders, 7* (9), 1–8.

Dykens, E. M., Shah, B., Sagun, J., Beck, T., & King, B. H. (2002). Maladaptive behavior in children and adolescents with Down syndrome. *Journal of Intellectual Disability Research, 46*, 484–492.

Edgin, J. O., Tooley, U., Demara, B., Nyhuis, C., Arnand, P., & Spano, G. (2015). Sleep disturbance and expressive language delays in preschool children with Down syndrome. *Child Development, 86*, 1984–1998.

*Eisenhower, A. S., Baker, B. L., & Blacher, J. (2005). Preschool children with intellectual disability: Syndrome specificity, behaviour problems, and maternal well-being. *Journal of Intellectual Disability Research, 49*(9), 657–671. doi:10.1111/j.1365–2788.2005.00699.x

Enea-Drapeau, C., Carlier, M., & Huguet, P. (2012). Tracking subtle stereotypes of children with Trisomy 21: From facial-feature-based to implicit stereotypes. *PLOS One, 7,* 4.

Enea-Drapeau, C., Huguet, P., & Carlier, M. (2014). Misleading face-based judgment of cognitive level in intellectual disability: The case of trisomy 21 (Down syndrome). *Research in Developmental Disabilities, 35,* 3598–3605.

Erickson, M., & Upshur, C. C. (1989). Caretaking burden and social support: Comparison of mothers of infants with and without disabilities. *American Journal on Mental Retardation, 94*(3), 25–258.

Fidler, D. J., & Hodapp, R. M. (1999). Craniofacial maturity and perceived personality in children with Down syndrome. *American Journal on Mental Retardation, 104,* 410–421.

*Fidler, D. J., Hodapp, R. M., & Dykens, E. M. (2000). Stress in families of young children with Down syndrome, Williams syndrome, and Smith-Magenis syndrome. *Early Education and Development, 11*(4), 395–406. doi:10.1207/s15566935eed1104_2

*Fidler, D. J., Most, D. E., Booth-LaForce, C., & Kelly, J. F. (1997). Temperament and behavior problems in young children with Down syndrome at 12, 30 and 45 months. *Down Syndrome Research and Practice, 10*(1), 23–29.

Fidler, D. J., Most, D., Booth-LaForce, C., & Kelly, J. F. (2006). Emerging social strengths in young children with Down syndrome. *Infants and Young Children, 21,* 207–220.

Foley, K.-R., Jacoby, P., Einfeld, S., Girdler, S., Bourke, J., Riches, V., & Leonard, H. (2014). Day occupation is associated with psychopathology for adolescents and young adults with Down syndrome. *BMC Psychiatry, 14,* (article 266).

Foley, K.-R., Taffe, J., Bourke, J., Einfeld, S. L., Tonge, B. J., Trollor, J., & Leonard, H. (2016). Young people with intellectual disability transitioning to adulthood: Do behavior trajectories differ in those with and without Down syndrome? *PLoS ONE, 11* (7), e0157667. doi:10.1371/journal.pone.0157667

Gibson, D. (1978). *Down's syndrome: The psychology of mongolism.* Cambridge, UK: Cambridge University Press.

*Glidden, L. M., Grein, K. A., & Ludwig, J. A. (2014). The Down syndrome advantage: It depends on what and when you measure. *American Journal on Intellectual and Developmental Disabilities, 119,* 389–404.

*Griffith, G. M., Hastings, R. P., Nash, S., & Hill, C. (2010). Using matched groups to explore child behavior problems and maternal well-being in children with Down syndrome and autism. *Journal of Autism and Developmental Disorders, 40*(5), 610–619. doi:10.1007/s10803-009-0906-1

*Hamlyn-Wright, S., Draghi-Lorenz, R., & Ellis, J. (2007). Locus of control fails to mediate between stress and anxiety and depression in parents of children with a developmental disorder. *Autism, 11*(6), 489–501. doi:10.1177/1362361307083258

*Hanson, M. J., & Hanline, M. F. (1990). Parenting a child with a disability: A longitudinal study of parental stress and adaptation. *Journal of Early Intervention, 14*(3), 234–248.

*Hayes, S. A., & Watson, S. L. (2012). The impact of parenting stress: A meta-analysis of studies comparing the experience of parenting stress in parents of children with and without autism spectrum disorder. *Journal of Autism and Developmental Disorders, 43,* 629–642.

Hodapp, R. M. (2007). Families of persons with Down syndrome: New perspectives, findings, and research and service needs. *Mental Retardation and Developmental Disabilities Research Reviews, 13,* 279–287.

Hodapp, R. M., Burke, M. M., Finley, C. I., & Urbano, R. C. (2016). Family caregiving of aging adults with Down syndrome. *Journal of Policy and Practice in Intellectual Disabilities, 13,* 181–189.

Hodapp, R. M., Burke, M. M., & Urbano, R. C. (2012). What's age got to do with it? Implications of maternal age on families of offspring with Down syndrome. *International Review of Research in Developmental Disabilities, 42,* 109–145.

Hodapp, R. M., Dykens, E. M., & Masino, L. L. (1997). Families of children with Prader-Willi Syndrome: Stress-support and relations to child characteristics. *Journal of Autism and Developmental Disorders, 27,* 11–24.

Hodapp, R. M., Ly, T. M., Fidler, D. J., & Ricci, L. (2001). Less stress, more rewarding: Parenting children with Down syndrome. *Parenting: Science and Practice, 1,* 317–337.

*Hodapp, R. M., Ricci, L. A., Ly, T. M., & Fidler, D. J. (2003). The effects of the child with Down syndrome on maternal stress. *British Journal of Developmental Psychology, 21*(1), 137–151. doi:10.1348/026151003321164672

Hodapp, R. M., & Urbano, R. C., &. (2007). Adult siblings of individuals with Down syndrome versus with autism: Findings from a large-scale American survey. *Journal of Intellectual Disability Research, 51*, 1018–1029.

Hodapp, R. M., & Urbano, R. C. (2008). Demographics of African-American and European-American mothers of newborns with Down syndrome. *Journal of Policy and Practice in Intellectual Disabilities, 5*, 187–193.

*Holmes, N., & Carr, J. (1991). The pattern of care in families of adults with a mental handicap: A comparison between families of autistic adults and Down syndrome adults. *Journal of Autism and Developmental Disorders, 21*(2), 159–176. doi:10.1007/BF02284757

Holroyd, J. (1987). *Questionnaire on resources and stress: For families with chronically ill or handicapped members.* Brandon, CT: Clinical Psychology Publishing.

*Holroyd, J., & McArthur, D. (1976). Mental retardation and stress on the parents: A contrast between Down's syndrome and childhood autism. *American Journal of Mental Deficiency, 80*(4), 431–436.

Hugenberg, K., & Wilson, J. P. (2013). Faces are central to social cognition. In D. E. Carlston (Ed.), *The Oxford handbook of social cognition* (pp. 167–193). Oxford, UK; Oxford University Press.

*Kasari, C., & Sigman, M. (1997). Linking parental perceptions to interactions in young children with autism. *Journal of Autism and Developmental Disorders, 27*(1), 39–57.

Kasari, C., & Freeman, S. F. N. (2001). Task-related social behavior in children with Down syndrome. *American Journal on Mental Retardation, 106*, 253–264.

*Lanfranchi, S., & Vianello, R. (2012). Stress, locus of control, and family cohesion and adaptability in parents of children with Down, Williams, Fragile X, Prader-Willi syndromes. *American Journal on Intellectual and Developmental Disabilities, 117*(3), 207–224. doi:10.1352/1944-7558-117.3.207

*Lewis, P., Abbeduto, L., Murphy, M., Richmond, E., Giles, N., Bruno, L., Schroeder, S., Anderson, J., & Orsmond, G. (2006). Psychological well-being of mothers of youth with fragile X syndrome: Syndrome specificity and within-syndrome variability. *Journal of Intellectual Disability Research, 50*(12), 894–904. doi:10.1111/j.1365–2788.2006.00907.x

Martin, T. F. (2018). Family Development Theory 30 years later. *Journal of Family Theory and Review, 10*, 49–69.

Massachusetts Department of Public Health (2014). *Massachusetts Births 2013.* Boston, MA: Office of Data Management and Outcomes Assessment, Massachusetts Department of Public Health.

Mathews, T. J., & Hamilton, B. E. (2002). *Mean age of mother, 1970–2000. National Vital Statistics Reports, 51*(2). Hyattsville, MD: National Center for Health Statistics.

Mathews, T. J., & Hamilton, B. E. (2016). *Mean age of mothers is on the rise: United States, 2000–2014. NCHS data brief, no. 232.* Hyattsville, MD: National Center for Health Statistics.

McLanahan, S. (2004). Diverging destinies: How children are faring under the second demographic transition. *Demography, 41*, 607–627.

McLanahan, S., & Jacobsen, W. (2015). Diverging destinies revisited. In P. R. Amato, A. Booth, S. M. McHale, & J. Van Hook (Eds.), *Families in an era of increasing inequality: Diverging destinies* (pp. 3–23). Cham, Switzerland: Springer International.

*Mitchell, D. B., Hauser-Cram, P., & Crossman, M. K. (2015). Relationship dimensions of the "Down syndrome advantage." *Journal of Intellectual Disability Research, 59*, 506–518.

*Noh, S., Dumas, J. E., Wolf, L. C., & Fisman, S. N. (1989). Delineating sources of stress in parents of exceptional children. *Family Relations: An Interdisciplinary Journal of Applied Family Studies, 38*(4), 456–461. doi:10.2307/585753

*Olsson, M. B., & Hwang, P. C. (2003). Influence of macrostructure of society on the life situation of families with a child with intellectual disability: Sweden as an example. *Journal of Intellectual Disability Research, 47*, 328–341.

Penrose, L. S. (1933). The relative effects of paternal and maternal age in Mongolism. *Journal of Genetics, 27*, 219–224.

Penrose, L. S. (1949). *The biology of mental defect.* London: Sidgwick & Jackson.

Penrose, L. S., & Smith, G. F. (1966). *Down's anomaly.* London: J. & A Churchill.

Pitcairn, T. K., & Wishart, J. G. (1994). Reactions of young children with Down's syndrome to an impossible task. *British Journal of Developmental Psychology, 12*, 485–489.

Rasmussen, S. A., Whitehead, N., Cottier, S. A., & Frias, J. L. (2008). Setting a public health research agenda for Down syndrome: Summary of a meeting sponsored by the Centers for Disease Control and Prevention and the National Down Syndrome Society. *American Journal of Medical Genetics, Part A, 146A*, 2998–3010.

*Roach, M. A., Orsmond, G. I., & Barrett, M. S. (1999). Mothers and fathers of children with Down syndrome: Parental stress and involvement in childcare. *American Journal of Mental Retardation, 104*, 422–436.

Roizen, N. (2010). Overview of health issues in Down syndrome. *International Review of Research in Mental Retardation, 39*, 3–33.

*Saunders, J. L., & Morgan, S. B. (1997). Family stress and adjustment as perceived by parents of children with autism or Down syndrome: Implications for intervention. *Child & Family Behavior Therapy, 19*(4), 15–32. doi:10.1300/J019v19n04_02

*Seltzer, M. M., Krauss, M. W., & Tsunematsu, N. (1993). Adults with Down syndrome and their aging mothers: Diagnostic group differences. *American Journal on Mental Retardation, 97*, 495–508.

Seltzer, M. M., & Ryff, C. D. (1994). Parenting across the life span: The normative and nonnormative case. *Life-Span Development and Behavior, 12*, 1–40.

Sheppardson, B. (1995). Two longitudinal studies of the abilities of people with Down's syndrome. *Journal of Intellectual Disability Research, 39*, 419–431.

Shilling, V., Morris, C., Thompson-Coon, J., Ukoumunne, O., Rogers, M., & Logan, S. (2013). Peer support for parents of children with chronic disabling conditions: A systematic review of quantitative and qualitative studies. *Developmental Medicine and Child Neurology, 55*, 602–609.

Shin, M., Besser, L. M., Kucik, J. E., Lu, C., Siffel, C., & Correa, A. (2009). Prevalence of Down syndrome among children and adolescents in 10 regions of the United States. *Pediatrics, 124*, 1565–1571.

*Shonkoff, J. P., Hauser-Cram, P., Krauss, M. W., & Upshur, C. C. (1992). Development of infants with disabilities and their families: Implications for theory and service delivery. *Monographs of the Society for Research in Child Development, 57*(6), v-153. doi:10.2307/1166087

*Siklos, S., & Kerns, K. A. (2006). Assessing need for social support in parents of children with autism and Down syndrome. *Journal of Autism and Developmental Disorders, 36*(7), 921–923. doi:10.1007/s10803-006-0129-7

*Smith, A. L., Romski, M., Sevcik, R. A., Adamson, L. B., & Barker, R. M. (2014). Parent stress and perceptions of language development: Comparing Down syndrome and other developmental disabilities. *Family Relations: An Interdisciplinary Journal of Applied Family Studies, 63*(1), 71–84. doi:10.1111/fare.12048

So, S. A., Urbano, R. C., & Hodapp, R. M. (2007). Hospitalizations for infants and young children with Down syndrome: Evidence from inpatient person-records from a statewide administrative database. *Journal of Intellectual Disability Research, 51*, 1030–1038.

Solomon, M., Pistrang, N., & Barker, C. (2001). The benefits of mutual support groups for parents of children with disabilities. *American Journal of Community Psychology, 29*, 113–132.

*Stoneman, Z. (2007). Examining the Down syndrome advantage: Mothers and fathers of young children with disabilities. *Journal of Intellectual and Developmental Disabilities, 51*, 1006–1017.

Stores, R., Stores, G., Fellows, B., & Buckley, S. (1998). Daytime behaviour problems and maternal distress in children with Down syndrome, their siblings, and their non-intellectually disabled peers. *Journal of Intellectual Disability Research, 42*, 221–237.

Will, G. (2007, January 29). The attack on children with Down syndrome. *Newsweek*.

Wishart, J. G., & Johnston, F. H. (1990). The effects of experience on attribution of a stereotyped personality to children with Down's syndrome. *Journal of Mental Deficiency Research, 34*, 409–420.

Zebrowitz, L. A., & Montepare, J. M. (1992). Impressions of babyfaced individuals across the lifespan. *Developmental Psychology, 28*, 1143–1152.

Zebrowitz, L. A. (1997). *Reading faces: Window to the soul?* Boulder, CO: Westview Press.

CHAPTER

6 Siblings' Influence on the Development of Individuals With Down Syndrome

Monica Cuskelly

Abstract

This chapter discusses the influences that siblings may have on developmental outcomes of children with Down syndrome including those related to cognition, language, self-regulation, social-emotional functioning, and identity formation. As there is very little research available that addresses sibling influences on individuals with Down syndrome, the literature related to sibling influence within sibships comprising typically developing children has been used to provide a starting point to the discussion. The influential roles of siblings may include teacher; model and social referent; friend and foe; contrast; and advocate, protector, and caregiver. The quality of the sibling relationship may also influence developmental outcomes. The few investigations that have been conducted suggest that siblings make an important contribution to developmental outcomes for individuals with Down syndrome. In conclusion, directions for future research are discussed.

Key Words: Down syndrome, siblings, brothers, sisters, family, sibship, development

Introduction

It is a truism that the sibling relationship is the longest relationship in one's life. While this relationship generally changes in fairly predictable ways across the lifespan, siblings typically remain connected to one another from birth until death (for a review, see Lanthier & Campbell, 2011). The intensity and longevity of this unique relationship means that it may play a central role across a number of life arenas. There is potential for this relationship to be more influential for children with Down syndrome than for children who do not have a disability, because their common experiences of social isolation and lack of acceptance in essential settings such as school (e.g., Schwab, Huber, & Gebhardt, 2016) may imbue considerably more potency to their interactions with their siblings.

This chapter is organized in four sections. The focus of the first is on the roles that siblings of an individual with Down syndrome may play in relation to their brother or sister. The second section is focused on the research regarding the quality of the relationship between those with Down syndrome and their siblings. Relationships that are positive are likely to create more opportunities for influential interactions among siblings. The foci of the third section are on areas of development of the individual with Down syndrome which may be open to the influence of siblings. The fourth section includes suggestions for research to advance our understanding of the mechanisms of influence that operate in sibships that include a member with Down syndrome, with the emphasis on the influence of siblings on the individual with Down syndrome. This chapter draws heavily on the research literature related to sibling influence in sibships involving only typically developing children to guide consideration of the potential mechanisms by which siblings influence each other's development and the areas in which sibling influence is likely to be most impactful. In order to avoid confusion, in this chapter, the term "sibling" will always refer to the typically developing member of the dyad.

Developmental Impact of Siblings

Research with typically developing children has shown that siblings influence the development of their brothers and sisters in multiple ways and that these influences may be direct or indirect (Brody, 2004; McHale, Updegraff, & Whiteman, 2012). Direct influences occur as siblings take on the roles of playmate, model, and sparring partner, while indirect influences occur when siblings influence the ways in which the family operates, such as when parents change their ways of interacting with a second child, based on their experiences with their firstborn. While sibling influences will, in part, be extensions of parental influence (e.g., parents set the "tone" of family interactions), siblings make a unique contribution to the developmental outcomes of their brothers and sisters. As an example, Padilla-Walker, Harper, and Jensen (2010) found that affection between siblings was predictive of a range of positive outcomes, including prosocial behavior and self-regulation, and that these associations were still apparent after the quality of parent-child relationships was accounted for.

Much of the research about the influence of siblings on developmental outcomes has been focused on structural aspects of the sibship, including number of siblings, sibling position (older vs. younger), and gender composition. The impact of these structural variables may differ, depending upon the aspect of functioning being considered, and they may not apply when one member of the sibship has Down syndrome. In sibling dyads with two typically developing members, there are somewhat predictable dynamics between the members, especially during the childhood period, but these are often overturned when one child has Down syndrome. As an example, in sibling dyads where both members are typically developing, the older child is usually the leader and is imitated by the younger sibling (Howe, Rosciszewska, & Persram, 2018), whereas when children with Down syndrome are the older member of the dyad, they are likely to be the imitator of their younger sibling (Gilmore, Ryan, Cuskelly, & Gavidia-Payne, 2016).

Siblings might be construed as a resource for their brothers or sisters as they can teach about the world, either explicitly or through being observed (Brody & Murry, 2001), and through their interactions with their brother or sister when they cooperate, share jokes, play tricks on, and argue with them (Chen, 2015). They may play a particularly important role for children with Down syndrome as they appear to be the drivers of interactions. In observational studies, Knott, Lewis, and Williams (2007) and Singh, Iacono, and Gray (2015) found that siblings were significantly more likely to initiate interactions with the child with Down syndrome than vice versa. Whereas Singh et al. (2015) collected data at one time point only, Knott et al. (2007) collected data on two occasions, 12 months apart. In Knott et al.'s (2007) study, the siblings initiated both positive and negative exchanges at almost twice the rate of their brother or sister with Down syndrome at both time points. Knott et al. (2007) suggested that the siblings were often the architects of interactions within the dyad—their initiations increased dramatically over the year, which provided increased prompts for responses from the child with Down syndrome.

While siblings themselves may be a resource, they reduce the parental resources available to the other children because parents will have less time to spend with each child the more children there are in the family (Lawson & Mace, 2009; Marjoribanks, 1991). Financial resources are also reduced. Reduction in these resources may impact negatively on outcomes such as academic achievement (Schmeer, 2009) and health (Lawson & Mace, 2008), although these effects are likely to be mitigated by the initial level of resources available in the family. Alternatively, competition for resources could result in skill development as children strive to meet their individual needs (Bjorkland & Pelligrini, 2011). To add to the difficulties in understanding sibling impacts, there may be different outcomes according to family position. As an example of this, Lawson and Mace (2010) found a negative impact on mental health for those who were older in larger sibships but positive impacts for those who were younger. Clearly, there are many complexities around the mechanisms by which siblings influence each other, and these may differ depending upon both the aspect of development being considered and the developmental stages of the children in the sibship.

Influential Roles

There are a number of potential roles to be filled by siblings in a family with a child with Down syndrome. I shall not be exhaustive here, as all are speculative at the moment; however, I have generally chosen to focus on roles for which there is evidence in typically developing dyads, such as teacher, model and social referent, friend, foe, and contrast. The exception is the role of advocate, protector, and caregiver, which may be found in sibships that include an individual with a disability but is not usually considered in the literature on typically developing sibships. All but this last role have been shown to be influential in child development in typically developing children and so may prove productive in understanding—and perhaps intervening in—the developmental trajectories of children with Down syndrome. The developmental impact of siblings will be influenced by the nature and level of engagement between them and their brother or sister, discussed further below, as well as by the personal characteristics of both members of the dyad.

Teacher

Children generally learn a great deal from their siblings, and while both younger and older siblings engage in teaching, older siblings undertake more teaching than their younger brothers or sisters (Abuhatoum, Howe, Della Porta, Recchia, & Ross, 2016; Howe, Della Porta, Recchia, Funamoto, & Ross, 2015). They provide explicit instruction, with this responsibility being observed in widely differing cultures (e.g., Rabain-Jamin, Maynard, & Greenfield, 2003). While sibling instruction will often be helpful, teaching that is too directive (i.e., not responsive to the needs of the child being taught) may undermine learning. Directive parenting has been found to be associated with reduced persistence in children with Down syndrome (Gilmore, Cuskelly, Jobling, & Hayes, 2009), and in a study of teaching in typically developing dyads, Howe, Recchia, Della Porta, and Funamoto (2012) found that directive teaching by a sibling led to disengagement from the activity by the learner partner.

There is a danger that siblings will engage in relatively high levels of directive behavior when teaching their brother or sister with Down syndrome. The siblings of children with Down syndrome were found to be significantly more likely to engage in interactions that were unequal (i.e., teaching, managing, helping) than children whose younger brother or sister was typically developing (Stoneman, Brody, Davis, & Crapps, 1989) and to be more directive in their communications (Singh et al., 2015). This is consistent with Floyd, Purcell, Richardson, and Kupersmidt's (2009) findings that the siblings of children with intellectual disability were more directive toward their brothers and sisters than were siblings of children who were developing typically. In Floyd et al.'s (2009) study, the siblings of the children with intellectual disability gave three times the number of commands to their brother or sister than they received, whereas the number of commands was relatively equal between the pair in the dyads in which both children were developing typically.

One reason that siblings may be more directive is that they perceive their brother or sister with Down syndrome to be relatively incompetent—for example, their language skills are likely to be poorer than those of age peers at most ages (Cuskelly, Povey, & Jobling, 2016). Klein, Feldman, and Zarur (2002) found that children's approaches to teaching were influenced by their beliefs about competence and they were more likely to draw on a smaller range of approaches to teaching with those they saw as less capable as opposed to more able. However, certain sibling characteristics may lessen the likelihood that they will adopt a directive approach to teaching, as those who are more sensitive to the needs of their brother or sister display more flexibility in their approaches to teaching (Prime, Perlman, Tackett, & Jenkins, 2014).

Some children are more sensitive to their brother's or sister's difficulty than are others, a characteristic that has been labeled "cognitive sensitivity" by Prime et al. (2014). Children with high cognitive sensitivity adjust their teaching to accommodate the abilities and knowledge of their sibling, for example by simplifying instructions or providing a demonstration, whereas those with low cognitive sensitivity might merely repeat the original instructions. This ability and willingness to be flexible in interactions has been observed in typically developing children. For example, Howe, Brody, and Recchia (2006) found that children used more demonstration and scaffolding with more difficult tasks when teaching their younger sibling and also employed more strategies with younger children. Cognitive sensitivity is likely to be useful if it means that sibling assistance is pitched at the correct level to enable the learner to improve in performance (referred to as working within the zone of proximal development, Vygotsky, 1978). However, if awareness of their brother's or sister's difficulty results in overprotectiveness or intrusive assistance, it may undermine the other's motivation and/or learning.

While the roles of teacher and learner are common in sibling interactions, this role sometimes becomes formalized in cases where one child has a disability. There have been a number of intervention studies in which siblings have been included as intervention agents (see Kim & Horn, 2010, for a review not specific to children with Down syndrome). As an example, Trent, Kaiser, and Wolery (2005) taught the older siblings of two girls with Down syndrome to use responsive behaviors when interacting with their sister with Down syndrome. Both siblings adopted the new behaviors and there were positive changes in the targeted behaviors of the young girls with Down syndrome. Recruiting siblings to the role of change agent may have unintended consequences, however. Having them take the role of teacher (at others' instigation) may emphasize the difficulties of the child with Down syndrome, increase perceptions of incompetence, and entrench directiveness in sibling interactions. Some consideration of these potential consequences needs to be built into interventions studies that use siblings as the agent of change, at least until researchers are certain that no inadvertent harm is caused.

Model and Social Referent

Children also learn from their siblings by observing them as they solve practical and social problems (e.g., Watson, Meeks, Dufrene, & Lindsay, 2002; Wishart, 1986). Siblings will be more effective models than adults with respect to many tasks because children are more likely to be influenced by those they see as similar to themselves (e.g., other children) than they are by those they perceive to be dissimilar (e.g., adults; Bandura, 1986; Barr & Hayne, 2003; Miltenberger, 2001). Modeling is the term most often used when discussing learning new skills through observation, but children also use others to provide information about how to respond to novel situations (e.g., with fear or openness) and how to manage their emotions. Sometimes known as social referencing, this can be seen in both immediate and deferred imitation, and may contribute to the similarities observed in the behaviors of siblings.

Imitation is one of the most important ways in which children learn from their siblings and is considered to be a relative strength for children with Down syndrome (Wright, Lewis, & Collins, 2006). Children with Down syndrome have been observed to use imitation in social and other situations (Wright et al., 2006), and have been found to be more likely to imitate their sibling than vice versa, regardless of whether they are the younger or older member of the dyad (Abramovitch, Stanhope, Pepler, & Corter, 1987). Knott et al. (2007) interpreted imitation by the child with Down syndrome as a strategy for maintaining the sibling interaction, and this view is supported by the finding reported by Howe et al. (2018) that imitation leads to increased warmth between typically developing siblings. Thus, imitation may well have multiple functions, including relationship building and developing competence. However, Cebula, Moore, and Wishart (2010) cautioned that imitation and social referencing may not always be used effectively by children with Down syndrome. They pointed to evidence that children with Down syndrome often choose to use imitation when a different strategy would be more appropriate for dealing with the problem confronting them, perhaps because social relationships are more motivating than other aspects of the problem situation. With respect to social referencing, Cebula et al. (2010) cited evidence that children with Down syndrome use "looks" to their parents less frequently than typically developing children. If this relative reduction in social referencing extends to others, including siblings, then the skills of children with Down syndrome will be diminished with respect to responding to situations in socially expected ways.

Friend and Foe

As in dyads where both siblings are developing typically, some sibships will generally be more amicable than others; however, all are likely to have times of harmony and of conflict. The impact of these relationship qualities on outcomes will largely be indirect as they act to amplify or decrease the effectiveness of the sibling as a teacher, model, and social referent (Whiteman, McHale, & Crouter, 2007). Siblings who have a positive, warm relationship are likely to choose to spend more time together than are those who experience a high degree of conflict (Noller, 2005) and are also likely to be more effective in the modeling role (Whiteman, Bernard, & McHale, 2010; Whiteman & Christiansen, 2008). Conversely, in cases of destructive conflict, siblings will avoid each other, thus lessening the opportunity for influences to flow between the members of the dyad.

High levels of conflict in the sibling relationship have been shown to be associated with poorer outcomes in social competence (Stormshak, Bellanti, & Bierman, 1996) and child adjustment (Dirks, Persram, Recchia, & Howe, 2015). Although children with Down syndrome are not exposed to more conflictual relationships with their brothers and sisters than are other children (Cuskelly & Gunn, 2003; Fisman et al., 1996), they are likely to experience some conflict with their siblings. Conflict is a normal part of the sibling relationship and can coexist with warmth. Conflict may be characterized as constructive or destructive (Howe, Rinaldi, Jennings, & Petrakos, 2002). Constructive conflicts are of low intensity and differences can usually be settled by negotiation while destructive conflicts are generally of high intensity, and resolution is likely to be through the use of power strategies such as coercion. An absence of *constructive* conflict in the relationship may reduce opportunities for the development of certain skills, such as negotiation, compromise, and understanding others' perspectives. This is supported by Floyd et al.'s (2009) finding that children with intellectual disability showed better social competence when their relationship with their sibling was characterized by either high warmth *or* high conflict. These findings suggest that both prosocial and constructively conflictual interactions between siblings will benefit the development of children with Down syndrome (see Kramer, 2014, for a review focused on typically developing children).

Contrast

One of the processes by which typically developing children develop the self that they present to the world is known as de-identification and involves differentiating themselves from their sibling. This process is seen to be particularly relevant for younger siblings as they attempt to carve out a niche for themselves that differs from that occupied by their older brother or sister. According to theories of de-identification, the process protects younger siblings from direct competition with their sibling and from the negative emotion that will sometimes be the consequence of upward social comparison, as occurs when children decide that someone else is better than they are in a certain respect (Whiteman et al., 2007).

Investigations of the role of siblings in helping to establish a "self" requires a developmental perspective because the roles that siblings play generally change with respect to how individuals understand themselves as they mature. With increasing age, differences in ability diminish and "roles" become more solidified. The trajectories of these changes are likely to differ in families with a child with Down syndrome. For example, the gap in competence between siblings will widen rather than narrow as both cognition and language develop at a slower rate in children with Down syndrome than in children who are typically developing (Couzens, Cuskelly, & Haynes, 2011; Cuskelly, Povey, et al., 2016). In some dyads in which the child with Down syndrome is older, there may be a crossover period as the younger sibling becomes the more capable. Thus, the processes of de-identification, with respect to the individual with Down syndrome, may be less intense than in typically developing children when the child with Down syndrome is younger, or more intense if they are the older child in the dyad.

There is some evidence that siblings are used for comparison purposes by individuals with Down syndrome, with parents reporting they were the most commonly used comparator (Cuskelly & Gordon, 2011; Glenn & Cunningham, 2004). Parents in the Glenn and Cunningham (2004) study reported that many of the young people in the study did not make downward (positive—"I am better") or upward (negative—"I am worse") comparisons with respect to their sibling but made explicit or implicit "lateral" comparisons where they described themselves as similar to, or wanting to be like, their sibling. The role that siblings play in the development of self-understanding of those with Down syndrome is a question that requires further investigation.

Advocate, Protector, and Caregiver

Siblings may take on a number of social roles in the lives of their brother or sister with Down syndrome. These have the potential to influence the quality of life experienced by the person with Down syndrome but are unlikely to impact developmental outcomes directly. Examples include the roles of advocate, protector, and caregiver. Acting as an advocate can occur during childhood as siblings assist their brother or sister to negotiate the complexities of playgrounds and school (Skotko & Levine, 2006). This role may become more formal as their brother or sister moves into the adult service system and decisions are made regarding occupation, housing, and health related matters. When discussing these concerns within the family, siblings may also take the role of advocate for their brother or sister if there are generational disagreements about what is possible and/or appropriate for the adult with Down syndrome. While the protector role has elements of advocacy attached to it, it is likely to be more personally demanding of siblings because it requires direct intervention including possible confrontations as siblings protect their brother or sister from taunts and unkindness from others (Skotko & Levine, 2006). Siblings have reported that they worry that their brother or sister will have unpleasant social experiences even though the vast majority also reported that their own friends were accepting of their brother or sister with Down syndrome (Skotko, Levine, & Goldstein, 2011).

Although siblings' contributions to the caregiving of their brother or sister with Down syndrome are not generally demanding during childhood (Cuskelly & Gunn, 2003), this may change as family members age. In Carr's (2005) longitudinal study of families with a child with Down syndrome in England, approximately 25 percent of mothers of adults with Down syndrome expected that the adult would live with a sibling, although the siblings themselves did not report on their intentions in this study. In a more recent study in Australia, plans to take a substantial caregiving role in adulthood were reported by a large proportion of young adult siblings (Cuskelly, 2016), although only some of these siblings expected to have the same level of responsibility as was taken by their parents. In an earlier North American study of adult siblings of individuals with intellectual disability (not specifically Down syndrome), Greenberg, Seltzer, Orsmond, and Krauss (1999) found higher rates of intention to take on primary caregiving responsibilities than those reported by either Carr (2005) or Cuskelly (2016). The differences apparent in these studies may reflect changes over time to social and family expectations about sibling responsibilities, may relate to the different ages of sibling respondents, or may reflect some aspect of family functioning related to Down syndrome (see Hodapp & Dykens, 2012, for a discussion).

There may also be country-based differences that reflect the type, quality, and accessibility of adult social services as well as cultural differences with respect to familial obligations.

The increasing longevity of adults with Down syndrome is likely to lead to changes in sibling roles as their brothers or sisters accompany them into old age (Hodapp, Burke, Finley, & Urbano, 2016). Of particular note in this regard are changes to health as adults with Down syndrome live longer than ever before. There is evidence of vulnerability to mental health problems in late adolescence and adulthood (Dykens et al., 2015; Mallardo, Cuskelly, White, & Jobling, 2014) and to dementia in middle to older adulthood (McCarron et al. 2017; Stancliffe et al., 2012). See Capone (in press, this volume) for further discussion. The sequelae of these illnesses may place increased demands on siblings to take an active role in the care and management of their brother's or sister's affairs, particularly as their parents age or experience poor health or death.

The Quality of the Sibling Relationship

The quality of the sibling relationship may act to magnify or diminish the developmental impact of siblings as it forms the context in which influential interactions occur. The sibling relationship determines, to some extent, the amount of the time the members of the sibship spend together and the nature of interactions between them. Most investigators of the relationship between individuals with Down syndrome and their siblings have reported that they are warm with low levels of conflict, regardless of whether the parents (Cuskelly & Gunn, 2003; Roper, Allred, Mandleco, Freeborn, & Dyches, 2014; Skotko, Levine, Macklin, & Goldstein, 2016) or the siblings (Cuskelly & Gunn, 2003; Kaminsky & Dewey, 2001; Pollard, Barry, Freedman, & Kotchick, 2013; Skotko et al., 2016) are the respondents. While positive relationships are the norm, not all children appear to share a positive relationship with their brother or sister with Down syndrome (e.g., Cunningham, 1996). In a study of 105 Korean mothers with a child with Down syndrome between the ages of 1 and 21 years and a typically developing sibling between the ages 4 to 19 years, Choi and Van Riper (2014) found that the mothers reported relationship difficulties between children with Down syndrome and their sibling. This is consistent with evidence from some other non-Western cultures that disability has different meanings from that attributed to it in the West (e.g., Grinker & Cho, 2013; Riany, Cuskelly, & Meredith, 2016), and these meanings will have an impact on the ways in which families, including siblings, respond to the individual with disability. Non-Western cultures are not all alike, of course, and even within a group of East Asian countries, Choi and Van Riper (2017) found different family responses to the presence of a child with Down syndrome.

In a study of the sibling relationship in adulthood, Cuskelly (2016) found that the siblings reported their relationship with their brother/sister to be moderately warm with low levels of conflict. Using an online questionnaire, Hodapp and Urbano (2007) also investigated adult relationships and found that siblings' reports of the relationship were very positive. Using a 6-point Likert scale (6 = most positive), item scores related to relationship quality ranged from 4.78 to 5.39. Hodapp and Urbano (2007) reported that the level of warmth of the relationship decreased as the members of the sibship moved into middle age, although the study was cross-sectional rather than longitudinal.

This reduction in warmth reflects that seen in dyads where both members are developing typically (Lanthier & Campbell, 2011). One explanation may be that contact reduces as adult siblings move into middle age, as found by Hodapp and Urbano (2007), a finding that mirrors relationship changes in sibling dyads in which both members are developing typically (White, 2001). A positive association has been reported between contact and the warmth of the sibling relationship in sibling dyads with a member with Down syndrome (Cuskelly, 2016; Hodapp & Urbano, 2007). Correlational associations are not causal, of course, and reductions in the frequency of contact and in sibling warmth may be the product of other variables. Middle adulthood is a very demanding life stage as offspring generally require a great deal of parental time and attention, and these demands may account for the observed reduction in contact and contribute to reduced emphasis on the relationship with siblings. As children mature to adulthood and move out of the parental home, contact between siblings of the parental generation often increases (Lanthier & Campbell, 2011), and these fluctuations may also occur in sibships with a member with Down syndrome.

Longitudinal studies are the most informative for understanding the natural history of sibling relationships, and Janet Carr's longitudinal study of families of child with Down syndrome provides some information relevant to sibling relationships in adulthood. Carr's population-based (a specified geographical area in England) longitudinal study of children with Down syndrome and their families was first described in 1975. In 2005, when the individuals with Down syndrome were 35 years old, she reported on contact between the adults with Down syndrome and their siblings. Based on maternal reports, she found that the siblings of 35-year-old adults with Down syndrome had substantially more contact with their brother or sister than did comparison siblings at the same age, although no information was available about whether the level of contact had changed over time as is usual in typically developing sibships.

A relationship, by definition, involves at least two parties; however, the studies of the relationship between individuals with Down syndrome and their siblings have generally only included the voice, or data, of the siblings. Only two studies were identified in which individuals with Down syndrome were asked to provide their perspective of the sibling relationship. Using the same method and instrument, Skotko et al. (2011) collected data from individuals with Down syndrome in the United States and Wakai et al. (2018) collected data in Japan. Skotko et al. (2011) developed the instrument and undertook a number of steps to ensure its reliability and validity for use with persons with Down syndrome; nonetheless, some individuals with Down syndrome still needed to be excluded from both studies as they were unable to understand the questions and/or the response choices. The participants in the study in the United States included 284 persons between the ages of 12 and 51 years (M = 23.4 years), and the participants in the study in Japan included 74 participants over 12 years of age. While Wakai et al. (2018) did not provide details of the average age of their sample, the Japanese sample was clearly older than the American group. The majority of respondents in both studies said they liked their sibling (United State, 97 percent; Japan 85 percent) and that they felt their sibling was a good friend (United States, 89 percent; Japan 67 percent). In the American study, those with more siblings were more likely to endorse this latter item. The percentages of Japanese individuals with Down syndrome agreeing with the positive statements about their feelings toward their siblings were significantly lower than in the sample from the United States (Wakai et al., 2018). Cultural differences were hypothesized to account for other differences between the two groups but no speculations were made about the differences with respect to sibling relationships. The associations between age and sibling relationships were not examined in either study, although this is a potential source of variation.

Aspects of Development Likely to Be Influenced by Siblings

Developmental areas in which siblings may have an impact include cognition and language, self-regulation, social-emotional competence, and identity formation. None of these areas develops in isolation from the others of course; for example, language experiences are central to social understanding (Milligan, Astington, & Dack, 2007) and both are important for social skill development (Girard, Pingault, Doyle, Falissard, & Tremblay, 2017; Mazza et al., 2017). While recognizing that these developmental domains are interrelated, for clarity they will be considered separately in the following discussion.

Cognition and Language

Cognitive development and academic skills have been the subject of substantial investigation with respect to the influence of siblings in typically developing children. However, this interest has generally focused on structural aspects such as number of siblings and birth order, rather than on the processes that might influence these. According to the Resource Dilution model (Blake, 1981; Downey, 2001), cognitive development is negatively affected by sibship size, as children with more siblings have lower achievement and children who are born later also fare more poorly (e.g., Steelman, Powell, Werum, & Carter, 2002). This association is explained by the reduction in parental resources available to individual children. For example, Workman (2017) found that older children received less parental time (e.g., storytelling and child care activities) when a new child was born into the family. In an investigation of this model at older ages, Jensen, Whiteman, Bernard, and McHale (2017) found that 77 percent of the second-born children in their study reported an increase in parental attention or material resources a year after the first born child left home (e.g., to attend college). Children who reported increases in paternal time also reported increased interest in math, and their achievement was significantly higher than in the previous year. There was a similar increase in interest in language arts subjects for those who reported an increase in maternal time but no corresponding improvement in grades.

A recent investigation of the Resource Dilution model by Osmanowski and Cardona (2016) found some evidence to support the model in families with children who were typically developing; however, it did not apply in all families. In single-child families, the birth of a second child increased maternal activities with the firstborn; in multiple-child families, an additional child decreased maternal activities. These contrasting effects indicate that siblings may act to positively or negatively impact the resources available, depending upon other family circumstances. One possibility in families who have a child with Down syndrome is that having multiple siblings may augment the capacity of a family to support the development of a child with Down syndrome through increased direct teaching, modeling, and providing practice in negotiation.

Changes in the average size of families in the developed world may render the question of the impact of the number of siblings on child development less compelling to researchers in these countries; however, not all children across the globe are born into small sibships. In addition, a focus purely on number of siblings overlooks the processes by which certain outcomes come about, and the Resource Dilution model provides one hypothesized mechanism. While no research has been conducted on these issues in families of a child with Down syndrome, it is an area that may be fruitful in understanding the impact of siblings and parental practices.

Sibling influence on the language development of typically developing children is unclear—some researchers cite benefits (Benigno, Clark, & Farrar, 2007) and others report negative impacts (Tompkins, Farrar, & Guo, 2013). This is somewhat surprising as it might be expected that language would be positively influenced by the presence of siblings because of the multiple opportunities for interaction that they provide. Understanding the impact of siblings on the language of children with Down syndrome would be very useful, as this area of development is an identified area of difficulty for them (Abbeduto, Warren, & Connors, 2007; Lee et al., 2017).

Self-Regulation

The ability to manage one's own behavior in pursuit of goals has been labeled self-regulation. It is a complex construct with multiple components and might be considered an umbrella term that incorporates a range of capabilities, including executive functioning, that need to be integrated to support effective performance across developmental domains (Lynn, Cuskelly, O'Callaghan, & Gray, 2011). Self-regulation develops as children mature and become increasingly able to set their own goals and to control their emotions and behaviors in pursuit of these. Cuskelly and colleagues (Cuskelly, Einam, & Jobling, 2001; Cuskelly, Gilmore, Glenn, & Jobling, 2016) have examined self-regulation in individuals with Down syndrome using the delay of gratification paradigm developed by Mischel and Baker (1975) in which individuals are asked to wait for a self-selected goal in the presence of an immediate, tempting alternative. Persons with Down syndrome appear to have a particular difficulty in self-regulation, over and above that caused by intellectual disability, with language problems being hypothesized to be a contributing factor (Cuskelly, Gilmore et al., 2016). While there were significant differences at the group level, some individuals demonstrated that they were able to self-regulate, waiting for 15 minutes to achieve their goal. The interactions that are a natural part of sibling relationships, along with the consequences for family routines that follow from having to accommodate the needs of more individuals, may act to assist with the development of self-regulation. Siblings with whom one needs to share, wait for, and resolve conflicts provide practice, models, and external support (e.g., parental instructions) for the multiple skills that contribute to self-regulation. This conjecture regarding the benefits of siblings in developing self-regulation is supported by studies of typically developing children (e.g., Brody & Murry, 2001; Downey & Condron, 2004) with these benefits lasting well into the school years (Downey, Condron, & Yucel, 2015). Downey et al. (2015) followed up with 11,820 children in fifth grade who were initially seen in kindergarten. Teachers provided the data on self-regulation. Children with one sibling increased their self-control more than those without siblings across the period, and existing deficits (observed in kindergarten) between those with no siblings and those with one or more siblings remained even after 5 years of interactions with peers.

Social-Emotional Competence

Social-emotional competence comprises a number of elements, including self-regulation of emotions and behavior as well as understanding of self and of others, that contribute to how effectively children operate in the social world. While no published studies examining the impact of siblings on the social skills of children with Down syndrome were able to be identified, there are some studies that provide evidence of a positive association for typically developing children (Downey et al., 2015) and individuals with other developmental difficulties (Ben-Itzchak, Nachson, & Zachor, 2019). Hughes, McHarg, and White (2018) provided a conceptual review of the ways in which siblings might contribute to the development of prosocial behavior in their brothers and sisters.

Despite views that children with Down syndrome have relatively strong skills in social relationships, Cebula et al. (2010) have pointed out a number of areas of difficulty in social cognition. One example is difficulty in the recognition and understanding of some emotions (e.g., Pochon & Declercq, 2014; Virji-Babul, Watt, Nathoo, & Johnson, 2012). These difficulties may be a barrier to positive peer and sibling relationships, as children with Down syndrome may not respond as expected to expressions of emotion such as sadness (Hippolyte, Barisnikov, Van der Linden, & Detraux, 2009) and anger (Goldman, Shulman, & Burack, 2018). The experience of having siblings could be expected to improve children's understanding of emotion, and there is some support for this expectation in families in which children are developing typically (Morand, 1999).

One central component of social-emotional competence, itself a multi-faceted, developmental construct, is theory of mind (ToM). ToM refers to the ability to "read" others' minds—to understand, for example, that others may have beliefs about a situation different from one's own or that they may not actually mean what they have said. ToM incorporates a range of abilities that are linked to understanding the mental state of self and of others which become more sophisticated as children mature and new abilities emerge. Skills in ToM assist children to understand others and thereby effectively respond in a range of social situations (Cutting & Dunn, 2006), for example by recognizing when a peer is joking or means what he or she is saying. Better ToM skills may also increase children's capacity to communicate about their own mental states, thus increasing their desirability as playmates. Social skills and ToM are positively correlated in typically developing children (Peterson, Slaughter, Moore, & Wellman, 2016; Weimer, Burleson, Stegall, & Eisenman, 2018). Investigations of ToM in children with Down syndrome provide evidence that ToM is more delayed than in children of the same mental age (Losh, Martin, Klusek, Hogan-Brown, & Sideris, 2012). While delayed, it does continue to develop (Amadó, Serrat, & Vallès-Majoral, 2016) and so may be open to influence by siblings.

Siblings are expected to be central to facilitating ToM because the relationship affords many opportunities for social interactions with a partner who is close in age. This repeated exposure allows children to develop an understanding of the connections between individuals' behaviors and their feelings and thoughts (Carpendale & Lewis, 2006; Howe, Ross, & Recchia, 2011). Larger sibships are likely to provide a more enriched "database" than smaller sibships as they provide multiple different examples. Positive sibling relationships have been found to be predictive of ToM in typically developing children (Hughes & Ensor, 2005), presumably because of increased exposure to another's way of understanding the world. However, children also experience conflict in their sibling relationships, and the negotiations required to resolve conflicts are also thought to contribute to ToM skills (Kramer, 2014). Older siblings have generally been found to benefit the development of ToM in their younger siblings (Derksen, Hunsche, Giroux, Connolly, & Bernstein, 2018; Kennedy, Lagattuta, & Sayfan, 2015). One potential reason for this advantage is the increased cognitive talk to which children with older siblings are exposed (Jenkins, Turrell, Takai, Lollis, & Ross, 2003). The contribution made by siblings to the social-emotional competence of children with Down syndrome is an area ripe for exploration.

Identity Formation

The elements of a robust self-identity comprise understanding and acceptance of one's strengths and limitations (i.e., self-knowledge) and a positive sense of self. Individuals with Down syndrome generally have a positive self-image (see Deakin, Moore, & Jahoda, 2018; Glenn & Cunningham, 2001). Siblings contribute to identity formation through the direct and indirect feedback they provide and through their role in social comparison processes. They contribute to the development of an understanding of self, in part by providing an "other," either to emulate or from which to try to differentiate (Davies, 2015; Wong, Branje, VanderValk, Hawk, & Meeus, 2010).

As most siblings feel warmly towards their brother or sister with Down syndrome (Skotko & Levine, 2006; Skotko et al., 2016), they are likely to provide affirmative feedback in their daily interactions. Positive sibling relationships contribute to healthy and positive self-views in typically developing adolescents (Milevsky & Levitt, 2005) and this is likely to also be the case for individuals with Down syndrome. As discussed previously, some individuals with Down syndrome engage in social comparison, with siblings the most common person used for this purpose (Cuskelly & Gordon, 2011; Glenn & Cunningham, 2001). There is a need to examine the contributions siblings make to the self-identify of their brothers and sisters with Down syndrome.

Directions for Future Research

The need for theory-driven research with respect to sibling influences on children with Down syndrome has been pointed out by Cebula et al. (2010). Bronfenbrenner's bioecological model of development (Bronfenbrenner, 2001; Bronfenbrenner & Morris, 2006) offers a useful overarching theory to guide research in this area because it focusses on children's proximal interactions (i.e., those that occur frequently and repeatedly) as the most important influences on development. The idea that sibling interactions are crucial drivers of development clearly fits well with this model, which also acknowledges the role of biological characteristics in influencing development. Thus, the model is able to accommodate the proposal that the characteristics associated with Down syndrome may elicit certain behaviors on the part of social partners (Hodapp & Dykens, 2012) as well as the possibility that certain aspects of development may be resistant to external influences. The bioecological model is able to encompass the impact of culture on the nature of sibling interactions and potential changes over time. In addition, Bronfenbrenner's broad theoretical model can accommodate other frameworks, such as the Resource Dilution model, with its focus on the number of siblings in the family (Downey, 2001) and changing impact of this family characteristic (Zajonc, 2001). Together these models may contribute a useful lens to understanding some of the links between siblings and the developmental outcomes of individuals with Down syndrome.

There are many challenges to undertaking research on sibling contributions to developmental outcomes because Down syndrome is a low-incidence condition with considerable within-group variability, including in areas of cognitive ability (e.g., Channell, Thurman, Kover, & Abbeduto, 2014) and language (e.g., Kaat-van den Os, Volman, Jongmans, & Lauteslager, 2017). A substantial proportion of children with Down syndrome have additional diagnoses, as they are at risk for visual (Duckman, 2014) and hearing problems (Nightengale, Yoon, Wolter-Warmerdam, Daniels, & Hickey, 2017) and for having co-morbid autism spectrum disorder (see, Reilly, 2009, for a review). These individual characteristics are likely to have some impact upon the influence of siblings on certain outcomes but may occur in a very small number of study participants.

Children with Down syndrome are born to parents in all socioeconomic groups, although research is somewhat hampered by the difficulty of recruiting and then maintaining families from across the entire spectrum, with reduced representation of families in the more disadvantaged groups (e.g., Couzens et al., 2011). Studies that are focused on sibling influences may also be affected by sampling bias because such studies may be more attractive to families in which the sibling relationship is positive than in those in which the relationship is acrimonious.

Parental characteristics and behaviors are likely to play a crucial role in the nature of sibling interactions and relationships (see, for example, Dawson, Pike, & Bird, 2015; Kretschmer & Pike, 2009). Parents of a child with Down syndrome are often identified as having higher levels of stress than parents whose children are developing typically and as parenting somewhat differently (e.g., Phillips, Conners, & Curtner-Smith, 2017). These aspects of family life should be incorporated into research on sibling influence because understanding the family context may help to explain variation in outcomes.

The indirect effects of sibling influence, through the impact on parental behavior, also need to be considered, and these considerations need to incorporate the reciprocal influences of siblings and the child with Down syndrome. Potential foci include whether parents parent differently if they have a typically developing child who is older than the child with Down syndrome in contrast to when the child with Down syndrome is first born, and the impact of a child with Down syndrome on the way that mothers and fathers parent their other children.

Siblings acting as intervention agents can be effective in changing the behavior of their brother or sister with Down syndrome (e.g., Trent et al., 2005), although these interventions may change the nature of the relationship between the members of the sibling dyad in ways that are not anticipated. Some changes may occur that are not positive. As examples, the increased responsibilities may increase sibling anxiety, and involvement in an explicit intervention program may introduce the idea that the child with Down syndrome is incompetent, thus changing the types and nature of interactions between the siblings. Alternatively, there may be positive changes in the relationship or other benefits to the sibling such as increased skills. Some consideration of these potential outcomes needs to be built into intervention studies that use siblings as the agent of change until the consequences for both children in the dyad are established.

Investigations of sibling influence will, on occasion, require input from participants with Down syndrome in order to obtain a complete understanding of the phenomenon. The difficulties inherent in research that aims to do this are evidenced by Skotko et al.'s (2011) attempt to develop an instrument to collect information from individuals with Down syndrome about their perspectives of the sibling relationship. Despite the rigorous approach in the construction of the questionnaire, some individuals were unable to respond due to their limitations in understanding the items. More needs to be done to ensure that there is a variety of methods appropriate to collecting information from as wide a range of persons with Down syndrome as possible. Without adequate data of their experience of sibling interactions and the impact of siblings on their behaviors from their perspective, we are limited in our understanding of the ways in which siblings impact their development.

As almost all of the research discussed in this chapter is based in the United States, Great Britain, or Australia, we need to also examine these issues in other cultures where expectations and engagement of siblings differ from those usual in Western cultures. Sibling obligations differ between cultures (Lauderdale-Littin & Blacher, 2017) as do community interpretations and understandings of disability (Riany et al., 2016). Our understanding of the roles that siblings can and do play in the development of their brother or sister with Down syndrome will be greatly enhanced with the recognition and consideration of differing cultural meanings of disability and sibling responsibility.

As argued throughout this chapter, siblings are likely to be crucial influences on developmental outcomes for individuals with Down syndrome. However, the mechanisms by which siblings contribute to positive growth in their brothers and sisters with Down syndrome may differ in important ways from those in typical sibships. There is very little research that has investigated these possibilities. This is an extraordinary oversight and one that demands the attention of researchers.

References

Abbeduto, L., Warren, S. E., & Connors, F. A. (2007). Language development in Down syndrome: From the prelinguistic period to the acquisition of literacy. *Mental Retardation and Developmental Disabilities Research Reviews, 13*, 247–261.

Abramovitch, R., Stanhope, L., Pepler, D., & Corter, C. (1987). The influence of Down's syndrome on sibling interaction. *Journal of Child Psychology and Psychiatry, 28*, 865–879.

Abuhatoum, S., Howe, N., Della Porta, S., Recchia, H., & Ross, H. (2016). Siblings' understanding of teaching in early and middle childhood: "Watch me and you'll know how to do it." *Journal of Cognition and Development, 17*, 180–196. doi:10.1080/15248372.2015.1042579

Amadó, A, Serrat, E., & Vallès-Majoral, E. (2016). The role of executive functions in social cognition among children with Down syndrome: Relationship patterns. *Frontiers in Psychology, 7*, Article 1363. doi:10.3389/fpsyg.2016.01363

Bandura, A. (1986). *Social foundations of thought and action: A social cognitive theory.* Englewood Cliffs, NJ: Prentice Hall.

Barr, R., & Hayne, H. (2003). It's not what you know, it's who you know: Older siblings facilitate imitation during infancy. *International Journal of Early Years Education, 11*, 7–21. doi:10.1080/09669760304714

Ben-Itzchak, E., Nachshon, N., & Zachor, D. A. (2019). Having siblings is associated with better social functioning in autism spectrum disorder. *Journal of Abnormal Child Psychology, 47*, 921–931. doi:10.1007/s10802-018-0473-z

Benigno, J. P., Clark, L., & Farrar, M. J. (2007). Three is not always a crowd: Contexts of joint attention and language. *Journal of Child Language, 34*, 175–187. doi:10.1017/S0305000906007732

Bjorkland, D. F., & Pelligrini, A. D. (2011). Evolutionary perspectives on social development. In P. K. Smith & C. H. Hart (Eds.). *The Wiley-Blackwell handbook of childhood social development* (2nd ed., pp. 64–81). London: Blackwell.

Blake, J. (1981). Family-size and the quality of children. *Demography, 18*, 421–442. doi:10.2307/2060941

Brody, G. H. (2004). Siblings' direct and indirect contributions to child development. *Current Directions in Psychological Science, 13*, 124–126.

Brody, G. H., & Murry, V. M. (2001). Sibling socialization of competence in rural, single-parent African American families. *Journal of Marriage and Family, 63*, 996–1008.

Bronfenbrenner, U. (2001). The bioecological theory of human development. In N. J. Smelser & P. B. Baltes (Eds.), *International encyclopedia of the social and behavioral sciences* (Vol. 10, pp. 6963–6970). New York: Elsevier.

Bronfenbrenner, U., & Morris, A. (2006). The bioecological model of human development. In R. M. Lerner (Ed.), *Theoretical models of human development. Vol. 1: Handbook of child psychology* (6th ed., pp. 793–828). Hoboken, NJ: Wiley.

Capone, G. (in press). Psychiatric comorbid conditions. In J. A. Burack, J. Edgin, & L. Abbeduto (Eds.), *Oxford handbook of Down syndrome and development*. Oxford: Oxford University Press.

Carpendale, J. I. M., & Lewis, C. (2006). *How children develop social understanding*. Malden, MA: Blackwell.

Carr J. (1975) *Young children with Down's syndrome: Their development, upbringing and effect on their families.* London: Butterworth.

Carr, J. (2005). Families of 30–35-year olds with Down's syndrome. *Journal of Applied Research in Intellectual Disabilities, 18*, 75–84.

Cebula, K. R., Moore, D. G., & Wishart, J. G. (2010). Social cognition in children with Down's syndrome: Challenges to research and theory building. *Journal of Intellectual Disability Research, 54*, 113–134. doi:10.1111/j.1365-2788.2009.01215.x

Channell, M. M., Thurman, A. J., Kover, S. T., & Abbeduto, L. (2014). Patterns of change in nonverbal cognition in adolescents with Down syndrome. *Research in Developmental Disabilities, 35*, 2933–2941. doi:10.1016/j.ridd.2014.07.014

Chen, W.-C. (2015). Academic performance of only children who monopolise parental resources: The case of Taiwan. *Sociological Perspectives, 58*, 609–626. doi:10.1177/0731121415578289

Choi, H., & Van Riper, M. (2014). Maternal perceptions of sibling adaptation in Korean families of children with Down syndrome. *Journal of Intellectual Disability Research, 58*, 962–977. doi:10.1111/jir12126

Choi, H., & Van Riper, M. (2017). Adaptation in families of children with Down syndrome in East Asia countries: An integrative review. *Journal of Advanced Nursing, 73*, 1792–1806. doi:10.1111/jan.13235

Couzens, D., Cuskelly, M., & Haynes, M. (2011). Cognitive development of individuals with Down syndrome: Age related change in subtest scores on the Stanford Binet: Fourth edition (SB:IV) between ages 4 and 30 years. *American Journal on Intellectual and Developmental Disabilities, 116*, 181–204. doi:10.1352/1944-7558-116.3.181

Cunningham, C. C. (1996). Families of children with Down syndrome. *Down Syndrome Research and Practice, 4*, 87–95.

Cuskelly, M. (2016). Contributors to adult sibling relationships and intention to care of siblings of individuals with Down syndrome. *American Journal on Intellectual and Developmental Disabilities, 121*, 204–218. doi:10.1352/1944-7558-121.3.204

Cuskelly, M., Einam, M., & Jobling, A. (2001). Delay of gratification in young adults with Down syndrome. *Down Syndrome Research and Practice, 7*, 60–67.

Cuskelly, M., Gilmore, L., Glenn, S., & Jobling, A. (2016). Delay of gratification: A comparison study of children with Down syndrome, moderate intellectual disability and typical development. *Journal of Intellectual Disability Research, 60*, 865–873. doi:10.111/jir.12262

Cuskelly, M., & Gordon, K. (2011). Social comparisons: Associations with psychosocial functioning in individuals with Down syndrome. *Down Syndrome Quarterly, 13*, 20–28.

Cuskelly, M., & Gunn, P. (2003). Sibling relationships of children with Down syndrome: Perspectives of mothers, fathers and siblings. *American Journal on Mental Retardation, 108*, 234–244. doi:10.1352/08958017(2003)108<234.SROCWD>2.0.CO;2

Cuskelly, M., Povey, J., & Jobling A. (2016). The developmental trajectory of receptive vocabulary in individuals with Down syndrome. *Journal of Policy and Practice in Intellectual Disabilities, 13*, 111–119. doi:10.1111/jppi.12151

Cutting, A. L., & Dunn, J. (2006). Conversations with siblings and with friends: Links between relationship quality and social understanding. *British Journal of Developmental Psychology, 24*, 73–87. doi:10.1348/026151005X70337

Davies, K. (2015). Siblings, stories and the self: The sociological significance of young people's sibling relationships. *Sociology, 49*, 679–695. doi:10.1177/0038038514551091

Dawson, A., Pike, A., & Bird, L. (2015). Parental division of household labour and sibling relationship quality: Family relationship mediators. *Infant and Child Development, 24*, 379–393. doi:10.1002/icd.1890

Deakin, K., Moore, D. G., & Jahoda, A. (2018). Children and young people with Down syndrome: Their awareness of Down syndrome and developing self-perceptions. *Journal of Applied Research in Intellectual Disabilities, 31*, 1197–1208. doi:10.1111/jar.12494

Derksen, D. G., Hunsche, M. C., Giroux, M. E., Connolly, D. A., & Bernstein, D. M. (2018). A systematic review of theory of mind's precursors and functions. *Zeitschrift für Psychologie*, 226, 87–97. doi:10.1027/2151-2604/a000325

Dirks, M. A., Persram, R., Recchia, H. E., & Howe, N. (2015). Sibling relationships as sources of risk and resilience in the development and maintenance of internalizing and externalizing problems during childhood and adolescence. *Clinical Psychology Review, 42*, 145–155. doi:10.1016/j.cpr.2015.07.003

Downey, D. B. (2001). Number of siblings and intellectual development: The resource dilution explanation. *American Psychologist, 56*, 497–504. doi:10.1037/0003-066X.56.6-7.497

Downey, D. B., & Condron, D. J. (2004). Playing well with others in kindergarten: The benefit of siblings at home. *Journal of Marriage and Family, 66*, 333–350.

Downey, D. B., Condron, D. J., & Yucel, D. (2015). Number of siblings and social skills revisited among American fifth graders. *Journal of Family Issues, 36*, 273–296. doi:10.1177/0192513X13507569

Duckman, R. H. (2014). Visual status of children with Down syndrome. *Optometry & Visual Performance, 2*, 240–243.

Dykens, E. M., Shah, B., Davis, B., Baker, C., Fife, T., & Fitzpatrick, J. (2015). Psychiatric disorders in adolescents and young adults with Down syndrome and other intellectual disabilities. *Journal of Neurodevelopmental Disorders, 7*, Article 9.

Fisman, S., Wolf, L., Ellison, D., Gillis, B., Freeman, T., & Szatmari, P. (1996). Risk and protective factors affecting the adjustment of siblings of children with chronic disabilities. *Journal of the American Academy of Child & Adolescent Psychiatry, 35*, 1532–1541. doi:10.1097/00004583-199611000-00023

Floyd, F. J., Purcell, S. E., Richardson, S. S., & Kupersmidt, J. B. (2009). Sibling relationship quality and social functioning of children and adolescents with intellectual disability. *American Journal on Intellectual and Developmental Disabilities, 114*, 110–127. doi:10.1352/2009.114:110-127

Gilmore, L., Cuskelly, M., Jobling, A., & Hayes, A. (2009). Maternal support for autonomy: Relationships with persistence for children with Down syndrome and typically developing children. *Research in Developmental Disabilities, 30*, 1023–1033. doi:10.1016/j.ridd.2009.02.005

Gilmore, L., Ryan, B., Cuskelly, M., & Gavidia-Payne, S. (2016). Understanding maternal support for autonomy in young children with Down syndrome. *Journal of Policy and Practice in Intellectual Disabilities, 13*, 92–101. doi:10.1111/jppi.12163

Girard, L. C., Pingault, J.-B., Doyle, O., Falissard, B., & Tremblay, R. E. (2017). Expressive language and prosocial behaviour in early childhood: Longitudinal associations in the UK Millennium Cohort Study. *European Journal of Developmental Psychology, 14*, 381–398. doi:10.1080/17405629.2016.1215300

Glenn, S., & Cunningham, C. (2001). Evaluation of self by young people with Down syndrome. *International Journal of Disability, Development and Education, 48*, 163–177. doi:10.1080/10349120120053649

Glenn, S., & Cunningham, C. (2004). Self-awareness in young adults with Down syndrome: II. Self-understanding. *International Journal of Disability, Development and Education, 51*, 363–381. doi:10.1080/1034912042000295026

Goldman, K. J., Shulman, C., & Burack, J. A. (2018). Inference from facial expressions among adolescents and young adults with Down syndrome. *American Journal on Intellectual and Developmental Disabilities, 123*, 344–358. doi:10.1352/1944-7558-123.4.344

Greenberg, J. S., Seltzer, M. M., Orsmond, G. I., & Krauss, M. W. (1999). Siblings of adults with mental illness or mental retardation: Current involvement and expectation of future caregiving. *Psychiatric Services, 50*, 1214–1219.

Grinker, R. R., & Cho, K. (2013). Border children: Interpreting autism spectrum disorder in South Korea. *Journal of the Society for Psychological Anthropology, 41*, 46–74. doi:10.1111/etho.12002

Hippolyte, L., Barisnikov, K., Van der Linden, M., & Detraux, J.-J. (2009). From facial recognition abilities to emotional attribution: A study in Down syndrome. *Research in Developmental Disabilities, 30*, 1007–1022. doi:10.1016/j.ridd.2009.02.004

Hodapp, R. M., Burke, M. M., Finley, C. I., & Urbano, R. C. (2016). Family caregiving of aging adults with Down syndrome. *Journal of Policy and Practice in Intellectual Disabilities, 13*, 181–189. doi:10.1111/jppi.12153

Hodapp, R. M., & Dykens, E. M. (2012). Genetic disorders of intellectual disability: Expanding our concepts of phenotype and of family outcomes. *Journal of Genetic Counseling, 21*, 761–769. doi:10.1007/s1089-012-9536-4

Hodapp, R. M., & Urbano, R. C. (2007). Adult siblings of individuals with Down syndrome versus with autism: Findings from a large-scale US survey. *Journal of Intellectual Disability Research, 51*(12), 1018–1029. doi:10.1111/j.1365-2788.2007.00994.x

Howe, N., Brody, M.-H., & Recchia, H. (2006). Effects of task difficulty on sibling teaching in middle childhood. *Infant and Child Development, 15*, 455–470. doi:10.1002/icd.470

Howe, N., Della Porta, S., Recchia, H., Funamoto, A, & Ross, H. (2015). "This bird can't do it 'cause this bird doesn't swim in water": Sibling teaching during naturalistic home observations in early childhood. *Journal of Cognition and Development, 16*, 314–332. doi:10.1080/15248372.2013.848869

Howe, N., Recchia, H., Della Porta, S., & Funamoto, A. (2012). "The driver doesn't sit, he stands up like the Flintstones!": Sibling teaching during teacher-directed and self-guided tasks. *Journal of Cognition and Development, 13*, 208–231. doi:10/1080/15248372.2011.57703

Howe, N., Rinaldi, C. M., Jennings, M., & Petrakos, H. (2002). "No! The lambs can stay out because they got cozies!": Constructive and destructive sibling conflict, pretend play, and social understanding. *Child Development, 73*, 1460–1473. doi:10.1111/1467-8624.00483

Howe, N., Rosciszewska, J., & Persram, R. J. (2018). "I'm an ogre so I'm very hungry!" "I'm assistant ogre": The social function of sibling imitation in early childhood. *Infant and Child Development, 27*, e2040. doi:10.1002/icd.2040

Howe, N., Ross, H., & Recchia, H. (2011). Sibling relations in early and middle childhood. In C. Hart & P. K. Smith (Eds.), *Wiley-Blackwell handbook of childhood social development* (pp. 356–372). New York: Wiley.

Hughes, C. & Ensor, R. (2005) Executive function and theory of mind in 2 year olds: A family affair? *Developmental Neuropsychology, 28*, 645–668. doi:10.1207/s15326942dn2802_5

Hughes, C., McHarg, G., & White, N. (2018). Sibling influences on prosocial behavior. *Current Opinion in Psychology, 20*, 96–101. doi:10.1016/j.copsyc.2017.08.015

Jenkins, J. M., Turrell, S., Takai, Y., Lollis, S., & Ross, H. S. (2003). Longitudinal investigation of the dynamics of mental state talk in families. *Child Development, 74*, 905–920. doi:10.1111/1467-8624.00575

Jensen, A. C., Whiteman, S. D., Bernard, J. M., & McHale, S. M. (2017). Family resource allocation after firstborns leave home: Implications for secondborns' academic functioning. *Family Process, 56*, 766–780. doi:10.1111/famp.12203

Kaat-van den Os, D. T., Volman, C., Jongmans, M., & Lauteslager, P. (2017). Expressive vocabulary development in children with Down syndrome: A longitudinal study. *Journal of Policy and Practice in Intellectual Disabilities, 14*, 311–318. doi:10.1111/jppi.12212

Kaminsky, L., & Dewey, D. (2001). Sibling relationships of children with autism. *Journal of Autism and Developmental Disorders, 31*, 399–410. doi:0162-3257/01/0800-0399

Kennedy, L., Lagattuta, K. H., & Sayfan, L. (2015). Sibling composition, executive function, and children's thinking about mental states. *Journal of Experimental Child Psychology, 132*, 121–139. doi:10.1016/j.jecp.2014.11.007

Kim, T., & Horn, E. (2010). Sibling-implemented intervention for skill development with children with disabilities. *Topics in Early Childhood Special Education, 30*, 80–90. doi:10.1177/0271121409349146

Klein, P. S., Feldman, R., & Zarur, S. (2002). Mediation in a sibling context: The relations of older siblings' mediating behaviour and younger siblings' task performance. *Infant and Child Development, 11*, 321–333. doi:10.1002/icd.261

Knott, R., Lewis, C., & Williams, T. (2007). Sibling interaction of children with autism: Development over 12 months. *Journal of Autism and Developmental Disabilities, 37*, 1987–1995. doi:10.1007/s10803-006-0347-z

Kramer, L. (2014). Learning emotional understanding and emotion regulation through sibling interaction. *Early Education and Development, 25*, 160–184. doi:10.1080/10409289.2014.838824

Kretschmer, T., & Pike, A. (2009). Young children's sibling relationship quality: Distal and proximal correlates. *Journal of Child Psychology and Psychiatry, 50*, 581–589. doi:10.1111/j.1469-7610.2008.02016.x

Lanthier, R. P., & Campbell, A. J. (2011). Sibling relationships as opportunities for development and learning is adulthood. In C. Hoare (Ed.), *The Oxford handbook of reciprocal adult development and learning* (2nd ed., pp. 381–395). New York: Oxford University Press.

Lauderdale-Littin, S., & Blacher, J. (2017). Young adults with severe intellectual disability: Culture, parent, and sibling impact. *Journal of Intellectual and Developmental Disability, 42*, 230–239. doi:10.3109/13668250.2016.1230843

Lawson, D. W., & Mace, R. (2008). Sibling configuration and childhood growth in contemporary British families. *International Journal of Epidemiology, 37*, 1408e1421.

Lawson, D. W., & Mace, R. (2009). Trade-offs in modern parenting: A longitudinal study of sibling competition for parental care. *Evolution and Human Behavior, 30*, 170–183. doi:10.1016/j.evolhumbehav.2008.12.001

Lawson, D. W., & Mace, R. (2010). Siblings and childhood mental health: Evidence of a later-born advantage. *Social Science & Medicine, 20*, 2061–2069. doi:10.1016/j.socscimed.2010.03.009

Lee, M., Bush, L., Martin, G. E., Barstein, J., Maltman, N., Klusek, J., & Losh, M. (2017). A multi-method investigation of pragmatic development in individuals with Down syndrome. *American Journal on Intellectual and Developmental Disabilities, 122*, 289–309. doi:10.1352/1944-7558-122.4.289

Losh, M., Martin, G. E., Klusek, J., Hogan-Brown, A. L., & Sideris, J. (2012). Social communication and theory of mind in boys with autism and fragile X syndrome. *Frontiers in Psychology, 3*, Article 266. doi:10.3389/fpsyg.2012.00266

Lynn, L. N., Cuskelly, M., O'Callaghan, M. J., & Gray, P. H. (2011). Self-regulation: A new perspective on learning problems experienced by children born extremely preterm. *Australian Journal of Educational and Developmental Psychology, 11*, 1–10.

Mallardo, M., Cuskelly, M., White, P., & Jobling, A. (2014). Mental health problems in adults with Down syndrome and their association with life circumstances. *Journal of Mental Health Research in Intellectual Disabilities, 7*, 229–245. doi:10.1080/19315864.2013.842622

Marjoribanks, K. (1991). The sibling resource dilution theory: An analysis. *The Journal of Psychology: Interdisciplinary and Applied*, 125, 337–346. doi:10.1080/00223980.1991.10543297

Mazza, M., Mariano, M., Peretti, S., Masedu, F., Pino, M. C., & Valenti, M. (2017). Role of theory of mind on social information processing in children with autism spectrum disorders: A mediation analysis. *Journal of Autism and Developmental Disorders, 47*, 1369–1379. doi:10.1007/s10803-017-3069-5

McCarron, M., McCallion, P., Reilly, E., Dunne, P., Carroll, R., & Mulryan, N. (2017). A prospective 20-year longitudinal follow-up of dementia in persons with Down syndrome. *Journal of Intellectual Disability Research, 61*, 843–852. doi:10.1111/jir.12390

McHale, S. M., Updegraff, K. A., & Whiteman, S. D. (2012). Sibling relationships and influences in childhood and adolescence. *Journal of Marriage and Family, 74*, 913–930. doi:10.1111/j.1741-3737.2012.01011.x

Milevsky, A., & Levitt, M. J. (2005). Sibling support in early adolescence: Buffering and compensation across relationships. *European Journal of Developmental Psychology, 2*, 299–320. doi:10.1080/17405620544000048

Milligan, K., Astington, J. W., & Dack, L. A. (2007). Language and theory of mind: Meta-analysis of the relation between language ability and false-belief understanding. *Child Development, 78*, 622–646. doi:10.1111/j.1467-8624.2007.01018.x

Miltenberger, R. G. (2001). *Behavior modification: Principles and procedures* (2nd ed.). Belmont CA: Wadsworth.

Mischel, W., & Baker, N. (1975). Cognitive appraisals and transformations in delay behaviour. *Journal of Personality and Social Psychology, 31*, 254–261.

Morand, D. A. (1999). Family size and intelligence revisited: The role of emotional intelligence. *Psychological Reports, 84*, 643–649.

Nightengale, E., Yoon, P., Wolter-Warmerdam, K., Daniels, D., & Hickey, F. (2017). Understanding hearing and hearing loss in children with Down syndrome. *American Journal of Audiology, 26*, 301–308. doi:10.1044/2017_AJA-17-0010

Noller, P. (2005). Sibling relationships in adolescence: Learning and growing together. *Personal Relationships, 12*, 1–22. doi:10.1111/j.13504126.2005.00099.x

Osmanowski M., & Cardona, A. (2016). Is less more? Number of siblings and frequency of maternal activities with preschool children. *Marriage & Family Review, 52*, 742–763. doi:10.1080/01494929.2016.1157557

Padilla-Walker, L. M., Harper, J. M., & Jensen, A. C. (2010). Self-regulation as a mediator between sibling relationship quality and early adolescents' positive and negative outcomes. *Journal of Family Psychology, 24*, 419–428. doi:10.1037/a0020387

Peterson, C., Slaughter, V., Moore, C., & Wellman, H. (2016). Peer social skills and theory of mind in children with autism, deafness, or typical development. *Developmental Psychology, 52*, 46–57. doi:10.1037/a0039833

Phillips, B. A., Conners, F., & Curtner-Smith, M. E. (2017). Parenting children with Down syndrome: An analysis of parenting styles, parenting dimensions, and parental stress. *Research in Developmental Disabilities, 68*, 9–19. doi:10.1016/j.ridd.2017.06.010

Pochon, R., & Declercq, C. (2014). Emotional lexicon understanding and emotion recognition: A longitudinal study in children with Down syndrome. *Journal of Developmental and Physical Disabilities, 26*, 549–563. doi:10.1007/s10882-01409380-6

Pollard, C. A., Barry, C. M., Freedman, B. H., & Kotchick, B. A. (2013). Relationship quality as a moderator of anxiety in siblings of children diagnosed with autism spectrum disorders or Down syndrome. *Journal of Child and Family Studies, 22*, 647–657. doi:10.1007/s10826-012-9618-9

Prime, H., Perlman, M., Tackett, J. L., & Jenkins, J. M. (2014). Cognitive sensitivity in sibling interactions: Development of the construct and comparison of two coding methodologies. *Early Education and Development, 25*, 240–258. doi:10.1080/10409289.2013.821313

Rabain-Jamin, J., Maynard, A. E., & Greenfield, P. (2003). Implications of sibling caregiving for sibling relations and teaching interactions in two cultures. *Ethos, 31*, 204–231. doi:10.1525/eth.2003.31.2.204

Reilly, C. (2009). Autism spectrum disorders in Down syndrome: A review. *Research in Autism Spectrum Disorders, 3*, 829–839. doi:10.1016/j.rasd.2009.01.012

Riany, Y. E., Cuskelly, M., & Meredith, P. (2016). Cultural beliefs about autism in Indonesia. *International Journal of Disability Development and Education, 63*, 1–18. doi:10.1080/1034912X.2016.1142069

Roper, S. O., Allred, D. W., Mandleco, B., Freeborn, D., & Dyches, T. (2014). Caregiver burden and sibling relationships in families raising children with disabilities and typically developing children. *Families, Systems, & Health, 32*, 241–246. doi:10.1037/fsh0000047

Schmeer, K. K. (2009). Changing sibship size and educational progress during childhood: Evidence from the Philippines. *Journal of Marriage and Family, 71*, 787–801. doi:10.1111/j.1741-3737.2009.00633.x

Schwab, S., Huber, C., & Gebhardt, M. (2016). Social acceptance of students with Down syndrome and students without disability. *Educational Psychology, 36*, 1501–1515, doi:10.1080/01443410.2015.1059924

Singh, S. J., Iacono, T., & Gray, K. M. (2015). Interactions of pre-symbolic children with developmental disabilities with their mothers and siblings. *International Journal of Language & Communication Disorders, 50*, 202–214. doi:10.1111/1460-6984.12128

Skotko, B. G., & Levine, S. P. (2006). What the other children are thinking: Brothers and sisters of persons with Down syndrome. *American Journal of Medical Genetics, 142C*, 180–186. doi:10.1002/ajmg.c.30101

Skotko, B. G., Levine, S. P., & Goldstein, R. (2011). Self-perceptions from people with Down syndrome. *American Journal of Medical Genetics Part A, 155*, 2360–2369. doi:10.1002/ajmg.a.34235

Skotko, B. G., Levine, S. P., Macklin, E. A., & Goldstein, R. D. (2016). Family perspectives about Down syndrome. *American Journal of Medical Genetics Part A, 170A*, 930–941. doi:10.1002/ajmg.a.37520

Stancliffe, R. J., Lakin, K. C., Larson, S. A., Engler, J., Taub, S., Fortune, J., & Bershadsky, J. (2012). Demographic characteristics, health conditions, and residential service use in adults with Down syndrome in 25 U.S. states. *Intellectual and Developmental Disabilities, 50*, 92–108. doi:10.1352/1934-9556-50.2.92

Steelman, L. C., Powell, B., Werum, R., & Carter, S. (2002). Reconsidering the effects of sibling configuration: Recent advances and challenges. *Annual Review of Sociology, 28*, 243–269. doi:10.1146/annurev.soc.28.111301.093304

Stoneman, Z., Brody, G. H., Davis, C. H., & Crapps, J. M. (1989). Role relations between children who are mentally retarded and their older siblings: Observations in three in-home contexts. *Research in Developmental Disabilities, 10*, 61–76.

Stormshak, E. A., Bellanti, C. J., & Bierman, K. L. (1996). The quality of sibling relationships and the development of social competence and behavioral control in aggressive children. *Developmental Psychology, 32*, 78089.

Tompkins, V., Farrar, M. J., & Guo, Y. (2013). Siblings, language and false belief in low-income children. *The Journal of Genetic Psychology: Research and Theory on Human Development, 174*, 457–463. doi:10.1080/00221325.2012.694918

Trent, J. A., Kaiser, A. P., & Wolery, M. (2005). The use of responsive interaction strategies by siblings. *Topics in Early Childhood Special Education, 26*, 107–123.

Virji-Babul, N., Watt, K., Nathoo, F., & Johnson, P. (2012). Recognition of facial expressions of emotion in adults with Down syndrome. *Physical and Occupational Therapy in Pediatrics, 32*, 333–343. doi:10.3109/01942638.2011.653626

Vygotsky, L. (1978). *Mind in society: The development of higher psychological processes*. Cambridge, MA: Harvard University Press.

Wakai, M., Takahashi, R., Higashigawa, S., Ikeda, M., Yotsumoto, J., & Numabe, H. (2018). Self-perceptions from people with Down syndrome in Japan. *Journal of Human Genetics, 63*, 669–672. doi:10.1038/s10038-018-0412-4

Watson, T. S., Meeks, C., Dufrene, B., & Lindsay C. (2002). Sibling thumb sucking: Effects of treatment for targeted and untargeted siblings. *Behavior Modification, 26*, 412–423, doi:10.1177/0145445502026003007

Weimer, A. A., Burleson, C., Stegall, S. E., & Eisenman, R. (2018). Theory of mind and social competence among school-age Latino children. *Early Child Development and Care*. doi:10.1080/03004430.2018.1499625

White, L. (2001). Sibling relationships over the life course: A panel analysis. *Journal of Marriage and Family, 63*, 555–568.

Whiteman, S. D., Bernard, J. M. B., & McHale, S. M. (2010). The nature and correlates of sibling influence in two-parent African American families. *Journal of Marriage and Family, 72*, 267–281. doi:10.1111/j.1741-3737.2010.00698.x

Whiteman, S. D., & Christiansen, A. (2008). Processes of sibling influence in adolescence: Individual and family correlates. *Family Relations, 57*, 24–34. doi:10.1111/j.1741-3729.2007.00480.x

Whiteman, S. D., McHale, S. M., & Crouter, A. C. (2007). Competing processes of sibling influence: Observational learning and sibling deidentification. *Social Development, 16*, 642–661. doi:10.1111/j.1467-9507.2007.00409.x

Wishart, J. G. (1986). Siblings as models in early infant development. *Child Development, 57*, 1232–1240.

Wong, T. M. L., Branje, S. J. T., VanderValk, I. E., Hawk, S. T., & Meeus, W. H. J. (2010). The role of siblings in identity development in adolescence and emerging adulthood. *Journal of Adolescence, 33*, 673–682. doi:10.1016/j.adolescence.2009.11.003

Workman, J. (2017). Sibling additions, resource dilution, and cognitive development during early childhood. *Journal of Marriage and Family, 79*, 462–474. doi:10.1111/jomf.12350

Wright, I., Lewis, V., & Collins, G. M. (2006). Imitation and representational development in young children with Down syndrome. *British Journal of Developmental Psychology, 24*, 429–450. doi:10.1348/026151005X51257

Zajonc, R. B. (2001). The family dynamics of intellectual development. *American Psychologist, 56*, 490–496. doi:10.1037/0003-066X.56-7.490

CHAPTER 7

From Transition Through Old Age: Caring for Adults With Down Syndrome

Robert M. Hodapp, Kelli A. Sanderson, *and* Maria Mello

Abstract

As adults with Down syndrome live longer lives, increased attention is being paid to their health, work, and living situations. In this chapter, we divide the adult years in Down syndrome into young adulthood—roughly from 20 through the late 40s—and older adulthood, from the late 40s until death in the late 50s or 60s. Many adults with Down syndrome are doing well during early adulthood, although concerns persist about their finding meaningful jobs, connecting to others in the community, and (sometimes) showing increased levels of depression. During later adulthood, changes emerge for many, including the onset of chronic "old-age" health problems during the 50s, as well as moving away from their parental homes (often occurring as late as the 40s). Despite 160 years of research on the syndrome, major gaps remain in our understanding of adulthood, especially concerning connections among the health, functioning, and work and residential status of the aging adult with Down syndrome, as well as the aging of their parents and their relationships with adult siblings.

Key Words: transition, premature aging, young adulthood, older adulthood, parental declines, sibling relationships, Down syndrome

Over the past few decades, research interest in adults with Down syndrome has increased enormously. Recent studies have begun to examine behavioral functioning among these adults, with a few even focused on the post-secondary transition period—roughly from the end of adolescence into the mid-20s. Combined with aging-related studies of health and Alzheimer's dementia (Zigman, 2013), we are gradually beginning to fill in the gaps in our knowledge about behavioral functioning in adults with Down syndrome.

This interest in Down syndrome adulthood also reflects the increasing life spans among persons with and without intellectual disability (ID). In the overall population of the United States, those born in 1900 could be expected to live until 47 years; for those born in 2017, life expectancy had reached almost 79 years (Arias & Xu, 2019). Across most industrialized countries, similar increases in life expectancy have also been noted for those with ID. Granted, exact numbers become complicated, as many surveys do not distinguish between those who have disabilities and are aging ("aging with disabilities") and those who acquire disabilities as they age ("disabilities with aging;" Heller & van Heumen, 2014). From the few available studies, however, increasing numbers of persons with disabilities seem to be reaching age 65 and beyond (Ouellette-Kunz, Martin, & McKenzie, 2015).

But lengthening life spans show a special twist in Down syndrome. Even compared to other groups of persons with ID, the increases in life spans among individuals with Down syndrome have been extreme and recent. The most extreme comparison may be to the early 20th century, when Penrose (1949) estimated that the average newborn with Down syndrome lived to only 9 years. Such increases have also occurred in more recent years. Compare, for example, Yang, Rasmussen, and Friedman's (2002) finding regarding median life spans from the mid-1980s (which were from 25–30 years) up through today's nearly 60-year life span. Such increases may even be continuing, with increasing numbers of adults with Down syndrome living into their 70s.

Yet, while the disability field has tracked the longevity of adults with Down syndrome for decades, the field has only begun to highlight practical implications of this change. To give one example, these adults are living longer, but they also often experience what might be called "old-age" health issues beginning in their late 40s (Torr, Strydom, Patti, & Jokinen, 2010). These older but more health-impaired adults with Down syndrome may, compared to same-aged adults with other forms of ID, also experience different caregiving arrangements, as well as different residential, employment, and leisure activities. In this chapter, we focus on these practical issues, as they concern the individuals with Down syndrome themselves, their parents and families, and their work and residential lives.

Before beginning, two themes must be noted. One, we as a field do not know nearly enough about the lives of adults with Down syndrome and their families. On many occasions, we rely on only a few studies to make larger, sweeping statements. Even these studies have often been performed many years (even decades) apart, often in one or only a few industrialized countries. A few are large in scale, but many involve smaller-scale examinations, most are cross-sectional, and many do not compare adults with Down syndrome to other groups, making it unclear whether findings are similar to or different from findings from others with ID more generally. As much as possible, we will try to specify a study's years, country, and methodology, but the field needs to know much more about these individuals and their families. Though partly explainable by the increasingly long lives of individuals with Down syndrome—and by how recently such changes have occurred—such gaps nevertheless remain troubling.

Two, the lives of adults with Down syndrome involve interactions with (and changes among) many different people, including the adult with Down syndrome, their parents and siblings, and the service system. To understand this multi-person story, one must cross many of the disability field's subdomains, ranging from aging and health, to adult family relationships, to characteristics of working and living. Historically, most studies have been focused on each aspect separately. Thus, we have studies on the health of aging adults with Down syndrome, some on their parents or adult siblings, and a few on their work, living, or recreational status. The field now needs to adopt a multi-person, multi-topical lens in life-span research in Down syndrome.

The Transition and Early Adult Years in Down syndrome

We begin by examining individuals with Down syndrome during the post-secondary transition years. Although the exact time period is debatable, transition years generally range from exiting high school to commencing adult life, roughly from 16 through 25 years. Even for many young adults without disabilities, the transition from high school to post-secondary life can be challenging. As high school ends, students leave behind the comfort of the school system, often moving away from the parental home for college or work in another town or to live in their own apartment. The transition period is also one in which the young adult, often for the first time, makes major life decisions regarding post-secondary education, living arrangements, and potential avenues of employment.

As might be expected, transition is a particularly difficult time for individuals with disabilities (Gil, 2007). While typically developing peers worry about which college offer to accept or who their future roommate might be, individuals with disabilities and their parents often struggle with finding meaningful employment; determining housing assistance; finding post-secondary education, job training, or day programs that fit their needs; and securing therapies, vocational rehabilitation, personal assistants, and/or supplemental security income (SSI) or other governmental programs. While difficulties in accessing adult services have been well documented for students with disabilities (Hanley-Maxwell, Whitney-Thomas, & Pogoloff, 1995; Shattuck, Wagner, Narendorf, Sterzing, & Hensley, 2011), details of this process are only now becoming known for young adults with Down syndrome and their families.

Transition Planning, Employment, and Leisure

With improved schooling and educational programs in recent decades, young adults with Down syndrome now have increased opportunities to learn academic and life skills during secondary school (Gothberg, Peterson, Peak, & Sedaghat, 2015; Jobling & Cuskelly, 2002). Secondary programs for this population typically focus on teaching life skills to promote a successful post-secondary transition, with literacy and numeracy instruction entwined throughout curricula.

Although in many countries federal laws foster student and parent participation in the transition planning process, the level of both student and parent participation might best be conceptualized as a continuum. According to Leonard et al.'s (2016) study of Australian secondary students with Down syndrome, the large majority of parents reported themselves extremely involved in decision making for their offspring's transition to adult life. In contrast, over 40 percent of their offspring—the students with Down syndrome—were not involved in this process. Given the benefits of student involvement, this pattern of parental—but not student—involvement is troubling; in addition, those young adults with Down syndrome who were extremely involved in decision making during transition were, after high school, more likely to work in open, or competitive, employment (Foley et al., 2012).

Although many factors play a role in the employment of young adults with Down syndrome, their levels of employment can vary widely. In her long-term British longitudinal study, Carr (2008) found that less than one-fourth of all adults with Down syndrome were ever employed at any point in their lifetimes. In contrast, Jobling and Cuskelly (2002) found that 65 percent of young Australian adults with Down syndrome were employed, with the majority working 20–40 hours per week (although see Kumin & Schoenbrodt, 2016, for lower percentages of US adults with Down syndrome who work 20 or more hours per week). The varied findings from these studies may reflect a changing societal landscape, wherein young adults with disabilities increasingly lead more fulfilling lives, including employment. Of those individuals who do work, most participate in some form of sheltered employment (Carr, 2008; Foley, Girdler, Downs et al., 2014; Jobling & Cuskelly, 2002), often isolated from the general working population and earning low levels of pay (Kregel & Dean, 2002).

A smaller portion of young adults with Down syndrome participate in open, or competitive, employment. These individuals and their families report several benefits from this type of employment experience. As a group, young adults with Down syndrome who work in open employment have higher levels of overall functioning, particularly in the areas of self-care, community, and communication skills (Foley et al., 2012), as well as fewer behavior problems (Foley, Jacoby, Einfeld et al., 2014). Additionally, their participation in open employment may positively influence the family's quality of life (Foley, Girdler, Downs et al., 2014).

Instead of directly entering the workplace upon exiting high school, some young adults in the United States participate in job training or postsecondary educational programs. Increasingly available for young people with significant disabilities, job training programs are typically offered within local community colleges or technical schools (Neubert, Moon, & Grigal, 2002). A smaller number of US young adults with Down syndrome participate in postsecondary education (PSE) programs. PSE programs, especially those at 4-year universities or community colleges, strive to provide age-appropriate services and promote community inclusion and independence. Across many industrialized countries, the numbers and types of such PSE programs have recently proliferated. According to Think College, an American organization focused on developing and improving postsecondary education for individuals with ID, across the country there were 293 college programs for individuals with ID for the 2019–2020 academic year (Think College, 2020).

Finally, upon exiting high school, many individuals with Down syndrome attend day recreation programs, or "day programs." Foley, Girdler, Downs, and colleagues (2014) found that approximately 20 percent of a sample of 180 Australian young adults with Down syndrome participated in day programs (Foley, Girdler, Downs et al., 2014). While day programs are meant to engage individuals with disabilities by promoting social inclusion through activities and outings, such programs may not be the best options for this population. Foley, Girdler, Downs et al. (2014) found that individuals with Down syndrome who attended 2 consecutive years of day programs "experienced an increase in range, intensity and overall behavior problems" (p. 5). Conversely, young adults who participated in open employment for 2 consecutive years experienced a decline in problem behavior. These findings suggest that day programs may not actually provide adequate stimulation for young adults with Down syndrome, resulting in increased problem behavior in an attempt to communicate unmet needs.

Recreation and leisure activities may be another way to provide mental and physical stimulation for young adults with Down syndrome. In fact, many young adults with Down syndrome are relatively active. Examining longitudinally a national sample of Norwegian adolescents with Down syndrome (beginning age = 14 years), Dolva, Kleiven, and Kollstad (2014) found that, with the support of their parents or other adults, almost all (97 percent) participated in both formal (organized) and informal leisure activities. Carr's (2008) longitudinal UK study also found that most adults with Down syndrome regularly played sports, read books or magazines, and attended events such as films, concerts, or plays. These activities may be especially important for the continued development of teens and young adults with the syndrome.

Though young adults with Down syndrome do engage in recreation and leisure activities, the parents of less than half report that their offspring has one good friend (Glenn, Cunningham, Nananidou, Prasher, & Glenholmes, 2013). The scarcity of such friendships may partly relate to immature friendship perceptions (Watt, Johnson, & Virj-Babul, 2010). Compared to both mental age- and chronological age-matched samples, a Canadian sample of adults with Down syndrome appeared to be less able to distinguish friends from non-friends, more often perceiving as friends their parents, siblings, or teachers (Watt et al., 2010; see also Freeman & Kasari, 2002). Additionally, as adults with Down syndrome get older, their numbers of typically developing friends dwindle and shared friends, often from their mother's friend group, increase (Carr, 2008).

Young adults with Down syndrome also experience a dearth of romantic relationships. Following a cohort of individuals with Down syndrome in the UK across many decades, Carr (2008) found that less than a quarter of adults in the sample reported being in a romantic relationship. This finding was consistent across time points, with 21 percent of participants reporting a romantic partner at 30 years, 24 percent at 35 years, and 24 percent at 40 years. However, although most adults with Down syndrome may not be in a romantic relationship, most do experience sexual desire. Bononi and colleagues (2009) interviewed 50 Brazilian teenagers with Down syndrome between the ages of 10 and 20 years. Of this sample, 50 percent acknowledged feeling sexual desire and 42 percent reported masturbating frequently. Almost half (43 percent) of the teens had kissed at least one person, with 12.9 years being the mean age of the first kiss. Because young adults with Down syndrome have sexual desires and are sexually active, they need sexual education to develop knowledge and skills that can lead to healthy sexual experiences, including consensual relationships (Wood, 2004).

Health, Psychopathology, and Well-Being

Although fairly healthy compared to other disability groups during the young adult years (Carr, 2008; Foley et al., 2012), many young adults with Down syndrome nevertheless experience health conditions (Bosch, 2003). Vision and hearing issues are common (Carr, 2008), with up to 90 percent of these individuals experiencing hearing loss (Bosch, 2003). Many young adults also experience obesity and musculoskeletal problems (Pikora, Bathgate, Foley, Lennox, Leonard, 2014), as well as one or more of the following: gastrointestinal problems, sleep apnea, cataracts, axial instability, dry skin, constipation, hypothyroidism, upper respiratory issues, and speech difficulties (Pueschel, 1996; Roizen, 2010). As individuals age, autoimmune issues can develop, including thyroiditis and alopecia. It is also estimated that 30–50 percent of individuals with Down syndrome have cardiovascular abnormalities (Bosch, 2003). These physical health impairments can impede the young adults' ability to work and may lead to stress for themselves and their families (Pikora et al., 2014).

Mental health issues are also prominent in young adults with Down syndrome. Rates of depression are elevated in this group, with up to 15 percent of these young adults experiencing depression (Bosch, 2003; Pikora et al., 2014), compared to approximately 9 percent of young adults without disabilities (Mojtabi, Olfson, & Han, 2016). Young adults with Down syndrome also demonstrate increased vulnerability to anxiety, obsessive compulsive behaviors, and cognitive regression (Devenny & Mathews, 2011; Dykens et al., 2015; Tasse et al., 2016). Such mental health issues may also manifest in other ways. Compared to age mates with ID, greater percentages of late teens and young adults with Down syndrome showed lower levels of outward sociability (Hodapp, Ricci, Ly, & Fidler, 2003) and more internalizing behavior (Dykens & Kasari, 1997; van Gameren-Oosterom et al., 2013).

Inverse relations may also occur between the amount of environmental stimulation and the presence of maladaptive behavior—psychopathology. Over a 2-year span in their Australian sample, Foley, Girdler, Downs et al. (2014) reported worsening behavior problems for those young adults with Down syndrome who attended relatively unstimulating day programs. Similarly, in a study of three groups of young adults with Down syndrome, Mallardo, Cuskelly, White, and Jobling (2014) found lower levels of engagement in everyday activities among those diagnosed with clinical depression, both compared to a non-depressed group and to another group with psychiatric diagnoses but not depression. Granted, psychopathology in Down syndrome likely has many contributing factors

(Dykens, 2007). Still, based on the few available studies and even compared to individuals with ID more generally, young adults with Down syndrome may especially benefit from being actively engaged (see also Sheppherdson, 1995).

Later Adulthood

In considering the years beyond the transition period, one needs to contrast early to later adulthood, essentially comparing the adult years up through the early 40s to the later adult years, beginning in the late 40s. As adults with Down syndrome increasingly live into their late 50s and 60s, with an occasional individual reaching 70 years of age (Krinsky-McHale et al., 2008), this fact hides the many changes that begin in the late 40s. Such changes relate to the health of these individuals and of their parents; their living and work situations; and sibling and family relations.

Life Spans and Health of Older Adults With Down syndrome

Over the past few decades, the life spans of individuals with Down syndrome have been increasing at rates beyond those witnessed in the larger population (Hodapp, Burke, & Urbano, 2012), with median life expectancies in the Down syndrome population now reaching almost 60 years (Zigman, 2013). But increasing life spans do not mean that these individuals are healthy during the decade preceding death. In the largest study of this issue, van Schrojenstein Lantman-deValk et al. (1997) examined 1,602 adults with intellectual disabilities—243 of whom had Down syndrome—who lived in two southern Dutch provinces. Comparing health conditions when adults with ID were in their 50s, percentages were higher among those persons with Down syndrome versus those without for visual impairments (DS = 59.1 percent; non-DS ID = 20.2 percent); hearing impairments (37.0 percent vs. 15.2 percent); and epilepsy (21.7 percent vs. 12.2 percent). These differences do not include Alzheimer's dementia, the main condition that occurred at much higher rates during the 50s among those with Down syndrome (45.7 percent) compared to those with non-Down syndrome ID (1.7 percent).

A recent US study replicated many of these health changes during the late 40s and throughout the 50s. Hodapp, Core, Burke, Mello, and Urbano (2019), studied this issue by using several large-scale US databases, one from the NIH-sponsored DSConnect project and another from the Tennessee portion of the National Core Indicators survey (Stancliffe et al., 2012). They found that many health problems occurred when adults with Down syndrome were in their 50s. Most notably, percentages of dementia rose from the 40s into the 50s but, depending on the database, percentages with seizures, diabetes, and other conditions sometimes also showed increases. Although limitations persist in such cross-sectional studies (including having parents, siblings, or other non-medical individuals as respondents), this study—as well as the earlier Dutch study by van Schrojenstein Lantman deValk et al. (1997)—highlight three main findings: high rates of several aging-related health problems among persons with Down syndrome; rates that are higher in the population with Down syndrome compared with others with ID; and (cross-sectionally determined) aging-related differences that always occur when adults with Down syndrome are in their 50s, sometimes when in their late 40s.

These health problems among older adults with Down syndrome also co-occur with health and adaptive declines of these adults' parents. Recall that in many English-speaking Western countries, mothers give birth to newborns with Down syndrome at a median age of 32 years, approximately 5 years older than parents of newborns in the general population, with or without disabilities. These findings, noted among births in the United States (Martin, Hamilton, Osterman, Curtin, & Mathews, 2015), Australia (Staples, Sutherland, Haan, & Clisby, 1991), and the United Kingdom (Congenital Anomaly Statistics, 2010), mean that the age differences between parents and their offspring with Down syndrome are large. As a result, when adults with Down syndrome reach their late 40s and begin to experience syndrome-related health and functional declines, their parents (if alive) may be in their 80s and older (Hodapp, Burke, Finley, & Urbano, 2016), making it difficult to provide appropriate care for their offspring.

This co-occurrence of parent and offspring declines has only begun to be appreciated. In one cross-sectional, US-based study, Hodapp, Perkins, Finley, and Urbano (2015) compared parent and offspring declines when the offspring had Down syndrome versus when the offspring had ID that was not associated with Down syndrome. Using the open-ended responses of the adult siblings, naïve raters coded responses as to whether the respondent mentioned problems—declines in the brother or sister with disabilities, or in either parent. Thus, they coded "yes" when adult siblings noted that "I worry for his health" (of the brother or sister with disabilities) or "[name of brother or sister with disabilities] has been living with me ever since my mother developed cancer." The health declines of the brother or sister with disability and of the parents were coded separately.

Differences between the Down syndrome and (non-Down syndrome) ID group were especially striking when individuals with disabilities were in their 40s. The respondents reported health or functional declines in either the brother or sister with Down syndrome or in their parent in 68 percent of cases, compared to only 40.6 percent of brothers/sisters or parents among the 40–49 year-old group with non-DS ID. Considered separately, when adults with disabilities were in their 40s, higher percentages of problems occurred in the Down syndrome versus heterogeneous intellectual disabilities groups among both the parents (DS = 55.0 percent; ID = 33.7 percent) and for the adults themselves (DS = 28.8 percent; ID = 11.9 percent).

In contrast, by the time that adults with disabilities were in their 50s, such age-related differences between the groups were more nuanced. For each of the two groups, siblings reported health problems or functional declines in over three-fourths of either their brothers or sisters with disabilities or their parents. Some between-group differences were noted, with much higher percentages of health problems in the 50–59 year old adults with Down syndrome (46.2 percent) versus the adults with intellectual disabilities not associated with Down syndrome (16.2 percent). Among the parents, high—but virtually identical—percentages showed health or functional declines, with health-functional declines noted among 68.0 percent of parents of the adults with Down syndrome and 66.2 percent of parents of the adults with intellectual disabilities not associated with Down syndrome. While aging eventually affects parents and offspring in both groups, these health-functional declines—in either the offspring or their parents—appeared earlier when offspring have Down syndrome.

Residential Status of Adults With Down syndrome

Two main issues characterize the residential status of adults with Down syndrome. One, compared to adults with non-Down syndrome ID, adults with Down syndrome show higher percentages who live in their family home as opposed to living independently or semi-independently. Two, the home-living percentages for adults with Down syndrome change across age-groups in adulthood, for example, among those in their 20s, 30s, 40s, and 50s.

In Table 7.1, we address both issues by summarizing findings from multiple datasets. Most prominently, these datasets include Stancliffe et al.'s (2012) data from the National Core Indicators (NCI) project, encompassing almost 1,200 adults with Down syndrome and 11,182 adults with non-Down syndrome ID from five US states. Although impressive, the NCI dataset includes only those adults who receive state-run disability services. Current estimates are that only about one fourth of all U.S. adults with intellectual disabilities receive such services (Hewitt, 2014), and it is difficult to ascertain the ways in which those who do and do not receive services differ. We present as well data from our own web-based survey of adult siblings of individuals with intellectual disabilities (Sanderson, Burke, Urbano, Arnold, & Hodapp, 2017), as well as a French study on aging and living status among adults with Down syndrome (Tsao, Kindelberger, Freminville, Touraine, & Bussy, 2015).

Taken together, these diverse sources inform us about these two main residential issues. One, across all datasets, high percentages of adults with Down syndrome live in their family homes. Overall, in these studies, the overall percentages of home-living individuals were higher in the Down syndrome group than in other groups with intellectual disabilities. Two, a clear decline occurs in percentages of home-living individuals from the 20s through each subsequent decade (see Hodapp et al., 2016 for a review). Some researchers (e.g., Carr, 2008; Stancliffe et al., 2012) found more gradual declines over the decades, whereas others (Sanderson et al., 2017; Tsao et al., 2015) showed more marked declines from when adults with Down syndrome are in their 30s versus in their 40s and 50s. As most of these studies were cross-sectional, we cannot rule out cohort effects. Still, compared to adults with intellectual disabilities, adults with Down syndrome seem more likely to reside with their families, and such group differences (i.e., DS vs. non-DS) may be most pronounced during the middle-adult years (e.g., 30s). Gradually, most members

Table 7.1. Overview of Living Arrangements for Participants With DS

Part One: Living in family home by age group for DS participants

Study	Participants	18–29 yrs	30–39 yrs	40–49 yrs	50–59 yrs	60+ yrs	Results/Comments
Carr (2008)	DS = 38	(21 years) 71%	(30 — 35 years) 60% — 54%	(40 years) 50%	N/A	N/A	Longitudinal study over 5 decades.
Sanderson et al. (2017)	DS = 102	45.1%	31.4%	19.6%	3.9%	0%	Cross-sectional study (adult sibling = reporter).
Stancliffe et al. (2012)	DS = 1,999	72.8%	50.9%	37.2%	18.0%	8.9%	NCI data from 5 states. Decreasing percentages living with family at each age period.
Hodapp et al. (2016)	DS = 284	81%	63.6%	24.2%	7.7%	NA	Sibling reporters; main decline from 30s to 40s and 50s.
Tsao et al. (2015)	DS = 120	78%	61.5%	21.5%	12%	NA	Study on the aging process for adults with DS who were dementia-free.

Part Two: Living in family home by comparison group

Study	Participants	Down Syndrome	Comparison Group	Results/Comments
Esbensen, Bishop, Seltzer, Greenberg, & Taylor (2010)	DS = 70 ASD & ID = 70	DS = 78.6% Mean age = 37 yrs	ASD & ID = 28.6% Mean age = 37 yrs	Adults with ASD (vs. DS) more likely to live away from family in community.
Stancliffe et al. (2012)	DS = 1,999 ID = 10,382	DS = 43.3% Mean age = 40.59 yrs	ID = 27.6% Mean age = 42.88 yrs	Higher proportion of people with DS lived in family home at ages 18–49 years.

of both groups move away from the family home (or in living with their families) as they proceed into the later adult years.

But why do such moves occur? Based on a large sample of American adults with heterogenous ID, Seltzer, Greenberg, Krauss, and Kim (1997) found that the main driver of leaving home was the mother's health and ability to care for the offspring with disabilities. Admittedly, that study was not limited to participants with Down syndrome, although adults with Down syndrome comprised 41 percent of the sample. Still, the role of maternal health functioning was instructive. Especially in groups with Down syndrome, the age of the parent may be most influential beginning when adults are in their 40s. In the Sanderson et al. (2017) dataset, for example, when adults with Down syndrome were aged 40 to 49, over three-fourths of their mothers (76 percent) were either over 80 years old or deceased, compared to less than half (46.4 percent) of mothers of 40–49 year old offspring with non-Down syndrome ID (Hodapp, Burke, & Urbano, 2016). Using several of the US databases noted above (DSConnect and several adult-sibling databases), Lee, Urbano, Burke, and Hodapp (2021) recently examined the living status of different-aged adults with Down syndrome, all of whom had mothers who were alive. Looking across adulthood, the best predictors of whether the person lived with their parents or in an out-of-home placement (several types) were the age of the adult with Down syndrome and, during the combined periods of adults in their 40s and 50s, the mother's health-functional levels. Especially concerning adults with Down syndrome in their 40s and 50s, parental health-functional declines often occurred and seemed a causal factor for these adults leaving the parental home.

An additional issue concerns where adults with Down syndrome live once they do leave their parents' homes. Although rarely examined, when parents have died or are no longer able to care for the offspring with disabilities, adult siblings may more often co-reside with their brothers or sisters with Down syndrome. In the sole study of this issue, Woodman, Mailick, Anderson, and Esbensen (2014) examined a group of adults with Down syndrome over a 20-year span (ending when adults with Down syndrome averaged 52 years). Across these two decades, high percentages of adults with Down syndrome were reported to subsequently reside with their siblings. Given that these adults were in their 50s at final testing, only 35 percent lived with family members (either parents or siblings). Of those who did live with relatives, however, half lived with adult siblings. This finding suggests that high percentages of adults with Down syndrome—probably between 10 and 20 percent—may ultimately live with one of their adult siblings.

Day Activities: Employment and Volunteering

Another age-related change concerns work, volunteer, and other daily activities. As with residential settings, few studies focus on different-aged adults with Down syndrome. Re analyzing our employment data from an earlier study (Taylor & Hodapp, 2012), we found that, when adults with Down syndrome were in their 20s and 30s, approximately one-third to one-half performed paid jobs in the community (with or without assistance). In contrast, among the 40-year-old group with Down syndrome (i.e., aged 40–49 years), only 20 percent held community-based jobs, and, among the 50-year-old group, no individuals held such community-based employment (0 percent; 0 of 26 individuals). Conversely, the percentages of adults with Down syndrome who participated in no daily activities whatsoever increased from below 5 percent of participants who were in their 20s and 30s, to 10 percent of 40-year-olds, to 20 percent of 50-year-olds. Such work declines, which may be related to functional declines tied to old-age health problems (Lin et al., 2015), were not nearly as marked among the 40- or 50-year-olds who had intellectual disabilities but not Down syndrome (see Figure 1 of Hodapp et al., 2016).

The Service System and Formal and Informal Supports

In contrast to the more available educational services during the childhood years, adult service systems in most industrialized countries are generally inadequate. Within the United States, for example, parents commonly decry the many difficulties in learning about, becoming eligible for, applying for, and receiving adult disability services (Hanley-Maxwell et al., 1995). They also note how such services are scattered and uncoordinated, with separate agencies (with different application and eligibility procedures) administering services in housing, work, post-secondary schooling, recreation, health, and insurance (e.g., Social Security Insurance—or SSI—and Social Security Disability Insurance, or SSDI). In addition, waiting lists for such services are common in most states, and national estimates are that approximately 2.0 to 2.4 million American adults with intellectual and developmental disabilities are on waiting lists for services (National Council on Disability, 2005). When it comes to receiving adult disability services, young adults with intellectual disabilities are, in most countries, "falling off a cliff."

Not all adults with disabilities experience similar service histories. Indeed, several studies focus on the service needs of adults with disabilities, with family factors included. In one study, Caserta, Connelly, Lund, and Paulton (1987) found that a higher proportion of adult service needs occurred when parents were in better health. In a more comprehensive study, Smith (1997) found that families of younger and female offspring received a greater number of formal services, whereas those of older offspring received greater numbers of informal services. The age of the mother and the mother's perception of caregiver burden also entered in, with more services reported by mothers who were better able to care for their offspring and who were in better health. In terms of unmet service needs, the other children in the family—the adult siblings—also seemed to matter; specifically, a negative relationship existed between sibling participation and unmet service needs.

When it comes to understanding care for adults with Down syndrome, then, we first need to distinguish between early and later adulthood, the period beginning in the late 40s and continuing until death in the late 50s and 60s. Especially at this later age period, adults with Down syndrome experience a confluence of changes, as they begin to have old-age health problems with accompanying vocational or other changes, even as they may more often live with their parents, who are themselves declining or deceased. In many cases, adult siblings may assume care of their brother or sister with Down syndrome, either in co-residing or in overseeing out-of-home care in group homes or other settings. This pattern, which occurs to some extent among aging adults with all types of intellectual and developmental disabilities, seems to occur earlier and be more pronounced in Down syndrome.

Looking to the Future: Caring for Adults With Down Syndrome Over the Adult Years

We end this chapter with a call for better understandings of—and appreciations for—the many issues involved in caring for adults with Down syndrome. But beyond the usual call that "more research is needed," we elaborate on what we need to know and to what effect. To us, two major themes arise in this future work, the need for better understanding of the issues and repercussions of aging in Down syndrome, and the need to incorporate multi-disciplinary and multi-person perspectives toward adults with Down syndrome.

The Need to Know More About Basic Issues of Aging in Down Syndrome

Given Down syndrome's 160-year research history, it might seem surprising that we often experience a lack of critical information. Nevertheless, we have major gaps in our knowledge of aging in this syndrome, even around seemingly basic issues. Consider the percentages of specific health problems present among adults with Down syndrome as they reach different ages. While many studies have been performed on the onset and course of Alzheimer's dementia in Down syndrome, most other health concerns have received little attention. Indeed, van Schrojenstein Lantman-deValk et al. (1997)—a Dutch study performed over 20 years ago—is among the few large-scale studies that examine the array of old-age health problems that arise in Down syndrome. A few, more recent studies have begun to appear (Hodapp, Core, Burke, Mello, & Urbano, 2019), but these studies are often limited in that they employ secondary datasets not originally (or optimally) designed to assess health conditions.

In other life aspects as well, we as a field know relatively little. While several researchers examine correlates of getting and keeping jobs among young adults with IDD, few focus on Down syndrome, fewer still on how job performance within the syndrome changes over the life span. Similarly, researchers are only beginning to note how different percentages of these adults live with their family members (Stancliffe et al., 2012). The family members themselves have also received short shrift, with few studies of how the effects of "advanced maternal age" persist into the later years of adults with Down syndrome. Researchers also need to examine more formally the siblings of these adults, especially as, compared to in other disability groups, sibling relationships in Down syndrome may be particularly close and these siblings may also more often assume long-term care of their brother-sister with disabilities (Hodapp, Sanderson, Meskis, & Casale, 2017).

To some extent, such neglect is understandable, as the life spans of individuals with Down syndrome have continued to lengthen in recent decades. As a result of such continually increasing life spans, recent generations constitute the first adults with Down syndrome who will outlive their parents. Compare, for example, today's individuals with Down syndrome versus those adults living during the 1980s. During that earlier time, life spans were thought to be in the 20s and 30s, with Yang et al. (2002) reporting that the median age at death in Down syndrome was 25 years in 1983. But, if adults with the syndrome now live until their late 50s or into their 60s (Zigman, 2013), then their parents (who were themselves more likely to be older at the birth of these offspring) will be either deceased or in their 80s or 90s. Down syndrome may have a long research history, but individuals who live with the syndrome today differ from those who reached adulthood several decades ago. Researchers are only now catching up.

The Need for Perspectives on Down Syndrome Aging That Are Multi-disciplinary and Involve Multiple Perspectives

In contemplating the care of aging adults with Down syndrome, one is confronted with the reality that the field is not "owned" by any single discipline. Researchers in this topic are interested in aging; in family functioning; in life-span change in cognitive, linguistic, and adaptive functioning; in dementia and associated medical conditions; in adult siblings and sibling caregiving; in residential and vocational changes; and in connections with (and effects of) various aspects of the adult disability service system. And yet, to examine caring for adults with Down syndrome, one must consider together all of these perspectives.

Such relations, in turn, operate both within the adult with Down syndrome and between the adult and the surrounding social environment. Within these adults themselves, aging-related health problems may impact cognitive, linguistic, and adaptive functioning, but such changes also likely influence changes in work or leisure activities during the older years. But within-person relationships are only part of the picture. Parental aging also factors in, but exactly how is only beginning to be understood. And although, compared to adults with autism, adults with Down syndrome experience better relationships with their adult siblings (Hodapp & Urbano, 2007), we continue to know little about whether, when, and how such close relationships translate into the care of the adult with Down syndrome, potentially as these adults move from parental care to sibling care. Also unknown are whether such family-care changes happen more often in Down syndrome and whether caregiving works differently when adults have Down syndrome as opposed to other IDD conditions (e.g., due to dementia or other medical complications).

Concluding Thoughts

The increasingly long life span in Down syndrome is among the most important of all advances in the field of developmental disabilities. And yet, while such a change is worthy of celebration, increasing life spans bring about a need to understand many aspects and components. In the case of adulthood in Down syndrome, some of this understanding relates to Alzheimer's dementia, but we also need to understand cognitive, adaptive, maladaptive, and other aging-related changes, even among those older adults with Down syndrome who do not show dementia. Beyond the individuals themselves, we need to understand co-occurring changes in their parents, the group that—in many cases—continues to provide day-to-day care within the family home. So too do we need to pay attention to the adult siblings who often take on care once parents can no longer do so.

Yet just as increasing longevity fosters research interest and leads to policy implications, so too do we need to connect longer lives to the adult's surrounding environments. From transition and early adulthood, to later aging while living with aging parents, adulthood in Down syndrome features certain aspects that are similar to—and others that differ from—adulthood among others with intellectual disability. It is time to fill in the many gaps in our knowledge, thereby helping these individuals and their families to experience more connected, fulfilled lives.

References

Arias, E., & Xu, J. (2019). United States life tables, 2017. *National Vital Statistics Reports, 68*(7).

Bononi, B. M., Sant'Anna, M. J. C., de Oliveira, A. C. V., Renattini, T. S., Pinto, C. F., Passarelli, M. L., . . . Omar, H. A. (2009). Sexuality and persons with Down syndrome: A study from Brazil. *International Journal of Adolescent Medicine and Health, 21*(3), 319–326.

Bosch, J. J. (2003). Health maintenance through the lifespan for individuals with Down syndrome. *Journal of the American Academy of Nurse Practitioners, 15*, 5–16.

Carr, J. (2008). The everyday life of adults with Down syndrome. *Journal of Applied Research in Intellectual Disability, 21*, 389–397.

Caserta, M. S., Connelly, J. R., Lund, D. A., & Paulton, J. L. (1987). Older adult caregivers of developmentally disabled household members: Service needs and fulfillment. *Journal of Gerontological Social Work, 10*, 35–50.

Congenital Anomaly Statistics, England and Wales (Series MB3). *Official National Statistics*, 2010. http://www.ons.gov.uk/ons/rel/vsob1/congenital-anomaly-statistics--england-and-wales--series-mb3-/no--23--2008/index.html. Accessed February 4, 2015.

Devenny, D. A., & Matthews, A. (2011). Regression: Atypical loss of attained functioning in children and adolescents with Down syndrome. *International Review of Research in Developmental Disabilities, 41*, 233–264.

Dolva, A.-S., Kleiven, J., & Kollstad, M. (2014). Actual leisure participation of Norwegian adolescents with Down syndrome. *Journal of Intellectual Disabilities, 18*, 159–175.

Dykens, E. M. (2007). Psychiatric and behavioral disorders in persons with Down syndrome. *Mental Retardation and Developmental Disabilities Research Reviews, 13*, 272–278.

Dykens, E. M., & Kasari, C. (1997). Maladaptive behavior in children with Prader-Willi syndrome, Down syndrome, and non-specific mental retardation. *American Journal on Mental Retardation, 102*, 228–237.

Dykens, E. M., Shah, B., Davis, B., Baker, C., Fife, T., & Fitzpatrick, J. (2015). Psychiatric disorders in adolescents and young adults with Down syndrome and other intellectual disabilities. *Journal of Neurodevelopmental Disorders, 7*, 1–8.

Esbensen, A., Bishop, S., Seltzer, M. M., Greenberg, J. S., & Taylor, J. L. (2010). Comparisons between individuals with Autism Spectrum Disorder and individuals with Down syndrome in adulthood. *American Journal of Intellectual and Developmental Disabilities, 115*, 277–290.

Foley, K.-R., Girdler, S., Downs, J., Jocoby, P., Bourke, J., Lennox, N., . . . Leonard, H. (2014). Relationship between family quality of life and day occupations of young people with Down syndrome. *Social Psychiatry, 49*, 1455–1465.

Foley, K.-R., Jacoby, P., Einfeld, S., Girdler, S., Bourke, J., Riches, V., & Leonard, H. (2014). Day occupation is associated with psychopathology for adolescents and young adults with Down syndrome. *BMC Psychiatry, 14*, no. 266.

Foley, K.-R., Jacoby, P., Girdler, S., Bourke, J., Pikora, T., Lennox, N., . . . Leonard, H. (2012). Functioning and post-school transition outcomes for young people with Down syndrome. *Child: Care, Health, and Development, 39,* 789–800.

Freeman, S. F. N., & Kasari, C. (2002). Characteristics and qualities of the play dates of children with Down syndrome: Emerging or true friendships? *American Journal on Mental Retardation, 107*, 16–31.

Gil, L. A. (2007). Bridging the transition gap from high school to college: Preparing students with disabilities for a successful postsecondary experience. *Teaching Exceptional Children, 40,* 12–15.

Glenn, S., Cunningham, C., Nananidou, A., Prasher, V., & Glenholmes, P. (2013). Using the strengths and difficulties questionnaire with adults with Down syndrome. *Research in Developmental Disabilities, 34,* 3343–3351.

Gothberg, J. E., Peterson, L. Y., Peak, M., & Sedaghat, J. M. (2015). Successful transition of students with disabilities to 21st century college and careers: Using triangulation and gap analysis to address nonacademic skills. *TEACHING Exceptional Children, 47*, 344–351.

Hanley-Maxwell, C., Whitney-Thomas, J., & Pogoloff, S. M. (1995). The second shock: A qualitative study of parents' perspectives and needs during their child's transition from school to adult life. *Journal of the Association for Persons with Severe Handicaps, 20*, 3–15.

Heller, T., & van Heumen, L. (2014). Aging with disability. In M. L. Wehmeyer (Ed.), *The Oxford handbook of positive psychology and disability* (pp. 409–423). Oxford, UK: Oxford University Press.

Hewitt, A. (2014). Embracing complexity: Community inclusion, participation, and citizenship. *Intellectual and Developmental Disabilities, 52*, 475–495.

Hodapp, R. M., Burke, M. M., Finley, C. I., & Urbano, R. C. (2016). Family caregiving of aging adults with Down syndrome. *Journal of Policy and Practice in Intellectual Disabilities, 13,* 181–189.

Hodapp, R. M., Burke, M. M., & Urbano, R. C. (2012). What's age got to do with it? Implications of maternal age on families of offspring with Down syndrome. *International Review of Research in Developmental Disabilities, 42,* 109–145.

Hodapp, R. M., Burke, M. M., & Urbano, R. C. (2016). *Aging adults with and without Down syndrome: Parental changes when offspring are in their 40s and 50s*. Presentation to the 49th Gatlinburg Conference on Research and Theory in Intellectual and Developmental Disabilities, San Diego, CA.

Hodapp, R. M., Core, R. E., Burke, M. M., Mello, M. P., & Urbano, R. C. (2019). Health issues across adulthood in Down syndrome: Juxtaposing multiple databases. *International Review of Research in Developmental Disabilities, 57*, 229–265.

Hodapp, R. M., Perkins, A. M., Finley, C. I., & Urbano, R. C. (2015). Growing old together: Similarities/differences in families of adults with and without Down syndrome. *International Review of Research in Developmental Disabilities, 49*, 151–189.

Hodapp, R. M., Ricci, L., Ly, T., & Fidler, D. (2003). The effect of the child with Down syndrome on maternal stress. *The British Journal of Developmental Psychology, 21*, 137–151.

Hodapp, R. M., Sanderson, K. A., Meskis, S. A., & Casale, E. G. (2017). Adult siblings of persons with intellectual disabilities: Past, present, and future. *International Review of Research in Developmental Disabilities, 53*, 163–202.

Hodapp, R. M., & Urbano, R. C., &. (2007). Adult siblings of individuals with Down syndrome versus with autism: Findings from a large-scale American survey. *Journal of Intellectual Disability Research, 51,* 1018–1029.

Jobling, A. & Cuskelly, M. (2002). Life styles of adults with Down syndrome living at home. In M. Cuskelly, A. Jobling, & S. Buckley (Eds.), *Down syndrome across the life span* (pp. 109–120). London, UK: Whurr Publishers.

Kregel, J. & Dean, D. H (2002). Sheltered vs. supported employment: A direct comparison of long-term earnings outcomes for individuals with cognitive disabilities. In J. Kregel, D. H. Dean, & P. Wehman (Eds.), *Achievements and challenges in employment services for people with disabilities: The longitudinal impact of workplace supports monograph.* https://vcurrtc.org/resources/viewcontent.cfm/151

Krinsky-McHale, S. J., Devenny, D. A., Gu, H., Jenkins, E. C., Kittler, P., Murty, V. V., . . . Silverman, W. (2008). Successful aging in a 70-year-old man with Down syndrome: A case study. *Intellectual and Developmental Disabilities, 46*, 215–228.

Kumin, L., & Schoenbrodt, L. (2016). Employment in adults with Down syndrome in the United States: Results from a national survey. *Journal of Applied Research in Intellectual Disabilities, 29*, 330–345.

Lee, C. E., Urbano, R. C., Burke, M. M., & Hodapp, R. M. (2021). Who lives where and why? Residential changes across adulthood in persons with Down syndrome. *Journal of Policy and Practice in Intellectual Disabilities*, 18, 151–161. Published online. doi: 10.1111/jppi.12364.

Leonard, H., Foley, K.-R., Pikora, T., Bourke, J., Wong, K., McPherson, L., Lennox, N., & Downs, J. (2016). Transition to adulthood for young people with intellectual disability: The experiences of families. *European Child & Adolescent Psychiatry, 25*, 1369–1381.

Lin, J. D., Lin, L. P., Hsu, S. W., Chen, W. X., Lin, F. G., Wu, J. S., & Chu, C. (2015). Are early onset aging conditions correlated to daily activity functions in youth and adults with Down syndrome? *Research in Developmental Disabilities, 36*, 532–536.

Mallardo, M., Cuskelly, M., White, P. & Jobling, A. (2014). Mental health problems in adults with Down syndrome and their association with life circumstances. *Journal of Mental Health Research in Intellectual Disabilities, 7*, 229–245.

Martin, J., Hamilton, B., Osterman, M., Curtin, M., & Mathews, M. (2015). *Births: Final data for 2013—Internet Tables*. In: *National Vital Statistics Reports*. Vol 1 (Supplement). http://www.cdc.gov/nchs/data/nvsr/nvsr64/nvsr64_01_tables.pdf. Accessed January 21, 2015.

Mojtabai, R., Olfson, M., & Han, B. (2016). National trends in the prevalence and treatment of depression in adolescents and young adults. *Pediatrics, 138*(6), e20161878. doi:10.1542/peds.2016–1878.

National Council on Disability. (2005). *The state of 21st century long-term services and supports: Financing and systems reform for Americans with disabilities*. Washington, DC: National Council on Disability.

Neubert, D. A., Moon, M. S., & Grigal, M. (2002). Postsecondary education and transition services for students age 18–21 with significant disabilities. *Focus on Exceptional Children, 34*, 1–11.

Ouellette-Kunz, H., Martin, L., & McKenzie, K. (2015). A review of health surveillance in older adults with intellectual and developmental disabilities. *International Review of Research in Developmental Disabilities, 48*, 151–194.

Penrose, L. S. (1949). The incidence of Mongolism in the general population. *Journal of Mental Science, 95*, 685–688.

Pikora, T. J., Bathgate, K., Foley, K. R., Lennox, N., & Leonard, H. (2014). Health conditions and their impact among adolescents and young adults with Down syndrome. *PLoS One, 9*(5): e96868.

Pueschel, S. M. (1996). Young people with Down syndrome: Transition from childhood to adulthood. *Mental Retardation and Developmental Disabilities, 2*, 90–95.

Roizen, N. (2010). Overview of health issues among persons with Down syndrome. *International Review of Research in Mental Retardation, 39*, 3–33.

Sanderson, K. A., Burke, M. M., Urbano, R. C., Arnold, C. K., & Hodapp, R. M. (2017). Who helps? Characteristics and correlates of informal supporters to adults with disabilities. *American Journal on Intellectual and Developmental Disabilities, 122*, 492–510.

Seltzer, M. M., Greenberg, J. S., Krauss, M. W., & Hong, J. (1997). Predictors and outcomes of the end of co-resident caregiving in aging families of adults with mental retardation or mental illness. *Family Relations, 46*, 13–22.

Shattuck, P. T., Wagner, M., Narendorf, S., Sterzing, P., & Hensley, M. (2011). Post-high school service use among young adults with an autism spectrum disorder. *Archives of Pediatric and Adolescent Medicine, 165*, 141–146.

Sheppherdson, B. (1995). Two longitudinal studies of the abilities of people with Down's syndrome. *Journal of Intellectual Disability Research, 39*, 419–431.

Smith, G. C. (1997). Aging families of adults with mental retardation: Patterns and correlates of service use, need, and knowledge. *American Journal on Mental Retardation, 102*, 13–26.

Stancliffe, R. J., Lakin, C. K., Larsen, S. A., Engler, J., Taub, S., Fortune, J., & Bershadsky, J. (2012). Demographic characteristics, health conditions, and residential service use in adults with Down syndrome in 25 U.S. states. *Intellectual and Developmental Disabilities, 50*, 92–108.

Staples, A. J., Sutherland, G. R., Haan, E. A., & Clisby, S. (1991). Epidemiology of Down syndrome in South Australia, 1960–89. *American Journal of Human Genetics, 49*, 1014–1024.

Tasse, M. J., Macho, P. N., Havercamp, S. M., Benson, B. A., Allain, D. C., Manikam, K., & Davis, S. (2016). Psychiatric conditions prevalent among adults with Down syndrome. *Journal of Policy and Practice in Intellectual Disabilities, 13,* 173–180.

Taylor, J. L., & Hodapp, R. M. (2012). Doing nothing: Adults with disabilities with no daily activities and their siblings. *American Journal of Intellectual and Developmental Disabilities, 117,* 67–79.

Think College. (2020). https://thinkcollege.net/college-search. Accessed November 2, 2020.

Torr, J., Strydom, A., Patti, P., & Jokinen, N. (2010). Aging in Down syndrome: Morbidity and mortality. *Journal of Policy and Practice in Intellectual Disabilities, 7,* 70–81.

Tsao, R., Kindelberger, C., Freminville, B., Touraine, R., & Bussy, G. (2015). Variability of the aging process in dementia-free adults with Down syndrome. *American Journal on Intellectual and Developmental Disabilities, 120,* 3–15.

van Gameren-Oosterom, H. B. M., Fekkes, M., van Wouwe, J. P., Detmar, S. B., Oudesluys-Murphy, A., & Verkerk, P. H. (2013). Problem behavior of individuals with Down syndrome in a nationwide cohort assessed in late adolescence. *The Journal of Pediatrics, 163,* 1396–1401.

van Schrojenstein Lantman-deValk, H. M. J., van den Akker, M., Maaskant, M. A., Haveman, M. J., Urlings, H. F. J., Kessels, A. G. H., & Crebolder, H. F. J. M. (1997). Prevalence and incidence of health problems in people with intellectual disability. *Journal of Intellectual Disability Research, 41,* 42–51.

Watt, K. J., Johnson, P., & Virj-Babul, N. (2010). The perception of friendship in adults with Down syndrome. *Journal of Intellectual Disability Research, 54,* 1015–1023.

Wood, A. (2004) Sexuality and relationships education for people with Down syndrome. *Down Syndrome News and Update, 4*(2), 42–51. doi:10.3104/practice.330.

Woodman, A. C., Mailick, M. R., Anderson, K. A., & Esbensen, A. (2014). Residential transitions among adults with intellectual disability across 20 years. *American Journal on Intellectual and Developmental Disabilities, 119,* 496–515.

Yang, Q., Rasmussen, S. A., & Friedman, J. M. (2002). Mortality associated with Down's syndrome in the USA from 1983 to 1997: A population-based study. *Lancet, 359,* 1019–1025.

Zigman, W. B. (2013). Atypical aging in Down syndrome. *Developmental Disabilities Research Reviews, 18,* 51–67.

SECTION 3

Cognition and Neuropsychology

CHAPTER

8 The Emerging Phenotype in Infants With Down Syndrome: Adaptations to Atypical Constraints

Hana D'Souza *and* Dean D'Souza

Abstract

The aim of this chapter is not just to present a selection of literature on early development in Down syndrome (DS), but also to integrate findings from across disciplines within an overarching framework. In this chapter, DS is viewed not as a collection of cognitive and motor deficits, nor as an assortment of relative strengths and weaknesses, but as a functioning adaptive system, albeit with a different start state (trisomy 21). According to this view, the emerging characteristics of DS are adaptations to atypical constraints and thus serve an immediate functional purpose—but these early adaptations will in turn act as new developmental constraints, and some of them may exacerbate the divergence of the DS trajectories. This chapter focuses on the first few years after birth, because to understand how the DS phenotype gradually emerges, it is important to focus on early developmental constraints. The chapter introduces DS as an adaptive system with trisomy 21, explains why a developmental systems approach is needed to understand it, and discusses how such an approach can be implemented in research. It then describes how trisomy 21 may constrain neural plasticity, which is likely to have cascading effects on the developmental process of specialization—contributing to less efficient information processing and atypical motor activity. The chapter then discusses how young children with DS may adapt to these challenges within the context of the social environment. Finally, this chapter points to future directions in theory, research, and intervention.

Key Words: Down syndrome, infancy, adaptive systems, developmental systems, neural plasticity, specialization, perception-action cycles, cognitive development, motor development, social development

> The study of Down's syndrome has become a fractionated business, each discipline pressing exclusive views about mechanisms and management. The result has been a confusing array of books, pamphlets and technical articles about Down's syndrome (close to 1000 published items to date on psychological matters alone) which mostly fail to enlighten.
>
> *(Gibson, 1978, p. xi)*

More than 40 years and over half a million academic papers and books later (according to a Google Scholar search), there seems to be an exponential tendency to review and meta-analyze findings in the Down syndrome (DS) field.[1] There is also growing recognition that DS is a multilevel, multisystem, neurodevelopmental disorder which needs to be understood by collating empirical findings across disciplines and across the lifespan (e.g., D'Souza, D'Souza, et al., 2017; D'Souza & Karmiloff-Smith, 2017). However, in order to understand these findings and move forward, it is necessary to cohere them into a single developmental story.

The aim of this chapter is not just to present a selection of the vast literature on individuals with DS, but to provide some clarity by integrating findings from across disciplines within an overarching approach or framework. The approach we take is to view DS not as a collection of cognitive and motor deficits, nor as an assortment of relative strengths and weaknesses, but as a *functioning adaptive system albeit with a different start state (trisomy 21)*. According to this view, the emerging characteristics of DS are adaptations to atypical constraints, and thus serve a functional purpose—and constrain later emerging skills. We focus on the first few years after birth, because to understand how the DS phenotype gradually emerges, it is important to focus on early developmental constraints (D'Souza & Karmiloff-Smith, 2016). We start by introducing DS as an adaptive system with trisomy 21 and explain why a developmental systems approach is needed to understand it. We continue by discussing how such an approach can be implemented in research. We then describe how trisomy 21 may constrain neural plasticity, which is likely to have cascading effects on the developmental process of specialization—contributing to less efficient information processing and atypical motor activity. We discuss how a young child may adapt to these challenges within their social environment. Finally, we point to future directions in theory, research, and intervention.

Down Syndrome: An Adaptive System With a Different Start State

Although the characteristics of DS vary across individuals in number and intensity (Dykens & Hodapp, 2001; Karmiloff-Smith et al., 2016), a widely accepted profile of individuals with DS has been described. In addition to general intellectual disability, the profile includes particular difficulties in motor ability, auditory processing, verbal short-term memory, and language ability (especially expressive language; e.g., Miller & Leddy, 1999); relative strengths in visuospatial processing and some aspects of social functioning (e.g., Cebula et al., 2010; Jarrold & Baddeley, 1997; Wishart & Johnston, 1990); and atypical motivation (Pitcairn & Wishart, 1994). However, most of what we know about this profile of individuals with DS comes from studies of older children and adults. Yet, the DS profile only gradually *emerges* over developmental time (e.g., Fidler, 2005; Fidler et al., 2008; Will et al., 2018). Studying infants with DS therefore affords a window onto this process.

Because DS is diagnosed by genetic testing, it is tempting to assume that the emergence of the DS phenotype—with its loose assemblage of relative strengths and weaknesses—is under the control of *genetic* activity (e.g., trisomy 21). However, there is now ample evidence that control is distributed among multiple, diverse, interconnected, and interdependent factors, many of which are external to the individual (for discussion, see D'Souza, D'Souza, et al., 2017). Therefore, DS is not a static *disorder* with deficits and areas of relative strengths, but an *adaptive system* with a different *start state*. Adaptive systems comprise manifold interdependent parts, which develop and give rise to new structures and functions by actively *adapting* to their environment. Each adaptive system begins from a slightly different start state, has a separate set of experiences, and thus develops different behaviors. But the behavior of these systems, including those with trisomy 21, are *adaptations—developmental* processes in which the system maximizes its fit to the environment under internal and external constraints (Johnson, 2017). Moreover, while internal/external factors (e.g., genes) influence developmental processes, developmental processes (e.g., neural reorganization) constrain the factors (e.g., genetic expression). In other words, development is produced by interacting factors across various levels (Fig. 8.1).

Take language, for example. If language development were under the control of genetic activity and pre-programmed, then we would expect that damage to classic language areas in the brain would cause irrecoverable damage to the language system (see D'Souza & Karmiloff-Smith, 2011, 2016, for discussion). However, if control is distributed and

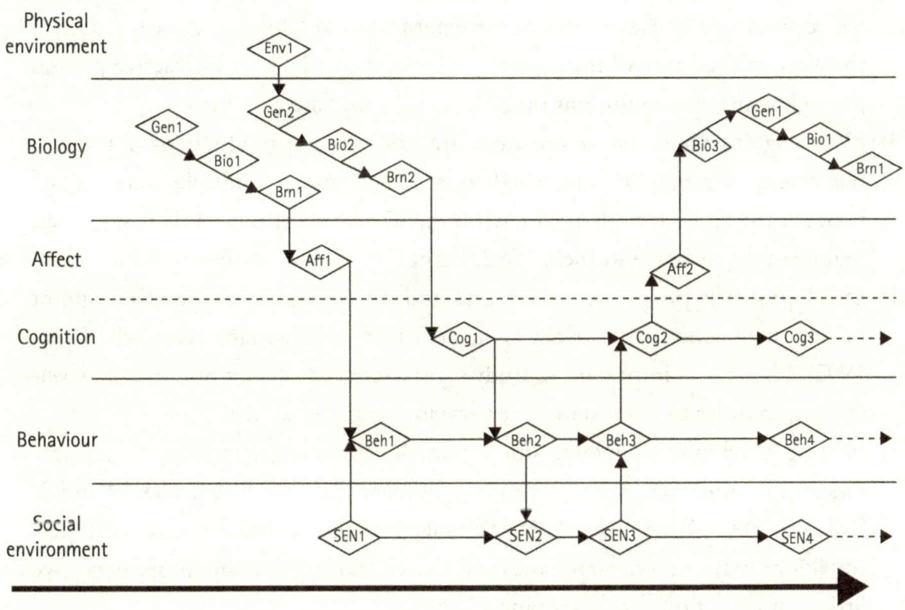

Figure 8.1. Illustration of cascading effects and the complexity of development across time (*x*-axis). Horizontal arrows = trajectories within a domain of functioning; diagonal arrows = causal pathways within levels of functioning; vertical arrows = effects between levels of functioning. Adapted from Moore & George (2015). Reproduced by permission of Taylor and Francis Group, LLC, a division of Informa plc.

language development is probabilistic, then we might expect that an adaptive system would have the flexibility to compensate for the injury. And, indeed, this is what seems to be the case; the literature is replete with examples of children with perinatal left-hemisphere brain damage who nevertheless acquire important age-appropriate language skills (e.g., Bates et al., 2001; see D'Souza & Karmiloff-Smith, 2016, for discussion). By the same token, in individuals with DS, language development has been shown to be a highly complex process that is contingent on multiple components, including nonverbal communication skills, motor skills, attentional abilities, face scanning, sleep, verbal short-term memory, visuospatial short-term memory, and family context (e.g., Chapman & Hesketh, 2001; Deckers et al., 2019; D'Souza et al., 2015; D'Souza, D'Souza, Horváth, et al., 2020; D'Souza, D'Souza, Jones, et al., 2020; D'Souza, Lathan, Karmiloff-Smith, et al., 2020; Edgin et al., 2015; Martin et al., 2009; Mason-Apps et al., 2018; Mundy et al., 1995).

The DS phenotype therefore seems to emerge through a cascade of interconnected and interdependent effects, which may reflect a more probabilistic than deterministic process (Gottlieb, 2007). According to this "developmental systems"[2] perspective:

(1) At conception, the organism "inherits" a wide range of interacting resources (genes, chromatin marks, endosymbionts, nutrients, a family, society, etc.—the "start state"), which affect, and are affected by, the infant's development (Oyama, 1985).
(2) The infant learns and develops through the *active* process of adapting its internal connectivity to the metrics of the external world (Buzsáki, 2006). Action is therefore at the heart of learning and development. It is an interactive process through which the conditions of the external world are also altered.
(3) Neurocognitive and motor processes are not the sole products of our genes, but emerge through self-organized interactions among multiple factors (e.g., between the child and physical environment) across various levels (e.g., genes, brain, family, society; Gottlieb, 1992; Lerner, 1978; also see Fig. 8.1).
(4) Development is progressive; structures and systems that emerge at one point in time may constrain later-emerging structures and systems (Gottlieb, 1970, 1992). Hence, it is important to study constraints and adaptations early in development in order to understand later developmental processes.
(5) Because development involves the interaction of diverse, interdependent factors over multiple timescales, it can be nonlinear (Buzsáki, 2004; McClelland & Vallabha, 2009; Rosenblatt, 1958; Schöner & Kelso, 1988). That is, small perturbations may result in large cascading effects, and large perturbations may have little or no effect on the developing system.

In other words, development is constrained (i.e., context-dependent and time-sensitive) and involves an active process of adapting to typical and atypical constraints.

An understanding of how the DS phenotype emerges, therefore, necessitates an understanding of how the system adapts to constraints across time, and especially to constraints in early development, as these early adaptations may constrain the emergence of later adaptations.

How to Implement a Developmental Systems Approach to Study Infants With DS

Although the principles of developmental systems are widely acknowledged, they are not often reflected in our current research practices. This is not surprising given the complexity of human development. How might we go about implementing a developmental systems approach in our research practice? On the practical side, we need to collect large datasets and use advanced analytical techniques to reveal the patterns concealed within (*big data*). This requires time, resources, and the opportunity to test many participants many times and over many timescales (from moment to moment to longitudinally). But big data is not sufficient. Identifying patterns, trends, and associations is an important step, but it does not elucidate how emergent dynamics (e.g., object exploration) arise from the underlying mechanistic dynamics (e.g., neuronal firing). An interdisciplinary approach is needed to integrate the data in order to understand how the whole system functions and develops. This is because different levels of description (genetic, neural, behavioral, societal, etc.; see Fig. 8.1) constrain each other. For example, the firing of a neuron is partly constrained by activity at the genetic level (gene expression), while the expression of a gene in a neuron is partly constrained by the firing pattern of that neuron (Flavell & Greenberg, 2008; Leslie & Nedivi, 2011; Tyssowski et al., 2018). Causality thus appears to be multidirectional and distributed across levels in complex systems. Therefore, it is important to study interactions *between* levels, rather than each level in isolation.

How can we piece together the many interactions that occur across different timescales both within and between different levels? We need to bring together different methodologies which have been applied to the DS field: neurobiological methods (including animal modelling, induced pluripotent stem cells (iPSC) research, and postmortem histology), human brain imaging, cognitive and behavioral experiments, observational studies, and computational modelling. Each method has its strengths and weaknesses. A range of cutting-edge techniques can be used to probe mechanistic pathways by manipulating variables such as gene expression. However, these tend to involve mouse models or human cells that have been developed in a lab environment. They may therefore generate findings that are not directly applicable to humans and need to be interpreted with caution. On the other hand, a number of methods can be used directly with humans, but for ethical reasons these rarely involve manipulations that elucidate mechanistic causes. It is therefore challenging—perhaps even impossible—to investigate different levels of description using a single method or a single population in order to understand how levels interact and what processes give rise to the DS phenotype. But it is possible to piece together evidence from different studies, disciplines, and techniques, capitalizing on their different strengths. And it is only through converging evidence (consilience) that we can begin to make sense of the field.

In this chapter, we try to bind evidence from different levels into a coherent developmental story. This will mean that parts of this chapter will be suggestive rather than explicit, based on tentative rather than conclusive pieces of evidence. But these parts are far from trivial. We include them because they highlight links between levels that need exploring. Our hope is that binding evidence from different disciplines may help us to grasp the bigger picture and/or generate new hypotheses. We focus on the first few years after birth in individuals with DS because in order to understand how the DS phenotype gradually emerges, it is important to focus on early developmental constraints (see D'Souza, D'Souza, et al., 2017, for discussion). Of course, it would be interesting to study developmental trajectories from the earliest moment, from conception. But practical and technological limitations currently make it very difficult to study and integrate information on the different levels prenatally. Thus, we offer a compromise. In this chapter, we seek to link information from different levels at the earliest possible time in development that we believe this can currently be attempted: *infancy*.

We start at the level of the genes (because DS is diagnosed on this level) and then move "up" the levels of organization. It is important to note that this does not mean that the genetic level is more fundamental or important than the "higher" levels (the word "hierarchy" is a misnomer in this context).[3] Another crucial point is that our use of the words "hierarchy" and "levels" do not imply unidirectional causality; the different levels constrain each other. Causality is distributed and multidirectional, and organisms adapt to the world through the feedback they receive from acting on it.

Trisomy 21 Constrains Neural Plasticity

The genetics and neurobiology of DS have been extensively reviewed elsewhere (e.g., Dierssen, 2020; Stagni et al., 2018; Vacca et al., 2019). Here we focus on connections *between* the different levels of description to understand how they constrain each other. The start state of DS includes the presence of a partial or complete triplication of chromosome 21 (trisomy 21; Reeves et al., 2001). Although chromosome 21 is the smallest human chromosome, making up only 1.5% of the human genome (Dierssen, 2012), the extra chromosome contributes to diffuse, widespread, and cascading atypicalities in brain and cognitive development. Not every gene on chromosome 21 is overexpressed in DS (Antonarakis, 2017), but dysregulation of genes such as *DYRK1A*, *APP*, *OLIG1*, *OLIG2*, and *RUNX1* is known to constrain cortical development (Sobol et al., 2019). For example, *DYRK1A* is involved in the production of an enzyme that regulates proteins involved in cell proliferation and differentiation (which, after cell migration, results in an accumulation of neurons in cerebral cortex by 20–21 weeks of gestation) (Nakano-Kobayashi et al., 2017; Park et al., 2009; Stagni et al., 2016). This process is atypical in individuals with

DS. For example, cell proliferation is reduced (Guidi et al., 2011; Larsen et al., 2008). Whereas typically developing (TD) fetuses at 19 weeks of gestation were found to have ~10.4 billion neocortical cells (neurons and glia), fetuses with DS at 19 weeks of gestation had only ~6.85 billion (Larsen et al., 2008). Moreover, neural progenitor cells in DS are less likely to acquire a neuronal phenotype and more likely to acquire an astrocytic phenotype (Stagni et al., 2018). More astrocytes in DS are likely to exacerbate overexpression of a gene located on chromosome 21 (*S100B*) whose product (the S100B protein) is secreted by astrocytes and which, unless suppressed, impairs neurogenesis and induces neuronal cell death in DS (Chen et al., 2014). Consequently, the brain in DS develops both fewer neocortical cells than the TD brain as well as fewer neurons relative to overall brain cells (Stagni et al., 2018).

The DYRK1A enzyme is also involved in regulating proteins that form dendrites and dendritic spines (neuronal outgrowths that enable the neuron to receive signals from other neurons) (Park et al., 2009). Infants with DS present with spine dysmorphology and have less dendritic arborization and fewer dendrites/spines than TD infants (Becker et al., 1986; Benavides-Piccione et al., 2004; Purpura, 1975; Takashima et al., 1981; Wisniewski & Schmidt-Sidor, 1989). The abnormalities in spine morphology and cell proliferation may explain another finding: cortical lamination (the 7- to 10-week-long process through which the cortical neurons rearrange to form layers) is delayed and atypical in DS, and several cortical areas show underdeveloped gyral patterns (Golden & Hyman, 1994).

In sum, the altered expression of genes on chromosome 21 has cascading effects on brain development, including cell development and cortical organization (for summary, see Fig. 8.2). While the impact of the atypicalities in cortical lamination on the developing system is unclear, fewer dendritic spines should result in less input from other neurons, which, in combination with fewer neurons, would lead to reduced neural signaling. Fewer dendritic spines may also contribute to inhibitory predominance. For instance, while the most common neurons (*principal cells*) excite each other via dendrites and dendritic spines, one family of neurons (*interneurons*) often control (inhibit) the activity of principal cells by targeting the cell body—that is, bypassing dendrites and spines (Buzsáki, 2006). Interneurons may therefore have more influence on brain function in DS. Indeed, there is evidence of increased inhibitory (relative to excitatory) activity in mouse models of DS (for a review, see Contestabile et al., 2017).

Inhibition is necessary for brain function. In its absence, sensory input generates similar widespread one-way patterns of activation (Buzsáki, 2006; Dichter & Ayala, 1987). Interneurons can stabilize activity (through feedback loops), dampen activity (feedforward loops), and segregate activity (by suppressing the activity of some neurons and not others) (see Buzsáki, 2006, for discussion). However, brain function requires an appropriate balance between excitation and inhibition (Haider et al., 2006). Inhibitory predominance and reduced signaling in DS are likely to affect how the neurons in a system self-organize and optimize their functionality. To adapt to the world, neurons require some degree

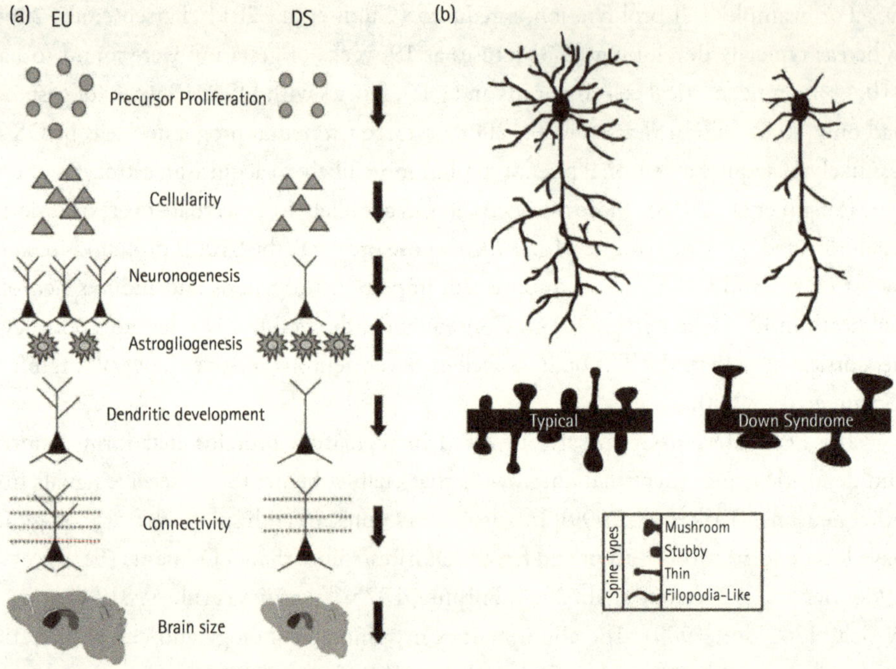

Figure 8.2. (a) Compared to typical development (EU = euploid mouse), a mouse model of DS (Ts65Dn) shows impairment in proliferation, reduced cellularity, decreased neurogenesis, increased astrogliogenesis, dendritic hypotrophy, reduced connectivity, and reduced brain size (as indicated by up/down arrows). Adapted from Bartesaghi et al. (2015); (b) Schematic representation of a neuron depicting atrophies in dendrite morphology in brains of individuals with DS (right) compared to TD individuals (left). Adapted from Kulkarni & Firestein (2012). The DS neuron contains fewer dendritic spines than the TD neuron. Also, dendritic spines in DS often have larger heads. Adapted from Phillips & Pozzo-Miller (2015). Image credit: Elsevier.

of flexibility (*plasticity*). They need to communicate with each other and connect to the external world in order to calibrate to it. Communication between neurons occurs via synapses between neurons, and most synapses are found on the neurons' dendritic spines. Synapses are thus the sites at which plasticity (learning) occurs at the level of the brain. As intimated previously, learning involves both the flow of information (through excitatory connections) and control of that flow through inhibition to form coalitions or specialized subsystems of neurons. Plasticity enables the developing system to learn from and adapt to the environment, even in the face of extreme adversity such as brain injury. However, if neural communication in DS is constrained by lack of synaptic resources and overinhibition, then flexibility (*synaptic plasticity*) and the ability of the system to adapt will be compromised (Buzsáki, 2006; see also Singer et al., 2019).

For learning to have a long-lasting effect (i.e., to be adaptive in the long term), it needs to be consolidated within the system. In the human brain, this process requires molecular and cellular stabilizing mechanisms. These stabilizing mechanisms include homeostatic negative feedback mechanisms (*homeostatic plasticity*) that are sensitive to, and regulate, the level of neural excitability (Turrigiano & Nelson, 2004). In this way, excitatory connections may lead to structural changes in postsynaptic material (e.g., dendritic spines) that are subsequently stabilized by genetic and molecular activity that is, in part, facilitated by inhibitory connections. We therefore speculate that inhibitory predominance in DS results in overregulation of neural excitability, further increasing the excitatory-inhibitory (E/I) imbalance and reducing the plasticity of the brain, and thus its capacity to adapt to the external world. This is consistent with the findings of a study that used single-cell-resolution intravital microscopy to monitor cortical tissue grafts derived from the skin fibroblasts of two individuals with DS (Real et al., 2018). Real and colleagues had reprogrammed the fibroblasts in vitro to form induced pluripotent stem cells (iPSCs), which were then differentiated into cortical neurons, labelled with fluorescent proteins (markers), and transplanted into the brains of mice. Longitudinal in vivo imaging of the markers revealed increased synaptic stability and reduced functional neural network activity (less oscillatory activity) in the DS neurons than in disomic clones without the extra copy of chromosome 21 (Real et al., 2018). Structural changes at the synapse were shown to be modifiable in three different DS mouse models (Tg, Ts65Dn, Dp1Yey) by inhibiting *DYRK1A* activity, which was associated with improved learning and memory (Nguyen et al., 2018).

Although this section of the chapter has described paths that branch out from trisomy 21 and overexpression of the *DYRK1A* gene through fewer neurons and synapses to inhibitory dominance and reduced plasticity, these paths are not unidirectional. As explained in the previous section, DS is a complex *adaptive* system. This means that the system and components of the system are constantly in flux, adjusting to new conditions. For example, while there is an initial paucity of early born neurons, increased production of later-born neurons has been described in a Ts65Dn mouse model (Chakrabarti et al., 2007). This could be the result of adaptive processes. However, complex adaptive systems are also *path dependent*. This means that the timing of interactions can impact the developmental trajectory of the system. By the time the extra neurons have thickened the neocortical wall, the sparse connections between the early-born neurons may already have affected the process of neocortical lamination, a process that relies on spontaneous neural activity and is observed to be both delayed and disorganized in DS (Golden & Hyman, 1994). To further illustrate the complexity of development, like most (if not all) parts of a complex adaptive system, the role of interneurons is not fixed: it is context dependent. For example, the major inhibitory neurotransmitter in the adult brain, γ-Aminobutyric acid (GABA), often acts through the chloride-dependent GABA type A ($GABA_A$) receptor. Intracellular chloride concentration is high prenatally and only drops during neonatal life (Cherubini et al., 1991). This means that many interneurons are initially excitatory and only switch to an inhibitory role later in development. It is possible that because neocortical lamination requires spontaneous neural activity, prenatal brain development requires more excitatory connections than inhibitory connections, while postnatal brain development requires an increase in inhibitory control to prune connections and hone neural networks through postnatal experience. The relatively late upsurge of neurogenesis in DS may therefore thicken the cortex but not necessarily correct important differences in early E/I ratios. Moreover, the postnatal structure (and thus contribution) of the GABAergic interneuron changes through interactions with the external environment (Donato et al., 2013), which highlights the complex interplay between the various levels. In sum, the path from genes to neural networks is not unidirectional; the developmental trajectory of the system is constrained by manifold interactions across levels of description and timing.

Neural Plasticity Constrains Specialization

What may reduced synaptic plasticity mean for infants with DS? Early in typical development, the brain is characterized by overproduction of unspecified synaptic connections (Bourgeois, 2001; Greenough et al., 1987). Thus, patterns of activation in the infant brain are more diffuse than those in the adult brain. Brain activation becomes increasingly specialized (and thus more efficient) over developmental time through interactions between various brain regions and the environment (Elman et al., 1996; Fair et al., 2007; Johnson, 2001, 2011). Indeed, the process of specialization has been identified in several developmental domains, including face perception (e.g., Pascalis et al., 2005), cognitive control (e.g., Crone, 2014), phoneme perception (e.g., Werker & Hensch, 2015), emotional reactivity and regulation (e.g., Somerville & Casey, 2014), and motor development (e.g., D'Souza, Cowie, et al., 2017).

In typical development, the number of synapses reaches its peak in early childhood (Huttenlocher, 1979; Huttenlocher & Dabholkar, 1997; Liu et al., 2012). Synapses are initially weak but some are strengthened through experience (Hebb, 1949). To reduce noise in the system and increase signal-to-noise ratio, unused synapses become weaker and are eventually pruned out (Colman et al., 1997; Navlakha et al., 2015; Sengpiel & Kind, 2002; Sretavan & Shatz, 1984). Whereas synaptogenesis provides the brain with plasticity (which enhances the influence of postnatal experience on neural circuitry), synaptic pruning stabilizes the experience-driven changes that occur when self-organizing neural circuitry specializes to its environment (Johnson, 2001, 2011). Fewer neurons and reduced synaptic plasticity in infants with DS are likely to lead to a worse signal-to-noise ratio. This may in turn make it more difficult for the DS brain to specialize to its environment (Rubenstein & Merzenich, 2003). Moreover, increased inhibition, sparser neurons/synapses, and spine dysmorphology may make excitatory synapses in DS more vulnerable during the pruning process. This is because pruning occurs through synaptic activity, and synaptic activity is constrained by inhibitory processes, the number of neurons/synapses, and spine morphology (Colman et al., 1997; Cowan, 1979). Indeed, the neuronal derivatives of trisomy-21-induced pluripotent stem cells (iPSCs) (the reprogrammed cells of two individuals with DS) showed less synaptic activity than an isogenic control that is disomic for human chromosome 21 (Weick et al., 2013). Furthermore, because inhibitory synapses are less affected by pruning processes than excitatory synapses (De Felipe et al., 1997), pruning may further disrupt E/I imbalance (increase inhibitory predominance) in persons with DS. Indeed, the rate of pruning of inhibitory synapses is disrupted in Ts65Dn mouse models, resulting in an increase of inhibition (Mitra et al., 2012). Thus, reduced plasticity may make it more difficult for the DS brain to specialize in the same way or to the same extent as the TD brain.

The process of specialization also requires long-range connectivity between brain regions. This is because learning and development involve interregional interactions as well as intraregional refinement (Bassett & Sporns, 2017; Johnson, 2001, 2011). Interregional communication depends on axonal processes that can reach considerable distances in the brain and fast transmission. To establish fast transmission, axons are wrapped in a lipid-rich substance called myelin (Waxman, 1980). Traditionally considered to be modifiable only by damage, it now appears to participate in brain plasticity and be at least partly regulated by experience: brain imaging studies suggest that changes in white matter (which reflect changes in myelination) correlate with learning, and cellular studies reveal that myelination is modulated by neural activity (Almeida & Lyons, 2017; Fields, 2015; McKenzie et al., 2014; Mount & Monje, 2017). Myelination therefore plays an important role in brain plasticity and specialization. Yet, hypomyelination is observed early in development in DS, as demonstrated by a multiregion transcriptome analysis of myelin protein expression (Olmos-Serrano et al., 2016), histological examination (Ábrahám et al., 2012; Wisniewski & Schmidt-Sidor, 1989), magnetic resonance imaging (MRI; Koo et al., 1992), and diffusion tensor imaging (DTI; Gunbey et al., 2017). Moreover, a small near-infrared spectroscopy study found reduced long-range functional connectivity in infants with DS (n = 5) compared to 27 chronological age-matched term or late preterm and early term TD controls (Imai et al., 2014). Emerging evidence suggests that the dysregulated (genetic and molecular) signaling pathways that affect neuronal proliferation and differentiation also disrupt the process through which progenitor cells differentiate into the cells that form myelin, oligodendrocytes (see Reiche et al., 2019, for review). Brain plasticity, neural connectivity, and specialization in DS may therefore be affected by hypomyelination as well as fewer neurons and fewer synapses.

Although functional communication within and between brain regions is atypical in young children with DS, the process of specialization has yet to be studied in these children (see Hamner et al., 2018, for a review of the sparse pediatric neuroimaging literature). There is, however, indirect evidence from the adult literature (for a review of functional magnetic resonance imaging (fMRI) studies in DS, see Carbó-Carreté et al., 2020). For example, brain activity during a passive listening task was studied in nine young adults with DS using fMRI (Reynolds Losin et al., 2009). While nine chronological age-matched TD comparison participants showed more activation (in classic receptive language areas) in response to language (forward speech) than nonlanguage (backward speech) stimuli, the individuals with DS showed almost no difference in activation patterns between the two. The individuals with DS also showed a more diffuse brain response than the TD individuals, with greater activation in cingulate gyrus and parietal lobes. This suggests that the DS brain had not specialized for hearing speech, at least not to the same extent as the TD brain. Furthermore, Anderson et al. (2013) measured the brain activity of young adults with DS watching cartoons, and found that activity in adjacent brain regions was more synchronized than in TD participants matched on chronological age, while the opposite was true for distant brain regions. Diffuse local connectivity and reduced long-range connectivity is a hallmark of early brain development. As the brain specializes over developmental time, short-range connectivity decreases and long-range connections increase (Fair et al., 2007, 2009; Moraczewski et al., 2018). Therefore, the data of Anderson et al. suggest that the DS brain has not specialized to the same extent as the TD brain.

Specialization Is Driven by Perception-Action Cycles

Specialization is not a passive process; the infant calibrates its internal operations to the external world by *actively* exploring (selecting, acting on) and sampling it (Buzsáki, 2006; Frankenhuis & Panchanathan, 2011; Held & Hein, 1963; Piaget, 1954). This is achieved through cycles of perceiving and acting (Edelman, 1987; Gibson, 1988; Gibson & Pick, 2000; Sporns & Edelman, 1993). As Ulrich (2010, p. 1871) explained:

> As newborns use their available eye muscle strength and control to attend to objects or people moving through their space, they push their systems, bit by bit, to go farther, to see more and longer. These repeated cycles of moving and perceiving the consequences lead, over time, to sufficient control of head and neck muscles to lift the head and eyes upward, leading to new, interesting things to explore. Their efforts have cascading effects, enabling more and longer movements through greater distances, toward objects, people, and sounds that attract them. Bit by bit, the foundation takes shape and expands for discovering new concepts, consistencies, and motor control.

From this, it follows that if an infant is exposed to an atypical environment that hampers exploration, or its capacity to explore or sample the environment is limited (as may be the case in infants with DS), then the process of specialization will be affected and the infant would be more likely to develop atypically (Frankenhuis & Panchanathan, 2011; Johnson et al., 2015; Karmiloff-Smith et al., 2012).

Perceptual and Attentional Constraints on Information Sampling in Infants With DS

In order for the organism to specialize, it must be able to sample information from the environment (Frankenhuis & Panchanathan, 2011). This process is constrained by the ability to sense and perceive information. Early in development, DS is associated with perceptual difficulties in a number of modalities, including visual (John et al., 2004), auditory (Roizen et al., 1993), and tactile (Brandt, 1996). Furthermore, infants and toddlers with

DS seem to struggle to integrate information from different modalities (multisensory/multimodal integration; D'Souza et al., 2016). Emerging evidence also points to lower responsivity in children with DS as reported by their caregivers on the Short Sensory Profile questionnaire (Bruni et al., 2010; Will et al., 2019). Taken together, it is possible that many infants with DS may not notice changes in the environment that TD infants would sample, learn about, and act on (e.g., Ulrich et al., 1997).

Even if young children with DS notice a change in the environment, there is evidence that they take longer than chronological and mental age-matched TD infants to orient their focus of attention toward it (D'Souza, D'Souza, Jones, et al., 2020). This means that they may sample less from (and learn less about) the environment than their TD peers. Furthermore, some fleeting events may be missed altogether, potentially involving a loss of some critical learning moments (e.g., the parent labelling an object). This is consistent with findings that faster attentional orienting is concurrently associated with better cognitive performance in 9-month-old infants with DS (Fidler, Schworer, Will, et al., 2019) and greater language ability in 15-month-olds (both with and without DS; D'Souza, D'Souza, Jones, et al., 2020).

Less Efficient Information Processing in Infants With DS

Once the infant has perceived and oriented to an external stimulus, they need to process the information more deeply. One of the earliest ways that infants process information sampled from their environment is through habituation. Habituation (a progressive reduction in response to a repeated stimulus) reflects the process through which an internal representation of a familiar stimulus is gradually built up; the end triggers a switch in attention from the familiar stimulus to a novel one (Bremner & Fogel, 2004). If there is inhibitory predominance and a lack of neurons in the DS brain (and thus a lack of plasticity), it may take longer for the brain to build up sufficiently detailed representations—and thus take longer for it to habituate to stimuli in the external world. Indeed, this seems to be the case. Whereas ten TD fetuses during the final trimester of pregnancy habituated to repeated presentations of an auditory stimulus, atypical habituation was observed in two fetuses with DS (Hepper & Shahidullah, 1992). One of the fetuses with DS failed to habituate; the other showed a slower rate of habituation than all ten TD comparisons. Sadly, the fetus that failed to habituate did not survive long after birth, hinting at a link between habituation and developmental outcomes. Indeed, in typical development, infant habituation patterns are predictive of later-emerging cognitive functions such as language development (Bornstein & Tamis-LeMonda, 1989; Ruddy & Bornstein, 1982) and childhood intelligence (Bornstein & Sigman, 1986; Kavšek, 2004; McCall & Carriger, 1993; Rose et al., 1986). Furthermore, 106 neonates born at risk of intellectual delay (including DS) successfully habituated to a verbal stimulus, but oriented less to a novel stimulus and, later, less to the reappearance of the familiar stimulus than 37 TD neonates, indicating atypical information processing as early as 41 weeks (± 3 weeks) gestational age (Zelazo et al., 1989).

Atypical habituation has also been described in infants with DS using electroencephalography (EEG), a measure of neurophysiological activity in the brain. Whereas TD 6- and 12-month-old infants who were presented with a repetitive auditory stimulus showed neural habituation through a progressive decrement in the amplitude of their auditory evoked responses (AER) (Barnet et al., 1971), 6- and 12-month-old infants with DS did not show this pattern of neural habituation; it was also not observed among 1-month-olds, either with or without DS (Barnet et al., 1971). These data hint that the ability to process auditory information changes over the first half year of postnatal life in typical development, but less so (or not at all) among infants with DS. Atypical neural habituation in the auditory domain has also been identified in studies of older children with DS (Díaz & Zurron, 1995; Seidl et al., 1997), supporting the notion that infants with DS are slower at building internal representations of auditory stimuli. Similar findings have also been reported in the visual domain. For example, using a visual oddball paradigm in which one face was presented for 80% of the trials and another face for 20% of the trials to measure face discrimination and EEG in 6-month-old infants, Hill Karrer and colleagues (1998) found that attenuation of brain activity in response to the repetitive face stimuli (habituation) was more gradual in the infants with DS than in chronological age-matched TD participants.

Less efficient or slower habituation mechanisms in infants with DS, which is consistent with difficulties in building internal representations, may help to explain a core characteristic of individuals with DS—experiencing more difficulty in processing verbal information than visual information. In a familiar environment, an infant is unlikely to need the same level of representational detail to be able to discriminate between naturally occurring visual stimuli than between auditory stimuli. For example, during social interaction a child may not need to discriminate every featural change it observes in the body or face of an interacting social agent, but it would need to discriminate featural changes in any accompanying speech stream. Furthermore, key physical properties of speech can change rapidly over the duration of an utterance. This makes speech discrimination a challenging task.

If habituation is less efficient or slower in DS, an infant with DS would require more exposure to a stimulus in order to form an internal representation of it. This dovetails with the finding that infants with DS are relatively slow at disengaging attention from a visual stimulus in order to redirect attention to a novel stimulus (D'Souza, D'Souza, Jones, et al., 2020). They may require more time to build up an internal representation of a visual stimulus and are thus slower at switching attention to other stimuli. Rather than being an impairment, the long disengagement latency might therefore be a useful adaptation: infants with DS might benefit more by *not* shifting attention quickly. There is always a trade-off, however. By spending more processing time on a single stimulus, the infant with DS is spending less time exploring the environment.

Less Motor Activity in Infants With DS

Information sampling is not a passive process. It usually involves motor activity. Indeed, motor activity has been proposed to be at the core of early development (Piaget, 1952; Thelen & Smith, 1994; Von Hofsten, 2004). Even young infants actively select aspects of their environment to focus on by moving their eyes, reaching toward people and objects, and locomoting to new locations. TD infants generate a large amount of activity. By 3.5 months, TD infants experience 3–6 million eye movements (Johnson et al., 2003). Around the first year of life, TD infants spend about half of their day manipulating objects (Karasik et al., 2011). Between 12 and 19 months, TD toddlers produce around 14,000 steps per day (in terms of distance, this is equivalent to walking the length of 46 American football fields) and fall around 100 times per day (Adolph et al., 2012). TD children therefore generate what seems to be an extensive amount of motor activity to develop their skills to adult-like levels. Because the DS brain is characterized by fewer neurons, inhibitory predominance, and a poor signal-to-noise ratio, it may require even more motor activity to adapt its neural circuitry to the external world than the TD brain. Yet, from very early on, infants with DS produce less spontaneous motor activity than TD infants of the same chronological age (Mazzone et al., 2004). Motor activity in infants with DS also differs from that of the TD infants in terms of intensity and complexity. Infants with DS produce more low-intensity and less high-intensity spontaneous leg motor activity than TD infants of the same chronological age (McKay & Angulo-Barroso, 2006). They also produce fewer complex leg movements (i.e., kicking patterns; Ulrich & Ulrich, 1995) in comparison to TD infants matched on chronological age and TD infants matched on motor age.

Why do we see these differences in motor activity? Motor ability relies on the interactions of multiple subsystems (Thelen & Smith, 1994), many of which are atypical in infants with DS. Reduced motor activity in DS is likely to be a consequence of perceptual difficulties, atypical neural constraints, and an adaptive response to muscular and skeletal differences, including low muscle tone (hypotonia), joint laxity, and hypermobility (Block, 1991; Cardoso et al., 2015; Cowie, 1970; Lott, 2012; Ulrich & Ulrich, 1993). Furthermore, common health-related issues may also play a role, including congenital heart disease (Alsaied et al., 2016; Pfitzer et al., 2017) and sleep difficulties (Hauck et al., 2018; McKay & Angulo-Barroso, 2006). A combination of these constraints may make it more challenging for the developing system with DS to generate motor activity. Thus, the developing system may end up producing less motor activity, which would lead to fewer experience-dependent changes, impacting the system's developmental trajectory. Indeed, individual differences in early motor activity has been linked to the development of motor milestones in young children with DS. Infants who are more active than the mean at 2 or 3 months of age achieve several prone and sitting skills earlier (Hauck et al., 2020). Furthermore, intensity of leg kicks predicts onset of walking in young children with DS, as infants who show more high-intensity leg motor activity at around 12 and 14 months of age start walking earlier than those who show less of this activity (Lloyd et al., 2010). Although one explanation may be that those children whose starting state is more typical tend to produce more motor activity and reach their developmental milestones earlier, a randomized controlled study suggests that facilitating early motor experience has a positive effect on the emergence of later motor skills (Ulrich et al., 2001). Specifically, Ulrich and colleagues (2001) showed that infants with DS who underwent a home-based stepping training intervention achieved independent walking by an average of 101 days earlier than infants with DS who were not part of this intervention. This suggests that despite their particular genetic and neurocognitive constraints, the infants with DS were able to benefit from the extra motor activity, altering their developmental pathways.

Motor activity in young children with DS does not only differ from typical development in onset and intensity, but also in the type of strategies employed to reach a particular motor state. "Symmetrical" strategies have been observed across a range of contexts in young children with DS. For example, some children with DS use a symmetrical strategy (i.e., they move their limbs symmetrically along the body midline) to lift themselves up from a prone position into a sitting position, which involves doing the splits (Lydic & Steele, 1979). Infants and toddlers with DS have also been reported to use a symmetrical strategy when rising up from the floor into a standing position; they tend to simultaneously use both hands and both feet to provide maximal support (Lauteslager, 1995). A symmetrical strategy for locomotion—bottom shuffling—has also been described in young children with DS (Robb, 2015). Although atypical, these symmetrical strategies seem to be adaptive strategies employed to compensate for hypotonia and hypermobility of joints (Åkerström & Sanner, 1993; Kugel, 1970) and/or reduced posture reactions (balance and self-righting; Haley, 1986).

Though adaptive (it is likely to be more adaptive, for example, to sit up by "doing the splits" than not to sit up at all), these symmetrical strategies are likely to constrain the type of activity and experiences that the developing system can generate in the future, taking the system down a different developmental path. Reliance on symmetrical strategies may lead to less sensorimotor experience with differentiated limbs. Consequently, regular use of symmetrical strategies may impact motor behavior in situations when the strategies are not adaptive, such as when postural stability is provided by a seat (for an example in TD infants, see Corbetta & Bojczyk, 2002). In other words, if infants with DS regularly use symmetrical strategies as adaptations, they may subsequently have difficulties decoupling their limbs in situations when it would have been possible and advantageous to do so. This may potentially affect the development of motor skills that require asymmetrical strategies, such as intermanual coordination (e.g., using one hand to hold a jar while the other hand twists the lid of the jar). This is consistent with behavioral findings in school-aged children and adults with DS which show that, although they face many motor challenges, intermanual coordination is particularly challenging for this population (Ringenbach et al., 2002; Spanò et al., 1999).

Early motor ability not only constrains future motor ability, but also impacts how infants explore and interact with the world around them, such as how they engage with objects. Differences in self-generated activity have been observed in the emergence of reaching for objects. De Campos and colleagues (2013) followed infants with DS and TD infants monthly, with a first assessment at the age of 4 months. As expected, the majority of TD infants were able to reach at the age of their first assessment (i.e., at 4 months; Spencer et al., 2000). They subsequently showed a gradual increase in number of reaches. The age at which the infants started reaching was a better predictor of later reaching behavior than chronological age. This suggests that reaching behavior is dependent on experience rather than on chronological age (Carvalho et al., 2008). This conclusion is in line with the proposal that TD infants act and select aspects of their environment as a function of their current level of abilities (Kidd et al., 2012; Rovee-Collier & Cuevas, 2009). TD infants spontaneously repeat their actions and, in so doing, practice new emerging skills (Adolph et al., 2012). De Campos et al. (2013) observed the same trend in infants with DS, with an increasing number of reaches after onset of reaching (even though reaching onset was delayed). However, the average number of reaches and subsequent object exploration was lower in the infants with DS. Thus, the children with DS both started reaching later and practiced their actions less frequently than the TD infants. Although some developmental delay may be expected, it is not obvious why the infants with DS produced less reaching. Less repetition may be due to the actions being more taxing to infants with DS compared to TD infants. Emerging motor actions, such as reaching in young infants, requires the coordination of many motor, perceptual, and cognitive resources (Berger et al., 2019; Boudreau & Bushnell, 2000; for a review, see Berger et al., 2018). Whereas in TD infants many of these resources are freed as movements become automatized over development (Berger et al., 2018) and as the motor system becomes specialized (D'Souza, Cowie, et al., 2017), these processes are possibly delayed in DS. Thus, motor performance may be drawing on diverse (and already limited) resources in DS for a longer developmental period. The adaptive response to taxing motor actions may be to produce less of them. Taken together, even though the exact reasons are unclear, infants with DS engage less with their physical environment than TD infants.

Less motoric engagement with the environment is likely to negatively impact the development of other domains in infants with DS. Several studies in TD infants have demonstrated cascading effects of the motor domain on other domains. Independent sitting and visual-manual exploration in 4.5- to 7.5-month-olds were found to be related to infants' 3-dimensional object completion abilities (Soska et al., 2010). Crawling experience was found to increase sensitivity to optic flow information for balance (Campos et al., 2000) as well as mental rotation abilities (Schwarzer et al., 2013). Motor development was also found to be associated with social development. Training 3-month-old infants to manipulate and reach for objects affects their visual exploration of social agents (Libertus & Needham, 2010, 2011). Furthermore, the transition from crawling to walking was found to change interactions between infants and their caregivers, increasing opportunities for more advanced social interactions (Clearfield et al., 2008; Karasik et al., 2011, 2014). This could potentially contribute to the positive association between walking and language development (Walle & Campos, 2014).

If different domains (e.g., motor and social development) are interconnected and interdependent, then a deficit in one domain (e.g., motor) may have cascading effects on other domains (e.g., social). However, this does not mean that a particular domain provides the necessary and sufficient conditions for the development of other domains (Campos et al., 2000; Iverson, 2010). For example, even though vision and locomotion may be associated with language development in TD children, it is clearly possible for a child to develop language even when they are unable to see or locomote. The components of the system would adapt to the constraints; an alternative pathway would emerge. However, due to other constraints such as reduced brain plasticity, an infant with DS may have fewer alternative pathways available to them than an infant with no or fewer atypical constraints. Thus, identifying *early* atypicalities in motor development in DS may be important because of their potential cascading effects on other domains. Indeed, there is some emerging evidence that such cascading effects may be operating in DS. Yamauchi and colleagues (2019) observed motor abilities to be positively associated with both cognitive and language abilities in 1- to 3-year-olds with DS. This association strengthened with increasing age. Furthermore, onset of walking was suggested to facilitate both cognitive and language development in DS (Yamauchi et al., 2019). Even though longitudinal and intervention studies are needed to further probe these cascades in DS, the study supports the idea that early atypicalities in the motor domain may cascade onto cognitive and language development in DS. This may be an important focus of research, as infants with DS show particularly pronounced difficulties in motor development early in life (e.g., Carr, 1970; Harris, 1981; LaVeck & LaVeck, 1977). Indeed, motor development in DS seems to be delayed even when compared to mental age-matched children with developmental delays (Fidler et al., 2008). This may result in a unique set of cascading effects, potentially contributing to a DS-specific developmental trajectory.

Perception-Action Cycles Are Embedded Within Social Contexts

As young infants improve their motor skills, they can reach further, move their bodies faster, and explore places and objects they could not before. But they do not do this in isolation; perception-action cycles are embedded within social contexts and are consequently constrained by interactions with parents, siblings, peers, and other social agents (Adolph & Hoch, 2019). For example, social agents are often useful sources of information and infants integrate social information to guide their perception-action cycles (Karasik et al., 2016; Tamis-LeMonda et al., 2008). In the following section, we discuss how the perception-action cycles may interact with social contexts in the infant with DS. Could one adaptive response to motor difficulties and less efficient information processing in infants with DS be an overreliance on social agents?

Overreliance on Social Agents as an Adaptive Strategy

At birth, visual acuity and the ability to physically interact with the external world is limited. This constrains the type of information that neonates can perceive and makes them largely dependent on their caregivers for visual input. What kinds of visual scenes do their caregivers create for them? A study using head-mounted cameras demonstrated that these mostly comprise their caregivers' faces (Fausey et al., 2016). As the infants' motor abilities develop, however, they take a more active role manipulating objects and locomoting—with their visual input shifting from faces to hands and objects (Fausey et al., 2016). If infants with DS present with motor delay and put their emerging motor abilities to use less than TD controls, then the nature of their visual input will likely change less over developmental time than for TD infants. Perhaps this could partly explain the findings that, even though mutual gaze with a caregiver is initially slower to develop in infants with DS, it remains high over the first year of life whereas declines are seen among TD infants (Berger & Cunningham, 1981; Carvajal & Iglesias, 2000). In another observational study, 6- and 9-month-old infants with DS spent almost half of their time looking at their caregiver during free play, which was nearly twice as much as TD infants of the same chronological age (Gunn et al., 1982). If infants with DS receive more visual input of their caregiver, this might bias them to overrely on this source of information. This may over time contribute to relative strengths in other social domains, such as joint attention (for a metaanalysis, see Hahn et al., 2018).

The possible social bias is in line with observations that imitation abilities are relatively strong in children with DS (Nielsen & Hudry, 2010; Vanvuchelen et al., 2011). As John Langdon Down (1867) noted in early work on DS, individuals with DS seem to possess "considerable power of imitation, even bordering on being mimics" (p. 122). Even though imitation often has negative connotations, it may in fact be a very successful adaptive strategy for individuals with DS, as social agents are often useful and trustworthy sources of information. Hence, by imitating social agents, infants with DS may achieve goals that they would not easily accomplish through other means. Imitating others may be easier than generating and initiating novel ideas and actions. In support of this hypothesis, Wright and colleagues (2006) found that toddlers with DS use imitative strategies to solve cognitive tasks, even when it would be more appropriate for them to use different cognitively driven strategies. So, they seem apt at copying what they see around them rather than generating their own actions.

Further evidence in support of this hypothesis comes from a study of children with DS interacting with their TD sibling. The children with DS often adopted the role of "learner," while their sibling took on the role of "teacher" or "manager" (Stoneman et al.,

1987), irrespective of who was older (Abramovitch et al., 1987). Furthermore, children with DS were less likely to initiate interaction and more likely to imitate their sibling than vice versa (Knott et al., 1995). This asymmetry in interactions may again be an adaptive strategy in DS, but it could nevertheless further exacerbate an overreliance on others.

Overreliance on others is likely to hinder the development of independent behavior. Indeed, toddlers with DS at 21 months of mental age showed significantly more help-seeking behavior during an object retrieval task than both TD children of the same mental age and a group of children with developmental disabilities of mixed or unknown etiology (Fidler et al., 2005). Furthermore, lower levels of task persistence and higher levels of off-task behavior in children with DS have been reported (Landry & Chapieski, 1989; Pitcairn & Wishart, 1994; Ruskin et al., 1994; Vlachou & Farrell, 2000). For example, 4-year-olds with DS have been found to engage in more off-task "party pieces" or charming behavior to socially engage the experimenter compared to chronological and mental age-matched TD groups (Pitcairn & Wishart, 1994). Anecdotally, during our testing sessions, young children with DS often attempt to terminate more challenging tasks by clapping to indicate that the tasks have somehow been completed. We rarely observe this behavior in children with other neurodevelopmental disorders. These are certainly very creative and charming adaptive strategies to ending challenging or less engaging tasks. If reinforced, it is not inconceivable that these behaviors could steer developmental trajectories. Seeking help and ending tasks may be adaptive in the short term, but if it occurs at the expense of practicing solving problems, then it may reduce skill development and independence in the long term. This is consistent with the finding that, later in life, individuals with disabilities are more likely to select easier problems to solve, seek help from others, and demonstrate less satisfaction when working on problems (for a review, see Bybee & Zigler, 1998).[4]

Although children with DS are often considered to be highly social, neither their sociability nor their overreliance on social agents necessarily mean that they interact optimally with social agents. For example, Krakow and Kopp (1982) found that 19- to 38-month-old toddlers with DS spent less time socially oriented (e.g., engaging their caregiver in play, handing toys to their mother, seeking assistance) and also less time exploring their environment (e.g., looking around at other people and/or distant toys) than mental age-matched TD children. That poses the question of what they were doing during those interactions: 50% of the toddlers with DS engaged in stereotypic activity such as throwing toys and 75% of them spent time totally unoccupied (e.g., staring into space) (Krakow & Kopp, 1982). The fact that the toddlers with DS demanded less interaction from their caregivers than did the TD children suggests that overreliance on external sources of information does not imply expertise in social interaction (see Cebula et al., 2010, for a review). Rather, less self-generated, exploratory, and social behaviors place a demand *on the caregiver* to initiate social exchanges and provide opportunities for exploration and learning.

Parental Behavior May Matter More for Infants With DS

If infants with DS are less likely to explore their environment and initiate social exchanges, then their caregivers may take a more active role. Even though findings on parenting styles in DS are mixed (for a review, see Daunhauer et al., 2017), a number of observations of parent-child interaction have revealed that parents of children with DS are more directive than parents of TD children matched on chronological age (Soukup-Ascencao et al., 2016), mental age (Cielinski et al., 1995; Schworer et al., 2018; Venuti et al., 2009), or both (Roach et al., 1998). This is not dissimilar to observations in the study of children with DS interacting with their TD sibling (see previous discussion; Stoneman et al., 1987). There is some evidence that parenting style is associated with individual differences in the DS phenotype. For example, Gilmore and colleagues (2009) compared children with DS (and their mothers) to TD children matched on mental age (24–36 months) (and their mothers). The children were presented with a problem-solving task, and the ensuing parent-child interactions were observed. Although mothers of children with DS are often reported to be more directive, maternal style did not significantly differ across groups in this study, and mothers in both groups used similar verbal strategies (Gilmore et al., 2009). However, whereas maternal style was unrelated to task persistence in the TD children, greater persistence when working independently on a challenging task was observed in the children with DS whose mothers were more supportive of their autonomy (Gilmore et al., 2009). This suggests that parenting style may have more impact on children with DS than on TD children of the same mental age.

Of course, causal relationships cannot be inferred from correlational studies. The development of persistence in children with DS may be driven by parenting style. Alternatively, children who are more dependent on others may be more likely to elicit directive parenting behavior than children who are more independent. In addition, persistence may emerge through interactions among multiple diverse factors, of which internal motivation and parenting style are only two among many. Regardless of how it emerges, persistence in early childhood is associated with persistence in early adolescence in individuals with DS (Gilmore & Cuskelly, 2009).

If children with DS are less active and their caregivers are more directive, then learning and development in DS may be largely driven by the caregiver's selection of tasks. If caregivers do have more impact on developmental processes in infants with DS as compared to TD children, then the beliefs that parents hold about their children are likely to affect children with DS more than TD children. Yet, obtaining a "true" picture of an infant's current level of abilities if that infant has DS may be more challenging because infants with DS often present with an uneven profile with particular difficulties in the motor domain. This may make it more difficult for the caregiver to evaluate their child's developmental level and provide them with an appropriate amount and level of challenges—both of which are required for optimal learning (akin to a *zone of proximal development*; Vygotsky, 1978). Indeed, even though a group of children with DS at 18 and 24 months of mental age did not show any differences in task-directed behavior as compared to TD children of the same mental age, Glenn and colleagues (2001) found that their parents rated them as scoring lower on object-oriented play and general competence. This is consistent with evidence from young children with motor delay (Wang et al., 2013). The potential mismatch between what the parent believes their child is capable of and what the child is actually capable of may further exacerbate the child's difficulties. Thus, even though an immediate adaptive response to the more passive behaviors of infants with DS may be more directive behavior in the caregiver, in the long term it may be more beneficial for the caregiver to encourage the child with DS to take a more active role; stimulate them to generate, plan, and initiate actions; and steer them away from relying on others for motivation and self-control (Glenn et al., 2001).

Future Directions

Embracing Complexity

It is clear from the previous section that more research on infants with DS is needed in order to understand their development. The question is: what *type* of research? Most research (including our own) comprises group comparisons between TD individuals and individuals with DS (and/or other neurodevelopmental disorders). Sometimes it consists of associations between variables within a particular DS group. When planning the studies, we often think: *If only we could measure more variables, we would finally understand how infants with DS develop.* So we try to collect more information about the infants and their environment longitudinally (e.g., infant chronological age, infant mental age, health comorbidities, parental education, parenting style, sibling age, sleep patterns, family income, vocabulary size, memory abilities, attentional abilities, motor abilities); and when possible manipulate variables in order to understand their role in development. Thus, we study DS by first decomposing the system into separate units (the variables), and then by measuring/manipulating these units in order to understand their contribution to the system. In doing so, we are assuming that the system is *complicated but understandable as the sum of its parts.* Metaphorically, it is like trying to understand how fabric is made by cutting it into pieces, and then trying to reconstruct how each fiber fits together. But by taking apart the fabric, we no longer see how the fibers are *woven*. Yet the structure and functional properties of a fabric (e.g., its strength, breathability, warmth) are contingent on how the individual fibers are woven together. Likewise, the structure and functional properties of a living system are contingent on how the individual units interact with each other. This is because the living system is not *complicated* but *complex* (for the importance of this distinction, see Den Hartigh et al., 2017).

Complex systems cannot be understood by studying their parts in isolation; complexity emerges through dynamic multicausal interactions between interdependent, always-adapting components. It is very difficult—perhaps even impossible—to study all these interactions as the system adapts to and changes its environment over developmental time. But it is something to strive for—because it may not be possible to understand complex adaptive systems by breaking them down to their component parts, assigning each part a function, and then recomposing the system in a linear fashion. Embracing complexity necessitates a study of *interactions* (between and within different levels) as they unfold moment by moment. Such an approach has provided unexpected insights into typical development (as we demonstrate in what follows using the example of word learning) and thus we believe it is a very promising avenue for understanding how infants with DS develop.

As discussed in earlier sections, action-perception cycles are at the core of early development (Piaget, 1952; Thelen & Smith, 1994; Von Hofsten, 2004) and these are deeply embedded in social context (Adolph & Hoch, 2019). In fact, one of the most common contexts in which the developing child actively learns is parent-child interaction. During this free-flowing activity, parents direct or react to their child, while their child—who is often surrounded by interesting objects and in pursuit of their own goals—directs, reacts to, or ignores the activity of their parent. How do children learn in this rich (and thus potentially confusing) context? Traditional developmental research has been unable to answer this question, because it has predominantly used methods that require young children to sit and look at a computer screen (Fig. 8.3a). However, some studies now consider the child's embodied experiences in interaction with their parent by measuring gaze using head-mounted cameras/eye-trackers (Suarez-Rivera et al., 2019; Yoshida & Smith, 2008; Yu & Smith, 2012, 2013, 2016; Fig. 8.3c). This technology allows researchers to investigate the dynamic interplay between various components of parent-child interaction (Fig. 8.3e)—eye movements (visually selecting an object), hand movements (grasping an

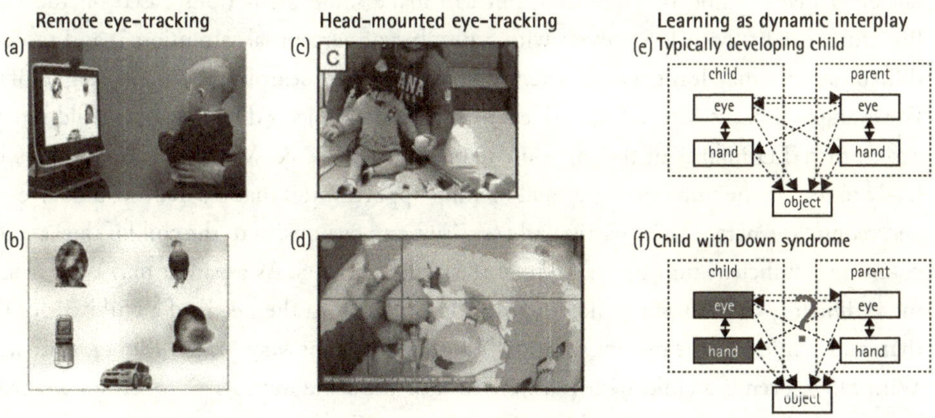

Figure 8.3. Comparison of (a) a remote eye-tracking setup with (c) a head-mounted eye-tracking setup. The remote eye-tracking setup allows researchers to track (b) the position of the eyes on a screen. Head-mounted eye-tracking enables researchers to record (d) the moment-by-moment gaze allocation of a child and a parent during naturalistic interaction, which captures (e) the dynamic interplay of various components in learning. Little is currently known about how learning unfolds moment by moment in (f) children with DS who often have perceptual, attentional, and motor difficulties. Image credit: (a) provided by Birkbeck Babylab; (b) modified from Task Engine—Face Popout (n.d.); (c) and (d) adapted from Slone et al. (2018); (e) and (f) modified from Yu & Smith (2013).

object), and speech (describing a grasped object)—which work together to form optimal learning moments in TD infants/toddlers (Yu & Smith, 2012).

Research on the interplay between different components of parent-child interaction (eyes, hands, speech) has been challenging fundamental assumptions about many aspects of early development, most notably word learning and language development in TD children. For example, from an adult's perspective it seems impossible for a child to learn the label for a single object in a cluttered visual scene containing multiple objects (the "referential ambiguity" problem; see Quine, 1960), yet researchers who take into account the children's perspective find that the problem of referential ambiguity disappears during parent-child interaction (Samuelson & McMurray, 2017; Yu & Smith, 2012). For example, Pereira and colleagues (2014) used a head-mounted camera to record gaze data from TD toddlers (16–25 months) as they played with novel objects while the parent spontaneously named them. They found that toddlers' allocation of attention is highly constrained by their hands/arms. Due to their limited reach, single objects often fill the toddler's field of view. Parents are sensitive to these moments and often provide labels for the object during them, eliminating the problem of referential ambiguity. In other words, in naturalistic settings, toddlers are not trying to learn labels by deducing what their caregivers are referring to; optimal word learning moments emerge from an interplay between eye movements (visually selecting an object), hand movements (grasping an object), and parental sensitivity (naming a grasped object) (Yu & Smith, 2012). This insight would have been missed had the variables been measured and analyzed separately.

How is this moment-by-moment learning constrained in infants with DS? We are currently investigating this question, but can make some predictions based on the DS literature. Infants with DS present with a number of perceptual, attentional, and motor difficulties that may limit the occurrence of optimal word learning moments (Fig. 8.3f). For example, infants with DS spend less time handling objects during parent-child interaction than TD infants of the same mental age (Legerstee & Weintraub, 1997). This is likely to reduce the number of optimal naming opportunities that a parent would have—and require the parent to be particularly sensitive and responsive to the child if they are to co-create a sufficient number of optimal learning moments. As a parent may experience more difficulty in evaluating and reacting appropriately to the needs of a child with DS than a TD child (see the previous section "Parental Behavior May Matter More for Infants With DS"), even if a child with DS were to hear the same number of tokens of a word, it may not occur during optimal learning moments. Furthermore, even if the child were to hear the word during an optimal learning moment, other processes necessary for word learning are often atypical in children with DS. As we mentioned previously, reduced neural plasticity and atypical information processing may mean that infants with DS require more repetition than is typically necessary (for a computational model showing an atypical associative learning mechanism in DS, see Tovar et al., 2018). Also sleep, which plays an important role in learning and memory (and thus in word learning), develops atypically in individuals with DS (D'Souza, D'Souza, Horváth, et al., 2020; Edgin et al., 2015; for discussion of other constraints on language learning in DS, see D'Souza, D'Souza, et al., 2017). To understand how infants with DS learn, it is thus necessary to embrace complexity and employ multiple methodologies (neuroimaging, head-mounted eye-tracking, movement sensors, etc.) across different timescales, with both the infant and their social partners as they interact in naturalistic settings. This approach could help us to understand why infants with DS diverge in their trajectories from TD infants and whether there is a DS-specific pathway.

Diverging Trajectories

As infants with DS get older, they seem to progressively diverge from their TD peers. For example, a decline in standardized cognitive and motor scores in children with DS, relative to TD children, was found in Carr's landmark longitudinal study of children who were tested at 6 weeks, 6 months, 10 months, 15 months, and 24 months of age (Carr, 1970).[5] This decline was particularly steep from 10 to 15 months of age. In other words, as children with DS develop, their standardized scores fall further behind those of their TD peers. This divergence is particularly pronounced for their areas of relative difficulties, giving rise to the classic profile associated with individuals with DS. Carr (1970) reported that from 6 months of age, mean standardized motor score was lower than mean standardized cognitive score in children with DS. A deceleration of development with increasing chronological age in children with DS has also been found in other studies, as has the finding that motor standardized scores lag behind cognitive standardized scores (Harris, 1981; LaVeck & LaVeck, 1977). Increased divergence over developmental time has also been found in expressive language, another area of relative difficulty in children with DS. While expressive language ability was at an appropriate level for almost 50% of 22-month-old children with DS given their mental age and receptive language ability, this was the case for only 21% of them 2 years later (Miller, 1992).

In order to understand why the trajectories of infants with DS diverge from those of TD infants, as well as how a DS-specific phenotype might emerge, the interactions of various constraints require longitudinal investigations across a range of domains. These investigations may benefit from comparing different disorders, as many constraints are unlikely to be specific to DS. In fact, it is likely that different disorders share similar constraints in early development, but particular clusters of constraints, or their intensity or co-occurrence, or the timing of the interactions between them, may increase the likelihood that disorder-specific phenotypes emerge. The converse may also apply: different constraints may give rise to similar phenotypes through common adaptations (Johnson, 2017; Oliver et al., 2000). For this reason, a multilevel, cross-syndrome, developmental approach to studying disorders is needed.

Individual Differences

Although a DS-specific phenotype has been described, individual differences in DS are vast on all levels of description (genetic, cellular, brain, cognition, behavior, social context; for examples, see Karmiloff-Smith et al., 2016). Large variability can already be detected early in development, including in the domains that at the group level have been identified as areas of relative difficulty. In the gross motor domain, while the average age of walking in TD children is 13 months and the age ranges from 9 to 17 months, most children with DS learn to walk between 18 and 36 months of age—with some DS children unable to walk even at 4 years of age (Palisano et al., 2001; see also Winders et al., 2019 for variability in motor development in children with DS). In the expressive language domain, in one longitudinal study of expressive vocabulary size in children with DS, the lowest-scoring child was nonverbal at 36 months, while the expressive vocabulary size of the highest-scoring child was close to the normal range (243 words; Zampini & D'Odorico, 2009). When the same children were assessed 6 months later, the nonverbal child remained nonverbal, while the child with the most developed language had doubled their expressive vocabulary size to nearly 500 words.

The fact that large variability exists in individuals with DS raises the question of whether it is possible to identify a single DS-specific profile. In other words, to what extent can the classic DS profile be applied to all young children with DS, when the individual differences seem so vast? Indeed, Tsao and Kindelberger (2009) identified four distinct cognitive profiles for children with DS between 6 and 11 years of age. Subgroups seem to be possible to detect even in infants with DS. Fidler, Schworer, Prince, and colleagues (2019) observed visual, manual, and oral exploration in 9-month-old infants with DS and found that they could differentiate between two subgroups: "active" and "passive". Subgrouping with a wider range of domains in younger children with DS may therefore be a fruitful approach—albeit a challenging one, as it would require large sample sizes with children of similar chronological age, ideally followed longitudinally at the same timepoints.

Although individual differences are often averaged out in DS studies in order to "extract" general developmental mechanisms, the individual differences themselves afford a window onto these mechanisms. For example, on the genetic level, while variability in the genetic origin of DS has been proposed to contribute to variation in the phenotype (e.g., mosaicism; for a review, see Papavassiliou et al., 2015), the contribution of genetic background effects (i.e., all the genes that infants with DS inherit from their parents) has received less focus. Would a child's genetic background have very little effect on the developmental path cleaved out by trisomy 21? Or can variation in this genetic background contribute to variation in the emerging DS phenotype? In older adults, variation in the apolipoprotein E (*APOE*) gene on chromosome 19 is related to variation in Alzheimer's disease (AD), both in individuals with DS (who are already at high risk for AD) and in the general population (Prasher et al., 2008; van der Lee et al., 2018). Interestingly, the *e4* allele of *APOE* (*APOE e4*) that relates to increased AD risk later in life is associated with an attentional *advantage* in early development in DS (D'Souza, Mason, et al., 2020), potentially through variation in myelination (Dean et al., 2014). Can these small but early differences in attentional abilities constrain the emergence of higher-level functions such as language in individuals with DS (D'Souza, D'Souza, et al., 2017; Karmiloff-Smith, 1998)? Indeed, we found that infants and toddlers (either with or without DS) with better attentional abilities demonstrate better language abilities than those whose attentional abilities are worse (D'Souza, D'Souza, Jones, et al., 2020). These findings dovetail with the perspective that higher-level functions (like language) gradually emerge through manifold interactions across levels and developmental time (roughly, from variation in genes, through variation in attention, to variation in language[6]). Although these studies are correlational, when taken together they illustrate how individual differences might be an important focus of research. A mechanistic understanding of the within-syndrome heterogeneity may thus provide us with greater power to predict outcomes and tailor interventions to individuals.

Getting the Interventions Right

If we view the DS phenotype as an adaptive response to atypical constraints, and take into consideration the fact that its divergence from the typical path becomes increasingly pronounced over time, with increases in individual differences over time too, it becomes apparent that early interventions are likely to have the most impact. Therefore, rather than building interventions around later-emerging relative strengths and weaknesses, a more useful strategy might be to alter constraints early in development to improve the child's present and future quality of life. This does not mean that interventions should aim to steer the child back toward the typical path, a process that might be neither possible nor desirable. It means that interventions should alter constraints to ensure that the system does not adapt in ways that might make life more difficult later on. Because development is constrained by factors across many interconnected domains, the most successful interventions are likely to be the ones that target multiple domains simultaneously.

Behavioral interventions: Early enough? Intense enough? The need for behavioral therapy programs to maximize developmental outcomes in infants with DS has been recognized across domains (e.g., speech and language therapy, physiotherapy, occupational therapy). It is crucial that these start early enough in development. For example, consider motor development, one of the earliest difficulties reported in children with DS. As we outlined previously, motor abilities constrain how infants interact with their environment, and difficulties in this area may have cascading effects on other domains such as social and language development. Therefore, infants must be engaged early in actively moving their bodies to build muscle strength and minimize motor delay. This is likely to increase self-driven exploration. Although it is difficult to establish the frequency and intensity of therapy required to significantly improve muscle strength and motor control in infants with DS, from what is known about TD infants, self-driven practice is extensive in typical development, as toddlers produce around 14,000 steps per day (Adolph et al., 2012). Young children with DS will likely require even more repetitions considering their reduced neural plasticity. How could such high-intensity intervention be feasibly delivered to infants with DS? Due to limited resources, the most viable pathway for delivering high intensity therapy is through engaging the caregivers. Ulrich and colleagues implemented this approach in a series of studies using a portable pediatric treadmill (Fig. 8.4a) to develop trunk and leg control and strength in infants with DS. Caregivers held their infants upright on a mini-treadmill for 8 minutes a day, 5 days a week. This amounted to an upper limit of about 960 steps per training session. This may be well short of the amount of activity spontaneously generated by TD children, yet this intervention was shown to reduce delay in walking onset in children with DS by an average of 3 months (Ulrich 2010; Ulrich et al., 2001). A more individually tailored version of this intervention, with the addition of small weights, led to even greater gains, bringing forward walking onset by 5 months (Angulo-Barroso et al., 2008; Ulrich et al., 2008). Although this may not seem much from the perspective of adult timescales, walking provides children with a very different set of experiences (Karasik et al., 2014), and every month spent not walking affects how the infant with DS interacts with the world, which may have cascading effects on other developing domains and alter the child's developmental trajectory (Yamauchi et al., 2019).

As the treadmill intervention demonstrated, therapies that are tailored to the needs of the individual seem to provide the largest effect. In the motor domain, a number of possible interventions have been developed which can be applied to different developmental stages, scaffolding development one step at a time. These include tummy time (Wentz, 2017), the Kick and Drive Gym (Lloyd & Ulrich, 2006), sticky mittens (Libertus et al., 2016; but cf. Corbetta et al., 2016), the Playskin Lift garment (Lobo et al., 2016), and the Go Baby Go car (Hospodar et al., 2021; Logan et al., 2017). When appropriate, a combination of these interventions may facilitate outcomes. For example, the treadmill may enable infants with DS to achieve a number of steps, or the type of step, they would not otherwise be able to self-generate, but it does not provide aspects of locomotion such

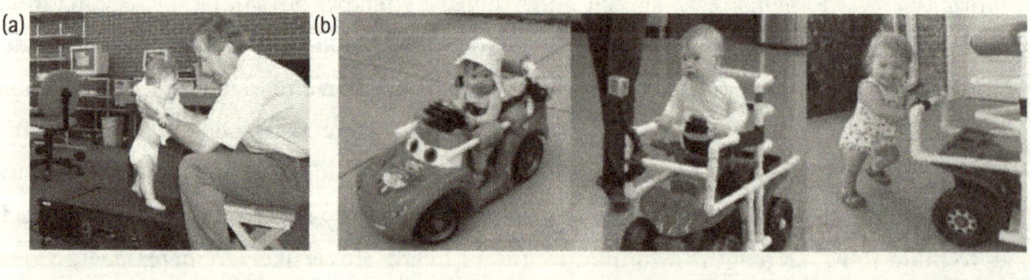

Figure 8.4. (a) Infant stepping during treadmill training. Photo provided by D. A. Ulrich. (b) Modified ride-on car which "grows" with the child. Adapted from Hospodar et al. (2021). Image credits: (a) D. A. Ulrich; (b) reproduced by permission of Taylor & Francis.

as visual flow or the experience of reaching new people and objects. This is something that Go Baby Go, a modified ride-on car, can provide. As the child grows, the car can be adjusted to "grow" with them, from seated, to standing, to walking (see Fig. 8.4b). This provides an experience that would be enjoyable and sufficiently challenging for the child to self-generate locomotion but not too challenging that it becomes discouraging. Therefore, a combined intervention utilizing both the motorized treadmill and self-generated ride-on car might enhance intervention gains.

It may also be advantageous to combine different types of interventions across domains. For example, as we discussed earlier in this chapter, motor activity is embedded in social interaction. Indeed, Ulrich (2010) notes that parents often reported enjoying treadmill intervention time, as it provided them with "face time" to spend in interaction with their infants. Therefore, as long as it is not too demanding on the child, one approach might be to integrate movement therapy with other types of therapies (e.g., speech and language therapy), rather than targeting each domain in separate sessions.

Ready for pharmacological interventions? The principle of behavioral intervention is to capitalize on brain plasticity by increasing stimulation. However, as noted earlier, plasticity itself is reduced in infants with DS. Therefore, preclinical research has often focused on identifying pharmacological targets for altering neural constraints (for a review, see the collection edited by Dierssen, 2020). However, translating preclinical research to human clinical trials presents some serious challenges (Lee et al., 2020; Zhu et al., 2019). One of them involves a lack of available tools that can accurately measure intervention-related changes across domains in individuals with DS (d'Ardhuy et al., 2015; Hedge et al., 2018). This is especially the case for studies involving infants and young children (D'Souza et al., 2021; Lee et al., 2020). Yet, obtaining accurate measurements across domains is crucial, as some pharmacological interventions (e.g., fluoxetine) have been suggested even for fetuses with DS (Bartesaghi et al., 2015; Guedj et al., 2014; Guidi et al., 2014; for an ethical discussion, see de Wert et al., 2017).[7] As discussed previously, because the developing system is highly interconnected, altering the chemical properties of one part may have unpredictable and widespread effects on the entire system. For example, it has been suggested that SSRI medications, which include fluoxetine, may have detrimental effects in pregnancy, including increased risk of heart defects, brain and craniofacial abnormalities, neonatal seizures, and changes in neurodevelopment and behavior (for review, see Ortega-Alves & Urato, 2016). Therefore, high quality outcome measures are needed both to capture domains in which gains would be expected (such as improved learning) and to reliably measure any negative effects a pharmacological intervention may have.

Conclusions

Compared to many other neurodevelopmental disorders, DS is often diagnosed—and therefore can be studied—very early in development. This provides us with a unique window onto early developmental processes. Rather than describing DS as a static assemblage of relative strength and difficulties, we have emphasized the importance of viewing DS as an adaptive system with a different start state (i.e., trisomy 21). We have argued that trisomy 21 has cascading effects on the adapting system, such as how it processes information and explores the environment. This may in turn lead to adaptations such as overreliance on social agents. These adaptations may be useful in the short term, but they are likely to constrain the emergence of functions later in development. Taking a developmental perspective may therefore help us to understand how the DS phenotype emerges, and what the best intervention approaches are likely to be.

Acknowledgments

Hana D'Souza is the Beatrice Mary Dale Research Fellow, supported by Newnham College (University of Cambridge) and the Isaac Newton Trust. Our work is further supported by the Waterloo Foundation and the Baily Thomas Charitable Fund.

Notes

1. In the past few years alone, there have been many reviews and meta-analyses in the DS field on topics such as pediatric brain development (Hamner et al., 2018), functional magnetic resonance imaging (fMRI) (Carbó-Carreté et al., 2020), the infant foundations of cognition (Fidler, Needham, et al., 2019), joint attention (Hahn et al., 2018), physical therapy (Ruiz-González et al., 2019), and memory (Godfrey & Lee, 2018), as well as a more general primer on DS (Antonarakis et al., 2020) and numerous reviews on neurobiological research and its implications for therapy (e.g., Lee et al., 2020; Stagni et al., 2018; Vacca et al., 2019; see also the collection edited by Dierssen, 2020).
2. Like Ulrich (2010), we (e.g., D'Souza & D'Souza, 2019) use the phrase "developmental systems" to refer to a cluster of (non-nativist) perspectives that share some (or all) of the core tenets of "developmental systems theory" (Ford & Lerner, 1992; Oyama, 1985; Oyama et al., 2001) and that view neurocognitive and motor development as the emergent functions of a complex adaptive system constrained by an intricate web of interactions between manifold factors (Blumberg, 2017). These perspectives include connectionism (Elman et al., 1996; McClelland & Vallabha, 2009; Rosenblatt, 1958), dynamic systems theory (Thelen, 1992; Thelen & Smith, 1994), and neuroconstructivism (Westermann et al., 2007).
3. We could have used the word "scale" instead of "levels," from small (genes) to large (society). We only use the word "level" because it is a familiar term, and one could argue that structures such as the brain and society emerge from more basic layers of organization such as atoms and molecules.
4. However, this may be highly constrained by the level of society and change with changing societal attitudes toward people with disabilities (Shogren et al., 2017).
5. These children have been followed across the life span (e.g., Carr & Collins, 2018).
6. One might then expect to find a relationship between *APOE e4* and language ability (for some suggestive analysis, see Thomas et al., 2020).
7. A pilot feasibility trial of perinatal fluoxetine treatment at the University of Texas was proposed in 2014 (as mentioned in Martínez Cué & Dierssen, 2020) but has yet to share any findings.

References

Ábrahám, H., Vincze, A., Veszprémi, B., Kravják, A., Gömöri, É., Kovács, G. G., & Seress, L. (2012). Impaired myelination of the human hippocampal formation in Down syndrome. *International Journal of Developmental Neuroscience, 30*(2), 147–158. https://doi.org/10.1016/J.IJDEVNEU.2011.11.005

Abramovitch, R., Stanhope, L., Pepler, D., & Corter, C. (1987). Influence of Down's syndrome on sibling interaction. *Journal of Child Psychology and Psychiatry, 28*(6), 865–879. https://doi.org/10.1111/j.1469-7610.1987.tb00675.x

Adolph, K. E., Cole, W. G., Komati, M., Garciaguirre, J. S., Badaly, D., Lingeman, J. M., Chan, G. L. Y., & Sotsky, R. B. (2012). How do you learn to walk? Thousands of steps and dozens of falls per day. *Psychological Science*, *23*(11), 1387–1394. https://doi.org/10.1177/0956797612446346

Adolph, K. E., & Hoch, J. E. (2019). Motor development: Embodied, embedded, enculturated, and enabling. *Annual Review of Psychology*, *70*(1), 141–164. https://doi.org/10.1146/annurev-psych-010418-102836

Åkerström, M. S., & Sanner, G. (1993). Movement patterns in children with Down's syndrome: A pilot study. *Physiotherapy Theory and Practice*, *9*(1), 33–41. https://doi.org/10.3109/09593989309036484

Almeida, R. G., & Lyons, D. A. (2017). On myelinated axon plasticity and neuronal circuit formation and function. *Journal of Neuroscience*, *37*(42), 10023–10034. https://doi.org/10.1523/JNEUROSCI.3185-16.2017

Alsaied, T., Marino, B. S., Esbensen, A. J., Anixt, J. S., Epstein, J. N., & Cnota, J. F. (2016). Does congenital heart disease affect neurodevelopmental outcomes in children with Down syndrome? *Congenital Heart Disease*, *11*(1), 26–33. https://doi.org/10.1111/chd.12322

Anderson, J. S., Nielsen, J. A., Ferguson, M. A., Burback, M. C., Cox, E. T., Dai, L., Gerig, G., Edgin, J. O., & Korenberg, J. R. (2013). Abnormal brain synchrony in Down syndrome. *NeuroImage: Clinical*, *2*, 703–715. https://doi.org/10.1016/j.nicl.2013.05.006

Angulo-Barroso, R., Burghardt, A. R., Lloyd, M. C., & Ulrich, D. A. (2008). Physical activity in infants with Down syndrome receiving a treadmill intervention. *Infant Behavior and Development*, *31*(2), 255–269. https://doi.org/10.1016/j.infbeh.2007.10.003

Antonarakis, S. E. (2017). Down syndrome and the complexity of genome dosage imbalance. *Nature Reviews Genetics*, *18*(3), 147–163. https://doi.org/10.1038/nrg.2016.154

Antonarakis, S. E., Skotko, B. G., Rafii, M. S., Strydom, A., Pape, S. E., Bianchi, D. W., Sherman, S. L., & Reeves, R. H. (2020). Down syndrome. *Nature Reviews Disease Primers*, *6*(1), 9. https://doi.org/10.1038/s41572-019-0143-7

Barnet, A. B., Elizabeth, Ohlrich S., & Shanks, B. L. (1971). EEG evoked responses to repetitive auditory stimulation in normal and Down's syndrome infants. *Developmental Medicine & Child Neurology*, *13*(3), 321–329. https://doi.org/10.1111/j.1469-8749.1971.tb03269.x

Bartesaghi, R., Haydar, T. F., Delabar, J. M., Dierssen, M., Martinez-Cue, C., & Bianchi, D. W. (2015). New perspectives for the rescue of cognitive disability in Down syndrome. *Journal of Neuroscience*, *35*(41), 13843–13852. https://doi.org/10.1523/JNEUROSCI.2775-15.2015

Bassett, D. S., & Sporns, O. (2017). Network neuroscience. *Nature Neuroscience*, *20*(3), 353–364. https://doi.org/10.1038/nn.4502

Bates, E. A., Reilly, J., Wulfeck, B., Dronkers, N., Opie, M., Fenson, J., Kriz, S., Jeffries, R., Miller, L., & Herbst, K. (2001). Differential effects of unilateral lesions on language production in children and adults. *Brain and Language*, *79*(2), 223–265. https://doi.org/10.1006/brln.2001.2482

Becker, L. E., Armstrong, D. L., & Chan, F. (1986). Dendritic atrophy in children with Down's syndrome. *Annals of Neurology*, *20*(4), 520–526. https://doi.org/10.1002/ana.410200413

Benavides-Piccione, R., Ballesteros-Yáñez, I., de Lagrán, M. M., Elston, G., Estivill, X., Fillat, C., Defelipe, J., & Dierssen, M. (2004). On dendrites in Down syndrome and DS murine models: A spiny way to learn. *Progress in Neurobiology*, *74*(2), 111–126. https://doi.org/10.1016/j.pneurobio.2004.08.001

Berger, J., & Cunningham, C. C. (1981). The development of eye contact between mothers and normal versus Down's syndrome infants. *Developmental Psychology*, *17*(5), 678–689. https://doi.org/10.1037/0012-1649.17.5.678

Berger, S. E., Harbourne, R. T., Arman, F., & Sonsini, J. (2019). Balancing act(ion): Attentional and postural control strategies predict extent of infants' perseveration in a sitting and reaching task. *Cognitive Development*, *50*, 13–21. https://doi.org/10.1016/J.COGDEV.2018.12.001

Berger, S. E., Harbourne, R. T., & Horger, M. N. (2018). Cognition–action trade-offs reflect organization of attention in infancy. *Advances in Child Development and Behavior*, *54*, 45–86. https://doi.org/10.1016/BS.ACDB.2017.11.001

Block, M. E. (1991). Motor development in children with Down syndrome: A review of the literature. *Adapted Physical Activity Quarterly*, *8*(3), 179–209. https://doi.org/10.1123/apaq.8.3.179

Blumberg, M. S. (2017). Development evolving: The origins and meanings of instinct. *Wiley Interdisciplinary Reviews: Cognitive Science*, *8*(1–2), e1371. https://doi.org/10.1002/wcs.1371

Bornstein, M. H., & Sigman, M. D. (1986). Continuity in mental development from infancy. *Child Development*, *57*(2), 251–274. https://doi.org/10.2307/1130581

Bornstein, M. H., & Tamis-LeMonda, C. S. (1989). Maternal responsiveness and cognitive development in children. *New Directions for Child and Adolescent Development, 1989*(43), 49–61. https://doi.org/10.1002/cd.23219894306

Boudreau, J. P., & Bushnell, E. W. (2000). Spilling thoughts: Configuring attentional resources in infants' goal-directed actions. *Infant Behavior and Development, 23*(3–4), 543–566. https://doi.org/10.1016/S0163-6383(01)00059-5

Bourgeois, J. P. (2001). Synaptogenesis in the neocortex of the newborn: The ultimate frontier for individuation? In C. A. Nelson & M. Luciana (Eds.), *Handbook of developmental cognitive neuroscience* (pp. 23–34). MIT Press. https://doi.org/https://doi.org/10.7551/mitpress/7437.001.0001

Brandt, B. R. (1996). Impaired tactual perception in children with Down's syndrome. *Scandinavian Journal of Psychology, 37*(3), 312–316. https://doi.org/10.1111/j.1467-9450.1996.tb00663.x

Bremner, J. G., & Fogel, A. (2004). *Blackwell handbook of infant development.* Blackwell Publishing Ltd. https://doi.org/10.1002/9780470996348

Bruni, M., Cameron, D., Dua, S., & Noy, S. (2010). Reported sensory processing of children with Down syndrome. *Physical & Occupational Therapy in Pediatrics, 30*(4), 280–293. https://doi.org/10.3109/01942638.2010.486962

Buzsáki, G. (2004). Large-scale recording of neuronal ensembles. *Nature Neuroscience, 7*(5), 446–451. https://doi.org/10.1038/nn1233

Buzsáki, G. (2006). *Rhythms of the brain.* Oxford University Press. https://doi.org/https://doi.org/10.1093/acprof:oso/9780195301069.001.0001

Bybee, J., & Zigler, E. (1998). Outerdirectedness in individuals with and without mental retardation: A review. In E. Zigler & D. Bennett-Gates (Eds.), *Handbook of mental retardation and development* (pp. 165–205). Cambridge University Press.

Campos, J. J., Anderson, D. D. I., Barbu-Roth, M. A., Hubbard, E. M., Hertenstein, M. J., & Witherington, D. (2000). Travel broadens the mind. *Infancy, 1*(2), 149–219. https://doi.org/10.1207/S15327078IN0102_1

Carbó-Carreté, M., Cañete-Massé, C., Peró-Cebollero, M., & Guàrdia-Olmos, J. (2020). Using fMRI to assess brain activity in people with Down syndrome: A systematic review. *Frontiers in Human Neuroscience, 14*, 147. https://doi.org/10.3389/fnhum.2020.00147

Cardoso, A. C., Campos, A. C., Santos, M. M., Santos, D. C., & Rocha, N. A. (2015). Motor performance of children with Down syndrome and typical development at 2 to 4 and 26 months. *Pediatric Physical Therapy, 27*(2), 135–141. https://doi.org/10.1097/pep.0000000000000120

Carr, J. (1970). Mental and motor development in young mongol children. *Journal of Mental Deficiency Research, 14*(3), 205–220. https://doi.org/https://doi.org/10.1111/j.1365-2788.1970.tb01116.x

Carr, J., & Collins, S. (2018). 50 years with Down syndrome: A longitudinal study. *Journal of Applied Research in Intellectual Disabilities, 31*(5), 743–750. https://doi.org/10.1111/jar.12438

Carvajal, F., & Iglesias, J. (2000). Looking behavior and smiling in Down syndrome infants. *Journal of Nonverbal Behavior, 24*(3), 225–236. https://doi.org/10.1023/A:1006693121491

Carvalho, R. P., Tudella, E., Caljouw, S. R., & Savelsbergh, G. J. P. (2008). Early control of reaching: Effects of experience and body orientation. *Infant Behavior and Development, 31*(1), 23–33. https://doi.org/10.1016/j.infbeh.2007.06.001

Cebula, K. R., Moore, D. G., & Wishart, J. G. (2010). Social cognition in children with Down's syndrome: Challenges to research and theory building. *Journal of Intellectual Disability Research, 54*(2), 113–134. https://doi.org/10.1111/j.1365-2788.2009.01215.x

Chakrabarti, L., Galdzicki, Z., & Haydar, T. F. (2007). Defects in embryonic neurogenesis and initial synapse formation in the forebrain of the Ts65Dn mouse model of Down syndrome. *Journal of Neuroscience, 27*(43), 11483–11495. https://doi.org/10.1523/JNEUROSCI.3406-07.2007

Chapman, R. S., & Hesketh, L. (2001). Language, cognition, and short-term memory in individuals with Down syndrome. *Down Syndrome Research and Practice, 7*(1), 1–7. https://doi.org/10.3104/reviews.108

Chen, C., Jiang, P., Xue, H., Peterson, S. E., Tran, H. T., McCann, A. E., Parast, M. M., Li, S., Pleasure, D. E., Laurent, L. C., Loring, J. F., Liu, Y., & Deng, W. (2014). Role of astroglia in Down's syndrome revealed by patient-derived human-induced pluripotent stem cells. *Nature Communications, 5*, 4430. https://doi.org/10.1038/ncomms5430

Cherubini, E., Gaiarsa, J. L., & Ben-Ari, Y. (1991). GABA: An excitatory transmitter in early postnatal life. *Trends in Neurosciences, 14*(12), 515–519. https://doi.org/10.1016/0166-2236(91)90003-d

Cielinski, K. L., Vaughn, B. E., Seifer, R., & Contreras, J. (1995). Relations among sustained engagement during play, quality of play, and mother-child interaction in samples of children with Down syndrome and normally developing toddlers. *Infant Behavior and Development, 18*(2), 163–176. https://doi.org/10.1016/0163-6383(95)90046-2

Clearfield, M. W., Osborne, C. N., & Mullen, M. (2008). Learning by looking: Infants' social looking behavior across the transition from crawling to walking. *Journal of Experimental Child Psychology, 100*(4), 297–307. https://doi.org/10.1016/j.jecp.2008.03.005

Colman, H., Nabekura, J., & Lichtman, J. W. (1997). Alterations in synaptic strength preceding axon withdrawal. *Science, 275*(5298), 356–361. https://doi.org/10.1126/science.275.5298.356

Contestabile, A., Magara, S., & Cancedda, L. (2017). The GABAergic hypothesis for cognitive disabilities in Down syndrome. *Frontiers in Cellular Neuroscience, 11*, 54. https://doi.org/10.3389/fncel.2017.00054

Corbetta, D., & Bojczyk, K. E. (2002). Infants return to two-handed reaching when they are learning to walk. *Journal of Motor Behavior, 34*(1), 83–95. https://doi.org/10.1080/00222890209601933

Corbetta, D., Williams, J. L., & Haynes, J. M. (2016). Bare fingers, but no obvious influence of "prickly" Velcro! In the absence of parents' encouragement, it is not clear that "sticky mittens" provide an advantage to the process of learning to reach. *Infant Behavior and Development, 42*, 168–178. https://doi.org/10.1016/j.infbeh.2015.05.001

Cowan, W. M. (1979). The development of the brain. *Scientific American, 241*(3), 113–133. https://doi.org/https://doi.org/10.1038/scientificamerican0979-112

Cowie, V. (1970). *A study of the early development of mongols*. Pergamon.

Crone, E. A. (2014). Cognitive control and affective decision making in childhood and adolescence. In M. S. Gazzaniga & G. R. Mangun (Eds.), *The cognitive neurosciences* (5th ed., pp. 23–32). MIT Press.

d'Ardhuy, X. L., Edgin, J. O., Bouis, C., de Sola, S., Goeldner, C., Kishnani, P., Nöldeke, J., Rice, S., Sacco, S., Squassante, L., Spiridigliozzi, G., Visootsak, J., Heller, J., & Khwaja, O. (2015). Assessment of cognitive scales to examine memory, executive function and language in individuals with Down syndrome: Implications of a 6-month observational study. *Frontiers in Behavioral Neuroscience, 9*, 300. https://doi.org/10.3389/fnbeh.2015.00300

D'Souza, D., & D'Souza, H. (2019). Emergent and constrained: Understanding brain and cognitive development. *Journal of Neurolinguistics, 49*, 228–231. https://doi.org/10.1016/j.jneuroling.2018.04.011

D'Souza, D., D'Souza, H., Horváth, K., Plunkett, K., & Karmiloff-Smith, A. (2020). Sleep is atypical across neurodevelopmental disorders in infants and toddlers: A cross-syndrome study. *Research in Developmental Disabilities, 97*, 103549. https://doi.org/10.1016/J.RIDD.2019.103549

D'Souza, D., D'Souza, H., Johnson, M. H., & Karmiloff-Smith, A. (2015). Concurrent relations between face scanning and language: A cross-syndrome infant study. *PLoS ONE, 10*(10), e0139319. https://doi.org/10.1371/journal.pone.0139319

D'Souza, D., D'Souza, H., Johnson, M. H., & Karmiloff-Smith, A. (2016). Audio-visual speech perception in infants and toddlers with Down syndrome, fragile X syndrome, and Williams syndrome. *Infant Behavior and Development, 44*, 249–262. https://doi.org/10.1016/j.infbeh.2016.07.002

D'Souza, D., D'Souza, H., Jones, E. J. H., & Karmiloff-Smith, A. (2020). Attentional abilities constrain language development: A cross-syndrome infant/toddler study. *Developmental Science, 23*(6), e12961. https://doi.org/10.1111/desc.12961

D'Souza, D., D'Souza, H., & Karmiloff-Smith, A. (2017). Precursors to language development in typically and atypically developing infants and toddlers: The importance of embracing complexity. *Journal of Child Language, 44*(3), 591–627. https://doi.org/10.1017/S030500091700006X

D'Souza, D., & Karmiloff-Smith, A. (2011). When modularization fails to occur: A developmental perspective. *Cognitive Neuropsychology, 28*(3–4), 276–287. https://doi.org/10.1080/02643294.2011.614939

D'Souza, D., & Karmiloff-Smith, A. (2016). Why a developmental perspective is critical for understanding human cognition. *Behavioral and Brain Sciences, 39*, e122. https://doi.org/10.1017/S0140525X15001569

D'Souza, H., Brady, D., Wiseman, F. K., Good, M. A., & Thomas, M. S. C. (2021). Aligning cognitive studies in mouse models and human infants/toddlers: The case of Down syndrome. In M. S. C. Thomas, D. Mareschal, & V. Knowland (Eds.), *Taking development seriously: A Festschrift for Annette Karmiloff-Smith: Neuroconstructivism and the multi-disciplinary approach to understanding the emergence of mind* (pp. 213–238). Routledge. https://doi.org/10.4324/9780429445590-16-16

D'Souza, H., Cowie, D., Karmiloff-Smith, A., & Bremner, A. J. (2017). Specialization of the motor system in infancy: From broad tuning to selectively specialized purposeful actions. *Developmental Science, 20*(4), e12409. https://doi.org/10.1111/desc.12409

D'Souza, H., & Karmiloff-Smith, A. (2017). Neurodevelopmental disorders. *Wiley Interdisciplinary Reviews: Cognitive Science, 8*(1–2), e1398. https://doi.org/10.1002/wcs.1398

D'Souza, H., Lathan, A., Karmiloff-Smith, A., & Mareschal, D. (2020). Down syndrome and parental depression: A double hit on early expressive language development. *Research in Developmental Disabilities, 100*, 103613. https://doi.org/10.1016/j.ridd.2020.103613

D'Souza, H., Mason, L., Mok, K. Y., Startin, C. M., Hamburg, S., Hithersay, R., Baksh, R. A. A., Hardy, J., Strydom, A., & Thomas, M. S. C. (2020). Differential associations of Apolipoprotein E ε4 genotype with attentional abilities across the life span of individuals with Down syndrome. *JAMA Network Open, 3*(9), e2018221. https://doi.org/10.1001/jamanetworkopen.2020.18221

Daunhauer, L. A., Schworer, E., & Howshar, M. (2017). Parenting matters: Parent–child interactions in Down syndrome and recommendations for future research. *International Review of Research in Developmental Disabilities, 53*, 1–43. https://doi.org/10.1016/BS.IRRDD.2017.08.003

de Campos, A. C., da Costa, C. S. N., Savelsbergh, G. J. P., & Rocha, N. A. C. F. (2013). Infants with Down syndrome and their interactions with objects: Development of exploratory actions after reaching onset. *Research in Developmental Disabilities, 34*(6), 1906–1916. https://doi.org/10.1016/j.ridd.2013.03.001

De Felipe, J., Marco, P., Fairén, A., & Jones, E. G. (1997). Inhibitory synaptogenesis in mouse somatosensory cortex. *Cerebral Cortex, 7*(7), 619–634. https://doi.org/10.1093/cercor/7.7.619

de Wert, G., Dondorp, W., & Bianchi, D. W. (2017). Fetal therapy for Down syndrome: An ethical exploration. *Prenatal Diagnosis, 37*(3), 222–228. https://doi.org/10.1002/pd.4995

Dean, D. C., Jerskey, B. A., Chen, K., Protas, H., Thiyyagura, P., Roontiva, A., O'Muircheartaigh, J., Dirks, H., Waskiewicz, N., Lehman, K., Siniard, A. L., Turk, M. N., Hua, X., Madsen, S. K., Thompson, P. M., Fleisher, A. S., Huentelman, M. J., Deoni, S. C. L., & Reiman, E. M. (2014). Brain differences in infants at differential genetic risk for late-onset Alzheimer disease. *JAMA Neurology, 71*(1), 11–22. https://doi.org/10.1001/jamaneurol.2013.4544

Deckers, S. R. J., Van Zaalen, Y., Van Balkom, H., & Verhoeven, L. (2019). Predictors of receptive and expressive vocabulary development in children with Down syndrome. *International Journal of Speech-Language Pathology, 21*(1), 10–22. https://doi.org/10.1080/17549507.2017.1363290

Den Hartigh, R. J. R., Cox, R. F. A., & Van Geert, P. L. C. (2017). Complex versus complicated models of cognition. In L. Magnani & T. Bertolotti (Eds.), *Springer handbook of model-based science* (pp. 657–669). Springer. https://doi.org/10.1007/978-3-319-30526-4_30

Díaz, F., & Zurron, M. (1995). Auditory evoked potentials in Down's syndrome. *Electroencephalography and Clinical Neurophysiology/Evoked Potentials Section, 96*(6), 526–537. https://doi.org/10.1016/0013-4694(95)00080-I

Dichter, M. A., & Ayala, G. F. (1987). Cellular mechanisms of epilepsy: A status report. *Science, 237*(4811), 157–164. https://doi.org/10.1126/science.3037700

Dierssen, M. (2012). Down syndrome: The brain in trisomic mode. *Nature Reviews Neuroscience, 13*(12), 844–858. https://doi.org/10.1038/nrn3314

Dierssen, M. (2020). Preclinical research in Down syndrome: Insights for pathophysiology and treatments. In Mara Dierssen (Ed.), *Progress in Brain Research* (Vol. 251, pp. 2–302). Elsevier B.V. https://www.sciencedirect.com/bookseries/progress-in-brain-research/vol/251

Donato, F., Rompani, S. B., & Caroni, P. (2013). Parvalbumin-expressing basket-cell network plasticity induced by experience regulates adult learning. *Nature, 504*(7479), 272–276. https://doi.org/10.1038/nature12866

Down, J. L. (1867). Observations on an ethnic classification of idiots. *Journal of Mental Science, 13*(61), 121–123. https://doi.org/10.1192/bjp.13.61.121

Dykens, E. M., & Hodapp, R. M. (2001). Research in mental retardation: Toward an etiologic approach. *Journal of Child Psychology and Psychiatry and Allied Disciplines, 42*(1), 49–71. https://doi.org/10.1017/S0021963001006540

Edelman, G. M. (1987). *Neural Darwinism: The theory of neuronal group selection.* Basic Books.

Edgin, J. O., Tooley, U., Demara, B., Nyhuis, C., Anand, P., & Spanò, G. (2015). Sleep disturbance and expressive language development in preschool-age children with Down syndrome. *Child Development, 86*(6), 1984–1998. https://doi.org/10.1111/cdev.12443

Elman, J. L., Bates, E. A., Johnson, M. H., Karmiloff-Smith, A., Parisi, D., & Plunkett, K. (1996). *Rethinking innateness: A connectionist perspective on development.* MIT Press. https://doi.org/https://doi.org/10.7551/mitpress/5929.001.0001

Fair, D. A., Cohen, A. L., Power, J. D., Dosenbach, N. U. F., Church, J. A., Miezin, F. M., Schlaggar, B. L., & Petersen, S. E. (2009). Functional brain networks develop from a "local to distributed" organization. *PLoS Computational Biology, 5*(5), e1000381. https://doi.org/10.1371/journal.pcbi.1000381

Fair, D. A., Dosenbach, N. U. F., Church, J. A., Cohen, A. L., Brahmbhatt, S., Miezin, F. M., Barch, D. M., Raichle, M. E., Petersen, S. E., & Schlaggar, B. L. (2007). Development of distinct control networks through segregation and integration. *Proceedings of the National Academy of Sciences, 104*(33), 13507–13512. https://doi.org/10.1073/pnas.0705843104

Fausey, C. M., Jayaraman, S., & Smith, L. B. (2016). From faces to hands: Changing visual input in the first two years. *Cognition, 152*, 101–107. https://doi.org/10.1016/j.cognition.2016.03.005

Fidler, D. J. (2005). The emerging Down syndrome behavioral phenotype in early childhood. *Infants & Young Children, 18*(2), 86–103. https://doi.org/10.1097/00001163-200504000-00003

Fidler, D. J., Hepburn, S. L., Mankin, G., & Rogers, S. J. (2005). Praxis skills in young children with Down syndrome, other developmental disabilities, and typically developing children. *American Journal of Occupational Therapy, 59*(2), 129–138. https://doi.org/10.5014/ajot.59.2.129

Fidler, D. J., Most, D. E., Booth-LaForce, C., & Kelly, J. F. (2008). Emerging social strengths in young children with Down syndrome. *Infants & Young Children, 21*(3), 207–220. https://doi.org/10.1097/01.IYC.0000324550.39446.1f

Fidler, D. J., Needham, A. W., & Schworer, E. (2019). Infant foundations in Down syndrome: Early constraints on cognitive skill acquisition. *International Review of Research in Developmental Disabilities, 56*, 41–65. https://doi.org/10.1016/BS.IRRDD.2019.06.008

Fidler, D. J., Schworer, E., Prince, M. A., Will, E. A., Needham, A. W., & Daunhauer, L. A. (2019). Exploratory behavior and developmental skill acquisition in infants with Down syndrome. *Infant Behavior and Development, 54*, 140–150. https://doi.org/10.1016/J.INFBEH.2019.02.002

Fidler, D. J., Schworer, E., Will, E. A., Patel, L., & Daunhauer, L. A. (2019). Correlates of early cognition in infants with Down syndrome. *Journal of Intellectual Disability Research, 63*(3), 205–214. https://doi.org/10.1111/jir.12566

Fields, R. D. (2015). A new mechanism of nervous system plasticity: Activity-dependent myelination. *Nature Reviews Neuroscience, 16*(12), 756–767. https://doi.org/10.1038/nrn4023

Flavell, S. W., & Greenberg, M. E. (2008). Signaling mechanisms linking neuronal activity to gene expression and plasticity of the nervous system. *Annual Review of Neuroscience, 31*(1), 563–590. https://doi.org/10.1146/annurev.neuro.31.060407.125631

Ford, D. H., & Lerner, R. M. (1992). *Developmental systems theory: An integrative approach.* Sage Publications, Inc.

Frankenhuis, W. E., & Panchanathan, K. (2011). Individual differences in developmental plasticity may result from stochastic sampling. *Perspectives on Psychological Science, 6*(4), 336–347. https://doi.org/10.1177/1745691611412602

Gibson, D. (1978). *Down's syndrome: The psychology of mongolism.* Cambridge University Press.

Gibson, E. J. (1988). Exploratory behavior in the development of perceiving, acting, and the acquiring of knowledge. *Annual Review of Psychology, 39*(1), 1–42. https://doi.org/10.1146/annurev.ps.39.020188.000245

Gibson, E. J., & Pick, A. D. (2000). *An ecological approach to perceptual learning and development.* Oxford University Press.

Gilmore, L., & Cuskelly, M. (2009). A longitudinal study of motivation and competence in children with Down syndrome: Early childhood to early adolescence. *Journal of Intellectual Disability Research, 53*(5), 484–492. https://doi.org/10.1111/j.1365-2788.2009.01166.x

Gilmore, L., Cuskelly, M., Jobling, A., & Hayes, A. (2009). Maternal support for autonomy: Relationships with persistence for children with Down syndrome and typically developing children. *Research in Developmental Disabilities, 30*(5), 1023–1033. https://doi.org/10.1016/J.RIDD.2009.02.005

Glenn, S., Dayus, B., Cunningham, C., & Horgan, M. (2001). Mastery motivation in children with Down syndrome. *Down's Syndrome, Research and Practice, 7*(2), 52–59. https://doi.org/10.3104/reports.114

Godfrey, M., & Lee, N. R. (2018). Memory profiles in Down syndrome across development: A review of memory abilities through the lifespan. *Journal of Neurodevelopmental Disorders, 10*(1), 5. https://doi.org/10.1186/s11689-017-9220-y

Golden, J. A., & Hyman, B. T. (1994). Development of the superior temporal neocortex is anomalous in trisomy 21. *Journal of Neuropathology & Experimental Neurology, 53*(5), 513–520. https://doi.org/10.1097/00005072-199409000-00011

Gottlieb, G. (1970). Conceptions of prenatal behavior. In L. R. Aronson, E. Tobach, D. S. Lehrman, & J. S. Rosenblatt (Eds.), *The significance of biology for human development: A developmental psychobiological systems view development and evolution of behavior* (pp. 111–137). Freeman.

Gottlieb, G. (1992). *Individual development and evolution: The genesis of novel behavior.* Oxford University Press. https://doi.org/https://doi.org/10.4324/9781410604422

Gottlieb, G. (2007). Probabilistic epigenesis. *Developmental Science, 10*(1), 1–11. https://doi.org/10.1111/j.1467-7687.2007.00556.x

Greenough, W. T., Black, J. E., & Wallace, C. S. (1987). Experience and brain development. *Child Development, 58*(3), 539–559. https://doi.org/10.2307/1130197

Guedj, F., Bianchi, D. W., & Delabar, J.-M. (2014). Prenatal treatment of Down syndrome. *Current Opinion in Obstetrics and Gynecology, 26*(2), 92–103. https://doi.org/10.1097/GCO.0000000000000056

Guidi, S., Ciani, E., Bonasoni, P., Santini, D., & Bartesaghi, R. (2011). Widespread proliferation impairment and hypocellularity in the cerebellum of fetuses with Down syndrome. *Brain Pathology, 21*(4), 361–373. https://doi.org/10.1111/j.1750-3639.2010.00459.x

Guidi, S., Stagni, F., Bianchi, P., Ciani, E., Giacomini, A., De Franceschi, M., Moldrich, R., Kurniawan, N., Mardon, K., Giuliani, A., Calzà, L., & Bartesaghi, R. (2014). Prenatal pharmacotherapy rescues brain development in a Down's syndrome mouse model. *Brain, 137*(2), 380–401. https://doi.org/10.1093/brain/awt340

Gunbey, H. P., Bilgici, M. C., Aslan, K., Has, A. C., Ogur, M. G., Alhan, A., & Incesu, L. (2017). Structural brain alterations of Down's syndrome in early childhood evaluation by DTI and volumetric analyses. *European Radiology, 27*(7), 3013–3021. https://doi.org/10.1007/s00330-016-4626-6

Gunn, P., Berry, P., & Andrews, R. J. (1982). Looking behavior of Down syndrome infants. *American Journal of Mental Deficiency, 87*(3), 344–347.

Hahn, L. J., Loveall, S. J., Savoy, M. T., Neumann, A. M., & Ikuta, T. (2018). Joint attention in Down syndrome: A meta-analysis. *Research in Developmental Disabilities, 78*, 89–102. https://doi.org/10.1016/J.RIDD.2018.03.013

Haider, B., Duque, A., Hasenstaub, A. R., & McCormick, D. A. (2006). Neocortical network activity in vivo is generated through a dynamic balance of excitation and inhibition. *Journal of Neuroscience, 26*(17), 4535–4545. https://doi.org/10.1523/JNEUROSCI.5297-05.2006

Haley, S. M. (1986). Postural reactions in infants with Down syndrome. Relationship to motor milestone development and age. *Physical Therapy, 66*(1), 17–22. https://doi.org/https://doi.org/10.1093/ptj/66.1.17

Hamner, T., Udhnani, M. D., Osipowicz, K. Z., & Lee, N. R. (2018). Pediatric brain development in Down syndrome: A field in its infancy. *Journal of the International Neuropsychological Society, 24*(9), 966–976. https://doi.org/10.1017/S1355617718000206

Harris, S. R. (1981). Effects of neurodevelopmental therapy on motor performance of infants with Down's syndrome. *Developmental Medicine & Child Neurology, 23*(5), 477–483. https://doi.org/10.1111/j.1469-8749.1981.tb02021.x

Hauck, J. L., Felzer-Kim, I. T., & Gwizdala, K. L. (2020). Early movement matters: Interplay of physical activity and motor skill development in infants with Down syndrome. *Adapted Physical Activity Quarterly, 37*(2), 160–176. https://doi.org/10.1123/apaq.2019-0012

Hauck, J. L., Zott, G. R., Felzer-Kim, I. T., & Adkins, C. M. (2018). A comparison of low-intensity physical activity, growth, and sleep behavior in 6-month old infants. *Infant Behavior and Development, 53*, 18–24. https://doi.org/10.1016/J.INFBEH.2018.09.013

Hebb, D. O. (1949). *The organization of behavior: A neuropsychological theory.* John Wiley & Sons, Inc. https://doi.org/https://doi.org/10.1002/sce.37303405110

Hedge, C., Powell, G., & Sumner, P. (2018). The reliability paradox: Why robust cognitive tasks do not produce reliable individual differences. *Behavior Research Methods, 50*(3), 1166–1186. https://doi.org/10.3758/s13428-017-0935-1

Held, R., & Hein, A. (1963). Movement-produced stimulation in the development of visually guided behavior. *Journal of Comparative and Physiological Psychology, 56*(5), 872–876. https://doi.org/10.1037/h0040546

Hepper, P. G., & Shahidullah, S. (1992). Habituation in normal and Down's syndrome fetuses. *The Quarterly Journal of Experimental Psychology Section B, 44*(3–4), 305–317. https://doi.org/10.1080/02724999208250617

Hill Karrer, J., Karrer, R., Bloom, D., Chaney, L., & Davis, R. (1998). Event-related brain potentials during an extended visual recognition memory task depict delayed development of cerebral inhibitory processes among 6-month-old infants with Down syndrome. *International Journal of Psychophysiology, 29*(2), 167–200. https://doi.org/10.1016/S0167-8760(98)00015-4

Hospodar, C. M., Sabet, A., Logan, S. W., Catena, M. A., & Galloway, J. C. (2021). Exploratory analysis of a developmentally progressive modified ride-on car intervention for young children with Down syndrome. *Disability and Rehabilitation: Assistive Technology, 16*(7), 749–757.

Huttenlocher, P. R. (1979). Synaptic density in human frontal cortex—Developmental changes and effects of aging. *Brain Research, 163*(2), 195–205. https://doi.org/10.1016/0006-8993(79)90349-4

Huttenlocher, P. R., & Dabholkar, A. S. (1997). Regional differences in synaptogenesis in human cerebral cortex. *Journal of Comparative Neurology, 387*(2), 167–178. https://doi.org/10.1002/(sici)1096-9861(19971020)387:2<167::aid-cne1>3.0.co;2-z

Imai, M., Watanabe, H., Yasui, K., Kimura, Y., Shitara, Y., Tsuchida, S., Takahashi, N., & Taga, G. (2014). Functional connectivity of the cortex of term and preterm infants and infants with Down's syndrome. *NeuroImage, 85*, 272–278. https://doi.org/10.1016/J.NEUROIMAGE.2013.04.080

Iverson, J. M. (2010). Developing language in a developing body: The relationship between motor development and language development. *Journal of Child Language, 37*(2), 229–261. https://doi.org/10.1017/S0305000909990432

Jarrold, C., & Baddeley, A. D. (1997). Short-term memory for verbal and visuospatial information in Down's syndrome. *Cognitive Neuropsychiatry, 2*(2), 101–122. https://doi.org/10.1080/135468097396351

John, F. M., Bromham, N. R., Woodhouse, J. M., & Candy, T. R. (2004). Spatial vision deficits in infants and children with Down syndrome. *Investigative Ophthalmology & Visual Science, 45*(5), 1566–1572. https://doi.org/10.1167/iovs.03-0951

Johnson, M. H. (2001). Functional brain development in humans. *Nature Reviews Neuroscience, 2*(7), 475–483. https://doi.org/10.1038/35081509

Johnson, M. H. (2011). Interactive specialization: A domain-general framework for human functional brain development? *Developmental Cognitive Neuroscience, 1*(1), 7–21. https://doi.org/10.1016/j.dcn.2010.07.003

Johnson, M. H. (2017). Autism as an adaptive common variant pathway for human brain development. *Developmental Cognitive Neuroscience, 25*, 5–11. https://doi.org/10.1016/j.dcn.2017.02.004

Johnson, M. H., Jones, E. J. H., & Gliga, T. (2015). Brain adaptation and alternative developmental trajectories. *Development and Psychopathology, 27*(2), 425–442. https://doi.org/10.1017/S0954579415000073

Johnson, S. P., Amso, D., & Slemmer, J. A. (2003). Development of object concepts in infancy: Evidence for early learning in an eye-tracking paradigm. *Proceedings of the National Academy of Sciences, 100*(18), 10568–10573. https://doi.org/10.1073/pnas.1630655100

Karasik, L. B., Tamis-LeMonda, C. S., & Adolph, K. E. (2011). Transition from crawling to walking and infants' actions with objects and people. *Child Development, 82*(4), 1199–1209. https://doi.org/10.1111/j.1467-8624.2011.01595.x

Karasik, L. B., Tamis-LeMonda, C. S., & Adolph, K. E. (2014). Crawling and walking infants elicit different verbal responses from mothers. *Developmental Science, 17*(3), 388–395. https://doi.org/10.1111/desc.12129

Karasik, L. B., Tamis-LeMonda, C. S., & Adolph, K. E. (2016). Decisions at the brink: Locomotor experience affects infants' use of social information on an adjustable drop-off. *Frontiers in Psychology, 7*, 797. https://doi.org/10.3389/fpsyg.2016.00797

Karmiloff-Smith, A. (1998). Development itself is the key to understanding developmental disorders. *Trends in Cognitive Sciences, 2*(10), 389–398. https://doi.org/10.1016/S1364-6613(98)01230-3

Karmiloff-Smith, A., Al-Janabi, T., D'Souza, H., Groet, J., Massand, E., Mok, K., Startin, C., Fisher, E., Hardy, J., Nizetic, D., Tybulewicz, V., & Strydom, A. (2016). The importance of understanding individual differences in Down syndrome. *F1000Research, 5*, 389. https://doi.org/10.12688/f1000research.7506.1

Karmiloff-Smith, A., D'Souza, D., Dekker, T. M., Van Herwegen, J., Xu, F., Rodic, M., & Ansari, D. (2012). Genetic and environmental vulnerabilities in children with neurodevelopmental disorders. *Proceedings of the National Academy of Sciences, 109*(Supplement 2), 17261–17265. https://doi.org/10.1073/pnas.1121087109

Kavšek, M. (2004). Predicting later IQ from infant visual habituation and dishabituation: A meta-analysis. *Journal of Applied Developmental Psychology, 25*(3), 369–393. https://doi.org/10.1016/J.APPDEV.2004.04.006

Kidd, C., Piantadosi, S. T., & Aslin, R. N. (2012). The Goldilocks effect: Human infants allocate attention to visual sequences that are neither too simple nor too complex. *PLoS ONE, 7*(5), e36399. https://doi.org/10.1371/journal.pone.0036399

Knott, F., Lewis, C., & Williams, T. (1995). Sibling interaction of children with learning disabilities: A comparison of autism and Down's syndrome. *Journal of Child Psychology and Psychiatry, 36*(6), 965–976. https://doi.org/10.1111/j.1469-7610.1995.tb01343.x

Koo, B. K., Blaser, S., Harwood-Nash, D., Becker, L. E., & Murphy, E. G. (1992). Magnetic resonance imaging evaluation of delayed myelination in Down syndrome: A case report and review of the literature. *Journal of Child Neurology, 7*(4), 417–421. https://doi.org/10.1177/088307389200700417

Krakow, J. B., & Kopp, C. B. (1982). Sustained attention in young Down syndrome children. *Topics in Early Childhood Special Education, 2*(2), 32–42. https://doi.org/10.1177/027112148200200208

Kugel, R. B. (1970). Combatting retardation in infants with Down's syndrome. *Children, 17*(5), 188–192.

Kulkarni, V. A., & Firestein, B. L. (2012). The dendritic tree and brain disorders. *Molecular and Cellular Neuroscience, 50*(1), 10–20. https://doi.org/10.1016/j.mcn.2012.03.005

Landry, S. H., & Chapieski, M. L. (1989). Joint attention and infant toy exploration: Effects of Down syndrome and prematurity. *Child Development, 60*(1), 103. https://doi.org/10.2307/1131076

Larsen, K. B., Laursen, H., Græm, N., Samuelsen, G. B., Bogdanovic, N., & Pakkenberg, B. (2008). Reduced cell number in the neocortical part of the human fetal brain in Down syndrome. *Annals of Anatomy—Anatomischer Anzeiger, 190*(5), 421–427. https://doi.org/10.1016/J.AANAT.2008.05.007

Lauteslager, P. E. M. (1995). Motor development in young children with Down syndrome. In A. Vermeer & W. E. Davis (Eds.), *Physical and motor development in mental retardation* (pp. 75–98). Karger. https://doi.org/https://doi.org/10.1159/000424520

LaVeck, B., & LaVeck, G. D. (1977). Sex differences in development among young children with Down syndrome. *The Journal of Pediatrics, 91*(5), 767–779. https://doi.org/10.1016/S0022-3476(77)81037-8

Lee, S. E., Duran-Martinez, M., Khantsis, S., Bianchi, D. W., & Guedj, F. (2020). Challenges and opportunities for translation of therapies to improve cognition in Down syndrome. *Trends in Molecular Medicine, 26*(2), 150–169. https://doi.org/10.1016/J.MOLMED.2019.10.001

Legerstee, M., & Weintraub, J. (1997). The integration of person and object attention in infants with and without Down syndrome. *Infant Behavior and Development, 20*(1), 71–82. https://doi.org/10.1016/S0163-6383(97)90062-X

Lerner, R. M. (1978). Nature, nurture, and dynamic interactionism. *Human Development, 21*(1), 1–20. https://doi.org/10.1159/000271572

Leslie, J. H., & Nedivi, E. (2011). Activity-regulated genes as mediators of neural circuit plasticity. *Progress in Neurobiology, 94*(3), 223–237. https://doi.org/10.1016/J.PNEUROBIO.2011.05.002

Libertus, K., Joh, A. S., & Needham, A. W. (2016). Motor training at 3 months affects object exploration 12 months later. *Developmental Science, 19*(6), 1058–1066. https://doi.org/10.1111/desc.12370

Libertus, K., & Needham, A. (2010). Teach to reach: The effects of active vs. passive reaching experiences on action and perception. *Vision Research, 50*(24), 2750–2757. https://doi.org/10.1016/j.visres.2010.09.001

Libertus, K., & Needham, A. (2011). Reaching experience increases face preference in 3-month-old infants. *Developmental Science, 14*(6), 1355–1364. https://doi.org/10.1111/j.1467-7687.2011.01084.x

Liu, X., Somel, M., Tang, L., Yan, Z., Jiang, X., Guo, S., Yuan, Y., He, L., Oleksiak, A., Zhang, Y., Li, N., Hu, Y., Chen, W., Qiu, Z., Pääbo, S., & Khaitovich, P. (2012). Extension of cortical synaptic development distinguishes humans from chimpanzees and macaques. *Genome Research, 22*(4), 611–622. https://doi.org/10.1101/gr.127324.111

Lloyd, M. C., Burghardt, A., Ulrich, D. A., & Angulo-Barroso, R. (2010). Physical activity and walking onset in infants with Down syndrome. *Adapted Physical Activity Quarterly, 27*(1), 1–16. https://doi.org/10.1123/apaq.27.1.1

Lloyd, M. C., & Ulrich, D. A. (2006). The use of the Kick and Drive Gym to increase kicking in infants with Down syndrome. *Journal of Sport and Exercise Psychology, S28*, 121. https://doi.org/https://doi.org/10.1123/jsep.28.s1.s23

Lobo, M. A., Koshy, J., Hall, M. L., Erol, O., Cao, H., Buckley, J. M., Galloway, J. C., & Higginson, J. (2016). Playskin Lift: Development and initial testing of an exoskeletal garment to assist upper extremity mobility and function. *Physical Therapy, 96*(3), 390–399. https://doi.org/10.2522/ptj.20140540

Logan, S. W., Feldner, H. A., Bogart, K. R., Goodwin, B., Ross, S. M., Catena, M. A., Whitesell, A. A., Zefton, Z. J., Smart, W. D., & Galloway, J. C. (2017). Toy-based technologies for children with disabilities simultaneously supporting self-directed mobility, participation, and function: A tech report. *Frontiers in Robotics and AI, 4*, 7. https://doi.org/10.3389/frobt.2017.00007

Lott, I. T. (2012). Neurological phenotypes for Down syndrome across the life span. *Progress in Brain Research, 197*, 101–121. https://doi.org/10.1016/B978-0-444-54299-1.00006-6

Lydic, J. S., & Steele, C. (1979). Assessment of the quality of sitting and gait patterns in children with Down's syndrome. *Physical Therapy, 59*(12), 1489–1494. https://doi.org/https://doi.org/10.1093/ptj/59.12.1489

Martin, G. E., Klusek, J., Estigarribia, B., & Roberts, J. E. (2009). Language characteristics of individuals with Down syndrome. *Topics in Language Disorders, 29*(2), 112–132. https://doi.org/10.1097/TLD.0b013e3181a71fe1

Martínez Cué, C., & Dierssen, M. (2020). Plasticity as a therapeutic target for improving cognition and behavior in Down syndrome. In M. Dierssen (Ed.), *Progress in Brain Research* (Vol. 251, pp. 269–302). Elsevier. https://doi.org/10.1016/bs.pbr.2019.11.001

Mason-Apps, E., Stojanovik, V., Houston-Price, C., & Buckley, S. (2018). Longitudinal predictors of early language in infants with Down syndrome: A preliminary study. *Research in Developmental Disabilities, 81*, 37–51. https://doi.org/10.1016/j.ridd.2017.12.021

Mazzone, L., Mugno, D., & Mazzone, D. (2004). The general movements in children with Down syndrome. *Early Human Development, 79*(2), 119–130. https://doi.org/10.1016/j.earlhumdev.2004.04.013

McCall, R. B., & Carriger, M. S. (1993). A meta-analysis of infant habituation and recognition memory performance as predictors of later IQ. *Child Development, 64*(1), 57–79. https://doi.org/10.1111/j.1467-8624.1993.tb02895.x

McClelland, J. L., & Vallabha, G. (2009). Connectionist Models of Development: Mechanistic Dynamical Models with Emergent Dynamical Properties. In J. P. Spencer (Ed.), *Toward a Unified Theory of Development Connectionism and Dynamic System Theory Re-Consider* (pp. 3–24). Oxford University Press. https://doi.org/10.1093/acprof:oso/9780195300598.003.0001

McKay, S. M., & Angulo-Barroso, R. M. (2006). Longitudinal assessment of leg motor activity and sleep patterns in infants with and without Down syndrome. *Infant Behavior and Development, 29*(2), 153–168. https://doi.org/10.1016/J.INFBEH.2005.09.004

McKenzie, I. A., Ohayon, D., Li, H., de Faria, J. P., Emery, B., Tohyama, K., & Richardson, W. D. (2014). Motor skill learning requires active central myelination. *Science, 346*(6207), 318–322. https://doi.org/10.1126/science.1254960

Miller, J. F. (1992). Lexical development in young children with Down syndrome. In R. Chapman (Ed.), *Processes in language acquisition and language disorders* (pp. 202–216). Mosby Year Book.

Miller, J. F., & Leddy, M. (1999). Verbal fluency, speech intelligibility, and communicative effectiveness. In J. F. Miller, M. Leddy, & L. A. Leavitt (Eds.), *Improving the communication of people with Down syndrome* (pp. 81–91). Brookes Publishing Co.

Mitra, A., Blank, M., & Madison, D. V. (2012). Developmentally altered inhibition in Ts65Dn, a mouse model of Down syndrome. *Brain Research, 1440*, 1–8. https://doi.org/10.1016/J.BRAINRES.2011.12.034

Moore, D. G., & George, R. (2015). ACORNS: A tool for visual modelling of causes and outcomes in neurodevelopmental disorders. In J. van Herwegen & D. M. Riby (Eds.), *Neurodevelopmental disorders: Research challenges and solutions* (pp. 93–113). Psychology Press.

Moraczewski, D., Chen, G., & Redcay, E. (2018). Inter-subject synchrony as an index of functional specialization in early childhood. *Scientific Reports, 8*(1), 2252. https://doi.org/10.1038/s41598-018-20600-0

Mount, C. W., & Monje, M. (2017). Wrapped to adapt: Experience-dependent myelination. *Neuron, 95*(4), 743–756. https://doi.org/10.1016/J.NEURON.2017.07.009

Mundy, P., Kasari, C., Sigman, M., & Ruskin, E. (1995). Nonverbal communication and early language acquisition in children with Down syndrome and in normally developing children. *Journal of Speech and Hearing Research, 38*(1), 157–167. https://doi.org/10.1044/jshr.3801.157

Nakano-Kobayashi, A., Awaya, T., Kii, I., Sumida, Y., Okuno, Y., Yoshida, S., Sumida, T., Inoue, H., Hosoya, T., & Hagiwara, M. (2017). Prenatal neurogenesis induction therapy normalizes brain structure and function in Down syndrome mice. *Proceedings of the National Academy of Sciences, 114*(38), 10268–10273. https://doi.org/10.1073/pnas.1704143114

Navlakha, S., Barth, A. L., & Bar-Joseph, Z. (2015). Decreasing-rate pruning optimizes the construction of efficient and robust distributed networks. *PLOS Computational Biology, 11*(7), e1004347. https://doi.org/10.1371/journal.pcbi.1004347

Nguyen, T. L., Duchon, A., Manousopoulou, A., Loaëc, N., Villiers, B., Pani, G., Karatas, M., Mechling, A. E., Harsan, L.-A., Limanton, E., Bazureau, J.-P., Carreaux, F., Garbis, S. D., Meijer, L., & Herault, Y. (2018). Correction of cognitive deficits in mouse models of Down syndrome by a pharmacological inhibitor of DYRK1A. *Disease Models & Mechanisms, 11*(9), dmm035634. https://doi.org/10.1242/dmm.035634

Nielsen, M., & Hudry, K. (2010). Over-imitation in children with autism and Down syndrome. *Australian Journal of Psychology, 62*(2), 67–74. https://doi.org/10.1080/00049530902758613

Oliver, A., Johnson, M. H., Karmiloff-Smith, A., & Pennington, B. (2000). Deviations in the emergence of representations: A neuroconstructivist framework for analysing developmental disorders. *Developmental Science, 3*(1), 1–23. https://doi.org/10.1111/1467-7687.00094

Olmos-Serrano, J. L., Kang, H. J., Tyler, W. A., Silbereis, J. C., Cheng, F., Zhu, Y., Pletikos, M., Jankovic-Rapan, L., Cramer, N. P., Galdzicki, Z., Goodliffe, J., Peters, A., Sethares, C., Delalle, I., Golden, J. A., Haydar, T. F., & Sestan, N. (2016). Down syndrome developmental brain transcriptome reveals defective oligodendrocyte differentiation and myelination. *Neuron, 89*(6), 1208–1222. https://doi.org/10.1016/j.neuron.2016.01.042

Ortega-Alves, M. V., & Urato, A. (2016). Making sense out of the controversy: Use of SSRIs in pregnancy. *Current Obstetrics and Gynecology Reports, 5*(3), 225–233. https://doi.org/10.1007/s13669-016-0173-z

Oyama, S. (1985). *The ontogeny of information.* Cambridge University Press.

Oyama, S., Griffiths, P., & Gray, R. D. (2001). *Cycles of contingency: Developmental systems and evolution.* MIT Press.

Palisano, R. J., Walter, S. D., Russell, D. J., Rosenbaum, P. L., Gémus, M., Galuppi, B. E., & Cunningham, L. (2001). Gross motor function of children with Down syndrome: Creation of motor growth curves. *Archives of Physical Medicine and Rehabilitation, 82*(4), 494–500. https://doi.org/10.1053/apmr.2001.21956

Papavassiliou, P., Charalsawadi, C., Rafferty, K., & Jackson-Cook, C. (2015). Mosaicism for trisomy 21: A review. *American Journal of Medical Genetics Part A, 167*(1), 26–39. https://doi.org/10.1002/ajmg.a.36861

Park, J., Song, W.-J., & Chung, K. C. (2009). Function and regulation of Dyrk1A: Towards understanding Down syndrome. *Cellular and Molecular Life Sciences, 66*(20), 3235–3240. https://doi.org/10.1007/s00018-009-0123-2

Pascalis, O., Scott, L. S., Kelly, D. J., Shannon, R. W., Nicholson, E., Coleman, M., & Nelson, C. A. (2005). Plasticity of face processing in infancy. *Proceedings of the National Academy of Sciences, 102*(14), 5297–5300. https://doi.org/10.1073/pnas.0406627102

Pereira, A. F., Smith, L. B., & Yu, C. (2014). A bottom-up view of toddler word learning. *Psychonomic Bulletin and Review, 21*(1), 178–185. https://doi.org/10.3758/s13423-013-0466-4

Pfitzer, C., Helm, P. C., Rosenthal, L.-M., Berger, F., Bauer, U. M. M., & Schmitt, K. R. (2017). Dynamics in prevalence of Down syndrome in children with congenital heart disease. *European Journal of Pediatrics, 177*(1), 107–115. https://doi.org/10.1007/s00431-017-3041-6

Phillips, M., & Pozzo-Miller, L. (2015). Dendritic spine dysgenesis in autism related disorders. *Neuroscience Letters, 601*, 30–40. https://doi.org/10.1016/j.neulet.2015.01.011

Piaget, J. (1952). *The origins of intelligence in children.* W. W. Norton & Co.

Piaget, J. (1954). *The construction of reality in the child.* Basic Books.

Pitcairn, T. K., & Wishart, J. G. (1994). Reactions of young children with Down's syndrome to an impossible task. *British Journal of Developmental Psychology, 12*(4), 485–489. https://doi.org/10.1111/j.2044-835X.1994.tb00649.x

Prasher, V. P., Sajith, S. G., Rees, S. D., Patel, A., Tewari, S., Schupf, N., & Zigman, W. B. (2008). Significant effect of APOE epsilon 4 genotype on the risk of dementia in Alzheimer's disease and mortality in persons with Down syndrome. *International Journal of Geriatric Psychiatry, 23*(11), 1134–1140. https://doi.org/10.1002/gps.2039

Purpura, D. P. (1975). Normal and aberrant neuronal development in the cerebral cortex of human fetus and young infant. In N. A. Buchwald & M. A. B. Brazier (Eds.), *Brain mechanisms in mental retardation* (Vol. 18, Issue 18, pp. 141–169). Academic Press. https://doi.org/https://doi.org/10.1016/B978-0-12-139050-1.50014-8

Quine, W. (1960). *Word and object.* MIT Press.

Real, R., Peter, M., Trabalza, A., Khan, S., Smith, M. A., Dopp, J., Barnes, S. J., Momoh, A., Strano, A., Volpi, E., Knott, G., Livesey, F. J., & De Paola, V. (2018). In vivo modeling of human neuron dynamics and Down syndrome. *Science, 362*(6416), eaau1810. https://doi.org/10.1126/science.aau1810

Reeves, R. H., Baxter, L. L., & Richtsmeier, J. T. (2001). Too much of a good thing: Mechanisms of gene action in Down syndrome. *Trends in Genetics*, *17*(2), 83–88. https://doi.org/10.1016/S0168-9525(00)02172-7

Reiche, L., Küry, P., & Göttle, P. (2019). Aberrant oligodendrogenesis in Down syndrome: Shift in gliogenesis? *Cells*, *8*(12), 1591. https://doi.org/10.3390/cells8121591

Reynolds Losin, E. A., Rivera, S. M., O'Hare, E. D., Sowell, E. R., & Pinter, J. D. (2009). Abnormal fMRI activation pattern during story listening in individuals with Down syndrome. *American Journal on Intellectual and Developmental Disabilities*, *114*(5), 369–380. https://doi.org/10.1352/1944-7558-114.5.369

Ringenbach, S. D., Chua, R., Maraj, B. K. V, Kao, J. C., & Weeks, D. J. (2002). Bimanual coordination dynamics in adults with Down syndrome. *Motor Control*, *6*(4), 388–407. https://doi.org/10.1123/mcj.6.4.388

Roach, M. A., Barratt, M. S., Miller, J. F., & Leavitt, L. A. (1998). The structure of mother–child play: Young children with Down syndrome and typically developing children. *Developmental Psychology*, *34*(1), 77–87. https://doi.org/10.1037/0012-1649.34.1.77

Robb, J. (2015). The delayed walker. In B. Joseph, J. Robb, R. T. Loder, & I. Torode (Eds.), *Paediatric orthopaedic diagnosis* (pp. 249–256). Springer India. https://doi.org/10.1007/978-81-322-2392-4_25

Roizen, N. J., Wolters, C., Nicol, T., & Blondis, T. A. (1993). Hearing loss in children with Down syndrome. *The Journal of Pediatrics*, *123*(1), S9–S12. https://doi.org/10.1016/S0022-3476(05)81588-4

Rose, D. H., Slater, A., & Perry, H. (1986). Prediction of childhood intelligence from habituation in early infancy. *Intelligence*, *10*(3), 251–263. https://doi.org/10.1016/0160-2896(86)90019-X

Rosenblatt, F. (1958). The perceptron: A probabilistic model for information storage and organization in the brain. *Psychological Review*, *65*(6), 386–408. https://doi.org/10.1037/h0042519

Rovee-Collier, C., & Cuevas, K. (2009). Multiple memory systems are unnecessary to account for infant memory development: An ecological model. *Developmental Psychology*, *45*(1), 160–174. https://doi.org/10.1037/a0014538

Rubenstein, J. L. R., & Merzenich, M. M. (2003). Model of autism: Increased ratio of excitation/inhibition in key neural systems. *Genes, Brain and Behavior*, *2*(5), 255–267. https://doi.org/10.1034/j.1601-183X.2003.00037.x

Ruddy, M. G., & Bornstein, M. H. (1982). Cognitive correlates of infant attention and maternal stimulation over the first year of life. *Child Development*, *53*(1), 183–188. https://doi.org/10.1111/j.1467-8624.1982.tb01306.x

Ruiz-González, L., Lucena-Antón, D., Salazar, A., Martín-Valero, R., & Moral-Munoz, J. A. (2019). Physical therapy in Down syndrome: Systematic review and meta-analysis. *Journal of Intellectual Disability Research*, *63*(8), 1041–1067. https://doi.org/10.1111/jir.12606

Ruskin, E. M., Kasari, C., Mundy, P., & Sigman, M. (1994). Attention to people and toys during social and object mastery in children with Down syndrome. *American Journal on Mental Retardation*, *99*(1), 103–111.

Samuelson, L. K., & McMurray, B. (2017). What does it take to learn a word? *Wiley Interdisciplinary Reviews: Cognitive Science*, *8*(1–2), e1421. https://doi.org/10.1002/wcs.1421

Schöner, G., & Kelso, J. A. (1988). Dynamic pattern generation in behavioral and neural systems. *Science*, *239*(4847), 1513–1520. https://doi.org/10.1126/science.3281253

Schwarzer, G., Freitag, C., Buckel, R., & Lofruthe, A. (2013). Crawling is associated with mental rotation ability by 9-month-old infants. *Infancy*, *18*(3), 432–441. https://doi.org/10.1111/j.1532-7078.2012.00132.x

Schworer, E., Fidler, D. J., Lunkenheimer, E., & Daunhauer, L. A. (2018). Parenting behaviour and executive function in children with Down syndrome. *Journal of Intellectual Disability Research*, *63*(4), 298–312. https://doi.org/10.1111/jir.12575

Seidl, R., Hauser, E., Bernert, G., Marx, M., Freilinger, M., & Lubec, G. (1997). Auditory evoked potentials in young patients with Down syndrome. Event-related potentials (P3) and histaminergic system. *Cognitive Brain Research*, *5*(4), 301–309. https://doi.org/10.1016/S0926-6410(97)00008-6

Sengpiel, F., & Kind, P. C. (2002). The role of activity in development of the visual system. *Current Biology*, *12*(23), R818–R826. https://doi.org/10.1016/S0960-9822(02)01318-0

Shogren, K. A., Wehmeyer, M. L., & Singh, N. N. (2017). *Handbook of positive psychology in intellectual and developmental disabilities*. Springer International Publishing. https://doi.org/10.1007/978-3-319-59066-0

Singer, W., Sejnowski, T. J., & Rakic, P. (2019). *The neocortex*. MIT Press. http://cognet.mit.edu/book/neocortex

Slone, L. K., Abney, D. H., Borjon, J. I., Chen, C., Franchak, J. M., Pearcy, D., Suarez-Rivera, C., Xu, T. L., Zhang, Y., Smith, L. B., & Yu, C. (2018). Gaze in action: Head-mounted eye tracking of children's dynamic visual attention during naturalistic behavior. *Journal of Visualized Experiments*, *141*, e58496. https://doi.org/10.3791/58496

Sobol, M., Klar, J., Laan, L., Shahsavani, M., Schuster, J., Annerén, G., Konzer, A., Mi, J., Bergquist, J., Nordlund, J., Hoeber, J., Huss, M., Falk, A., & Dahl, N. (2019). Transcriptome and proteome profiling of neural induced pluripotent stem cells from individuals with Down syndrome disclose dynamic dysregulations of key pathways and cellular functions. *Molecular Neurobiology, 56*(10), 7113–7127. https://doi.org/10.1007/s12035-019-1585-3

Somerville, L. H., & Casey, B. J. (2014). Emotional reactivity and regulation across development. In M. S. Gazzaniga & G. R. Mangun (Eds.), *The cognitive neurosciences* (5th ed., pp. 731–739). MIT Press.

Soska, K. C., Adolph, K. E., & Johnson, S. P. (2010). Systems in development: Motor skill acquisition facilitates three-dimensional object completion. *Developmental Psychology, 46*(1), 129–138. https://doi.org/10.1037/a0014618

Soukup-Ascencao, T., D'Souza, D., D'Souza, H., & Karmiloff-Smith, A. (2016). Parent-child interaction as a dynamic contributor to learning and cognitive development in typical and atypical development. *Infancia y Aprendizaje, 39*(4), 694–726. https://doi.org/10.1080/02103702.2016.1221054

Spanò, M., Mercuri, E., Randò, T., Pantò, T., Gagliano, A., Henderson, S., & Guzzetta, F. (1999). Motor and perceptual-motor competence in children with Down syndrome: Variation in performance with age. *European Journal of Paediatric Neurology, 3*(1), 7–14. https://doi.org/10.1053/ejpn.1999.0173

Spencer, J. P., Vereijken, B., Diedrich, F. J., & Thelen, E. (2000). Posture and the emergence of manual skills. *Developmental Science, 3*(2), 216–233. https://doi.org/10.1111/1467-7687.00115

Sporns, O., & Edelman, G. M. (1993). Solving Bernstein's problem: A proposal for the development of coordinated movement by selection. *Child Development, 64*(4), 960–981. https://doi.org/10.1111/j.1467-8624.1993.tb04182.x

Sretavan, D., & Shatz, C. J. (1984). Prenatal development of individual retinogeniculate axons during the period of segregation. *Nature, 308*, 845–848. https://doi.org/10.1038/308845a0

Stagni, F., Giacomini, A., Emili, M., Guidi, S., & Bartesaghi, R. (2018). Neurogenesis impairment: An early developmental defect in Down syndrome. *Free Radical Biology and Medicine, 114*, 15–32. https://doi.org/10.1016/J.FREERADBIOMED.2017.07.026

Stagni, F., Giacomini, A., Emili, M., Trazzi, S., Guidi, S., Sassi, M., Ciani, E., Rimondini, R., & Bartesaghi, R. (2016). Short- and long-term effects of neonatal pharmacotherapy with epigallocatechin-3-gallate on hippocampal development in the Ts65Dn mouse model of Down syndrome. *Neuroscience, 333*, 277–301. https://doi.org/10.1016/J.NEUROSCIENCE.2016.07.031

Stoneman, Z., Brody, G. H., Davis, C. H., & Crapps, J. M. (1987). Mentally retarded children and their older same-sex siblings: Naturalistic in-home observations. *American Journal on Mental Retardation, 92*(3), 290–298.

Suarez-Rivera, C., Smith, L. B., & Yu, C. (2019). Multimodal parent behaviors within joint attention support sustained attention in infants. *Developmental Psychology, 55*(1), 96–109. https://doi.org/10.1037/dev0000628

Takashima, S., Becker, L. E., Armstrong, D. L., & Chan, F. (1981). Abnormal neuronal development in the visual cortex of the human fetus and infant with Down's syndrome. A quantitative and qualitative golgi study. *Brain Research, 225*(1), 1–21. https://doi.org/10.1016/0006-8993(81)90314-0

Tamis-LeMonda, C. S., Adolph, K. E., Lobo, S. A., Karasik, L. B., Ishak, S., & Dimitropoulou, K. A. (2008). When infants take mothers' advice: 18-month-olds integrate perceptual and social information to guide motor action. *Developmental Psychology, 44*(3), 734–746. https://doi.org/10.1037/0012-1649.44.3.734

Task Engine—Face popout. (n.d.). [MATLAB software]. Retrieved June 30, 2020, from https://sites.google.com/site/taskenginedoc/task-packages/face-popout

Thelen, E. (1992). Development as a dynamic system. *Current Directions in Psychological Science, 1*(6), 189–193. https://doi.org/10.1111/1467-8721.ep10770402

Thelen, E., & Smith, L. B. (1994). *A dynamic systems approach to the development of cognition and action.* MIT Press.

Thomas, M. S. C., Ojinaga Alfageme, O., D'Souza, H., Patkee, P. A., Rutherford, M. A., Mok, K. Y., Hardy, J., & Karmiloff-Smith, A. (2020). A multi-level developmental approach to exploring individual differences in Down syndrome: Genes, brain, behaviour, and environment. *Research in Developmental Disabilities, 104*, 103638. https://doi.org/10.1016/j.ridd.2020.103638

Tovar, Á. E., Westermann, G., & Torres, A. (2018). From altered synaptic plasticity to atypical learning: A computational model of Down syndrome. *Cognition, 171*, 15–24. https://doi.org/10.1016/J.COGNITION.2017.10.021

Tsao, R., & Kindelberger, C. (2009). Variability of cognitive development in children with Down syndrome: Relevance of good reasons for using the cluster procedure. *Research in Developmental Disabilities, 30*(3), 426–432. https://doi.org/10.1016/J.RIDD.2008.10.009

Turrigiano, G. G., & Nelson, S. B. (2004). Homeostatic plasticity in the developing nervous system. *Nature Reviews Neuroscience, 5*(2), 97–107. https://doi.org/10.1038/nrn1327

Tyssowski, K. M., DeStefino, N. R., Cho, J.-H., Dunn, C. J., Poston, R. G., Carty, C. E., Jones, R. D., Chang, S. M., Romeo, P., Wurzelmann, M. K., Ward, J. M., Andermann, M. L., Saha, R. N., Dudek, S. M., & Gray, J. M. (2018). Different neuronal activity patterns induce different gene expression programs. *Neuron, 98*(3), 530–546.e11. https://doi.org/10.1016/J.NEURON.2018.04.001

Ulrich, B. D. (2010). Opportunities for early intervention based on theory, basic neuroscience, and clinical science. *Physical Therapy, 90*(12), 1868–1880. https://doi.org/10.2522/ptj.20100040

Ulrich, B. D., & Ulrich, D. A. (1993). Dynamic systems approach to understanding motor delay in infants with Down Syndrome. In G. J. P. Savelsbergh (Ed.), *Advances in psychology* (Vol. 97, pp. 445–459). Elsevier. https://doi.org/10.1016/S0166-4115(08)60963-2

Ulrich, B. D., & Ulrich, D. A. (1995). Spontaneous leg movements of infants with Down syndrome and nondisabled infants. *Child Development, 66*(6), 1844–1855. https://doi.org/10.1111/j.1467-8624.1995.tb00969.x

Ulrich, B. D., Ulrich, D. A., Angulo-Kinzler, R., & Chapman, D. D. (1997). Sensitivity of infants with and without Down syndrome to intrinsic dynamics. *Research Quarterly for Exercise and Sport, 68*(1), 10–19. https://doi.org/10.1080/02701367.1997.10608862

Ulrich, D. A., Lloyd, M. C., Tiernan, C. W., Looper, J. E., & Angulo-Barroso, R. M. (2008). Effects of intensity of treadmill training on developmental outcomes and stepping in infants with Down syndrome: A randomized trial. *Physical Therapy, 88*(1), 114–122. https://doi.org/10.2522/ptj.20070139

Ulrich, D. A., Ulrich, B. D., Angulo-Kinzler, R. M., & Yun, J. (2001). Treadmill training of infants with Down syndrome: Evidence-based developmental outcomes. *Pediatrics, 108*(5), e84. https://doi.org/10.1542/peds.108.5.e84

Vacca, R. A., Bawari, S., Valenti, D., Tewari, D., Nabavi, S. F., Shirooie, S., Sah, A. N., Volpicella, M., Braidy, N., & Nabavi, S. M. (2019). Down syndrome: Neurobiological alterations and therapeutic targets. *Neuroscience & Biobehavioral Reviews, 98*, 234–255. https://doi.org/10.1016/J.NEUBIOREV.2019.01.001

van der Lee, S. J., Wolters, F. J., Ikram, M. K., Hofman, A., Ikram, M. A., Amin, N., & van Duijn, C. M. (2018). The effect of APOE and other common genetic variants on the onset of Alzheimer's disease and dementia: A community-based cohort study. *The Lancet Neurology, 17*(5), 434–444. https://doi.org/10.1016/S1474-4422(18)30053-X

Vanvuchelen, M., Feys, H., & De Weerdt, W. (2011). Is the good-imitator-poor-talker profile syndrome-specific in Down syndrome?: Evidence from standardised imitation and language measures. *Research in Developmental Disabilities, 32*(1), 148–157. https://doi.org/10.1016/J.RIDD.2010.09.010

Venuti, P., de Falco, S., Esposito, G., & Bornstein, M. H. (2009). Mother–child play: Children with Down syndrome and typical development. *American Journal on Intellectual and Developmental Disabilities, 114*(4), 274–288. https://doi.org/10.1352/1944-7558-114.4:274-288

Vlachou, M., & Farrell, P. (2000). Object mastery motivation in pre-school children with and without disabilities. *Educational Psychology, 20*(2), 167–176. https://doi.org/10.1080/713663715

Von Hofsten, C. (2004). An action perspective on motor development. *Trends in Cognitive Sciences, 8*(6), 266–272. https://doi.org/10.1016/j.tics.2004.04.002

Vygotsky, L. S. (1978). *Mind in society: The development of higher psychological processes*. Harvard University Press.

Walle, E. A., & Campos, J. J. (2014). Infant language development is related to the acquisition of walking. *Developmental Psychology, 50*(2), 336–348. https://doi.org/10.1037/a0033238

Wang, P.-J., Morgan, G. A., Hwang, A.-W., & Liao, H.-F. (2013). Individualized behavioral assessments and maternal ratings of mastery motivation in mental age-matched toddlers with and without motor delay. *Physical Therapy, 93*(1), 79–87. https://doi.org/10.2522/ptj.20120068

Waxman, S. G. (1980). Determinants of conduction velocity in myelinated nerve fibers. *Muscle & Nerve, 3*(2), 141–150. https://doi.org/10.1002/mus.880030207

Weick, J. P., Held, D. L., Bonadurer, G. F., Doers, M. E., Liu, Y., Maguire, C., Clark, A., Knackert, J. A., Molinarolo, K., Musser, M., Yao, L., Yin, Y., Lu, J., Zhang, X., Zhang, S.-C., & Bhattacharyya, A. (2013). Deficits in human trisomy 21 iPSCs and neurons. *Proceedings of the National Academy of Sciences, 110*(24), 9962–9967. https://doi.org/10.1073/pnas.1216575110

Wentz, E. E. (2017). Importance of initiating a "tummy time" intervention early in infants with Down syndrome. *Pediatric Physical Therapy, 29*(1), 68–75. https://doi.org/10.1097/PEP.0000000000000335

Werker, J. F., & Hensch, T. K. (2015). Critical periods in speech perception: New directions. *Annual Review of Psychology, 66*(1), 173–196. https://doi.org/10.1146/annurev-psych-010814-015104

Westermann, G., Mareschal, D., Johnson, M. H., Sirois, S., Spratling, M. W., & Thomas, M. S. C. (2007). Neuroconstructivism. *Developmental Science, 10*(1), 75–83. https://doi.org/10.1111/j.1467-7687.2007.00567.x

Will, E. A., Caravella, K. E., Hahn, L. J., Fidler, D. J., & Roberts, J. E. (2018). Adaptive behavior in infants and toddlers with Down syndrome and fragile X syndrome. *American Journal of Medical Genetics Part B: Neuropsychiatric Genetics, 177*(3), 358–368. https://doi.org/10.1002/ajmg.b.32619

Will, E. A., Daunhauer, L. A., Fidler, D. J., Raitano Lee, N., Rosenberg, C. R., & Hepburn, S. L. (2019). Sensory processing and maladaptive behavior: Profiles within the Down syndrome phenotype. *Physical & Occupational Therapy In Pediatrics, 39*(5), 461–476. https://doi.org/10.1080/01942638.2019.1575320

Winders, P., Wolter-Warmerdam, K., & Hickey, F. (2019). A schedule of gross motor development for children with Down syndrome. *Journal of Intellectual Disability Research, 63*(4), 346–356. https://doi.org/10.1111/jir.12580

Wishart, J. G., & Johnston, F. H. (1990). The effects of experience on attribution of a stereotyped personality to children with Down's syndrome. *Journal of Intellectual Disability Research, 34*(5), 409–420. https://doi.org/10.1111/j.1365-2788.1990.tb01551.x

Wisniewski, K. E., & Schmidt-Sidor, B. (1989). Postnatal delay of myelin formation in brains from Down syndrome infants and children. *Clinical Neuropathology, 8*(2), 55–62. http://www.ncbi.nlm.nih.gov/pubmed/2524302

Wright, I., Lewis, V., & Collis, G. M. (2006). Imitation and representational development in young children with Down syndrome. *British Journal of Developmental Psychology, 24*(2), 429–450. https://doi.org/10.1348/026151005X51257

Yamauchi, Y., Aoki, S., Koike, J., Hanzawa, N., & Hashimoto, K. (2019). Motor and cognitive development of children with Down syndrome: The effect of acquisition of walking skills on their cognitive and language abilities. *Brain and Development, 41*(4), 320–326. https://doi.org/10.1016/J.BRAINDEV.2018.11.008

Yoshida, H., & Smith, L. B. (2008). What's in view for toddlers? Using a head camera to study visual experience. *Infancy, 13*(3), 229–248. https://doi.org/10.1080/15250000802004437

Yu, C., & Smith, L. B. (2012). Embodied attention and word learning by toddlers. *Cognition, 125*(2), 244–262. https://doi.org/10.1016/j.cognition.2012.06.016

Yu, C., & Smith, L. B. (2013). Joint attention without gaze following: Human infants and their parents coordinate visual attention to objects through eye-hand coordination. *PLoS ONE, 8*(11), e79659. https://doi.org/10.1371/journal.pone.0079659

Yu, C., & Smith, L. B. (2016). The social origins of sustained attention in one-year-old human infants. *Current Biology, 26*(9), 1235–1240. https://doi.org/10.1016/j.cub.2016.03.026

Zampini, L., & D'Odorico, L. (2009). Communicative gestures and vocabulary development in 36-month-old children with Down's syndrome. *International Journal of Language & Communication Disorders, 44*(6), 1063–1073. https://doi.org/10.1080/13682820802398288

Zelazo, P. R., Weiss, M. J., Papageorgiou, A. N., & Laplante, D. P. (1989). Recovery and dishabituation of sound localization among normal-, moderate-, and high-risk newborns: Discriminant validity. *Infant Behavior and Development, 12*(3), 321–340. https://doi.org/10.1016/0163-6383(89)90042-8

Zhu, F., Nair, R. R., Fisher, E. M. C., & Cunningham, T. J. (2019). Humanising the mouse genome piece by piece. *Nature Communications, 10*(1), 1845. https://doi.org/10.1038/s41467-019-09716-7

CHAPTER

9

The Developing Brain in Down Syndrome: Lessons From In Vivo Magnetic Resonance Neuroimaging

Nancy Raitano Lee, Manisha D. Udhnani, *and* Taralee Hamner

Abstract

Research on the developing brain in persons with Down syndrome has grown in recent years thanks to advances in neuroimaging approaches that are safe for pediatric populations. This literature documents global reductions in total brain volume as well as specific alterations in both cortical and subcortical structures. These include reductions in hippocampal and cerebellar volumes (that are in excess of reduced total brain volume) as well as abnormalities in frontal and temporal lobe anatomy. Recent neuroimaging research has highlighted the importance of using fine-grained approaches to characterizing cortical and subcortical anatomy in persons with Down syndrome as well as interpreting these findings within the context of research on typical brain development. In the current review, we attempt to synthesize this literature from a developmental perspective. Our hope is that this developmental focus will lead to discoveries about the biological underpinnings and unfolding of the learning difficulties associated with Down syndrome.

Key Words: Down syndrome, trisomy 21, neural, morphometry, cortex, hippocampus, cerebellum

Introduction

Since the turn of the 21st century, research on the developing brain in youth with Down syndrome (DS) has been steadily increasing. Apart from three studies published in the 1990s (Jernigan & Bellugi, 1990; Jernigan, Bellugi, Sowell, Doherty, & Hesselink, 1993; Wang, Doherty, Hesselink, & Bellugi, 1992), all of what we know about the developing brain in DS from neuroimaging studies has been amassed since the year 2000. Given that DS is the most common genetic cause of intellectual disability (ID; Parker et al., 2010) and is associated with high rates of precocious-onset Alzheimer's disease (for a review, see Head, Silverman, Patterson, & Lott, 2012), a great deal can be learned from pediatric neuroimaging research with this population. For example, pediatric imaging studies of DS may provide insights into atypicalities in the brain that are likely to play a role in the presentation of early manifestations of the DS cognitive-behavioral phenotype, including delays in language (for reviews, see Abbeduto, Arias-Trejo, Thurman,

Ramos-Sanchez, & del Hoyo Soriano, this volume; Abbeduto, Warren, & Conners, 2007), motor skills (Malak, Kostiukow, Krawczyk-Wasielewska, Mojs, E., & Samborski, 2015), and executive functions (Lanfranchi, Jerman, Dal Pont, Alberti, & Vianello, 2010; Lee et al., 2011; for a review, see Fidler, Daunhauer, Schworer, & Patel this volume). In addition, by studying individuals with DS long before the onset of Alzheimer's dementia, pediatric neuroimaging studies may provide a benchmark against which studies of neurodegeneration in DS may be compared. Thus, developmental neuroimaging in DS may provide important clues about neuroanatomy that are relevant to clinical care and our scientific understanding of the syndrome across the lifespan.

While the increase in DS pediatric imaging research has significantly grown in recent years, we are only beginning to learn about how the brain develops or changes during childhood and adolescence in this group. As researchers of typically developing children and adolescents describe the first three decades of life as a time of dynamic changes in the brain (see Giedd et al., 2009 for a review), we hope that this chapter will draw attention to the need for more research on the developing brain in persons with DS. Such investigations may provide important information about key windows of opportunity for biological and educational interventions in youth with DS during a period in which the brain is generally believed to be more plastic than it is during adulthood.

In this chapter, we review the small but growing literature on brain anatomy studied in vivo from childhood through young adulthood in individuals with DS. As this chapter is focused on development, we will begin by providing a summary of what is known about the typically developing brain based on studies from the structural neuroimaging literature. We provide this as a backdrop for interpreting existing neuroimaging study findings in persons with DS and as a means of highlighting directions for future research.

Overview of Early Typical Brain Development

Brain development, once thought to be linear and immutable with little variation in typical development, is now understood to be a unique process of dynamic growth and change with various individual differences contributing to development throughout the life span (Stiles & Jernigan, 2010). In the past, research on the brain was almost exclusively completed postmortem (i.e., after an individual has died) or through studies of brain and behavior focused on patients with different brain lesions. Significant advances in imaging have afforded unprecedented capacity for safe and feasible longitudinal investigations of pediatric populations, as concerns with radiation (which characterize imaging modalities like positron emission tomography, PET) were eliminated with the introduction of magnetic resonance imaging technology (Bunge & Kahn, 2009). This improved the field's ability to describe the *typically* developing brain, as researchers could readily view brains *in vivo* (i.e., in the living individual), a significant advantage over *ex vivo* (i.e., outside of the living individual) studies that have limited generalizability (due to possible pathologies that may have contributed to the death of the individual being studied, particularly in pediatric samples).

To statistically identify and characterize structural brain differences in vivo, tools have been developed to mathematically quantify anatomical features of the brain through modern neuroimaging technologies. A few of the more common methods to evaluate brain morphometry include surface-based morphometry, voxel-based morphometry, and deformation-based morphometry (Bunge & Kahn, 2009). Through the application of these technologies, brain structures and developmental changes have been mapped in great detail, producing distinct growth trajectories for different brain regions, with a particular emphasis on the developing cerebral cortex (e.g., Giedd et al., 1999; Gogtay et al., 2004).

The human brain is thought to be composed of roughly 85–100 billion neurons (Azevedo et al., 2009) that are responsible for transmitting and storing information. Whereas the bulk of neurons and rudimentary neural pathways are produced by the end of the second trimester (Kostovic & Jovanov-Milosevic, 2006; Rakic, 1995), infancy and very early childhood are characterized by so-called "synaptic exuberance" (Stiles & Jernigan, 2010), that is, the production of synaptic connections that afford the opportunity for neuronal communication. During infancy and early childhood, synaptogenesis occurs at an unparalleled rate (Moore, Persaud, & Torchia, 2015; Petanjek et al., 2011), resulting in an overabundance of synaptic connections. Through an experience-driven process, excess or redundant connections are thought to be pruned while critical connections are strengthened. During childhood and adolescence, approximately 40 percent of synapses are pruned in order to reach adult levels (for a review, see Webb, Monk, & Nelson, 2001). Thus, while the prenatal period is characterized by neural proliferation and the formation of basic neural pathways, infancy, childhood, and adolescence are characterized by synaptic exuberance and subsequent pruning. These processes permit the development of neural networks that are believed to underlie higher-level cognitive abilities (Innocenti & Price, 2005; O'Leary, 1992).

Structural Neuroimaging Studies of Typically Developing Youth

In the sections that follow, we describe what is known about the typically developing brain in childhood and adolescence from studies using magnetic resonance imaging (MRI) technology. MRI permits detailed descriptions of brain tissue (Bunge & Kahn, 2009). However, the resolution of MR imaging only allows descriptions of the brain at the level of the voxel (i.e., a discrete three-dimensional space that often ranges from 1–3 ml, though sizes are decreasing with advancing technology; Giedd, 2008). Voxels are believed to include thousands of neurons (Hassabis et al., 2009) or more. Thus, when interpreting MRI data, we need to acknowledge the (relatively) low degree of resolution it affords and the fact that this low resolution results in the need to make inferences about the cellular content of the images yielded from MRI investigations.

Descriptions of Total-Brain, Gray, and White-Matter Volumes

Total brain volume (TBV) is a global measure of brain size that typically describes cortical (i.e., the exterior surface of the brain) and subcortical (i.e., interior regions of the brain that are below the cerebral cortex) tissue. It is about 95 percent of its adult size in early childhood (Caviness, Kennedy, Richelme, Rademacher, & Filipek, 1996) but continues to undergo age-related changes well into adolescence. TBV has been linked to various cognitive capacities. For example, based on a meta-analysis including 1530 individuals amassed from 37 studies, McDaniel (2005) reported correlations, albeit modest ones, between TBV and measures of intelligence (r =0.33).

In the imaging literature, TBV is often divided into measures of total gray matter (GM) and total white matter (WM). As reviewed by Stiles and Jernigan (2010), GM is primarily composed of neuronal bodies, their dendrites (neuronal branches that receive information from other neurons), and synapses (gaps where electrical and chemical communication between neurons takes place). It also contains glial (support) cells and capillaries, as well as some axons. The outermost layer of the cerebrum, underneath the pial (i.e., outer) surface, is known as the cerebral cortex and is composed of GM. GM is also found deep within the brain (e.g., hippocampus, amygdala, hypothalamus, thalamus, basal ganglia) and in the cerebellum.

Stiles and Jernigan (2010) also note that WM is composed of bundles of myelinated axons, or tracts, found beneath the outer surface of the brain. These tracts form neural networks composed of vast webs of connections between various cortical and subcortical brain regions. By linking distal cell bodies within GM, WM tracts transport signals between different regions of the brain.

During infancy and very early childhood, GM is believed to increase across the brain, after which GM begins to decrease. This phenomenon is sometimes referred to as the inverted U-shaped trajectory (Giedd et al., 1999; Jernigan & Tallal, 1990; Sowell et al., 2003). In contrast, WM increases throughout childhood and into adulthood (Barnea-Goraly et al., 2005; Lenroot et al., 2007; Schmithorst, Wilke, Dardzinski, & Holland, 2002, when it begins to decline after age 40 years (Gunning-Dixon, Brickman, Cheng, & Alexopoulos, 2009).

In the next section, we will provide more nuanced descriptions of GM with a summary of what is known about the development of *subcortical* and *cortical* structures. The distinction between subcortical and cortical structures is an important one, because of the different evolutionary histories (Tuller, Kupiec, & Ruppin, 2008) and genetic contributions (Wen et al., 2016) to these structures. We start with descriptions of the evolutionarily "older" subcortex and then transition to summarizing the larger corpus of literature on the evolutionarily "newer" cortex.

Descriptions of subcortical structures. The subcortical structures reviewed in this section include the amygdala, hippocampus, various subdivisions of the basal ganglia, and the cerebellum. A part of the limbic system, the amygdala is involved in regulating emotions, memory, and survival instincts (McDonald, 1998). The amygdala experiences a rapid, nonlinear increase of volume after age 4, reaching peak volume between 9-11 years of age (Uematsu et al., 2012). The hippocampus is a subcortical structure recognized for its role in memory (Squire, 1992). Within the developing brain, age-related nonlinear increases of the hippocampus have been widely observed (Dennison et al., 2013; Giedd et al., 1996; Ostby et al., 2009; Sussman, Leung, Chakravarty, Lerch, & Taylor, 2016; Uematsu et al., 2012). Similar to the amygdala, peak volume of the hippocampus has been reported to be between 9–11 years of age (Uematsu et al., 2012).

The caudate nucleus and the putamen are components of the basal ganglia that form the dorsal striatum. They are separated by the internal capsule, a large WM tract that extends to the cerebral cortex. The caudate is believed to contribute to goal-directed behavior, executive function, and memory (Levy, Friedman, Davachi, & Goldman-Rakic, 1997). The putamen is associated with coordinating movement of the limbs (Crutcher & DeLong, 1984) as well as various cognitive functions, including executive functions (Sullivan, De La Paz, Zipursky, & Pfefferbaum, 1991) and implicit learning abilities (Reber, 2013). The volume of both the caudate and the putamen have been found to decrease during childhood and adolescence (Ostby et al., 2009; Sussman et al., 2016).

The cerebellum, which is Latin for "little brain" (Mendoza & Foundas, 2008), is located below the cerebrum (in an area sometimes referred to as an infratentorial region) and is a part of the hindbrain. Although once thought to contribute only to motor development, the cerebellum is now believed to be important for higher-order cognitive functioning (Middleton & Strick, 2001; Ramnani, 2006). Much like the overall curve of cortical development, the cerebellum is believed to follow an inverted U-shaped trajectory over childhood and adolescence (Tiemeier et al., 2010).

Descriptions of cortical structures. The cerebral cortex is characterized by a distinctive folded pattern of peaks (gyri) and ridges (sulci). It is believed to have evolved to maximize the total surface area of this neuron-rich part of the human brain (Hoffman, 1989; Todd, 1985) and to be a key contributor to the higher-level cognitive capacities that differentiate humans and other mammals (Rakic, 2009). The cerebral cortex is divided into four lobes—frontal, temporal, parietal, and occipital.

The maturation of the GM across the lobes of the cerebral cortex is heterogeneous, with different cortical regions maturing or reaching "peak volumes" at different times. GM maturation appears to follow a nonlinear trajectory with evolutionarily older areas of the cortex maturing before newer ones (Gogtay et al., 2004). Specifically, Gogtay et al. (2004) provided evidence that lower-order somatosensory (posterior frontal and anterior/superior parietal lobes) and visual (occipital lobe) regions (i.e., regions of the brain that are central to the development of abilities that emerge during infancy and the toddler years such as motor and visual development, respectively) are among the earliest to develop in childhood. The maturation of these regions is believed to precede the maturation of regions of the brain thought to be central to the execution of higher-level cognitive abilities, such as language, reasoning, and problem-solving abilities. These regions include higher-order association areas, such as prefrontal and superior temporal regions of the brain.

Complementing the studies of cortical volume in typically developing youth, researchers have employed surface-based morphometric approaches to neuroimaging to dissect the cortical mantle into its two constituent parts of cortical surface area and cortical thickness (Im et al., 2008). Cortical thickness represents the distance between the pial surface of the cortex (i.e., the surface that interfaces with cerebral spinal fluid) and the WM surface. These genetically (Panizzon et al., 2009) and evolutionarily (Rakic, 1995) distinct morphometric features appear to also be characterized by distinct developmental trajectories (Raznahan et al., 2011).

Now that we have provided a background on typical brain development, we turn to the literature on the development of the brain in persons with DS. In the sections that follow, we provide a brief overview of what is known about the brains of persons with DS during prenatal and infant development. We then turn our focus to studies of children, adolescents, and young adults with DS.

Early Brain Development in Persons With DS

Atypicalities in brain development in persons with DS have been reported during the prenatal period, infancy, childhood, and adolescence. While the focus of the current chapter is on in vivo neuroimaging investigations conducted during childhood and adolescence, we provide a brief summary of what is known about prenatal and infant brain development in persons with DS that was acquired from postmortem investigations of brain tissue from fetuses and infants. In particular, abnormalities have been found in both subcortical and cortical structures. Specifically, reductions in hippocampal (Guidi et al., 2008) and cerebellar (Guidi, Ciani, Bonasoni, Santini, & Bartesaghi, 2011) cell number have been reported in studies of fetuses. Moreover, cortical abnormalities have been noted, including both delayed and atypical cortical lamination (Golden & Hyman, 1994). Further, significantly reduced dendritic spine density and synaptogenesis have been reported during the prenatal period (Weitzdoerfer, Dierssen, Fountoulakis, & Lubec, 2001).

Consistent with the child structural neuroimaging literature which will be described next, gross morphological differences in the brains of infants with DS are observed prior to 6 months of age. These include decreased fronto-occipital length and a narrowed superior temporal gyrus (Schmidt-Sidor, Wisniewski, Shepard, & Sersen, 1990). Additionally, atypical cortical layering as well as reduced arborization (the branching of dendrites) and number of dendritic spines have been found within the visual cortex of fetuses and infants with DS (Takashima, Becker, Armstrong, & Chan, 1981). Delays in the myelination of intercortical fibers of the frontal and temporal lobes are also noted in infancy and very early childhood (Wisniewski & Schmidt-Sidor, 1989).

Structural Neuroimaging Studies of Youth With DS

Early literature on brain development in youth with DS studied in vivo using MRI focused on descriptions of gross anatomical differences between youth with DS and their typically developing peers (Jernigan & Bellugi, 1990; Jernigan et al., 1993; Kates, Folley, Lanham, Capone, & Kaufmann, 2002; Pinter, Brown, et al., 2001; Pinter, Eliez, Schmitt, Capone, & Reiss, 2001). As the literature has grown in the past 5–10 years, more nuanced descriptions of brain morphometry have been provided, including two studies in which voxel-based morphometry was used to describe fine-grained whole-brain structural differences in the developing brain in youth with DS (Carducci et al., 2013; Menghini, Costanzo, & Vicari, 2011) and one surface-based morphometric study in which vertex-level (~80,000 points bilaterally) deviations in cortical thickness and surface area in children, adolescents, and young adults with DS were reported (Lee et al., 2016). Moreover, detailed descriptions of WM architecture are beginning to emerge, with one study of toddlers with DS (Gunbey et al., 2017) in which diffusion tensor imaging (DTI) technology (a technique which measures diffusion of water in brain tissue to provide "maps" of WM tracks) revealed atypicalities in WM structures.

In this section, we compile the findings from structural neuroimaging studies of children, adolescents, and young adults with DS that (a) included a typically developing comparison group matched on chronological age (CA), and (b) reported on a DS sample with a mean age of 30 years or below. The rationale for imposing these inclusion criteria were as follows. One, we only included studies that compared youth with DS to a group of typically developing comparison participants so that we could provide the reader with a description of how the brain in DS differs from what is *typically expected* for individuals of a similar age. We chose not to focus on studies that compared participants with DS to other syndromes, as this would not allow us to speak to how the brains of persons with DS differ from typical age expectations. The studies reviewed in this chapter are focused on comparisons between participants with DS and CA-matched comparison participants. This is the case, as no published structural neuroimaging studies of youth with DS have included a mental age (MA) matched comparison group (a practice which is standard in the cognitive behavioral research literature on persons with DS and other syndromes associated with ID; for reviews, see Burack, Evans, Klaiman, & Iarocci, 2001; Burack, Russo, Flores, Iarocci, & Zigler, 2012; Godfrey & Lee, 2018). Use of a CA-matched comparison group in developmental neuroimaging investigations of atypical child development, including studies on attention deficit/hyperactivity disorder, autism, and childhood onset schizophrenia (for a review, see Shaw, Gogtay, & Rapoport, 2010), is standard practice. This practice also appears to have been adopted by researchers using structural neuroimaging to characterize the developing brain in youth with DS (however, for a discussion of the pitfalls of this approach, see Burack, Russo, Gordon Green, Landry, & Iarocci, 2016).

Regarding the second inclusion criterion, we imposed the upper age limit of 30 years for our review for two reasons. One, because virtually all adults with DS will present with the neuropathology associated with Alzheimer's disease by approximately 40 years of age (Mann, 1988), we elected to exclude studies with participants who may already be experiencing early Alzheimer's-related neurodegeneration (even if they do not behaviorally present with the symptoms of dementia). Thus, we selected a conservative age cutoff of 30 years to avoid describing studies of neurodegeneration rather than neurodevelopment in this group. Two, studies of the effects of aging on the brain in DS were excluded as they are discussed elsewhere in this volume (see Helman, Van Pelt, Schmitt, & Head, this volume).

These inclusion criteria for our review yielded a total of 14 studies published between the years 1990 and 2017. Details about the study designs, including numbers and ages of participants, MRI scanner, and the procedures used to quantify brain morphometry are provided in Table 9.1. The findings across studies of volumetric differences in whole-brain, cortical, and subcortical structures in youth with DS relative to typically developing comparison participants are summarized in Table 9.2. The studies in which nonvolumetric techniques were used are described below in the text only.

Descriptions of Total-Brain, Gray, and White-Matter Volumes

There is substantial empirical support that youth and young adults with DS present with smaller TBV than same age peers. As can be seen in Table 9.2, reduced TBV among youth with DS relative to typically developing comparison participants has been reported in six studies (Kates et al., 2002; Lee et al., 2016; Menghini et al., 2011; Pinter, Brown, et al., 2001; Pinter, Eliez, et al., 2001; Smigielska-Kuzia et al., 2011). Consistent with these findings, the evidence indicates reduced total GM and WM volumes in studies of children and adolescents with DS (Lee et al., 2016; Menghini et al., 2011; Pinter, Eliez, et al., 2001; but see Gunbey et al., 2017 for disparate findings in toddlers with DS).

In order to provide a more nuanced description of the developing brain in persons with DS, we now refine our focus and describe the literature on subcortical and cortical brain morphometry. Prior to reviewing this literature, though, we briefly highlight differences in the ways in which investigators quantify specific neuroanatomical differences in DS relative to typically developing comparison participants. More specifically, because of robust differences in TBV in youth with DS, some investigators deem it important to describe deviations in specific neuroanatomic structures *after accounting for overall reductions in TBV*—that is, after covarying for TBV in analyses. However, this is not a universal practice and some investigators do not adjust for reduced TBV. Some report results for raw/unadjusted volumes as well as adjusted volumes. Some describe findings when controlling for GM or WM specifically, and some report findings controlling for intracranial volume (ICV; i.e., the volume of the cranial vault). Thus, when summarizing results in the text and in Table 9.2, we make an effort to indicate whether the findings describe raw anatomical differences or differences in volumes after adjustment for some global measure of brain volume. This distinction is necessary because the former refers to absolute differences between the participants with DS and participants in the comparison group, whereas the latter refers to proportional differences. In this latter scenario, even though a structure may be

Table 9.1. Magnetic Resonance Imaging Studies of Individuals with DS between the Ages of 2 and 30 Years Organized Chronologically

Study ID	Authors	Year	Title	Groups (n)	Mean Ages (years)	Scanner Strength	Method Used to Quantify Brain Morphometry
1	Jernigan & Bellugi	1990	Anomalous brain morphology on magnetic resonance images in Williams syndrome and Down syndrome	DS (3) WS (6) TD (14)	DS (16) WS (15.8) TD (19)	1.5T	Manual tracing
2	Wang et al.	1992	Callosal morphology concurs with neurobehavioral and neuropathological findings in two neurodevelopmental disorders	DS (7) WS (11) TD (17)	no mean age given; age range 10-20	1.5T	Manual tracing
3	Jernigan et al.	1993	Cerebral morphologic distinctions between Williams and Down syndromes	WS (9) DS (6) TD (21)	DS (15.5) WS (14.7)TD (14.5)	1.5T	Computerized segmentation; of GM, WM, CSF; manual tracing of structures
4	Pinter et al.	2001	Amygdala and hippocampal volumes in children with Down syndrome: A high-resolution MRI study	DS (16) TD (15)	DS (11.3) TD (11.9)	1.5T	Semi-automated with manual tracing of amygdala and hippocampus
5	Pinter et al.	2001	Neuroanatomy of Down's syndrome: A high-resolution MRI study	DS (16) TD (15)	DS (11.3) TD (11.9)	1.5T	Semi-automated with some manual tracing
6	Kates et al.	2002	Cerebral growth in fragile X syndrome: Review and comparison with Down syndrome	DS (12) FXS (33) DLD (15) TD (8)	M~5-6	1.5T	Computerized segmentation of GM, WM, CSF; manual tracing of structures
7	Kaufmann et al.	2003	Specificity of cerebellar vermian abnormalities in autism: A quantitative magnetic resonance imaging study	DS (11) DS+ASD (16) FXS (9) FXS+ASD (13) ASD (10) TD (22)	DS (7.2) DS+ASD (7.0) FXS (5.3) FXS+ASD (5.7) ASD (6.9) TD (8.3)	1.5T	Semi-automated; manual delineation of midline structures and quantification with BrainImage

(*continued*)

Table 9.1. *Continued*

Study ID	Authors	Year	Title	Groups (n)	Mean Ages (years)	Scanner Strength	Method Used to Quantify Brain Morphometry
8	Carter et al.	2008	Neuroanatomic correlates of autism and stereotypy in children with Down syndrome	DS (15) TD (22) DS+ ASD (15)	DS (9.1) TD (10.3) DS+ASD (7.9)	1.5T	Automated parcellation
9	Menghini et al.	2011	Relationship between brain and cognitive processes in Down syndrome	DS (12) TD (12)	DS (16) TD (15.9)	1.5T	Automated parcellation using voxel-based morphometry
10	Smigielska-Kuzia et al.	2011	A volumetric magnetic resonance imaging study of brain structures in children with Down syndrome	DS (23) TD (26)	DS (6.7) TD (8.3)	1.5T	Manual tracing
11	Carducci et al.	2013	Whole-brain voxel-based morphometry study of children and adolescents with Down syndrome	DS (21) TD (27)	DS (10.5) TD (10.7)	1.5T	Automated parcellation using voxel-based morphometry
12	Lee et al.	2016	Dissociations in cortical morphometry in youth with Down syndrome: Evidence for reduced surface area but increased thickness	DS (31) TD (45)	DS (15.2) TD (15.7)	3T	Automated parcellation of volumes and surface-based measurements of cortical thickness & surface area using CIVET pipeline
13	Fujii et al.	2017	A small pons as a characteristic finding in Down syndrome: A quantitative MRI study	DS (32) TD (32)	DS (3) TD (3)	1.5T	Manual tracing of height, width and area of brain stem structures
14	Gunbey et al.	2017	Structural brain alterations of Down's syndrome in early childhood evaluation by DTI and volumetric analyses	DS (10) TD (8)	DS (2.6) TD (2.5)	1.5T	Automated measurement of diffusion using FMRIB's diffusion toolbox

Key: ASD=Autism Spectrum Disorder; DLD=Developmental Language Delay; DS=Down syndrome; FXS=Fragile X syndrome; T=Tesla (magnet strength); TD=typically developing; WS=Williams syndrome

Table 9.2. Volumetric Findings for DS Neuroimaging Studies Summarized and Numbered in Table 1

	Raw (Unadjusted Volumes)		Adjusted Volumes		
	DS < TD	DS ~ TD	DS < TD	DS ~ TD	DS > TD
Total Tissue Measures					
Total Brain	**4, 5, 6, 9, 10, 12**				
Total WM	**5, 9, 12**	**14**		**12^**	
Total GM	**5, 9, 12**	**14**		**12^**	
Cerebrum	**3, 5**				
Cerebral GM	**3, 5**				
Cerebral WM	**5**				
Subcortical GM	**14**	**5**			
Total Cortical	**1, 6**				
Cortical GM	**6, 12, 14**				**12^**
Cortical WM	**6, 12**			**12^**	
Subcortical Structures					
Basal Ganglia					
Putamen	**14L**	**14R**			
Caudate	**14**			**3@**	
Pallidum	**14L**	**14R**			
Limbic Structures					
Hippocampus	**10**	**14**	**4^**		
Amygdala	**10**	**14**		**4^**	
Thalamus	**14**				
Infratentorial Structures					
Total Cerebellar	**1, 3**		**5^**		
Cerebellar GM	**14**		**5***		
Cerebellar WM	**14R**		**5$**		
Vermis I-V	**1**				
Vermis VI-VII		**1**			
Brainstem	**14**				
Cortical Structures					
Total Frontal	**10**	**6**		**5^**	
Frontal GM	**12**	**6**		**12^**	
Frontal WM	**12**	**6**	**12^**		

(continued)

Table 9.2. *Continued*

	Raw (Unadjusted Volumes)		Adjusted Volumes		
	DS < TD	DS ~ TD	DS < TD	DS ~ TD	DS > TD
Total Temporal	**6, 10**			**$5^{\wedge}$**	
Temporal GM	**6,12**			**5^{*}**	**$12^{\wedge}$**
Temporal WM	**6,12**				**$5^{\$}$, $12^{\wedge}$**
Total Parietal	**6**			**$5^{\wedge}$**	
Parietal GM		**6, 12**			**5^{*}, $12^{\wedge}$**
Parietal WM	**6, 12**			**$5^{\$}$**	**$12^{\wedge}$**
Total Occipital		**6**		**$5^{\wedge}$**	
Occipital GM	**12**	**6**			**$12^{\wedge}$**
Occipital WM	**12**	**6**		**$12^{\wedge}$**	

Key:

L=left

R=right

Numbers correspond to "Study ID" in Table 9.1.

Please note that superscripts denote that the study adjusted for:

^ TBV; @ cerebral GM volume; * total GM volume; $ total WM

absolutely smaller for the participants with DS, it may be proportionally larger than that observed in comparison participants once reductions in TBV are controlled.

Descriptions of subcortical structures. As can be seen in Table 9.2, there is consistent evidence for reductions in the volume of the hippocampus in youth with DS, both when raw (unadjusted) volumes are considered (Pinter, Brown, et al., 2001; Smigielska-Kuzia et al., 2011) and when TBV-adjusted hippocampal volumes (Pinter, Brown, et al., 2001) are examined. These findings converge with postmortem human investigations (Contestabile et al., 2007; Guidi et al., 2008). Similarly, reductions in unadjusted amygdala volumes have been reported in school-age children with DS (Pinter, Brown, et al., 2001; Smigielska-Kuzia et al., 2011). However, unlike the hippocampus, reductions in the amygdala do not survive adjustment for reduced TBV in school-aged children with DS (Pinter, Brown, et al., 2001), thus suggesting greater impacts to the hippocampus than the amygdala in DS.

With regard to infratentorial subcortical structures, the cerebellum has garnered much attention in the literature on the effects of trisomy 21 on the brain. This literature includes studies of individuals with DS as well as studies that have utilized animal models to help illuminate atypicalities in the cerebellum (Haydar & Reeves, 2012; Aziz & Haydar, this volume; Moyer and Reeves, this volume). Studies with pediatric populations provide converging evidence for reductions in total cerebellar volume both with (Pinter, Eliez, et al., 2001) and without (Jernigan & Bellugi, 1990; Jernigan et al., 1993) adjustment for TBV. Specific reductions have also been noted in cerebellar GM and WM volumes (Gunbey et al., 2017; Pinter, Eliez, et al., 2001), and in some cerebellar vermal structures (Jernigan & Bellugi, 1990).

Findings from voxel-based morphometric studies in which group differences are described at the level of voxel confirm atypicalities in the above-mentioned subcortical structures. For example, Carducci et al. (2013) reported reduced GM density (after correcting for differences in total intracranial volume) in regions of the hippocampus as well as multiple regions in the anterior and posterior cerebellum in children with DS. They also reported reduced WM density in regions of the pons (part of the brainstem) and both the anterior and posterior cerebellum. Consistent with these findings, Menghini et al. (2011) reported reduced GM density in regions of the posterior cerebellum and the hippocampus in youth with DS.

Complementing these studies are two recent studies of toddlers with DS. In a study focused on the brainstem, Fujii et al. (2017) reported reductions in the width and area of the midbrain; the height, width, and area of the pons; and the area of the medulla oblongata in toddlers with DS. In the only pediatric DTI investigation published to date, Gunbey et al. (2017) reported reduced fractional anisotropy (FA; i.e., directional water diffusion in brain tissue) in several WM bundles in toddlers with DS, suggesting atypical WM structure. These included the right cerebral peduncle, right anterior limb of the internal capsule, the uncinate fasciculus, the inferior longitudinal and inferior fronto-occipital fasciculi, and the body of the corpus callosum.

Descriptions of cortical structures. Table 9.2 summarizes studies in which the volume of the four cortical lobes are quantified, including findings when raw, unadjusted values and TBV-adjusted values are considered. As can be seen, statistically significant reductions in the volumes of all four lobes have been reported in several investigations. However, results vary by whether the researchers adjusted for overall TBV as well as what tissue type is considered—GM vs. WM. In addition, it is important to note that many of the studies published as of this writing focused on small samples of individuals with DS, resulting in limited power to detect statistically significant differences between groups. Our recent review of the DS pediatric neuroimaging literature revealed that most studies of cortical lobar anatomy in DS indicate group differences that are medium to large in effect; however, not all studies were sufficiently powered to detect these differences (Hamner, Udhnani, Osipowicz, & Lee, 2018).

Of the four lobes, the most consistent evidence for reduced volume of large effect comes from studies of the frontal lobe. Collapsed across studies that compared a group of persons/children with DS to an age-matched typically developing comparison group (Carter, Capone, & Kaufman, 2008; Kates et al., 2002; Lee et al., 2016; Pinter, Eliez, et al., 2001), the mean effect size for group differences in total frontal volume or frontal GM and WM calculated using Cohen's *d* formula (DS group mean—comparison group mean/pooled standard deviation; Cohen, 1988) is -1.73 (range = -1.13 to -2.62). Consistent with these findings is evidence from a voxel-based morphometric investigation that revealed reductions in GM density in multiple frontal regions in persons with DS after controlling for total intracranial volume (Carducci et al., 2013) as well as reductions in WM density (after controlling for reduced intracranial volume; Carducci et al., 2013). Similarly, Lee et al. (2016) reported reductions in cortical surface area in much of the frontal lobe, with particularly significant reductions in dorsal medial regions after adjusting for reductions in TBV. These reductions in surface area in Lee et al. (2016) were alongside *increases* in cortical thickness in the frontal lobes. See Figure 9.1 for a reproduction of the results from Lee et al. (2016).

For the temporal, parietal, and occipital lobes, reduced lobar volumes with mean effect sizes of -1.43 (range: -0.54 to -3.1), -1.27 (range: -0.2 to -1.92), and -1.38 (range: -0.34 to -2.37), respectively, have been found across studies (Carter et al., 2008; Kates et al., 2002; Lee et al., 2016; Pinter, Eliez, et al., 2001). These lobar-level findings are complemented by findings from voxel-based morphometric studies that have reported reduced GM density in the medial (Carducci et al., 2013; Menghini et al., 2011) and inferior (Menghini et al., 2011) temporal lobe, as well as regions of the parietal lobe (Menghini et al., 2011). These reductions were accompanied by increases in GM density in regions of the medial

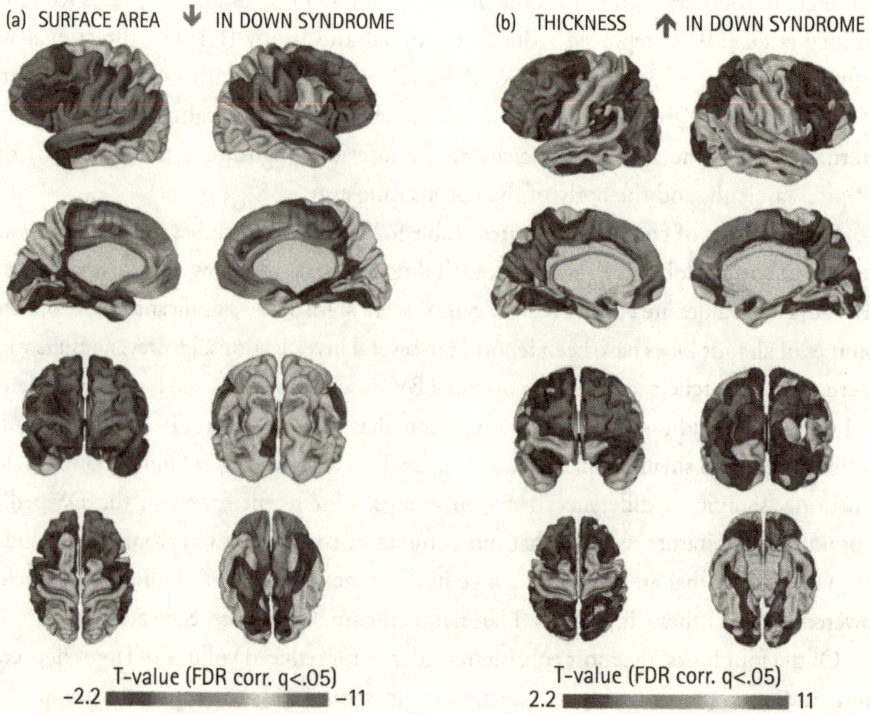

Figure 9.1. Decreases in cortical surface area (panel a) and increases in cortical thickness (panel b) in a pediatric brain imaging sample from Lee et al. (2016). Reductions in cortical surface area and increases in cortical thickness in DS relative to typical controls. A series of regression analyses were completed at 40,962 vertices in each hemisphere using the following regression equation: Cortical thickness or surface area ($vertex_i$) ~ intercept + β1(sex) + β2 (age centered) + β3 (group). T-statistics associated with the group term that exceeded the FDR-corrected threshold of ±2.2 were projected onto the cortex. Panel (a) displays surface area findings; panel (b) displays cortical thickness findings. Note that the range of T-values for surface area is negative 2.2 to negative 11 while the range for thickness is positive 2.2 to positive 11. This is because DS is associated with largely decreased surface area relative to controls but largely increased cortical thickness. To identify regions in which cortical surface area and thickness were most deviant from controls, the t-scores associated with the group term in the regression equation were ranked and those vertices above the 90th percentile for thickness and below the 10th percentile for surface area were identified. The approximate locations of the peak vertices within these regions are marked with small red circles in panels (a) and (b). *Reference:* Image and caption taken from Lee et al. (2016).

temporal lobe. With regard to WM density, Carducci et al. (2013) reported reductions in WM in multiple regions of the parietal lobes as well as increases in some regions of the temporal lobes including the parahippocampal gyrus.

In summary, widespread differences in the cerebral cortex have been reported for children and young adults with DS relative to same age peers. While studies of the frontal lobes reveal consistently large effect sizes relative to CA-matched comparison participants, all of the cortical lobes have been reported to differ from same age peers, with mean effect sizes collapsing across investigations falling into the large range. In the section that follows, we synthesize the structural neuroimaging literature reviewed thus far within the context of what is known about the cognitive-behavioral phenotype of persons with DS. We also integrate findings from functional neuroimaging investigations of DS. We then review the neuroimaging literature through a developmental lens and note trends in more recent publications that may provide clues to the developmental unfolding of the DS neuroanatomical and cognitive phenotypes.

Cognitive-Behavioral Synthesis

The hallmark of the DS cognitive-behavioral phenotype is ID, with the vast majority (Gibson, 1978), but not all (Epstein, 1989), persons with DS having varying degrees of ID. In addition to global intellectual impairments, DS is associated with deficits in language comprehension and expression that far exceed general cognitive delays. These include impaired articulation (Dodd, 1975) and syntactic weaknesses (Fowler, Gelman, & Gleitman, 1994), as well as significant deficits in verbal short-term memory (for reviews, see Baddeley & Jarrold, 2007; Smith & Jarrold, this volume). Impairments in multiple domains of executive function are also reported, with the most consistent deficits reported for working memory and cognitive flexibility (see Lee, Maiman, & Godfrey, 2016; Fidler et al., this volume, for reviews). In addition, impairments on explicit long-term memory tasks, such as paired associates learning, spatial memory, and delayed recall tasks are a prominent feature among those with DS (Edgin, Pennington, & Mervis, 2010; Pennington, Moon, Edgin, Stedron, & Nadel, 2003). In contrast, implicit memory abilities (Vicari, Verucci, & Carlesimo, 2007) and some aspects of visual-spatial processing (for a review, see Yang, Conners, & Merrill, 2014) have been reported to be closer to MA expectations, although still below expectations for CA.

Neuroanatomical regions relevant to the DS cognitive-behavioral phenotype. We now highlight what is known about the neural correlates of (a) intellectual abilities, (b) speech and language skills, (c) explicit memory, and (d) executive function from the literature on individuals with typical development and those with other developmental disorders or acquired brain injuries to hypothesize about the neural underpinnings of cognitive difficulties that are commonly reported in individuals with DS.

Intellectual ability. Research from studies of typically developing adults has provided evidence for a modest positive correlation between TBV and intellectual abilities (for a review and meta-analysis, see McDaniel, 2005). Further research should explore whether this association extends to those with intellectual disabilities, particularly DS. Complementing these studies are those documenting relations between cortical volume (Jung & Haier, 2007), thickness (Shaw et al., 2006), and surface area (Schnack et al., 2015) of the frontal and parietal lobes with intellectual functioning in typically developing individuals. Group differences in frontal and parietal lobe volumes have been reported in persons with DS relative to typically developing controls (see Hamner et al., 2018 for a review). In addition, prominent atypicalities in cortical thickness have been noted in the frontal and parietal lobes in youth with DS (Lee et al., 2016). These findings suggest that future research should be focused on the relations between frontal and parietal anatomy/physiology and intellectual functioning in persons with DS in order to begin to understand the neural underpinnings of reduced intellectual ability in this population.

Speech and language functioning. With regard to more specific aspects of the DS cognitive-behavioral phenotype including the prominent speech and language challenges faced by persons with DS (see Martin et al., 2009 for a review), we turn to the literature on idiopathic speech and language disorders (i.e., speech and language disorders without an identified cause) to identify regions of interest for understanding the neural correlates of these challenges among persons with DS. In a review of this literature, Liégeois, Mayes, and Morgan (2014) highlighted volumetric differences in the superior temporal gyrus (for the speech disorders), the inferior frontal gyrus (for language disorders), and the temporo-parietal junction (for both speech and language disorders). Complementing this literature is research emerging over the past decade that has drawn attention to the cerebellum as a key brain structure involved with language functioning, including both articulation and broader language function (for a review, see Mariën et al., 2014). Given evidence for atypical frontal, temporal, and cerebellar development in DS, atypicalities in these regions (among others) likely contribute to the prominent speech and language impairments faced by individuals with DS.

Memory abilities. Research on the neural correlates of explicit memory abilities such as those tapped by list learning or paired associates learning tasks have repeatedly been tied to the functioning of the medial temporal lobes and hippocampal formation structures in particular (for a review, see Jabès & Nelson, 2015). As summarized above, the hippocampal formation and related medial temporal lobe structures have been the focus of much research, with converging evidence from pediatric and adult neuroimaging, postmortem investigations of children and adults with DS, as well as animal models documenting atypical development (see Clark, Fernandez, Sakhon, Spanò, & Edgin, 2017 for a review). In contrast, implicit memory abilities, which have been found to be MA-appropriate in DS (Vicari et al., 2007), have been tied to the basal ganglia among other structures (Reber, 2013), which, at least in the neuroimaging literature with adults with DS, have been reported to be similar in volume to that of typically developing comparison participants (Raz et al., 1995); however, see Gunbey et al., (2017) in which lateralized reductions in basal ganglia structures were noted in preschoolers with DS.

Executive functions. With regard to executive function, and in particular, impairments in working memory and cognitive flexibility that are often reported for persons with DS (for reviews, see Smith & Jarrold, this volume; Fidler et al., this volume), a large body of research implicates the prefrontal cortex and its widespread neural connections with both working memory (for a review, see D'Esposito & Postle, 2015) and cognitive flexibility (for a review, see Dajani & Uddin, 2015). In addition, networks that connect the cerebellum to the frontal and parietal lobes are likely to be a source of variability in executive function and other complex cognitive skills (for a review, see Stoodley, 2012). Given evidence suggesting strong ties between working memory and fluid intelligence (Engle, Tuholski, Laughlin, & Conway, 1999), research on the factors that contribute to the atypical development and connectivity of the frontal lobes and cerebellum in DS may be fruitful for augmenting our understanding of the biological underpinnings of not only executive function impairments, but also global learning challenges experienced by individuals with DS.

Functional neuroimaging studies of persons with DS. Though functional neuroimaging comprises methods such as PET, electroencephalography (EEG), magnetoencephalography (MEG), and functional magnetic resonance imaging (fMRI), we will focus our brief review on the fMRI literature only (for a more detailed review of functional imaging in DS, including EEG investigations, see Burack et al., 2016). Unlike structural MRI, that is used to quantify deviations in neuroanatomy in DS, fMRI is used to describe deviations in neurophysiology both globally and locally when individuals are at rest or engaged in tasks. The primary variable of interest in fMRI investigations is the blood oxygen level dependent (BOLD) signal. It is a measurement of variations in oxygenated blood that is believed to be an indirect estimate of neural activity (for a review, see Brown, Perthen, Liu, & Buxton, 2007). While many associate fMRI with task-based measurements of the BOLD-signal (i.e., changes in BOLD signal in different brain regions as a function of completion of a cognitive or other task), there has been an increasing interest over the past several years in resting state fMRI (for a review of resting state methods, see Smitha et al., 2017). This latter method is concerned with measuring coordinated fluctuations in the BOLD signal in different brain regions while the subject is at rest (or engaging in some passive experience) in order to identify networks of brain regions that are thought to work in unison in order to complete different cognitive tasks.

We include studies in which both task-based and resting-state techniques are used in order to characterize the DS neurophysiological phenotype. The studies reviewed are focused on the neurophysiological correlates of global learning difficulties (IQ) and adaptive function impairments, story listening, and semantic classification/object recognition. Analogous to the prior section, we begin our review with the neurophysiological correlates of global abilities, such as IQ and adaptive functioning. We then narrow our discussion to examine specific cognitive skills.

Resting state functional connectivity studies of DS. In the first study on widespread neural synchrony in the brains of persons with DS using fMRI, Anderson et al. (2013)

reported higher levels of synchrony between short-distance brain regions alongside lower levels of synchrony between long-distance brain regions in persons with DS relative to typically developing comparison participants. Anderson et al. suggested that the reduced long-distance connectivity (i.e., correlated activity) may contribute to an impaired ability to integrate information collected from distant brain areas to provide a cohesive network necessary for higher-level cognitive function. This suggestion fits with the developmental literature on "functional brain networks" in which long-distance, functionally related connections are believed to develop later and underlie higher-level cognitive abilities that emerge over childhood and adolescence (Fair et al., 2009). Fair et al. (2007) hypothesized that, as functional networks develop, correlations within networks increase while those between networks decrease. Consistent with this developmental framework, Anderson et al. (2013) reported that individuals with DS with lower intellectual abilities (as assessed by nonverbal IQ) demonstrated the weakest within-network correlations, suggesting "less mature" neural synchrony.

Similar to Anderson et al. (2013), Pujol et al. (2015) reported that individuals with DS demonstrated anomalous functional connectivity relative to comparison participants matched on age and sex. Specifically, higher global connectivity (i.e., correlated activity) was reported in the ventral anterior cingulate cortex (ACC), while lower global connectivity was reported in the dorsal ACC/medial frontal cortex, dorsal prefrontal cortex, left posterior insula cortex, and poster cingulate cortex. Moreover, these functional connectivity disturbances were associated with performance on the Adaptive Behavior Assessment System, Second Edition (ABAS-II; Harrison & Oakland, 2006), a commonly used questionnaire that assesses adaptive functioning skills. Both the increases and decreases in connectivity within these regions were associated with individual differences in adaptive skills, suggesting that widespread disturbances in connectivity patterns may contribute to difficulties completing activities of daily living by persons with DS.

Task-based functional neuroimaging studies of DS. Two fMRI studies of the neural correlates of story listening revealed abnormal activation patterns among adolescents and young adults with DS (Jacola et al., 2014; Losin, Rivera, O'Hare, Sowell, & Pinter, 2009). In the first study, Losin et al. (2009) examined neural activation in young adults with DS relative to a typically developing comparison participants matched roughly on CA, ~22 and 18 years, respectively, when passively listening to a story (forward speech), listening to the story read backwards (backward speech), and at rest. They reported lower levels of activation for the participants with DS as compared to the typically developing comparison participants within language comprehension regions of the brain, including the superior and middle temporal gyri, during story listening. They also reported that when forward speech (i.e., language) and backward speech (nonlanguage) conditions were compared within the DS group only, they showed almost no differences in activation patterns for the two conditions. These results suggest that there may be less specialization for language processing in the brains of young people with DS as compared to their peers of the same CA in the general population. However, this reduced specialization may not relate to DS specifically but rather may be associated more generally with lower MA or overall developmental level (for further discussion of differences in the interpretation of findings relative to CA vs. MA matched peers, see Burack et al., 2016).

In the second study of story comprehension, Jacola et al. (2014) compared neural activation during story listening of adolescents and young adults (ages 12–26 years) with DS to that of both CA- and MA-matched typically developing comparison participants. Consistent with Losin et al. (2009), they found atypical neural activation in the participants in the DS group relative to CA-matched controls. In addition to reduced activation in the superior and middle temporal gyri relative to the comparison participants, those with DS exhibited abnormally greater activation in the middle frontal and posterior cingulate gyrus. Novel to this study, Jacola et al. (2014) also reported atypical neural activation in DS relative to MA-matched comparison participants. Group differences observed relative to the MA-matched comparison group suggest that the atypical neural processing reported for individuals with DS in this study cannot be accounted for entirely by generally lower developmental levels, as those with DS differed from peers matched not only on chronological age but also on overall developmental level (i.e., the MA-matched comparison group). Thus, it appears that neural processing differences may be reflective of atypical neural development (rather than "less mature" neural functioning). Without the inclusion of a comparison group with a different neurodevelopmental disorder, we are unable to conclude, however, whether these neural processing differences are due to DS specifically or to atypical brain development more generally.

In the last fMRI study to be reviewed, we turn to a study of semantic processing in persons with DS. Specifically, Jacola et al. (2011) investigated the neural correlates of object recognition and semantic classification among adolescents and young adults with DS and those with typical developmental histories matched on CA. Visual object recognition and semantic classification were assessed with a task in which the participants pressed a button if the target animal lived on a farm. The brain regions activated in response to the task differed by group, with greater bilateral activation of the occipital cortex, anterior and posterior cingulate gyri, and middle and inferior temporal gyri among the typically developing comparison participants relative to the participants with DS. Greater activation of the right fusiform gyrus and the left inferior and superior frontal gyri were also seen in those with typical development. Jacola et al. (2011) noted that these structures have been implicated in visual processing, object encoding, and recognition, as well as semantic selection and decision making. In comparison, the individuals with DS demonstrated increased activity in the middle frontal gyrus, lateral portions of the superior frontal gyrus, and the left inferior parietal lobe. These differences suggest that those with DS present with atypical neural activation patterns when engaging in semantic classification tasks, which in addition to tapping semantic classification also involve visual processing, object recognition, and decision-making abilities.

Taken together, the results of fMRI investigations suggest that the brains of young people with DS may be characterized by less efficient neural processing. Moreover, there appears to be support for atypical neural activation patterns during the completion of language processing tasks in those with DS. Specifically, fMRI studies suggest less specialized neural processing of language. These findings will be discussed further in the developmental synthesis below.

Developmental Synthesis

While there are twice as many brain imaging studies of adults with DS than pediatric and young adult populations (Hamner et al., 2018), there appears to be a growing interest in pediatric neuroimaging of children with DS, as evidenced by the publication of several pediatric neuroimaging studies in the last 5 years. This progress is exciting, as these studies are contributing to the field's understanding of the *developing* brain in DS. In this section, we begin to conceptualize some of the more recent neuroimaging studies focused on persons with DS through a developmental lens.

To date, no longitudinal neuroimaging studies of children with DS have been published and studies of children with DS of different ages are extremely limited. To stimulate further thinking and research about brain development in DS, we focus this section on two recent studies of persons with DS that involved advanced neuroimaging methods and conceptualized findings within the context of what is known about brain maturation in individuals with typical development.

First, we turn to our research in which we described paradoxically *increased* cortical thickness in adolescents with DS despite overall reductions in cortical volume (Lee et al., 2016). Data from this study revealed dramatic reductions in cortical surface area (which was highly correlated with cortical volume in the sample) in the face of increased cortical thickness. These cortical thickness findings, when reviewed against the backdrop of what is known about the trajectory of cortical thickness over the course of childhood and adolescence (for a review, see Raznahan et al., 2011), could be interpreted as reflecting a developmentally "less mature" cortex, as late childhood and adolescence are periods of time characterized by significant cortical *thinning*. This cortical thinning in typical development has been hypothesized to be the result of experience-dependent synaptic pruning that occurs during late childhood and adolescence (Whitford et al., 2007) and has been found to be associated with improvements in cognitive function observed during this developmental period (Squeglia, Jacobus, Sorg, Jernigan, & Tapert, 2013). Thus, it may be that having a thicker cortex, as is the case for persons with DS, is disadvantageous for cognitive maturation in childhood and adolescence. However, this suggestion must be considered only speculation at this time.

The lack of longitudinal structural neuroimaging data precludes any conclusions regarding whether the cortex thins at a slower rate in individuals with DS or if static differences in the neural structure of the cortex underlie the increased cortical thickness findings. This is a question for future research that has implications both for understanding the development of children with DS and for children with other neurodevelopmental disorders characterized by ID. More specifically, research on the cortex of individuals with Williams syndrome has also noted increased cortical thickness in the face of reduced total brain volume (Green et al., 2016; Meda, Pryweller, & Thornton-Wells, 2012; Thompson et al., 2005). This similarity across conditions suggest that clues to understanding the neural underpinnings of ID may lie in future investigations of the *development* of the cortex in youth with DS and other neurodevelopmental disorders, particularly using longitudinal methodologies.

Consistent with the hypothesis that the thicker cortex in persons with DS may be conceptualized as a less "mature" cortex, the neural network structure of adolescents and adults with DS has been described as "simplified" and reflecting a greater degree of local connectivity (Anderson et al., 2013). The increased local connectivity described in Anderson et al. (2013) was accompanied by underconnectivity in a small number of long-range connections. As brain development in the typical population is characterized by reduced local connectivity and increased "distributed" connectivity (Fair et al., 2009), studies of the *development* of functional connectivity in DS are greatly needed. As the research on functional network structure in persons with DS is not longitudinal and it is limited in scope, a strong developmental conceptualization of this literature cannot be made at this time. Longitudinal neuroimaging research (both functional and structural) in concert with developmentally focused postmortem investigations of brain morphology are needed to provide a comprehensive synthesis of brain development in DS.

Conclusion

Over the past decade, we have witnessed a dramatic increase in structural neuroimaging research focused on children and adolescents with DS. Moreover, the first functional neuroimaging studies of DS were published in the past decade. These developments are exciting, as advances in neuroimaging technologies are allowing researchers to provide finer grained descriptions of the brain in individuals with DS across the lifespan. In addition, the emerging field of developmental neuroimaging provides a powerful backdrop with which to interpret findings from the DS pediatric neuroimaging literature. Moreover, it provides an impetus to begin truly studying the *developing* brain in DS—that is, studies focused on relations between age and neuroimaging findings rather than studies focused on static snapshots of differences in brain anatomy or physiology between children or adolescents with DS and same-age typically developing peers studied at one point in time.

The field is at an essential crossroads in our search for answers about the neural underpinnings of the cognitive challenges experienced by individuals with DS. We are hopeful that recent scientific advances will spur further neuroimaging research, particularly longitudinal studies of infants, children, and adolescents with DS. Such research can provide important clues about points in which the neural trajectory for children with DS deviates more or less from typically developing peers, possibly revealing windows of opportunity in which both educational/behavioral and pharmaceutical interventions may be optimally efficacious. There is still much to be done, but recent advances suggest that great opportunities lie ahead that have the potential to improve quality of life for individuals with DS and their families.

References

Abbeduto, L., Arias-Trejo, N., Thurman, A. J., Ramos-Sanchez, J., & del Hoyo Soriano, L. (in press). Language development in Down syndrome. In J. A. Burack, J. O. Edgin, & L. Abbeduto (Eds.), *Oxford Handbook of Down Syndrome and Development*. New York, NY: Oxford University Press.

Abbeduto, L., Warren, S. F., & Conners, F. A. (2007). Language development in Down syndrome: From the prelinguistic period to the acquisition of literacy. *Mental retardation and developmental disabilities research reviews, 13*(3), 247–261.

Anderson, J. S., Nielsen, J. A., Ferguson, M. A., Burback, M. C., Cox, E. T., Dai, L., . . . Korenberg, J. R. (2013). Abnormal brain synchrony in Down Syndrome. *Neuroimage Clinical, 2*, 703–715. https://doi.org/10.1016/j.nicl.2013.05.006

Azevedo, F. A., Carvalho, L. R., Grinberg, L. T., Farfel, J. M., Ferretti, R. E., Leite, R. E., . . . Herculano-Houzel, S. (2009). Equal numbers of neuronal and nonneuronal cells make the human brain an isometrically scaled-up primate brain. *Journal of Comparative Neurology, 513*(5), 532–541. https://doi.org/10.1002/cne.21974

Aziz, N. M., & Haydar, T. F. (in press). Cellular and molecular brain development in Down syndrome. In J. A. Burack, J. O. Edgin, & L. Abbeduto (Eds.), *Oxford Handbook of Down Syndrome and Development*. New York, NY: Oxford University Press.

Baddeley, A., & Jarrold, C. (2007). Working memory and Down syndrome. *Journal of Intellectual Disability Research, 51*(Pt 12), 925–931.

Barnea-Goraly, N., Menon, V., Eckert, M., Tamm, L., Bammer, R., Karchemskiy, A., . . . Reiss, A. L. (2005). White matter development during childhood and adolescence: A cross-sectional diffusion tensor imaging study. *Cerebral Cortex, 15*(12), 1848–1854. https://doi.org/10.1093/cercor/bhi062

Brown, G. G., Perthen, J. E., Liu, T. T., & Buxton, R. B. (2007). A primer on functional magnetic resonance imaging. *Neuropsychology Review, 17*(2), 107–125. https://doi.org/10.1007/s11065-007-9028-8

Bunge, S. A., & Kahn, I. (2009). Cognition: An overview of neuroimaging techniques. *Encyclopedia of Neuroscience, 2*, 1063–1067.

Burack, J. A., Evans, D. W., Klaiman, C., & Iarocci, G. (2001). The mysterious myth of attention deficits and other defect stories: Contemporary issues in the developmental approach to mental retardation. In L. M. Glidden (Ed.), *International Review of Research in Mental Retardation* (Vol. 24, pp. 299–320). San Diego: Academic Press.

Burack, J. A., Russo, N., Flores, H., Iarocci, G., & Zigler, E. (2012). The more you know the less you know, but that's OK: Developments in the developmental approach to intellectual disability. In J. A. Burack, N. Russo, H. Flores, G. Iarocci & E Zigler (Eds.), *The Oxford handbook of intellectual disability and development*, 3–10.

Burack, J. A., Russo, N., Gordon Green, C., Landry, O., & Iarocci, G. (2016). Developments in the developmental approach to intellectual disability. In D. Cicchetti (Ed.), *Developmental psychopathology: Maladaptation and psychopathology* (Vol. 3, pp.1–67). New York, NY: Wiley.

Carducci, F., Onorati, P., Condoluci, C., Di Gennaro, G., Quarato, P. P., Pierallini, A., . . . Albertini, G. (2013). Whole-brain voxel-based morphometry study of children and adolescents with Down syndrome. *Functional Neurology, 28*(1), 19–28.

Carter, J. C., Capone, G. T., & Kaufmann, W. E. (2008). Neuroanatomic correlates of autism and stereotypy in children with Down syndrome. *Neuroreport, 19*(6), 653–656.

Caviness, V. S., Jr., Kennedy, D. N., Richelme, C., Rademacher, J., & Filipek, P. A. (1996). The human brain age 7–11 years: A volumetric analysis based on magnetic resonance images. *Cerebral Cortex, 6*(5), 726–736.

Clark, C. A., Fernandez, F., Sakhon, S., Spanò, G., & Edgin, J. O. (2017). The medial temporal memory system in Down syndrome: Translating animal models of hippocampal compromise. *Hippocampus, 27*(6), 683–691.

Cohen, J. (1988). *Statistical power analysis for the behavioral sciences*. Hilsdale, NJ: Erlbaum.

Contestabile, A., Fila, T., Ceccarelli, C., Bonasoni, P., Bonapace, L., Santini, D., . . .& Ciani, E. (2007). Cell cycle alteration and decreased cell proliferation in the hippocampal dentate gyrus and in the neocortical germinal matrix of fetuses with Down syndrome and in Ts65Dn mice. *Hippocampus, 17*(8), 665–678.

Crutcher, M. D., & DeLong, M. R. (1984). Single cell studies of the primate putamen. II. Relations to direction of movement and pattern of muscular activity. *Experimental Brain Research, 53*(2), 244–258.

Dajani, D. R., & Uddin, L. Q. (2015). Demystifying cognitive flexibility: Implications for clinical and developmental neuroscience. *Trends in Neurosciences, 38*(9), 571–578.

D'Esposito, M., & Postle, B. R. (2015). The cognitive neuroscience of working memory. *Annual Review of Psychology, 66*, 115–142. https://doi.org/10.1146/annurev-psych-010814-015031

Dennison, M., Whittle, S., Yucel, M., Vijayakumar, N., Kline, A., Simmons, J., & Allen, N. B. (2013). Mapping subcortical brain maturation during adolescence: Evidence of hemisphere- and sex-specific longitudinal changes. *Developmental Science, 16*(5), 772–791. https://doi.org/10.1111/desc.12057

Dodd, B. (1975). Recognition and reproduction of words by Down's syndrome and non-Down's syndrome retarded children. *American Journal of Mental Deficiency, 80*(3), 306–311.

Edgin, J. O., Pennington, B. F., & Mervis, C. B. (2010). Neuropsychological components of intellectual disability: The contributions of immediate, working, and associative memory. *Journal of Intellectual Disability Research, 54*(5), 406–417. https://doi.org/10.1111/j.1365-2788.2010.01278.x

Engle, R. W., Tuholski, S. W., Laughlin, J. E., & Conway, A. R. (1999). Working memory, short-term memory, and general fluid intelligence: A latent-variable approach. *Journal of Experimental Psychology-General, 128*(3), 309–331.

Epstein, C. J. (1989). Down syndrome. In C. R. Scriver, A. L. Beaudet, W. S. Sly, & P. Valle (Eds.), *The metabolic basis of inherited disease* (pp. 291-396). New York, NY: McGraw.

Fair, D. A., Cohen, A. L., Power, J. D., Dosenbach, N. U., Church, J. A., Miezin, F. M., . . . Petersen, S. E. (2009). Functional brain networks develop from a "local to distributed" organization. *PLoS Computational Biology, 5*(5), e1000381. https://doi.org/10.1371/journal.pcbi.1000381

Fair, D. A., Dosenbach, N. U., Church, J. A., Cohen, A. L., Brahmbhatt, S., Miezin, F. M., . . . Schlaggar, B. L. (2007). Development of distinct control networks through segregation and integration. *Proceedings of the National Academy of Sciences of the United States of America, 104*(33), 13507–13512. https://doi.org/10.1073/pnas.0705843104

Fidler, D. J., Daunhauer, L. A., Schworer, E., & Patel, L. (in press). Executive function in Down syndrome: Links to adaptation and treatment implications. In J. A. Burack, J. O. Edgin, & L. Abbeduto (Eds.), *Oxford Handbook of Down Syndrome and Development.* New York, NY: Oxford University Press.

Fowler, A. E., Gelman, R., & Gleitman, L. A. (1994). The course of language learning in children with Down syndrome: Longitudinal and language level comparisons with young normally developing children. In H. Tager-Flusberg (Ed.), *Constraints on language acquisition* (pp. 91–140). Hillsdale, NJ: Erlbaum.

Fujii, Y., Aida, N., Niwa, T., Enokizono, M., Nozawa, K., & Inoue, T. (2017). A small pons as a characteristic finding in Down syndrome: A quantitative MRI study. *Brain and Development, 39*(4), 298–305.

Gibson, D. (1978). *Down syndrome: The psychology of mongolism.* London: Cambridge University Press.

Giedd, J. N. (2008). The teen brain: Insights from neuroimaging. *Journal of Adolescent Health, 42*(4), 335–343. https://doi.org/10.1016/j.jadohealth.2008.01.007

Giedd, J. N., Blumenthal, J., Jeffries, N. O., Castellanos, F. X., Liu, H., Zijdenbos, A., . . . Rapoport, J. L. (1999). Brain development during childhood and adolescence: A longitudinal MRI study. *Nature Neuroscience, 2*(10), 861–863.

Giedd, J. N., Lalonde, F. M., Celano, M. J., White, S. L., Wallace, G. L., Lee, N. R., & Lenroot, R. K. (2009). Anatomical brain magnetic resonance imaging of typically developing children and adolescents. *Journal of the American Academy of Child and Adolescent Psychiatry, 48*(5), 465–470. https://doi.org/10.1097/CHI.0b013e31819f2715

Giedd, J. N., Vaituzis, A. C., Hamburger, S. D., Lange, N., Rajapakse, J. C., Kaysen, D., . . . Rapoport, J. L. (1996). Quantitative MRI of the temporal lobe, amygdala, and hippocampus in normal human development: Ages 4–18 years. *Journal of Comparative Neurology, 366*(2), 223–230. https://doi.org/10.1002/(SICI)1096-9861(19960304)366:2<223::AID-CNE3>3.0.CO;2-7

Godfrey, M., & Lee, N. R. (2018). Memory profiles in Down syndrome across development: A review of memory abilities through the lifespan. *Journal of Neurodevelopmental Disorders, 10(5),* 1–31.

Gogtay, N., Giedd, J. N., Lusk, L., Hayashi, K. M., Greenstein, D., Vaituzis, A. C., . . . Thompson, P. M. (2004). Dynamic mapping of human cortical development during childhood through early adulthood. *Proceedings of the National Academy of Sciences of the United States of America, 101*(21), 8174–8179. https://doi.org/10.1073/pnas.0402680101

Golden, J. A., & Hyman, B. T. (1994). Development of the superior temporal neocortex is anomalous in trisomy 21. *Journal of Neuropathology & Experimental Neurology, 53*(5), 513–520.

Green, T., Fierro, K. C., Raman, M. M., Saggar, M., Sheau, K. E., & Reiss, A. L. (2016). Surface-based morphometry reveals distinct cortical thickness and surface area profiles in Williams syndrome. *American Journal of Medical Genetics—Part B Neuropsychiatric Genetics, 171B*(3), 402–413. https://doi.org/10.1002/ajmg.b.32422

Guidi, S., Bonasoni, P., Ceccarelli, C., Santini, D., Gualtieri, F., Ciani, E., & Bartesaghi, R. (2008). Neurogenesis impairment and increased cell death reduce total neuron number in the hippocampal region of fetuses with Down syndrome. *Brain Pathology, 18*(2), 180–197. https://doi.org/10.1111/j.1750-3639.2007.00113.x

Guidi, S., Ciani, E., Bonasoni, P., Santini, D., & Bartesaghi, R. (2011). Widespread proliferation impairment and hypocellularity in the cerebellum of fetuses with down syndrome. *Brain Pathology, 21*(4), 361–373. https://doi.org/10.1111/j.1750-3639.2010.00459.x

Gunbey, H. P., Bilgici, M. C., Aslan, K., Has, A. C., Ogur, M. G., Alhan, A., & Incesu, L. (2017). Structural brain alterations of Down's syndrome in early childhood evaluation by DTI and volumetric analyses. *European radiology, 27*(7), 3013–3021.

Gunning-Dixon, F. M., Brickman, A. M., Cheng, J. C., & Alexopoulos, G. S. (2009). Aging of cerebral white matter: A review of MRI findings. *International Journal of Geriatric Psychiatry, 24*(2), 109–117. https://doi.org/10.1002/gps.2087

Hamner, T., Udhnani, M. D., Osipowicz, K. Z., & Lee, N. R. (2018). Pediatric brain development in Down syndrome: A field in its infancy. *Journal of the International Neuropsychological Society, 24,* 1–11.

Harrison, P., & Oakland, T. (2006). Adaptive Behavior Assessment System, Second Edition (ABAS-II.). San Antonio, TX: Harcourt Assessment.

Hassabis, D., Chu, C., Rees, G., Weiskopf, N., Molyneux, P. D., & Maguire, E. A. (2009). Decoding neuronal ensembles in the human hippocampus. *Current Biology, 19*(7), 546–554. https://doi.org/10.1016/j.cub.2009.02.033

Haydar, T. F., & Reeves, R. H. (2012). Trisomy 21 and early brain development. *Trends in Neurosciences, 35*(2), 81–91. https://doi.org/10.1016/j.tins.2011.11.001

Head, E., & Helman, A. (in press). Brain aging and Alzheimer's disease. In J. A. Burack, J. O. Edgin, & L. Abbeduto (Eds.), *Oxford Handbook of Down Syndrome and Development.* New York, NY: Oxford University Press.

Head, E., Silverman, W., Patterson, D., & Lott, I. T. (2012). Aging and down syndrome. *Current Gerontology and Geriatrics Research, 2012,* Art. 412536. https://doi.org/10.1155/2012/412536

Hoffman, M. A. (1989). On the evolution and geometry of the brain in mammals. *Progress in neurobiology, 32,* 137–158.

Im, K., Lee, J. M., Lyttelton, O., Kim, S. H., Evans, A. C., & Kim, S. I. (2008). Brain size and cortical structure in the adult human brain. *Cerebral Cortex, 18*(9), 2181–2191.

Innocenti, G. M., & Price, D. J. (2005). Exuberance in the development of cortical networks. *Nature Reviews Neuroscience, 6*(12), 955.

Jabès, A., & Nelson, C. A. (2015). The ontogeny of human memory: A cognitive neuroscience perspective," where are we? *International Journal of Behavioral Development, 39,* 293–303.

Jacola, L. M., Byars, A. W., Chalfonte-Evans, M., Schmithorst, V. J., Hickey, F., Patterson, B., . . . Schapiro, M. B. (2011). Functional magnetic resonance imaging of cognitive processing in young adults with Down syndrome. *American Journal on Intellectual and Developmental Disabilities, 116*(5), 344–359. https://doi.org/10.1352/1944-7558-116.5.344

Jacola, L. M., Byars, A. W., Hickey, F., Vannest, J., Holland, S. K., & Schapiro, M. B. (2014). Functional magnetic resonance imaging of story listening in adolescents and young adults with Down syndrome: Evidence for atypical neurodevelopment. *Journal of Intellectual Disability Research, 58*(10), 892–902. https://doi.org/10.1111/jir.12089

Jernigan, T. L., & Bellugi, U. (1990). Anomalous brain morphology on magnetic resonance images in Williams syndrome and Down syndrome. *Archives of Neurology, 47*(5), 529–533.

Jernigan, T. L., Bellugi, U., Sowell, E., Doherty, S., & Hesselink, J. R. (1993). Cerebral morphologic distinctions between Williams and Down syndromes. *Archives of Neurology, 50*(2), 186–191.

Jernigan, T. L., & Tallal, P. (1990). Late childhood changes in brain morphology observable with MRI. *Developmental Medicine and Child Neurology, 32*(5), 379–385.

Jung, R. E., & Haier, R. J. (2007). The Parieto-Frontal Integration Theory (P-FIT) of intelligence: Converging neuroimaging evidence. *Behavioral and Brain Sciences, 30*(2), 135–154; discussion 154–187.

Kates, W. R., Folley, B. S., Lanham, D. C., Capone, G. T., & Kaufmann, W. E. (2002). Cerebral growth in fragile X syndrome: Review and comparison with Down syndrome. *Microscopy Research and Technique, 57*(3), 159–167.

Kaufmann, W. E., Cooper, K. L., Mostofsky, S. H., Capone, G. T., Kates, W. R., Newschaffer, C. J., . . . Lanham, D. C. (2003). Specificity of cerebellar vermian abnormalities in autism: A quantitative magnetic resonance imaging study. *Journal of Child Neurology, 18*(7), 463–470.

Kostovic, I., & Jovanov-Milosevic, N. (2006). The development of cerebral connections during the first 20–45 weeks' gestation. *Seminars in Fetal & Neonatal Medicine, 11*(6), 415–422. https://doi.org/10.1016/j.siny.2006.07.001

Lanfranchi, S., Jerman, O., Dal Pont, E., Alberti, A., & Vianello, R. (2010). Executive function in adolescents with Down syndrome. *Journal of Intellectual Disability Research, 54*(4), 308–319.

Lee, N. R., Adeyemi, E. I., Lin, A., Clasen, L. S., Lalonde, F. M., Condon, E., . . . Giedd, J. N. (2016). Dissociations in cortical morphometry in youth with Down Syndrome: Evidence for reduced surface area but increased thickness. *Cerebral Cortex, 26*(7), 2982–2990. https://doi.org/10.1093/cercor/bhv107

Lee, N. R., Fidler, D. J., Blakeley-Smith, A., Daunhauer, L., Robinson, C., & Hepburn, S. L. (2011). Caregiver report of executive functioning in a population-based sample of young children with Down syndrome. *American Journal on Intellectual and Developmental Disabilities, 116*(4), 290–304.

Lee, N. R., Maiman, M., & Godfrey, M. (2016). What can neuropsychology teach us about intellectual disability? Searching for commonalities in the memory and executive function profiles associated with Down, Williams, and fragile X syndromes. In R. M. Hodapp & D. J. Fidler (Eds.), *International Review of Research in Developmental Disabilities* (Vol. 51, pp. 1–40). https://doi.org/10.1016/bs.irrdd.2016.07.002

Lenroot, R., Gogtay, N., Greenstein, D., Wells, G. L., Wallace, L. S., Clasen, L., . . . Giedd, J. (2007). Sexual dimorphism of brain development trajectories during childhood and adolescence. *Neuroimage, 36*(4), 1065–1073. https://doi.org/10.1016/j.neuroimage.2007.03.053

Levy, R., Friedman, H. R., Davachi, L., & Goldman-Rakic, P. S. (1997). Differential activation of the caudate nucleus in primates performing spatial and nonspatial working memory tasks. *Journal of Neuroscience, 17*(10), 3870–3882.

Liégeois, F., Mayes, A., & Morgan, A. (2014). Neural correlates of developmental speech and language disorders: Evidence from neuroimaging. *Current Developmental Disorders Reports, 1*(3), 215–227.

Losin, E. A., Rivera, S. M., O'Hare, E. D., Sowell, E. R., & Pinter, J. D. (2009). Abnormal fMRI activation pattern during story listening in individuals with Down syndrome. *American Journal on Intellectual and Developmental Disabilities, 114*(5), 369–380.

Malak, R., Kostiukow, A., Krawczyk-Wasielewska, A., Mojs, E., & Samborski, W. (2015). Delays in motor development in children with Down syndrome. *Medical Science Monitor: International Medical Journal of Experimental and Clinical Research, 21*, 1904.

Mann, D. M. (1988). Alzheimer's disease and Down's syndrome. *Histopathology, 13*(2), 125–137.

Mariën, P., Ackermann, H., Adamaszek, M., Barwood, C. H., Beaton, A., Desmond, J., . . . & Leggio, M. (2014). Consensus paper: Language and the cerebellum: An ongoing enigma. *The Cerebellum, 13(3),* 386–410.

Martin, G. E., Klusek, J., Estigarribia, B., & Roberts, J. E. (2009). Language characteristics of individuals with Down syndrome. *Topics in Language Disorders, 29*(2), 112.

McDaniel, M. A. (2005). Big-brained people are smarter: A meta-analysis of the relationship between in vivo brain volume and intelligence. *ScienceDirect, 33*(4), 337–346. https://doi.org/10.1016/j.intell.2004.11.005

McDonald, A. J. (1998). Cortical pathways to the mammalian amygdala. *Progress in Neurobiology, 55*(3), 257–332.

Meda, S. A., Pryweller, J. R., & Thornton-Wells, T. A. (2012). Regional brain differences in cortical thickness, surface area and subcortical volume in individuals with Williams syndrome. *PLoS One, 7*(2), e31913. https://doi.org/10.1371/journal.pone.0031913

Mendoza, J. E., & Foundas, A. L. (2008). *Clinical neuroanatomy: A neurobehavioral approach.* New York, NY: Springer.

Menghini, D., Costanzo, F., & Vicari, S. (2011). Relationship between brain and cognitive processes in Down syndrome. *Behavior Genetics, 41*(3), 381–393. https://doi.org/10.1007/s10519-011-9448-3

Middleton, F. A., & Strick, P. L. (2001). Cerebellar projections to the prefrontal cortex of the primate. *Journal of Neuroscience, 21*(2), 700–712.

Moore, K. L., Persaud, T. V. N., & Torchia, M. G. (2015). *The developing human: Clinically oriented embryology* (10th ed.) . Philadelphia, PA: Elsevier.

O'Leary, D. D. (1992). Development of connectional diversity and specificity in the mammalian brain by the pruning of collateral projections. *Current Opinion in Neurobiology, 2*(1), 70–77.

Ostby, Y., Tamnes, C. K., Fjell, A. M., Westlye, L. T., Due-Tonnessen, P., & Walhovd, K. B. (2009). Heterogeneity in subcortical brain development: A structural magnetic resonance imaging study of brain maturation from 8 to 30 years. *Journal of Neuroscience, 29*(38), 11772–11782. https://doi.org/10.1523/JNEUROSCI.1242-09.2009

Panizzon, M. S., Fennema-Notestine, C., Eyler, L. T., Jernigan, T. L., Prom-Wormley, E., Neale, M., . . . Kremen, W. S. (2009). Distinct genetic influences on cortical surface area and cortical thickness. *Cerebral Cortex, 19*(11), 2728–2735. https://doi.org/10.1093/cercor/bhp026

Parker, S. E., Mai, C. T., Canfield, M. A., Rickard, R., Wang, Y., Meyer, R. E., . . . National Birth Defects Prevention Network. (2010). Updated national birth prevalence estimates for selected birth defects in the United States, 2004–2006. *Birth Defects Research Part A: Clinical and Molecular Teratology, 88*(12), 1008–1016. https://doi.org/10.1002/bdra.20735

Pennington, B. F., Moon, J., Edgin, J., Stedron, J., & Nadel, L. (2003). The neuropsychology of Down syndrome: Evidence for hippocampal dysfunction. *Child Development, 74*(1), 75–93.

Petanjek, Z., Judas, M., Simic, G., Rasin, M. R., Uylings, H. B., Rakic, P., & Kostovic, I. (2011). Extraordinary neoteny of synaptic spines in the human prefrontal cortex. *Proceedings of the National Academy of Sciences, 108*(32), 13281–13286. https://doi.org/10.1073/pnas.1105108108

Pinter, J. D., Brown, W. E., Eliez, S., Schmitt, J. E., Capone, G. T., & Reiss, A. L. (2001). Amygdala and hippocampal volumes in children with Down syndrome: A high-resolution MRI study. *Neurology, 56*(7), 972–974.

Pinter, J. D., Eliez, S., Schmitt, J. E., Capone, G. T., & Reiss, A. L. (2001). Neuroanatomy of Down's syndrome: A high-resolution MRI study. *American Journal Of Psychiatry, 158*(10), 1659–1665.

Pujol, J., del Hoyo, L., Blanco-Hinojo, L., de Sola, S., Macia, D., Martinez-Vilavella, G., . . . de la Torre, R. (2015). Anomalous brain functional connectivity contributing to poor adaptive behavior in Down syndrome. *Cortex, 64*, 148–156. https://doi.org/10.1016/j.cortex.2014.10.012

Rakic, P. (1995). A small step for the cell, a giant leap for mankind: A hypothesis of neocortical expansion during evolution. *Trends in Neuroscience, 18*(9), 383–388.

Rakic, P. (2009). Evolution of the neocortex: A perspective from developmental biology. *Nature Reviews Neuroscience, 10*(10), 724–735. https://doi.org/10.1038/nrn2719

Ramnani, N. (2006). The primate cortico-cerebellar system: Anatomy and function. *Nature Reviews Neuroscience, 7*(7), 511–522. https://doi.org/10.1038/nrn1953

Raz, N., Torres, I. J., Briggs, S. D., Spencer, W. D., Thornton, A. E., Loken, W. J., . . . Acker, J. D. (1995). Selective neuroanatomical abnormalities in Downs syndrome and their cognitive correlates—Evidence from MRI morphometry. *Neurology, 45*(2), 356–366.

Raznahan, A., Shaw, P., Lalonde, F., Stockman, M., Wallace, G. L., Greenstein, D., . . . Giedd, J. N. (2011). How does your cortex grow? *Journal of Neuroscience, 31*(19), 7174–7177. https://doi.org/10.1523/JNEUROSCI.0054-11.2011

Reber, P. J. (2013). The neural basis of implicit learning and memory: A review of neuropsychological and neuroimaging research. *Neuropsychologia, 51*(10), 2026–2042. https://doi.org/10.1016/j.neuropsychologia.2013.06.019

Schmidt-Sidor, B., Wisniewski, K. E., Shepard, T. H., & Sersen, E. A. (1990). Brain growth in Down syndrome subjects 15 to 22 weeks of gestational age and birth to 60 months. *Clinical Neuropathology, 9*(4), 181–190.

Schmithorst, V. J., Wilke, M., Dardzinski, B. J., & Holland, S. K. (2002). Correlation of white matter diffusivity and anisotropy with age during childhood and adolescence: A cross-sectional diffusion-tensor MR imaging study. *Radiology, 222*(1), 212–218. https://doi.org/10.1148/radiol.2221010626

Schnack, H. G., van Haren, N. E., Brouwer, R. M., Evans, A., Durston, S., Boomsma, D. I., . . . Hulshoff Pol, H. E. (2015). Changes in thickness and surface area of the human cortex and their relationship with intelligence. *Cerebral Cortex, 25*(6), 1608–1617. https://doi.org/10.1093/cercor/bht357

Shaw, P., Gogtay, N., & Rapoport, J. (2010). Childhood psychiatric disorders as anomalies in neurodevelopmental trajectories. *Human Brain Mapping, 31*(6), 917–925.

Shaw, P., Greenstein, D., Lerch, J., Clasen, L., Lenroot, R., Gogtay, N., . . . Giedd, J. (2006). Intellectual ability and cortical development in children and adolescents. *Nature, 440*(7084), 676–679.

Smigielska-Kuzia, J., Bockowski, L., Sobaniec, W., Sendrowski, K., Olchowik, B., Cholewa, M., . . . Lebkowska, U. (2011). A volumetric magnetic resonance imaging study of brain structures in children with Down syndrome. *Neurologia Neurochirurgia Polska, 45*(4), 363–369.

Smith, E. A., & Jarrold, C. (in press). Working memory and Down syndrome. In J. A. Burack, J. O. Edgin, & L. Abbeduto (Eds.), *Oxford Handbook of Down Syndrome and Development*. New York, NY: Oxford University Press.

Smitha, K. A., Akhil Raja, K., Arun, K. M., Rajesh, P. G., Thomas, B., Kapilamoorthy, T. R., & Kesavadas, C. (2017). Resting state fMRI: A review on methods in resting state connectivity analysis and resting state networks. *The Neuroradiology Journal, 30*(4), 305–317.

Sowell, E. R., Peterson, B. S., Thompson, P. M., Welcome, S. E., Henkenius, A. L., & Toga, A. W. (2003). Mapping cortical change across the human life span. *Nature Neuroscience, 6*(3), 309–315. https://doi.org/10.1038/nn1008

Squeglia, L. M., Jacobus, J., Sorg, S. F., Jernigan, T. L., & Tapert, S. F. (2013). Early adolescent cortical thinning is related to better neuropsychological performance. *Journal of the International Neuropsychological Society, 19*(9), 962.

Squire, L. R. (1992). Memory and the hippocampus: A synthesis from findings with rats, monkeys, and humans. *Psychological Review, 99*(2), 195–231.

Stiles, J., & Jernigan, T. L. (2010). The basics of brain development. *Neuropsychology Review, 20*(4), 327–348. https://doi.org/10.1007/s11065-010-9148-4

Stoodley, C. J. (2012). The cerebellum and cognition: Evidence from functional imaging studies. *Cerebellum, 11*(2), 352–365. https://doi.org/10.1007/s12311-011-0260-7

Sullivan, E. V., De La Paz, R., Zipursky, R. B., & Pfefferbaum, A. (1991). Neuropsychological deficits accompanying striatonigral degeneration. *Journal of Clinical and Experimental Neuropsychology, 13*(5), 773–788. https://doi.org/10.1080/01688639108401089

Sussman, D., Leung, R. C., Chakravarty, M. M., Lerch, J. P., & Taylor, M. J. (2016). Developing human brain: Age-related changes in cortical, subcortical, and cerebellar anatomy. *Brain and Behavior, 6*(4), e00457. https://doi.org/10.1002/brb3.457

Takashima, S., Becker, L. E., Armstrong, D. L., & Chan, F. (1981). Abnormal neuronal development in the visual cortex of the human fetus and infant with Down's syndrome. A quantitative and qualitative Golgi study. *Brain research, 225*(1), 1–21.

Thompson, P. M., Lee, A. D., Dutton, R. A., Geaga, J. A., Hayashi, K. M., Eckert, M. A., . . . Reiss, A. L. (2005). Abnormal cortical complexity and thickness profiles mapped in Williams syndrome. *Journal of Neuroscience, 25*(16), 4146–4158. https://doi.org/10.1523/JNEUROSCI.0165-05.2005

Tiemeier, H., Lenroot, R. K., Greenstein, D. K., Tran, L., Pierson, R., & Giedd, J. N. (2010). Cerebellum development during childhood and adolescence: A longitudinal morphometric MRI study. *Neuroimage, 49*(1), 63–70. https://doi.org/10.1016/j.neuroimage.2009.08.016

Todd, P. H. (1985). Gaussian curvature as a parameter of biological surface growth. *Journal of Theoretical Biology, 113*(1), 63–68.

Tuller, T., Kupiec, M., & Ruppin, E. (2008). Evolutionary rate and gene expression across different brain regions. *Genome Biology, 9*(9), R142. https://doi.org/10.1186/gb-2008-9-9-r142

Uematsu, A., Matsui, M., Tanaka, C., Takahashi, T., Noguchi, K., Suzuki, M., & Nishijo, H. (2012). Developmental trajectories of amygdala and hippocampus from infancy to early adulthood in healthy individuals. *PLoS One, 7*(10), e46970. https://doi.org/10.1371/journal.pone.0046970

Vicari, S., Verucci, L., & Carlesimo, G. A. (2007). Implicit memory is independent from IQ and age but not from etiology: Evidence from Down and Williams syndromes. *Journal of Intellectual Disability Research, 51*(Pt. 12), 932–941. https://doi.org/10.1111/j.1365-2788.2007.01003.x

Wang, P. P., Doherty, S., Hesselink, J. R., & Bellugi, U. (1992). Callosal morphology concurs with neurobehavioral and neuropathological findings in two neurodevelopmental disorders. *Archives of Neurology, 49*(4), 407–411.

Webb, S. J., Monk, C. S., & Nelson, C. A. (2001). Mechanisms of postnatal neurobiological development: Implications for human development. *Developmental Neuropsychology, 19*(2), 147–171. https://doi.org/10.1207/S15326942DN1902_2

Weitzdoerfer, R., Dierssen, M., Fountoulakis, M., & Lubec, G. (2001). Fetal life in Down syndrome starts with normal neuronal density but impaired dendritic spines and synaptosomal structure. In G. Lubec (Ed.), *Protein expression in Down syndrome brain* (pp. 59–70). Vienna: Springer.

Wen, W., Thalamuthu, A., Mather, K. A., Zhu, W., Jiang, J., de Micheaux, P. L., . . . Sachdev, P. S. (2016). Distinct genetic influences on cortical and subcortical brain structures. *Scientific Reports, 6*, 32760. https://doi.org/10.1038/srep32760

Whitford, T. J., Rennie, C. J., Grieve, S. M., Clark, C. R., Gordon, E., & Williams, L. M. (2007). Brain maturation in adolescence: Concurrent changes in neuroanatomy and neurophysiology. *Human Brain Mapping, 28*(3), 228–237. https://doi.org/10.1002/hbm.20273

Wisniewski, K. E., & Schmidt-Sidor, B. (1989). Postnatal delay of myelin formation in brains from Down syndrome infants and children. *Clinical neuropathology, 8*(2), 55–62.

Yang, Y., Conners, F. A., & Merrill, E. C. (2014). Visuo-spatial ability in individuals with Down syndrome: Is it really a strength?. *Research in developmental disabilities, 35*(7), 1473–1500.

CHAPTER

10 Sensory and Perceptual Abilities in People With Down Syndrome

Armando Bertone, Jacalyn Guy, *and* Christina Marcone

Abstract

During typical development, the efficiency with which distinct image attributes, objects such as faces, and emotions are analyzed depends on the development of ocular functioning (sensory level) and brain mechanisms mediating perceptual abilities (neural level). Compared to typically developing individuals, ocular differences are more frequent in persons with Down syndrome (DS) and include an increased incidence of refractive errors, i.e. hyperopia and myopia, and difficulties with accommodation (focusing up close). In most cases, these conditions can be corrected with bifocals, resulting in greatly improved literary skills that underlie reading, particularly for younger persons with DS. In addition, individuals with DS seem to benefit from the spatially structured presentation of visual material when learning, another accommodation that can be implemented during instruction. Finally, although not specific to DS, young children and adults with DS generally identify and recognize emotions less efficiently than do persons without DS. However, among persons with DS, these difficulties seem to be more pronounced for more intense emotions, including fear and anger. In sum, visual profiles based on sensory and perceptual performance can advance our understanding of atypical information processing among persons with DS, as well as provide practical information aimed at improving learning and instruction.

Key Words: Down syndrome, vision, sensory, perception, development, optical, face perception

Introduction

Vision is intricately integrated into developing systems underlying other functions that mediate behavior, including cognition, language, attention, and motor skills. The ability to efficiently differentiate, identify, and recognize visual stimuli in our surroundings enables us to create an easily interpretable veridical internal representation of our external environment that guides our behavior (Berk, 2000). Differences or impairments in even the most basic visual processes can have considerable effects on how one perceives and interacts within the immediate surroundings. In addition to having a significant impact on visually related motor skills such as reaching, grasping, and fixating, visual functioning is also significantly related to higher levels of cognitive processes such as attention, learning, and reading (Braddick & Atkinson, 2011, Atkinson & Braddick, 2013). For these reasons, an understanding of both sensory and perceptual processes is especially critical for accommodating the specific needs of individuals who develop atypically, including those with Down syndrome (DS). Much research has been centered around describing the physical abnormalities of the eyes of individuals with DS, and defining the neurocognitive profiles in persons with DS. However, much less is known about the sensory abilities of individuals with DS and how these abilities interact with other cognitive functions. In this chapter, we first outline differences in basic visual functions in terms of optical factors, such as the ability for focus; second, we address the process of simple visual information, such as perceiving color; and third, we turn to later stages of perceptual processing and highlight the strengths and challenges that individuals with DS have in perceiving and interpreting more complex information, such as that related to social communication and behavior. The data considered are relevant to developing appropriate learning strategies and cognitive interventions aimed at improving the outcomes of individuals with DS based on their visuo-sensory and perceptual profiles.

Optical Factors

Down syndrome is associated with several physical abnormalities specific to the eyes, including folding at the upper eyelids as well as the presence of slanted eyes and colored spots on the iris of the eye, or brushfield spots (Bull, 2011). These physical characteristics are common among people with DS. In addition, optical atypicalities affect the majority of individuals with DS, from the cornea through the retina (de Cuhna & Moreira, 1996). Individuals with DS experience difficulties in vision, especially at its most basic level (Watt, Robertson, & Jacobs, 2015), especially with ocular atypicalities, including differences in refractive error, acuity (i.e., detailed vision), and accommodation (focusing up close).

Refractive Errors

Refractive errors occur when the eye cannot clearly focus the images from the outside world, resulting in a blurred vision. The main types of refractive errors are myopia (nearsightedness), hyperopia (farsightedness), presbyopia (loss of near vision with age), and astigmatism. Although refractive errors are not preventable, they can be diagnosed by an eye examination and treated with corrective glasses, contact lenses, or refractive surgery. Refractive errors are particularly common among persons with DS (Haugen, Høvding, & Lundström, 2001). In a review, Watt et al. (2015) reported that approximately 50 to 80 percent of individuals with DS experience refractive errors, including difficulties focusing up close (hyperopia) and at a distance (myopia). Additional difficulties in focusing, such as astigmatism, are also frequent among persons with DS. These visual impairments are largely the same as those affecting typically developing individuals, but their presence and severity are greater among persons with DS. For example, as compared to typically developing children, children with DS show an increase in refractive errors that fail to improve naturally without corrective lenses throughout the preschool years, as they do in typically developing children. The reasons why this occurs are unknown, but some researchers suggest that the natural correction of the atypical physical development of the eye—referred to as emmetropisation—may be a contributing factor (Watt et al., 2015). A failure to outgrow such impairments explains why more children with DS are required to wear glasses with corrective lenses (Haugen et al., 2001; see Watt et al., 2015 for review).

Acuity

In terms of acuity, individuals with DS also show differences relative to their typically developing peers. A consensus in the literature is that children with DS have poorer visual acuity than their typically developing peers (reviewed in Watt et al., 2015). For example, using clinical screening charts, Woodhouse et al. (1996) showed that from the age of 2 years, children with DS have poorer visual acuity. Using similar stimuli, Courage, Adams, and Hall (1997) measured full contrast sensitivity functions (CSF's) in infants and children with DS and reported lower levels of sensitivity across all spatial frequencies relative to typically developing participants. They further noted that these differences were most apparent at high spatial frequencies, a finding that may underlie difficulties in detailed visual processing. Furthermore, Little, Woodhouse, Lauritzen, and Saunders (2007) demonstrated reduced levels of acuity in 9- to 16-year-olds with DS relative to typically developing children.

Felius et al. (2014) examined whether poor visual acuity in individuals with DS was the result of an inability to fixate, caused by a visual condition called nystagmus, in which the eyes make repetitive, involuntary eye movements. The inability to fixate is detrimental to acuity since stabilizing an image on the retina is essential for normal vision. Felius et al. (2014) found that, although not an exclusive cause, fixation instability could account for a significant proportion of visual acuity deficits in persons with DS. Such findings are important as congenital visual conditions, such as nystagmus, can affect the precision of visual acuity assessment of individuals with DS. In addition, studies involving clinical acuity charts rely heavily on the cognitive abilities of participants and, therefore, present additional challenges for individuals with DS. As discussed by Watt et al. (2015), poor performances in individuals with DS can relate to cognitive difficulties, such as those in recognizing letters or symbols, which in turn can lead to low levels of motivation and possibly lapses in attention during visual acuity assessments. For these reasons, acuity deficits in persons with DS are difficult to interpret because reliable measures of vision are difficult to obtain using clinical screening charts.

To circumvent issues related to cognition and/or motivation during visual acuity measures, assessments with more minimal cognitive demands can be used, such as when participants are asked to detect, rather than identify (i.e., read), visual targets during an optometric testing. A more passive approach can also be employed whereby the person's acuity can be assessed in a nonverbal manner, thus circumventing challenges patients may have with regards to cognition and/or motivation. In one example. John, Bromham, Woodhouse, and Candy (2004) used an electroencephalographic technique called visual evoked potentials (VEPs) in which brain activity is measured in the visual brain areas while stimuli of specific sizes and spatial frequencies (i.e., spatial detail) are presented to the participant. They found reduced visual acuity for participants with DS aged from 2 through 14 years, when using both behavioral tests (i.e., acuity charts) and physiological responses to the visual stimuli as compared to typically developing children. John et al. concluded that deficits in acuity for children and adolescents with DS are either perceptual or neurological in origin and not due to cognitive difficulties since the visual evoked potential approach used in their study minimized cognitive processes (i.e., reading, attention, task comprehension, etc.). Similarly, Krinsky-McHale (2014) found an overall reduction of sensitivity across spatial frequencies among adults with DS on a behavioral task. This reduction was especially marked at high spatial frequencies, which convey fine details.

Accommodation

In addition to acuity, individuals with DS show striking differences in accommodation, or the ability of the eye to focus over a range of distances. Approximately 55 to76 percent of children with DS are thought to underaccommodate and have difficulty focusing on visual information presented near their eyes (e.g., at arm's length when reading; reviewed in Little, 2015). There is a suggestion that the high co-occurrence of accommodative deficits and refractive errors in DS may be of etiological importance. For example, mechanical factors of the cornea have been suggested to be considered as a main etiological aspect in persons with DS due to the right-left specificity of astigmatic eyes (Haugen et al., 2001). When assessing objective measures of both static (e.g., accommodative response) and dynamic (e.g., microfluctuations) aspects of accommodation in individuals with DS, Anderson et al. (2011) found that the primarily motor aspects of accommodation did not differ between mental age-matched participants (MA) with and without DS, whereas the primarily sensory and sensory-motor aspects of accommodation were poorer among the participants with DS. These findings are therefore more congruent with a sensory, rather than motor, pathway deficit for accommodative function. However, the exact origin of the accommodative dysfunction in persons with DS is not yet fully understood, given the large degree of variability regarding accommodative function in this group originating from different sources, including refractive error, binocular perception, and level of cognitive functioning (Anderson et al., 2011).

Despite the unknown origin of accommodative difficulties in persons with DS, there is now good evidence to show that by wearing bifocals children with DS show dramatic improvements in near focus. For example, Stewart, Woodhouse, and Trojanowska (2005) and Nandakumar and Leat (2009) both studied the efficacy of bifocals in correcting near focus in children with DS and found that the children who wore bifocals displayed improvements in accommodation, particularly in terms of near focus. Nandakumar and Leat (2009) also found that the children who wore bifocals improved in perceptual and literacy skills, suggesting a direct benefit of bifocal wear for educational outcomes (see also Nandakumar et al., 2011). In addition to improving learning and more general activities of daily living, wearing bifocals has also been suggested as a treatment for reducing accommodation deficits among persons with DS (Al-Bagdady, Stewart, Watts, Murphy, & Woodhouse, 2009), although there is no clear consensus of whether this treatment reliably recovers accommodative function in children with DS (see Little, 2015; Nandakumar & Leat, 2009). Thus, school-aged children with DS appear to focus poorly at near distances and under-accommodate, leaving them at a disadvantage for conventional schoolwork and reading.

Visual Perception

In the following sections, summaries of perceptual abilities among persons with DS that are mediated by the visual brain (rather than the eye) at different levels of visual analysis will be presented, starting with the most basic of perceptual visual functions (i.e., perceiving color), followed by other more complex visual processes such as recognizing faces and emotions. Defining and understanding the visuo-perceptual profiles of children and adults with DS in such a systematic manner will lead to a better understanding of visual strengths and challenges specific to persons with DS and inform the development of appropriate educational approaches, accommodations, and practices.

Low-Level Perception in DS

Low-level perception refers to information processing that occurs in early visual centers (i.e., primary and secondary visual cortices). Though broad, this definition includes the processing of basic visual attributes such as luminance (contrast), texture, and color, in addition to simple dynamic and static stimuli. In the one study with a comprehensive assessment of low-level visual perceptual functions, Krinsky-McHale (2014) examined spatio-temporal contrast sensitivity, stereopsis, vernier acuity, and color vision and reported overall reductions in performance in adults aged from 28 through 48 years with DS relative to younger (16–28 years old) and older adults (51–61 years old) without intellectual disability. Sensitivity was reduced across all spatial frequencies and temporal modulation rates, suggesting poorer visual acuity at the level of the primary visual cortex (De Valois et al., 1982; De Valois & De Valois, 1988). Stereopsis, or depth perception, was also diminished in the participants with DS, as was vernier acuity, a measure of spatial relations. The participants with DS further showed a decreased ability to discriminate color. Krinsky-McHale noted that this pattern of findings was similar to that seen in individuals with Alzheimer's disease (AD) and suggested a possible common neuropathology as a disproportionate number of individuals with DS go on to develop AD (Head, Powell, Gold, & Schmitt, 2012). Future research in this area is imminent as many individuals with DS now have much longer life expectancies with improved care and intervention (Head, Silverman, Patterson, & Lott, 2012; Helman et al., this volume).

Higher-Level Perception of Nonsocial Information in DS

The most common method of assessing higher-level visual perception of nonsocial information in clinical populations is to measure the sensitivity to static and dynamic information using "global motion/global form" paradigms (see Atkinson et al., 1997). In these paradigms, individual dots are presented to the observer either moving in a specific direction (global motion) or spatially presented in a specific form (circle). The coherence of the dots (i.e., the percentage moving in a certain direction or in the shape of a circle) is manipulated until a certain direction (left vs. right) or form (circle vs. square) is detected or identified. In order to do so, the individual dots must be integrated across time and/or space, a process considered to be a robust measure of visual integration. In addition, it has been argued that the ability to perceive global motion and form information reflects the functional integrity of specialized visual areas comprising the dorsal and ventral visual pathways, respectively (see Atkinson et al., 1997; Braddick et al., 2003; see also Braddick, et al., 2000).

Del Viva et al. (2015) assessed global motion perception in a group of adults with DS (mean age of 26 years) by measuring their sensitivity to optic flow stimuli (random dots moving in radial, rotational, and translational trajectories), and found a significant decrease in optic flow sensitivity for participants with DS as compared to mental age-matched typically developing participants. They interpreted these findings as evidence of a higher-level perceptual deficit that is contingent on the efficient integration of local, dynamic information in persons with DS. However, group differences in performance were not found for luminance-defined sinewave gratings, a dynamic stimulus that targets mechanisms operating in lower-level, primary visual areas. The findings of Del Viva et al. (2015) can be interpreted as evidence for a specific impairment in higher-level perception among persons with DS for nonsocial, dynamic information. This interpretation is consistent with other findings suggesting that the sensitivity to other types of complex motion requiring the integration of local moving parts, such as those produced by point-light walkers, or biological motion (BM; Johansson, 1973)—is also less efficient among both adults (Riddell et al., 2017) and children (Virji-Babul et al., 2006) with DS. However, since BM paradigms are also used to measure the ability to perceive information that communicates social information (Blakemore & Decety; 2001; Pelphrey et al., 2003), an alternative explanation for decreased BM sensitivity among persons with DS originating from a "social-impairment" optic can also be posited. Specifically, less efficient processing of such social stimuli may at least in part be attributable to decreased social functioning and understanding among persons with DS, rather than a perceptual, visuo-integrative origin per se (Næss et al., 2017). Future research can address this issue by simultaneously assessing the sensitivity to higher-level motion by using stimuli that do (e.g., biological motion) and do not (e.g., optic flow stimuli) contain social information so as to isolate and assess the origin of impaired complex motion perception in persons with DS.

With regard to higher-level, spatial visual information, individuals with DS are thought to generally show particular strengths in visuo-spatial abilities, especially when compared to their significant difficulty in verbal skills (e.g., Silverman, 2007). However, in an extensive review, Yang, Conners, and Merrill (2014) questioned this notion. In their evaluation of studies of a variety of skills including mental rotation, visual-spatial construction, visual-spatial memory, closure, and wayfinding, they failed to find consistent evidence of a particular strength in any of these abilities among persons with DS relative to their general cognitive ability. Rather, they suggested that most of these abilities are areas of weaknesses among individuals with DS in relation to MA-matched typically developing individuals, with the exception of spatial sequential memory as measured by the Corsi block task. Yang et al. emphasize that variations in how relative strengths are defined contribute to the inconsistencies in the literature. For example, when compared to verbal abilities or other neurodevelopmental groups, such as persons with Williams syndrome, visual spatial skills are indeed a relative strength among persons with DS.

Another approach for assessing higher-level perception in persons with DS is to use standardized test batteries that provide profiles of perceptual functions across a range of visually based tasks; the Developmental Test of Visual Perception (DTVP; Hammill, Pearson, & Voress, 1993) and the Test of Visual Perceptual Skill-3rd edition (TVPS-3; Martin, 2006) are among the most commonly cited. For example, Yang et al. (2014) used the TPVS-3 to examine performances of children with DS on visual discrimination, memory, spatial relationships, form constancy, sequential memory, figure-ground, and closure tasks. They reported that across all of the tasks, the performances of the children with DS were significantly poorer than those of MA-matched typically developing children, but not of those of others with intellectual disability (ID); performances correlated positively with age across all groups. This latter finding highlights an important caveat with this type of approach: the associations with age suggest that this standardized battery, like many others, may rely too heavily on other cognitive functions, such as language. Therefore, perception might be best measured using tasks with minimal verbal demands to better understand the profiles of strengths and weaknesses among persons with DS. In using a similar approach to measure perceptual abilities in adults with other forms of ID and DS using the Developmental Test of Visual Perception (DTVP) battery, Ikeda et al. (2013) found that adults with DS performed poorer on subtests of form perception and position in spatial referencing, suggesting weaknesses in object categorization and visuo-spatial orientation. However, like adults with ID associated with different etiologies, the adults with DS also showed strengths in subtests requiring eye-hand coordination and the ability to distinguish target figures from the background. This uneven profile suggests that some, but not all, visuo-perceptual functions are atypical among persons with DS, and it highlights the importance of comparison groups when interpreting perceptual strengths and challenges for a given profile.

Defining and understanding the visuo-perceptual abilities of individuals with DS can also directly benefit teaching and instruction by adapting the manner with which material is presented to individuals with DS during learning. In one example, Carretti and Lanfranchi (2010) used an experimental passive memory task during which school-aged children had to memorize and recall spatial positions in a sequence under structured and unstructured conditions. They found that the individuals with DS benefited significantly from structured material when performing spatial-simultaneous working memory tasks. The findings from this study, as with others relevant to defining perceptual abilities in persons with DS, are of relevance to the clinical and educational context of persons with DS, informing how best to intervene and teach individuals with DS based on their perceptual profiles.

High-Level Perception of Socially Relevant Information in DS

Studies assessing face perception—the most commonly used visual metric of social functioning—are based on the premise that a decreased or atypical ability to efficiently recognize, discriminate, match, identify, or decode visual facial information translates to, at least in part, atypical social behavior. Assessing face perception in persons with DS is therefore relevant because many children with DS manifest challenges with different aspects of social cognition—including joint attention, imitation, and social referencing (understanding their emotions and intentions). At a neural level, social cognition is mediated by the functioning of the social brain network (Adolphs et al., 2003; Allison et al., 2000), which consists of several interrelated brain regions—including the amygdala, superior-temporal sulcus, and, most importantly, the fusiform face area—that are specifically sensitive to different types of social information. Dysfunction in one or more of these regions, or in the communication between them, can result in social cognition deficits, and changes in the functioning of face-specific brain areas have been identified as potentially causal (Powell et al., 2018). The function of such brain areas can be assessed using targeted behavioral paradigms that target the functional integrity of underlying brain mechanisms within the social brain network, which includes those specialized for face information processing, such as the fusiform face area (FFA), and possibly limbic structures mediating the emotional content contained in face information (Adolphs et al., 2003; Johnson et al., 2005). In addition, face perception paradigms are also often used to assess "holistic processing," as the ability to discriminate, recognize, and/or identify the information communicated by face stimuli can be mediated by manipulating the features of the face stimuli (Farah et al., 1998). When assessed, the face perception ability in persons with DS is often (a) examined within the context of emotion recognition, (b) compared to that of other neurodevelopmental conditions (cross-syndrome assessment), and (c) used as a "control performance" for other individuals with other neurodevelopmental conditions with lower cognitive abilities (i.e., MA matched).

In an initial study of face perception among youth with DS, Annaz et al. (2009) compared the typical development of holistic face processing in school-aged children (aged between 5 and 12 years) with age-matched children diagnosed with Williams syndrome, DS, or high- or low-functioning autism. In addition to measures of receptive vocabulary and spatial ability, face recognition was also assessed across all groups using the Benton Facial Recognition Test (Benton et al., 1983). Annaz et al. found that chronologically age-matched participants with DS performed significantly worse compared to typically developing participants on facial recognition tasks, but they performed comparably to that of the lower- but not the higher-functioning participants with autism. As Annaz et al. (2009) noted, this result is of interest because persons with DS are not typically thought to display a significant deficit in social cognition in contrast to persons with autism (Kent, Evans, Paul, & Sharp, 1999). The participants also completed a modified version of Tanaka and Farah's (1993) part-whole face paradigm in which the participants were asked whether a face or a feature (e.g., eyes) was similar to that of a target face or feature (Farah et al., 1998). Developmental trajectories (trajectory analyses in a cross-sectional design) were then constructed associating part-whole performance either to chronological age or to other cognitive measures (receptive vocabulary, visuo-spatial construction, and the Benton Facial Recognition Test). Although the overall performance of the persons with DS did not improve with age across the face conditions tested (as was the case with the participants with WS and LFA), the children with DS discriminated features more efficiently when presented in a *whole* face than when presented in isolation. Annaz et al. interpreted this finding as evidence for a holistic rather than featural processing strategy among persons with DS, at least within the context of the part-whole face paradigm used.

In a follow-up study of the same populations, Dimitriou et al. (2015) also assessed featural and configural processing using a different recognition task (Jane task; Mondloch et al., 2002), which can be used to assess face perception/recognition strategies in terms of a preference for using either featural (individual analysis of either eyes, nose, or mouth) or configural processes (analysis of spatial relationship between face features) during face perception. Configural processing has for the most part been found to be disrupted (it is more difficult) when an entire face stimulus is presented upside-down, or inverted, whereas inverting an individual feature of a face is not as detrimental to recognizing a face. This effect, called the "face-inversion effect" (see Rakover, 2002; Valentine et al., 1991; and Yin, 1969; for reviews), has been widely used to assess face perception strategies across a variety of neurodevelopmental conditions. Dimitriou et al. (2015) used this approach to assess featural and configural face processing by asking participants with DS to either detect a difference between two simultaneously presented faces while manipulating either featural or configural aspects of the face stimuli; this was done for upright and inverted faces. Overall, the performance of the participants with DS, unlike that of the TD group, did not improve with age for either the featural or configural conditions. In addition, the expected face-inversion effect was not demonstrated by the participants with DS in the configural condition. Dimitriou et al. (2015) interpreted these findings as evidence for poorer face recognition abilities (generally considered to reflect a configural process) among persons with DS despite previous suggestions that individuals with DS prefer a holistic or global processing (and less featural) strategy for nonsocial visuo-spatial information (Bellugi et al., 2000).

High-Level Perception of Socially Relevant Information

The ability to identify and recognize emotions conveyed in face stimuli is especially pertinent when assessing visually related "social cognition," particularly since atypical social interaction is manifested, albeit in different manners, across many neurodevelopmental syndromes. In general, atypical social behavior is thought to be associated with dysfunctional neural mechanisms that normally process emotions in face stimuli, which in turn results in maladaptive behavior in response to emotionally salient information. Furthermore, these deficits acting through the course of development may result in affected individuals manifesting difficulties understanding the emotional states of others.

Wishart and Pitcairn (2000) used a facial-recognition task to assess the understanding of emotion in school-aged children with DS, with the participants being asked to match photographs of unfamiliar adults on the basis of either facial identity or facial expression conveying different emotions (e.g., happiness, sadness, anger, surprise, fear, and disgust). Compared to typically developing children of a similar MA and a comparison group of children with nonspecific intellectual disability of comparable chronological age (CA), the participants with DS made significantly more expression- and identity-matching errors, particularly when the face stimuli conveyed anger and fear. Although performance was significantly correlated with CA for both of the MA and CA comparison groups, performance was not associated with age across the 6-year age span among the group of participants with DS. Wishart and Pitcairn interpreted this finding as evidence for a ceiling effect of ability that is specific to persons with DS.

A specific difficulty for persons with DS with certain emotions more than others was also demonstrated by Kasari et al. (2001), who used a puppet paradigm to assess the recognition of happiness, fear, sadness, and anger in a group (mean MA of 40 months) of young children with DS. Kasari et al. (2001) demonstrated that, compared to MA- and CA-matched typically developing comparison groups, the children with DS displayed specific impairments in recognizing fear and anger. In addition, Kasari et al. (2001) also highlighted the finding that the children with DS did not differ from the MA-matched groups in the ability to recognize emotion at 3 years, but did so at 4 years, as they showed relatively little improvement despite their increased MA. Among the possible explanations, Kasari et al. suggested that this developmental-specific group difference may be related to language development given the nature of the task used (i.e., discerning the emotion from a story read to the child) and suggest that future studies should assess the effect of language development, in addition to cognitive status, when assessing the development of emotion recognition in youth with DS.

These and other considerations were addressed by Williams et al. (2005) in a very comprehensive assessment of emotion recognition among persons with DS. They assessed the performance of 34 participants with DS aged between 7 and 17 years (CA) on identity- and emotion-matching tasks as compared to that of participants with nonspecific intellectual disability and typically developing children. All of the participants were also assessed for cognitive ability, language comprehension and expression, adaptive behavior, and face identification ability using the Benton Facial Recognition Test (Benton et al., 1983). The performance of the participants with DS was significantly lower than that of the TD group (but similar to that of the nonspecific intellectual disability group) on both identity- and emotion-matching tasks. According to a post hoc analysis, the persons with DS had specific difficulty recognizing fear. In addition, face-task performance was not found to be correlated with the other measures collected from the persons with DS, leading Williams et al. (2005) to argue that cognitive ability, language comprehension and expression, and adaptive behavior are not related to the emotion-recognition difficulties among school-aged children with DS. In sum, children with DS appear to have emotion-recognition difficulties, with particular challenges for the recognition of face stimuli conveying fear, surprise, and anger (Goldman et al., 2018; Kasari et al., 2001; Williams et al., 2005; Wishart & Pitcairn 2000).

In one study of recognition abilities among *adults* with DS, Hippolyte et al. (2008) used a variety of experimental tasks that assessed performance in matching and identifying face stimuli with (Emotion Identification, Match and Recognition and Intensity Attribution Tests) and without (Identity Matching Test) emotional content (Bruce et al., 2000; Rojahn, Rabold, & Schneider, 1995). As compared to a comparison group matched on receptive vocabulary task performance, the adults with DS were less able to match face stimuli with emotional content, with specific difficulty for those conveying neutral and surprised expressions, consistent with the evidence from children with DS (Williams et al., 2005; Wishart & Pitcairn, 2000). This finding is consistent with that of Conrad et al. (2007), who also suggested that children with DS experience emotions more intensely, reflecting a possible "emotion-specific" face processing difficulty.

Summary and Synthesis

As with other neurodevelopmental conditions, atypical optical and perceptual functions and abilities are present in children, adolescents, and adults with DS. At an optical level, many of these abnormalities are similar to those present in typically developing children, but their prevalence and severity appear to be higher in persons with DS. These include, for example, errors of refraction and acuity and poor accommodation. One finding that seems to be specific to children with DS is that over time, these difficulties do not ameliorate naturally as they do among typically developing children, which explains at least in part why a greater proportion of children with DS wear corrective lenses. This is an important finding since optically related visual functions, including acuity and accommodation, are crucial for optimal learning and literary abilities. As these optical functions do not improve over time, they should be assessed early and often in persons with DS, particularly during the preschool-age years in order to maximize learning at home and within the classroom environment. In order to obtain the most accurate measures of ocular function (i.e., acuity) in DS, nonverbal or adapted approaches can be used (such as asking patients to detect instead of identifying targets) during optometric testing in order to minimize potential cognitive or motivational factors that may affect assessment outcome.

Just as optical factors are important considerations for learning and classroom environments, so too are perceptual processes. For example, in addition to research suggesting that individuals with DS are visual learners, at least some findings also suggest that presenting visual information in a structured manner may be especially beneficial for learners with DS. An increased understanding of such favorable perceptual environments is thus crucial for optimizing strength-based interventions and, most importantly, academic achievement among persons with DS. With regards to understanding social behavior among persons with DS, empirical studies assessing higher-level processes such as face perception in children and adults with DS demonstrate diminished efficiency in identifying and recognizing emotions, particularly for fear and anger. These findings suggest that inappropriate social behavior in DS may stem from atypical information processing that has a neurological basis. A greater understanding of social information processing may have a significant impact on managing behaviors for younger and older individuals with DS, as well as potentially developing behavioral interventions that are specific for individuals with DS.

References

Adolphs, R. (2003). Cognitive neuroscience of human social behaviour. *Nature Reviews: Neuroscience, 4*, 165–178. https://doi.org/10.1038/nrn1056

Al-Bagdady, M., Stewart, R. E., Watts, P., Murphy, P. J., & Woodhouse, J. M. (2009). Bifocals and Down's syndrome: Correction or treatment? *Ophthalmic and Physiological Optics, 29*(4), 416–421. https://doi.org/10.1111/j.1475-1313.2009.00646.x

Allison, T., Puce, A., & McCarthy, G. (2000). Social perception from visual cues: Role of the STS region. *Trends in Cognitive Science, 4*(7), 267–278. https://doi.org/10.1016/s1364-6613(00)01501-1

Anderson, H. A., Manny, R. E., Glasser, A., & Stuebing, K. K. (2011). Static and dynamic measurements of accommodation in individuals with Down syndrome. *Investigative Ophthalmology & Visual Science, 52*(1), 310–317. https://doi.org/10.1167/iovs.10-5301

Annaz, D., Karmiloff-Smith, A., Johnson, M. H., & Thomas, M. S. (2009). A cross-syndrome study of the development of holistic face recognition in children with autism, Down syndrome, and Williams syndrome. *Journal of Experimental and Child Psychology, 102*(4), 456–486. https://doi.org/10.1016/j.jecp.2008.11.005

Atkinson, J., & Braddick, O. (2013). Visual development. In P. D. Zelazo (Ed.), *The Oxford handbook of developmental psychology: Vol. 1. Body and mind* (pp. 271–309). New York, NY: Oxford University Press.

Atkinson, J., King, J., Braddick, O., Nokes, L., Anker, S., & Braddick, F. (1997). A specific deficit of dorsal stream function in Williams' syndrome. *Neuroreport, 8*(8), 1919–1922. https://doi.org/10.1097/00001756-199705260-00025

Bellugi, U., Lichtenberger, L., Jones, W., Lai Z., & St. George, M. (2000). The neurocognitive profile of Williams syndrome: A complex pattern of strengths and weaknesses. *Journal of Cognitive Neuroscience, 12*(1), 7–29. https://doi.org/10.1162/089892900561959

Benton, A. L., Sivan, A. B., de Hamsher, S. K., Varney, N. R., & Spreen, O. (1983). *Benton Facial Recognition Test.* New York, NY: Oxford University Press.

Berk, L. E. (2000). *Child development.* Boston, MA: Allyn and Bacon.

Blakemore, S.-J., Decety, J. (2001). From the perception of action to the understanding of intention. *Nature Reviews Neuroscience, 2*, 561–567. https://doi.org/10.1038/35086023

Braddick, O., & Atkinson, J. (2011). Development of human visual function. *Vision Research, 51*, 1588–1600. https://doi.org/10.1016/j.visres.2011.02.018

Braddick O., Atkinson, J., & Wattam-Bell, J. (2003). Normal and anomalous development of visual motion processing: Motion coherence and "dorsal-stream vulnerability." *Neuropsychologia, 41*(13), 1769–1784. https://doi.org/10.1016/s0028-3932(03)00178-7

Braddick O., O'Brien, J. M., Wattam-Bell, J., Atkinson, J., & Turner, R. (2000). Form and motion coherence activate independent, but not dorsal/ventral segregated, networks in the human brain. *Current Biology, 10*(12), 731–734. https://doi.org/10.1016/s0960-9822(00)00540-6

Bruce, V., Campbell, R. N., Doherty-Sneddon, G., Import, A., Langton, S., McAuley, S., & Wright, R. (2000). Testing face processing skills in children. *British Journal of Developmental Psychology, 18*(3), 319–333. https://doi.org/10.1348/026151000165715

Bull, M. J. (2011). Health supervision for children with Down syndrome. *Pediatrics, 128*(2), 393–406. https://doi.org/10.1542/peds.2011-1605

Carretti, B., & Lanfranchi, S. (2010). The effect of configuration on VSWM performance of Down syndrome individuals. *Journal of Intellectual Disability Research, 54*(12), 1058–1066. https://doi.org/10.1111/j.1365-2788.2010.01334.x

Conrad, N. J., Schmidt, L. A., Niccols, A., Polak, C. P., Riniolo, T. C., & Burack, J. A. (2007). Frontal electroencephalogram asymmetry during affective processing in children with Down syndrome: a pilot study. *Journal of Intellectual Disability Research, 51*(12), 988–995. https://doi.org/10.1111/j.1365-2788.2007.01010.x

Courage, M. L., Adams, R. J., & Hall, E. J. (1997). Contrast sensitivity in infants and children with Down syndrome. *Vision Research, 37*(11), 1545–1555. https://doi.org/10.1016/s0042-6989(96)00304-5

da Cunha, R. P., Moreira, J. B. (1996). Ocular findings in Down's syndrome. *American Journal of Ophthalmology, 122*(2), 236–244. https://doi.org/10.1016/s0002-9394(14)72015-x

Del Viva, M. M., Tozzi, A., Bargagna, S., & Cioni, G. (2015). Motion perception deficit in Down Syndrome. *Neuropsychologia, 75*, 214–220. https://doi.org/10.1016/j.neuropsychologia.2015.06.005

De Valois, R. L., Albrecht, D. G., & Thorell, L. G. (1982). Spatial frequency selectivity of cells in macaque visual cortex. *Vision Research, 22*(5), 545–559.

De Valois, L & De Valois, K. K. (1988). *Spatial vision.* New York, NY: Oxford University Press.

Dimitriou, D., Leonard, H. C., Karmiloff-Smith, A., Johnson, M. H., & Thomas MS. (2015). Atypical development of configural face recognition in children with autism, Down syndrome and Williams syndrome. *Journal of Intellectual Disability Research, 59*(5), 422–38. https://doi.org/10.1111/jir.12141

Farah, M. J., Wilson, K. D., Drain, M., & Tanaka, J. W. (1998). What is "special" about face perception. *Psychological Review, 105*, 482–498. https://doi.org/10.1037/0033-295X.105.3.482

Felius, J., Beauchamp, C. L., & Stager, D. R. Sr. (2014). Visual acuity deficits in children with nystagmus and Down syndrome. *American Journal of Ophthalmology, 157*(2), 458–463. https://doi.org/10.1016/j.ajo.2013.09.023

Goldman, K. J., Shulman, C., & Burack, J. A. (2018). Inference from facial expressions among adolescents and young adults with Down syndrome. *American Journal on Intellectual and Developmental Disabilities, 123*(4), 344–358. https://doi.org/10.1352/1944-7558-123.4.344

Hammill, D.D., Pearson, N.A., & Voress, J.K. (1993). *Developmental Test of Visual Perception: DTVP-2* (2nd ed.). Austin, TX: Pro-Ed, @1993.

Haugen, O. H., Høvding, G., & Lundström, I. (2001). Refractive development in children with Down's syndrome: A population based, longitudinal study. *British Journal of Ophthalmology, 85*(6), 714–719. https://doi.org/10.1136/bjo.85.6.714

Head, E., Powell, D., Gold, B. T., & Schmitt, F. A. (2012). Alzheimer's disease in Down syndrome. *European Journal of Neurodegenerative Disease, 1*(3), 353.

Head, E., Silverman, W., Patterson, D., & Lott, I. T. (2012). Aging and down syndrome. *Current Gerontology and Geriatrics Research*, Article 412536. https://doi.org/10.1155/2012/412536

Hippolyte, L., Barisnikov, K., & van der Linden, M. (2008). Face processing and facial emotion recognition in adults with Down syndrome. *American Journal of Mental Retardation, 113*(4), 292–306. https://doi.org/10.1352/0895-8017

Ikeda, K., Kasugai, H., Yamaguchi, A., Uchino, Y., Katase, H., & Kanno, A. (2013). Visual perceptual strengths and weaknesses in adults with intellectual disabilities compared with a birth year-matched norm. *Journal of Intellectual Disability Research, 57*(1), 67–79. https://doi.org/10.1111/j.1365-2788.2011.01516.x

Johansson, G. (1973). Visual perception of biological motion and a model for its analysis. *Perception & Psychophysics, 14*(2), 201–211. https://doi.org/10.3758/BF03212378

John, F. M., Bromham, N. R., Woodhouse, J. M., & Candy, T. R. (2004). Spatial vision deficits in infants and children with Down syndrome. *Investigative Ophthalmology & Visual Science, 45*(5), 1566–1572. https://doi.org/10.1167/iovs.03-0951

Johnson, M. H., Griffin, R., Csibra, G., Halit, H., Farroni, T., de Haan, M., Tucker, L.A., Baron-Cohen, S., & Richards, J. (2005). The emergence of the social brain network: Evidence from typical and atypical development. *Developmental Psychopathology, 17*(3), 599–619. https://doi.org/10.1017/S0954579405050297

Kasari, C., Freeman, S. F., & Hughes, M. A. (2001). Emotion recognition by children with Down syndrome. *American Journal of Mental Retardation, 106*(1), 59–72.

Kent, L., Evans, J., Paul, M., & Sharp, M. (1999). Comorbidity of autistic spectrum disorders in children with Down syndrome. *Developmental Medicine & Child Neurology, 41*(3),153–158. 10.1017/s001216229900033x.

Krinsky-McHale, S. J., Silverman, W., Gordon, J., Devenny, D. A., Oley, N., & Abramov, I. (2014). Vision deficits in adults with Down syndrome. *Journal of Applied Research in Intellectual Disabilities, 27*(3), 247–263. https://doi.org/10.1111/jar.12062

Little, J.-A. (2015). Accommodation deficit in children with Down syndrome: Practical considerations for the optometrist. *Clinical Optometry, 7*, 81–89. https://doi.org/10.2147/OPTO.S63351

Little, J.-A., Woodhouse, J. M., Lauritzen, J. S., & Saunders, K. J. (2007). The impact of optical factors on resolution acuity in children with Down syndrome. *Investigative Ophthalmology & Visual Science, 48*(9), 3995–4001. https://doi.org/10.1167/iovs.06-1387

Martin, N. A. (2006). *Test of visual perceptual skills* (3rd ed.). Novato, CA: Academic Therapy Publications.

Mondloch C. J., Le Grand R., & Maurer D. (2002). Configural face processing develops more slowly than featural face processing. *Perception, 31*, 553–566. https://doi.org/10.1068/p3339

Næss, K. B., Nygaard, E., Ostad, J., Dolva, A. S., & Lyster, S. H. (2017). The profile of social functioning in children with Down syndrome. *Disability and Rehabilitation, 39*(13), 1320–1331.

Nandakumar, K., Evans, M. A., Briand, K., & Leat, S. J. (2011). Bifocals in Down Syndrome Study (BiDS): analysis of video recorded sessions of literacy and visual perceptual skills. *Clinical and Experimental Optometry, 94*(6), 575–585. https://doi.org/10.1111/j.1444-0938.2011.00650.x

Nandakumar, K., & Leat, S. J. (2009). Bifocals in Down Syndrome Study (BiDS): Design and baseline visual function. *Optometry and Vision Science, 86*(3), 196–207. https://doi.org/10.1097/OPX.0b013e318196cd93

Pelphrey, K. A., Mitchell, T. V., McKeown, M. J., Goldstein, J., Allison, T., & McCarthy, G. (2003). Brain activity evoked by the perception of human walking: Controlling for meaningful coherent motion. *Journal of Neuroscience, 23*(17), 6819–6825. https://doi.org/10.1523/JNEUROSCI.23-17-06819.2003

Powell, L. J., Kosakowski, H. L., & Saxe, R. (2018). Social origins of cortical face areas. *Trends in Cognitive Science, 22*(9), 752–763. https://doi.org/10.1016/j.tics.2018.06.009

Rakover, S. S. (2002). Featural vs. configural information in faces: A conceptual and empirical analysis. *British Journal of Psychology, 93*, 1–30.

Riddell, H., Tolentino-Castro, J. W., Wagner, H., & Lappe, M. (2017). Impairments in the visual processing of global biological motion cues in Down syndrome. *Perception, 46*, 1283–1297. https://doi.org/10.1177/0301006617718716

Rojahn, J., Rabold, D. E., & Schneider, F. (1995). Emotion specificity in mental retardation. *American Journal on Mental Retardation, 99*, 477–486.

Silverman, W. (2007). Down syndrome: Cognitive phenotype. *Mental Retardation and Developmental Disabilities Research Reviews, 13*, 228–236. http://dx.doi.org/10.1002/mrdd.20156

Stewart, R. E., Woodhouse, J. M., & Trojanowska, L. D. (2005). In focus: The use of bifocals for children with Down syndrome. *Ophthalmic and Physiological Optics*, *25*, 514–522. https://doi.org/10.1111/j.1475-1313.2005.00326.x

Tanaka, J. W., & Farah, M. J. (1993). Parts and wholes in face recognition. *The Quarterly Journal of Experimental Psychology Section A*, *46*(2), 225–245. https://doi.org/10.1080/14640749308401045

Watt, T., Robertson, K., & Jacobs, R. J. (2015). Refractive error, binocular vision and accommodation of children with Down syndrome. *Clinical & Experimental Optometry*, *98*(1), 3–11. https://doi.org/10.1111/cxo.12232

Williams K. R., Wishart J. G., Pitcairn T. K., & Willis D. S. (2005). Emotion recognition by children with Down syndrome: Investigation of specific impairments and error patterns. *American Journal on Mental Retardation*, *110*, 378–392. https://doi.org/10.1352/0895-8017(2005)110[378:ERBCWD]2.0.CO;2

Wishart, J., & Pitcairn, T. (2000). Recognition of identity and expression in faces by children with Down syndrome. *American Journal of Mental Retardation*, *105*, 466–479. https://doi.org/10.1352/0895-8017(2000)105<0466:ROIAEI>2.0.CO;2

Valentine, T. (1991). A unified account of the effects of distinctiveness, inversion, and race in face recognition. *Quarterly Journal of Experimental Psychology*, *43*(2), 161–204. https://doi.org/10.1080/14640749108400966

Virji-Babul, N., Kerns, K., Zhou, E., Kapur, A., & Shiffrar, M. (2006). Perceptual-motor deficits in children with Down syndrome: Implications for intervention. *Down Syndrome Research and Practice*, *10*(2), 74–82. https://doi.org/10.3104/reports.308

Woodhouse, J. M., Pakeman, V. H., Saunders, K. J., Parker, M., Fraser, W. I., Lobo, S., & Sastry, P. (1996). Visual acuity and accommodation in infants and young children with Down's syndrome. *Journal of Intellectual Disability Research*, *40*(1), 49–55.

Yang, Y., Conners, F. A., & Merrill, E. C. (2014). Visuo-spatial ability in individuals with Down syndrome: Is it really a strength? *Research in Developmental Disabilities*, *35*(7), 1473–500. https://doi.org/10.1016/j.ridd.2014.04.002

Yin, R. K. (1969). Looking at upside-down faces. *Journal of Experimental Psychology*, *81*(1), 141–145. https://doi.org/10.1037/h0027474

CHAPTER 11

The Development of Attention Among Persons With Down Syndrome

Elizabeth A. Kaplan-Kahn, Elizabeth P. McKernan, Justin B. Kopec,
Erin Matsuba, *and* Natalie Russo

Abstract

Clinical reports of persons with Down Syndrome (DS) generally include descriptions of attentional challenges, which in some cases are diagnosed as attention-deficit/hyperactivity disorder (ADHD). While the rates of diagnosable disorders of attentional function are important considerations for clinicians, educators, researchers, and stakeholders, so too is an understanding of strengths and weaknesses in the development of different facets of attention that may not rise to the level of a psychological disorder but nonetheless adversely affect daily functioning. Attentional challenges among persons with DS must be understood, both clinically and empirically, within a developmental context that considers an individual's relative strengths and weaknesses, as well how, and in relation to whom, comparisons are being made. The purpose of this chapter is to critically assess and synthesize the research on attentional processes among persons with DS, focusing on the development of attentional orienting as well as selective and sustained attention. Findings are contextualized with respect to contemporary definitions of attention, and their development among typically developing persons, and yield a fairly consistent profile of strengths and weaknesses in attentional function among persons with DS across the lifespan. Conclusions focus on recommendations for future research including clinical implications and considerations.

Key Words: Down Syndrome, attention, development, attention-deficit/hyperactivity disorder, clinical psychology

Clinical observations that people with Down Syndrome (DS) experience attentional challenges have permeated descriptions of the phenotype of DS for several decades and include reports of distractible children who are sometimes impulsive and fidgety (Capone et al., 2006; Ekstein et al., 2011; Oxelgren et al., 2017). In some cases, these behaviors are significant enough to impede functioning and can lead to a comorbid diagnosis of attention-deficit/hyperactivity disorder (ADHD), a neurodevelopmental disorder characterized by inattention and/or hyperactivity (American Psychiatric Association, 2013). Prevalence estimates for ADHD among persons with DS range broadly from around 40% (Ekstein et al., 2011; Gath & Gumley, 1986; Määttä et al., 2006) to as low as 6.1%

(Myers & Pueschel, 1991). Even conservative estimates of the rates of ADHD among persons with DS are higher than in the general population (estimated to be 5%; American Psychiatric Association, 2013), with recent reports that a lower gestational age is associated with a higher likelihood of ADHD symptoms among persons with DS (del Hoyo Soriano et al., 2020). The rates of diagnosable disorders of attentional function are important considerations for clinicians, educators, researchers, and stakeholders. However, so too is an understanding of strengths and weaknesses in the development of different facets of attention that may not rise to the level of psychological disorder but may nonetheless adversely affect daily functioning. Further, areas of strength in attentional function, if identified, could help to compensate for weakness and be leveraged in the development of educational, behavioral, or occupational interventions.

Historically, the study of attention among persons with DS has proceeded along two parallel lines of inquiry. One, clinical in nature, focused on identifying and remediating deficits in attentional function, usually in support of academic learning. The second was focused on the basic sciences, aimed at understanding the underlying causes or profiles of cognitive deficits in individuals with DS and other populations of persons with intellectual disability (ID). Both of these lines of inquiry attempted to measure attention in relation to some sort of metric or expectation, usually the performance or functioning of individuals who were typically developing (TD). These two lines of inquiry also faced similar challenges, including how to operationalize and measure the construct of attention; how to understand the relationship between attention, cognitive ability, and daily function; and, critically, how to contextualize these with respect to development.

The construct of attention and its underlying development are complex and dynamic, and the study of how these processes unfold among persons with DS is even more intricate. It requires not only a clear understanding of typical developmental trajectories of attention, but also considerations of, at the very least, the roles that age, experience, overall cognitive ability, and their potential dissociations might play in shaping developmental trajectories among persons with DS. While seemingly obvious, these considerations are often ignored in both clinical and research enterprises. This oversight occurs clinically when individuals with DS (or their parents) are asked to complete psychological assessments that have not been specifically validated for populations with intellectual disability, and it is compounded when these assessments are then scored in relation to how other individuals of the same age perform. This occurs empirically when the performance of a group of individuals with DS is compared to that of a group of individuals of the same chronological age. In both of those cases, one will likely find the obvious—that those with lower cognitive abilities perform more poorly than those with higher cognitive abilities (for reviews, see Burack, Russo, et al., 2012; Flanagan et al., 2008). This approach, referred to as the deficit model, is contrasted with a developmental approach (Burack et al., 2021; Cicchetti et al., 1982; Hodapp et al., 1990; Hodapp & Zigler, 1995), which attempts to account for discrepancies among those with DS between their chronological ages and developmental levels through the conduct and interpretation of clinical evaluations and research. Ignoring the developmental considerations has the potential to negatively impact our field, our profession, and our ability to identify discrepancies in performance and to intervene respectfully and appropriately with persons with DS and their families when supports are needed. In one related example from a different population, Lane et al. (2014) challenged prevailing notions of attentional deficits among children with fetal alcohol spectrum disorder (FASD) by contrasting findings of clinically significant levels of attentional problems as rated by parents, which were scored according to age-based norms for the general population, with better-than-expected performance on a standardized measure of attention that was scored in relation to the children's developmental level. This contrast between findings of deficit versus findings of strength in attention within the same group of children puts into sharp relief the critical role of approaching the interpretation of clinical and research findings within the context of a developmental lens.

In this chapter, we attempt to make sense of empirical research focused on the development of attention among persons with DS. In so doing we keep at the forefront the changing landscape of how we define and measure attention. Additionally, we interpret research findings through the lens offered by the developmental approach. A summary of each of the studies presented in this chapter, including the mental and chronological ages of the participants, matching strategies (including whether participants were matched on verbal or nonverbal abilities), and study findings, are presented in Table 11.1. A summary of findings as a function of attentional construct and developmental stage are presented in Table 11.2.

How Do We Understand Attention?

> "Everyone knows what attention is. . . . It is the taking possession by the mind, in clear and vivid form, of one out of what may seem several simultaneously possible objects or trains of thought. . . . It implies withdrawal from some things in order to deal effectively with others.
>
> *James, 1890*

William James' ubiquitous quote still serves as a good heuristic for our understanding of attention, though the field of attention research has grown tremendously over the last 130 years. Attention was once considered a static discrete mental mechanism that could be localized in a specific brain structure (Posner et al., 1988; Posner & Petersen, 1990) and was invariant across both individuals and contexts (for a review, see Ristic & Enns, 2015). However, according to contemporary perspectives, attention is seen as a multifaceted cognitive process (Enns, 1993; Petersen & Posner, 2012) that changes dynamically with changes in the individual and their environmental context (Burack et al., 2017; Ristic & Enns, 2015), such as emotional cues (Fulcher et al., 2008; Hoehl et al., 2008;

Table 11.1. Summary of Empirical Studies Organized by Chronological Age of Participants

Authors (Year)	Group(s)	Mean CA of Groups	Matching Measure	Mean MA of Groups	Type of Attention Task	Characterization of Stimuli	Results
Landry & Chapieski (1989)							
	14 DS 14 MA Controls	12.8 mo. (SD = 0.8 mo.) 14.5 mo. (SD = 0.5 mo.)	BSID (full scale)	10.5 mo. (SD = 1.0 mo.) 11.2 mo. (SD = 1.1 mo.)	10 min. mother-infant interaction session	Toys (ecologically valid)	DS group less likely to shift attention to new toys, but attention behaviors impacted by mother interactions
Brown et al. (2003)							
Experiment 1	13 WS 19 DS 17 CA Controls 15 MA Controls	29 mo. (range: 23–37 mo.) 29 mo. (range: 24–37 mo.) 30 mo. (range: 23–37 mo.) 15 mo. (range: 12–21mo.)	BSID-II (full scale)	101.43 (SD: 10.00) 100.89 (SD: 9.96) 146.76 (SD: 9.30) 99.44 (SD: 10.81)	Visual orienting to exogenous stimuli	Squares on computer screen (not ecologically valid)	DS group performed similarly to CA and MA groups
Experiment 2	Same as Experiment 1	Same as Exp. 1	BSID-II (full scale)	Same as Exp. 1	Sustained attention, parents instructed to not interact with child	Toys (ecologically valid)	DS group exhibited shorter total duration periods of sustained attention
Krakow & Kopp (1982)							
Experiment 1	16 DS 40 MA Controls	29 mo. (range: 45–73 mo.) 15 mo. (range: 12–18 mo.)	GDS (full scale)	17 mo. (n.r.) 17 mo. (n.r.)	Sustained attention, parents instructed not to interact with child	Toys (ecologically valid)	DS group performed similarly to MA group
Experiment 2	15 DS 17 MA Controls	Range: 3–4 years Range: 2–2.5 years	n.r.	29 mo. (n.r.) 29 mo. (n.r.)	Sustained attention, parents instructed not to interact with child	Toys (ecologically valid)	DS group exhibited more repetitive play and fewer social bids than MA group

Cornish et al. (2007)							
Experiment 1	8 FXS 8 WS 8 DS 40 MA Controls	43 mo. (range: 34–50 mo.) 46 mo. (range: 37–50 mo.) 63 mo. (range: 56–72 mo.) 35 mo. (range: 28–48 mo.)	BSID-II (full scale)	29 mo. (range: 23–36 mo.) 29 mo. (range: 18–49 mo.) 36 mo. (range: 28–45 mo.) Range: 18–49 mo.	Visual selective attention to exogenous stimuli	Circles on computer screen with faces underneath (minimal ecological validity)	DS group performed similarly to MA group
Experiment 2	25 FXS 25 DS 50 MA Controls	11 yrs. (range: 8–15 yrs.) 11 yrs. (range: 7–15 yrs.) 8 yrs. (range: 5–10 yrs.) * same participants as Munir et al. (2000)	BPVS (receptive language)	7 yrs. (range: 4–11 yrs.) 6 yrs. (range: 3–9 yrs.) 7 yrs. (range: 5–10 yrs.)	Selective, sustained & inhibition tasks of TEA-Ch	Computer tasks intended to be games (minimal ecological validity)	DS group performed significantly worse than FXS and MA groups on measure of selective attention, but performed similarly to MA group on measures of sustained attention and inhibition
Shalev et al. (2019)							
	18 DS 25 WS 31 MA Controls	7.2 yrs. (range: 4–8 yrs.) 6.6 yrs. (range: 5–8 yrs.) 3.8 yrs. (range: n.r.)	British Ability Scales II (full scale) & BPVS-II (receptive language)	3.3 yrs. (n.r.) 3.2 yrs. (n.r.) 4.1 yrs. (n.r.)	Sustained attention on a continuous performance task	Computer tasks intended to be games (minimal ecological validity)	DS group performed similarly to MA group and better than the WS group in their sensitivity to the task; the DS group demonstrated a similar pattern of performance to the TD group

(*continued*)

Table 11.1 *Continued*

Authors (Year)	Group(s)	Mean CA of Groups	Matching Measure	Mean MA of Groups	Type of Attention Task	Characterization of Stimuli	Results
Breckenridge, Braddick, Anker, et al. (2013)							
	32 WS 32 DS	8 yrs. (range: 5–16 yrs.) 10 yrs. (range: 5–15 yrs.)	WPPSI (full scale)	5 yrs. (range: 4–6 yrs.) 5 yrs. (range: 3–6 yrs.)	Selective, sustained, & executive control tasks of ECAB scaled based on MA	Computer tasks intended to be games (minimal ecological validity)	DS group performed as well as or better than WS group on all ECAB tasks, DS group scale scores were lower than MA comparisons for visual search and executive control tasks but were similar to or higher than MA comparisons on all other ECAB scores
Goldman et al. (2005)							
	12 DS 13 MA Controls	15.0 yrs. (SD = 2.93 yrs.) 5.6 yrs. (SD = 0.45 yrs.)	Leiter K-BIT (matrices) (nonverbal)	5.6 yrs. (SD = 0.64 yrs.) n.r.	Visual orienting	Computer task intended to be a game (minimal ecological validity)	DS group exhibited faster reaction times than MA-matched controls across conditions, though patterns of performance were similar for both groups
Brodeur et al. (2013)							
	13 DS 13 MA Controls	15.1 yrs. (SD = 3.4 yrs.) 5.2 yrs. (SD = 0.54 yrs.)	Leiter-R (nonverbal)	5.4 yrs. (SD = 0.75 yrs.) 5.5 yrs. (SD = 0.76 yrs.)	Sustained attention—multiple object tracking	Computer tasks intended to be games (minimal ecological validity)	DS group performed similarly to MA group on static object identification but significantly worse than MA controls on multiple object tracking

Costanzo et al. (2013)							
	18 WS 15 DS 17 MA Controls	17.6 yrs. (SD = 7.4 yrs.) 14.5 yrs. (SD = 3.7 yrs.) 7.4 yrs. (SD = 0.8 yrs.)	Leiter-R (nonverbal)	6.7 yrs. (SD = 0.9 yrs.) 6.2 yrs. (SD = 0.9 yrs.) 6.9 yrs. (SD = 0.7 yrs.)	Selective and sustained attention tasks of BVN, TEA-Ch, and BELLS	Listening to words and tones and searching for visual targets on paper (minimal ecological validity)	DS group performed similarly to MA group on auditory selective task and visual sustained tasks, but significantly worse than MA controls on visual selective tasks
Lanfranchi et al. (2010)							
	15 DS 15 MA Controls	15 yrs. (range: 11–18 yrs.) 5 yrs. (range: 4–7yrs.)	Logical Operations Test (nonverbal)	6 yrs. (range: 4–7 yrs.) n.r.	Sustained attention	Pointing to pictures on pages (minimal ecological validity)	DS group performed similarly to MA group for total measure, but exhibited significantly more errors
Munir et al. (2000)							
	25 FXS 25 DS 25 "poor attention" MA Controls 25 "good attention" MA Controls	11 yrs. (range: 8–15 yrs.) 11 yrs. (range: 7–15 yrs.) 8 yrs. (range: 5–10 yrs.) 8 yrs. (range: 5–10 yrs.) * same participants as Cornish et al. (2007)	BPVS (receptive language)	7 yrs. (SD = 1.6 yrs.) 6 yrs. (SD = 1.5 yrs.) 7 yrs. (SD = 1.4 yrs.) 8 yrs. (SD = 1.6 yrs.)	Selective, divided, and sustained attention tasks of the WATT and TEA-Ch	Computer tasks intended to be games (minimal ecological validity)	DS group performed worse than MA groups on selective and divided attention tasks, DS group performed similarly to "poor attention" MA controls on sustained attention task
Randolph & Burack (2000)							
	20 DS 20 MA Controls	20 yrs. (SD = 6.8 yrs.) 5.5 yrs. (SD = 0.9 yrs.)	KBIT (nonverbal)	5.3 yrs. (SD = 0.9 yrs.) 5.4 yrs. (SD = 0.8 yrs.)	Visual filtering and orienting	Computer task intended to be a game (minimal ecological validity)	DS group performed similarly to MA group

(*continued*)

Table 11.1. *Continued*

Authors (Year)	Group(s)	Mean CA of Groups	Matching Measure	Mean MA of Groups	Type of Attention Task	Characterization of Stimuli	Results
Cornish et al. (2001)							
	15 FXS 15 DS 15 MA Controls n.r.	23 yrs. (range: 18–28 yrs.) 24 yrs. (range: 18–27 yrs.) 13 yrs. (range: 12–15 yrs.)	BPVS (verbal)	Individual MAs n.r.	Selective and sustained attention tasks of TEA	Searching a map and counting tones on an "elevator" (minimal ecological validity)	DS group performed significantly worse than MA controls on both tasks, but similar to FXS group

Note: WS = persons with Williams syndrome; DS = persons with Down syndrome; CA = chronological age matched comparisons; MA = mental age matched comparisons; FXS = persons with Fragile X Syndrome; n.r. = not reported

Table 11.2. Summary of Empirical Literature

Facet of Attention	Early Childhood		Middle Childhood & Adolescence		Adulthood	
	Typical Attention	Atypical Attention	Typical Attention	Atypical Attention	Typical Attention	Atypical Attention
Orienting	Brown et al. (2003)		Goldman et al. (2005)		Randolph & Burack (2000)	
Visual Selective	Cornish et al. (2007)			Cornish et al. (2007); Munir et al. (2000); Breckenridge et al. (2013); Costanzo et al. (2013)		Cornish et al. (2001)
Visual Sustained	Krakow & Kopp (1982)	Brown et al. (2003); Landry & Chapieski (1989)	Cornish, Scerif, & Karmiloff-Smith (2007); Munir et al. (2000); Breckenridge et al. (2013); Costanzo et al. (2013); Lanfranchi et al. (2010); Brodeur et al. (2013) – Static task Shalev et al. (2019);	Brodeur et al. (2013) – MOT task		
Auditory Sustained			Breckenridge et al. (2013)	Costanzo et al. (2013)		Cornish et al. (2001)

LoBue, 2009) and sociocultural factors (Gavrilov et al., 2012). While there are longstanding debates about how best to study attention and how it develops (Mirsky et al., 1991; Posner et al., 1988; Steele et al., 2012), the idea that the components that serve attention are comprised of separable functions has achieved a consensus among researchers (e.g., Corbetta & Shulman, 2002; Plebanek & Sloutsky, 2019; Posner & Petersen, 1990). These functions are (a) the *orienting* function, which involves shifting one's eyes or mind toward an environmental stimulus; (b) the *selection function*, which involves *filtering* irrelevant information and *searching* for targeted information; and (c) the *sustained* function, which involves maintaining a vigilant state over a period of time.

Each of these three broad functions of attention are influenced, or cued, by a combination of exogenous (e.g., an externally produced stimulus) and endogenous (e.g., an internal process) factors. These functions are governed by different, but interconnected, brain networks and triggered or influenced by the functional salience of stimuli. For example, environmental inputs that are more socially, emotionally, or evolutionarily salient (e.g., faces, spiders, etc.) capture our attention and are processed in a fundamentally different manner than stimuli without such natural importance (e.g., shapes, arrows, etc.; Ristic & Enns, 2015). Further, a person's current state of mind, which includes factors such as anxiety, hunger, fatigue, and also more fundamental processes such as oscillatory brain dynamics (Fiebelkorn et al., 2018; Fiebelkorn, Saalmann, et al., 2013; Fiebelkorn, Snyder, et al., 2013), influences what we attend to in any moment. That is, attention is dynamic, changes moment to moment and context to context, and is inherently influenced by both external and internal factors and experiences (e.g., Ristic & Enns, 2015).

Challenges in Understanding Attention Among Persons With DS

Clinical and empirical conceptualizations of attention often differ. Clinicians typically focus their diagnostic lens on whether individuals with DS experience attentional challenges that rise to the level of a potentially comorbid diagnosis of ADHD. They do so by determining whether an individual meets a certain threshold or number of symptoms that reflect attentional deficits. For example, the "inattentive" symptoms of ADHD include a persistent pattern of inattention, reflected in difficulty sustaining attention to a particular task, difficulty paying attention to details, or struggling to filter out distractions to a degree that interferes with functioning. These are often defined contextually with respect to day-to-day life, such as "often fails to give close attention to details or makes careless mistakes in schoolwork, at work, or during other activities" (American Psychiatric Association, 2013). In contrast, empirical conceptualizations of attention are concerned more with what attention is and how it works than in determining whether it is problematic, highlighting a significant divide between the clinical disciplines and the cognitive sciences. The differences between these conceptualizations and foci make it difficult to bridge the gap between these two areas of inquiry, despite them being mutually informative (Burack, 2016; Burack et al., 2016; Burack, Dawkins, et al., 2012; Burack, Russo, et al., 2012; Cicchetti, 1984; Jaswal et al., 2016).

While contemporary definitions and research focused on typical development are beginning to embrace the complexity and dynamic nature of attention, research on attention in persons with DS has been mostly focused on static facets of attention, and, again with some exceptions, uses nonaffective or nonsocial stimuli, limiting the conclusions that can be drawn regarding the state of attention among those with DS. Three additional challenges that, while not unique to the study of attention in DS, relate to the study of most groups of individuals with an ID deserve mention. The first is that findings from most lab-based studies are limited with regard to power because of the challenges associated with participant recruitment and retention. Accordingly, the number of participants with DS in any one of these studies is around 20, and usually the chronological ages of participants also vary considerably, making it difficult to disentangle how life experience and current contexts influence task performance. This makes developing a clear picture of attentional development among persons with DS challenging, as individual differences carry more weight when the number of participants is small.

Second, the performance of individuals with DS is generally compared to another participant group anchored on some metric. Some standardized tests, such as the Leiter-R (Roid & Miller, 1997), provide growth scores as one way to approach characterizing changes in cognitive ability level over time in a way that does not require a comparison group. While this approach shows promise (Channell et al., 2014), none of the studies reviewed here adopted this approach. Rather, most group comparisons of ability involved consideration of task performance in relation to developmental level, operationalized as mental age (MA), where MA = CA (chronological age) * IQ/100. While matching on the basis of MA is not a panacea, as it does not account for differences in life experiences between the groups (among other things), it does provide a more useful metric for determining whether there are meaningful differences in specific attentional function between those with and without DS in a way that considers *a priori* differences in general levels of cognitive functioning (see Russo et al., 2021, for an examination of the limits of various tests in measuring MA at different ages).

The composition of the comparison group and its interaction with researchers' choice of matching measures need to be considered in the interpretation of research findings. For example, individuals with DS, as a group, tend to have relative strengths in their nonverbal learning and memory and relative weaknesses in verbal abilities (e.g., Grieco et al., 2015), while those with Williams syndrome (WS) tend to have the opposite cognitive profile of strengths and weaknesses (e.g., Mervis et al., 2000). Thus, matching these two groups on verbal abilities and testing their attention skills might yield different findings than having participants complete the same attentional task but matching them on nonverbal abilities. These differences would likely have nothing to do with attentional function but instead would be attributable to differences in cognitive profiles and matching strategies. Therefore, depending on the type of experimental task, considerations of the measures on which participants are matched and how differences in profiles of cognitive strengths and weaknesses might impact task performance are informative (e.g., Burack et al., 2004). Of the studies reviewed for this chapter, most involved matching on full-scale IQ (FSIQ) or nonverbal/performance IQ (PIQ), with only three studies (by the same group) matching on the basis of verbal abilities (Cornish, et al., 2007, experiment 2; Munir, et al., 2000; & Shalev et al., 2019; see Table 11.1).

With these challenges in mind, our review is broadly organized by attentional component and developmentally (based on the chronological ages of participants) within each of the components of attention. Understanding the development of attention among persons with DS can help us not only determine whether, how, and/or when development attentional preferences or abilities differ between those with and without DS but also provide us with insights into the unique attentional profiles of persons with DS by considering the impact that different experimental conditions have on performance within participant groups. This understanding could provide critical information regarding how those with DS construct and make sense of the world around them, because the features of the environment that are, or become salient, capture attention, or distract an individual over both immediate and developmental time, have a tremendous impact on behavior, learning, and how the brain self-organizes. Further, because attention mediates memory, spatial navigation, language, numerical processing (Ansari et al., 2007; Shaywitz et al., 2001), object recognition, and complex learning (Dayan et al., 2000; Treisman, 1998), it is a crucial component of nearly all cognitive processes that are shaped by and shape an individual's developmental trajectory. While we have defined each of the components of attention quite broadly in this introduction, we will delve more deeply into their definition and function in each of the relevant sections.

Orienting

Orienting is the process of directing one's attention to a specific stimulus. This process can be engaged reflexively, which happens, for example, when we turn toward a flash of light or a loud sound. This stimulus of abrupt or unexpected onset automatically captures our attention and often leads to an overt behavior such as turning our eyes, ears, or body towards it. Our attentional response can also be covert, in that we tune our mind's eye to the stimulus that elicited our attention without making an overt response. Overt and covert orienting responses often work together to increase our perception of an event, but covert attention can be engaged without an overt response, and these two processes, while they share some neural features, do not have completely overlapping brain circuits (Fairhall et al., 2009).

In addition to this distinction between overt and covert orienting, exogenous orienting, which is under stimulus control, and endogenous orienting, which is goal directed, can also be distinguished. For example, when an event (e.g., a flash of light) captures our attention and leads to a covert orienting response, we are faster to respond to items that occur at that same location than we are to items cued at a different location. We can also choose to attend to a particular location or object in a goal-directed manner, such as deliberately listening to the subway loudspeaker to learn the next station. This endogenous orienting process also enhances our perception of the event to which we are attending. In the lab, orienting tasks that map onto exogenous, reflexive attention and/or endogenous goal-directed attention are used to compare accuracy and/or reaction times between trials in which a target appears in the same or a different location than either an endogenous or exogenous predictive cue (see Fig. 11.1a). Findings in these studies are two-fold: (a) targets that appear at cued locations are processed more quickly and accurately than those at un-cued locations, and (b) the time-course of exogenous attention is faster (100ms) and shorter lasting (100–200ms) than endogenous attention, which is slower to engage (300ms) but whose effects can last up to several minutes. While exogenous and endogenous cues both receive and send inputs to and from sensory cortices, these two processes engage different neural pathways (e.g., Fiebelkorn & Kastner, 2020).

The Development of Orienting

While the orienting process can be engaged by sound and touch (e.g., McDonald et al., 2000; Reece et al., 2016; Spence et al., 1998; Tummeltshammer & Amso, 2018), we know most about the development of orienting in response to visual stimuli (e.g., Farroni et al., 2000; Hood et al., 1998b; Johnson et al., 1991; Richards, 2001; Tummeltshammer & Amso, 2018). Reflexive orienting, as measured by infant analogues of the orienting tasks presented in Figure 11.1a, is established by approximately 3 months of age, with improvements in the speed of these processes over the first year of life. By around 5 months of age, infants orient to a target more quickly when it is preceded by a valid cue than when it is preceded by a nonvalid cue (e.g., Johnson et al., 1991; Richards, 2001), right around the same time as they will shift their attention to a location that has been cued by adult eye gaze (e.g., Farroni et al., 2000; Hood et al., 1998b). While the data suggest that reflexive or overt exogenous orienting is present, and adult-like in these first months of life, the development of endogenous aspects of attentional orienting continue to develop until well into early childhood (e.g., Enns & Brodeur, 1989; Wainwright & Bryson, 2002) and become adult-like on simple tasks between 8 and 10 years of age (e.g., Enns & Akhtar, 1989; Leclercq & Siéroff, 2013; though see Ristic & Kingstone, 2009 for a different perspective).

The foregoing lab-based studies of TD infants are critical to our understanding of the development of attention in DS; however, a couple of general points are worth mentioning here. First, while lab-based experiments provide evidence for "reaction time" facilitation and cue validity effects emerging around 4 months, orienting responses are established well before 4 months, as days-old infants preferentially orient to social stimuli such as

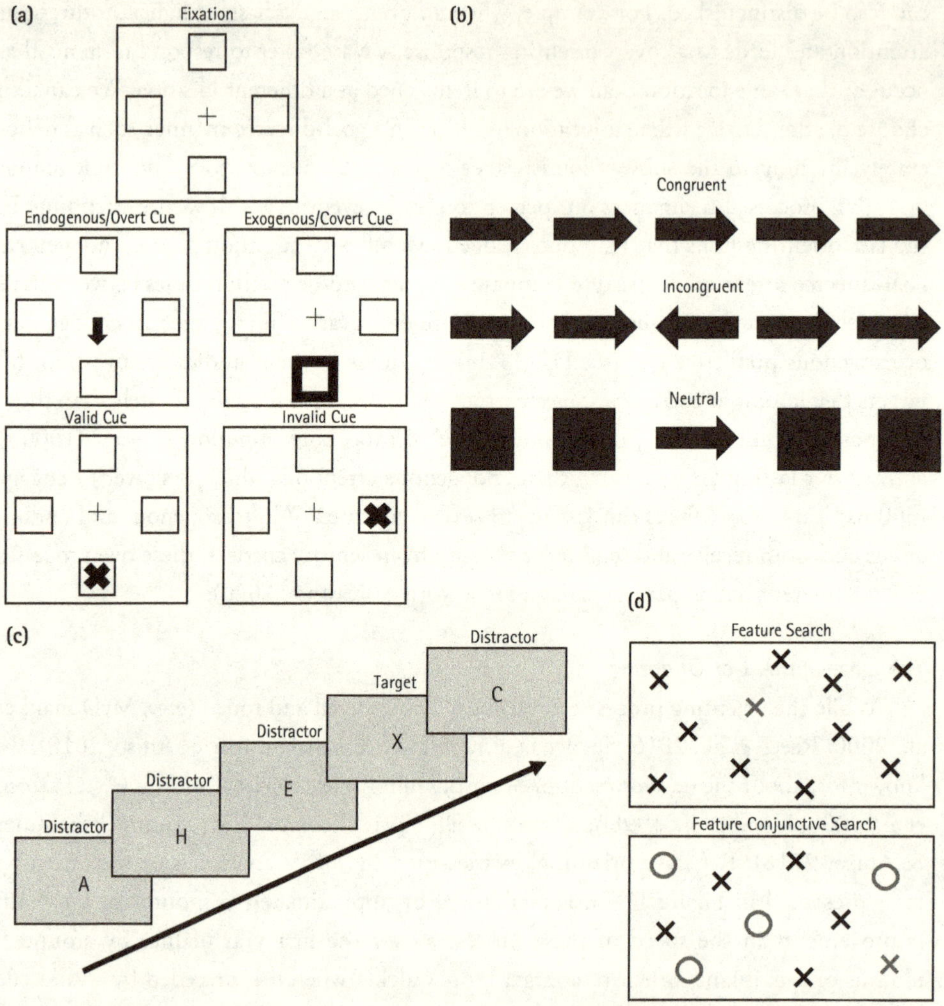

Figure 11.1. Popular paradigms used to study visual attention Researchers typically measure behavioral outcomes such as response time and accuracy as indices of performance. (a) Orienting task in which participants initially fixate on a mark (plus sign). Subsequently, either an endogenous/overt or exogenous/covert cue directs their attention toward the target (valid cue) or not (invalid cue). (b) Eriksen and Eriksen flanker task (1974) in which participants use a button press to identify the direction of the central (target) arrow. The central target can be flanked by congruent, incongruent, or neutral shapes. (c) Continuous performance task (Rosvold et al., 1956) where participants are asked to respond to an infrequently presented target (X) and inhibit responses to distractors. (d) Visual search paradigm in which participants are asked to locate either a unique target (red X) in a feature search or a target which shares some commonality with other distractors (red distractor Os and red target X) in a feature conjunctive search.

their primary caregiver's voice and smell (DeCasper & Fifer, 1980; Kisilevsky et al., 2003; Porter & Winberg, 1999). Second, and somewhat paradoxically, while we know that infants orient to and develop a preference for social stimuli that include familiar faces and voices, and that social and nonsocial functions are served by different brain mechanisms in the adult brain, it remains unclear if the developmental trajectories of social and nonsocial attention are identical, and how interdependent they are in the infant brain. Some researchers argue that we should be moving away from this commonly stated social/nonsocial distinction (e.g., Birmingham & Kingstone, 2009; Duncan & Barrett, 2007) and toward understanding attention in context (Ristic & Enns, 2015) as the salience of a social or nonsocial stimulus depends on what is happening in the moment (e.g., what are the other stimuli in the environment; what demands are being placed endogenously or exogenously on the attender; Beck & Kastner, 2009; Buschman & Kastner, 2015; Reynolds & Desimone, 2003; Yantis, 2005).

Orienting Among Individuals With Down Syndrome

Orienting among individuals with DS has been addressed in only three studies that meet the methodological requirements we established for review. Each of these were focused on a different age range providing a snapshot of the development of orienting across the lifespan. Whereas, all of these studies were focused on nonsocial visual stimuli, they differed with regard to focus on exogenous (Brown et al., 2003; Randolph & Burack, 2000) or endogenous (Goldman et al., 2005) aspects of overt (Brown et al., 2003) and covert (Goldman et al., 2005; Randolph & Burack, 2000) orienting.

Orienting in Early Childhood

Brown et al. (2003) assessed the exogenous overt orienting abilities to two sequentially presented targets among toddlers with DS and WS of the same mental and chronological ages (see Table 11.1), and two groups of TD children, one matched on CA (around 30 months), and one on MA (around 15 months). Toddlers' attention was first captured by a fixation stimulus, and once they were attending to the fixation stimulus, two targets, appearing rapidly one after another on opposite sides of the screen (i.e., up and down or left and right), were presented. The participants' eye gaze patterns were recorded to determine whether and how quickly they oriented to the rapidly presented images. Brown et al. reported no group differences in baseline performance, indicating that all of the groups were able to attend to the fixation stimulus. Toddlers with DS performed similarly to the CA- and MA-matched toddlers, and better than the toddlers with WS, in their visual orienting to the first target and used similar gaze patterns to both TD groups to orient to the second target. These findings suggest no exogenous orienting deficits in toddlers with DS. Their abilities appear to be in line with TD toddlers of the same CA and MA (the performance of the latter two groups did not differ from one another, suggesting this ability is well established by 15 months among TD children).

Orienting in Middle Childhood and Adolescence

Goldman et al. (2005) compared endogenous covert visual orienting abilities to an arrow cue in a group of children and adolescents with DS (mean CA = 15 years; mean

MA = 5.6 years) and an MA-matched TD comparison group (mean CA = 5.6 years; mean MA = not reported) using a standard Posner task (see Fig. 11.1a). As expected, invalidly cued trials resulted in longer reaction times than valid cues, and this was true for both groups. Further, and perhaps owing to their higher CA, the participants with DS demonstrated overall faster reaction times than the MA-matched TD participants. These results suggest that endogenous, covert visual orienting abilities of children and adolescents with DS are commensurate with their developmental level through middle childhood and adolescence.

Orienting in Adulthood

Randolph and Burack (2000) studied exogenous covert orienting in adults with DS relative to TD individuals of a similar MA. The participants fixated on the center of a screen and then a brief flash was used to capture attention exogenously. This was followed by the presentation of a target that was either in the same or a different location as the cue. As expected, reaction times were slower when targets were preceded by invalid cues, and this was true for both groups. These similar patterns of visual orienting and filtering across individuals matched on MA suggest that these abilities develop in a similar manner and at a rate commensurate with their overall cognitive development for adults with DS (Randolph & Burack, 2000).

The orienting studies reviewed here point to findings of similar task performance that is commensurate with developmental expectations. All of the studies were in the visual modality, leaving open the question of whether typical orienting abilities would be noted for hearing or touch. In addition, we do not yet have clear data on the endogenous orienting abilities of those with DS in toddlerhood or adulthood nor do we have data on exogenous orienting in childhood; thus, we cannot draw firm conclusions about the general developmental trajectory of different facets of orienting among persons with DS. Nonetheless we tentatively conclude that attentional orienting does not appear to be an area of deficit among persons with DS.

Selective Attention

In addition to its orienting function, attention also serves as a filter, inhibiting or suppressing "unimportant, or extraneous" stimuli so that one can more attend to what is important in the moment. For example, attentional filtering allows us to quickly scan our bookshelves in search of a particular text or allows us to pay attention to one conversation and ignore the surrounding noise when at a cocktail party. In coordination with filtering functions of attention, searching functions allow us to scan and select relevant stimuli in our environment. For example, searching facilitates a deployment of attentional resources over space and time such that we can find a friend in a crowd of people or a particular color crayon in a crayon box. Filtering and searching go hand-in-hand and reflect selective aspects of attention.

Filtering

Auditory filtering is often measured through dichotomous listening tasks in which individuals must pay attention to information presented in one ear and ignore information presented simultaneously to the other ear. Visual filtering is usually measured through variations on the Eriksen flanker task (Eriksen & Eriksen, 1974), in which a centrally presented target (e.g., an arrow pointing left) is flanked by distractors that are either congruent (facing the same direction) or incongruent (facing the opposite direction) with the target (Fig. 11.1b). Participants must respond to the direction of the central target. On these tasks, incongruent flankers slow reaction time and accuracy relative to neutral (e.g., squares) and congruent targets (see Fig. 11.1b). For both auditory and visual filtering tasks, filtering efficiency is measured by examining the "cost" of the distracting information (e.g., the auditory stimuli in the other ear for auditory tasks and the incongruent flankers in visual tasks) on task performance.

Searching

Most studies of attentional search are conducted in the visual domain. Visual search abilities are often measured through feature or conjunctive search tasks that differ in their complexity and developmental trajectories. For example, in Fig. 11.1d, finding a red target X among black distractor Xs is easy because the target only shares one feature with the distractors and thus pops out (feature search). In contrast, when the distractors are composed of red Os and black Xs, such as in Figure 11.1d, the target, which shares features with both distractor types, is much more difficult to find (conjunctive search). In the first instance, one searches serially from item to item and adding more distractors does not really impair performance, as the target pops out regardless of the number of distractors on the screen. However, in the second instance, one must search all of the items in parallel, which is a much more arduous attentional process. In the lab, these parallel searches are slower than serial searches, and increasing the number of distractors also slows performance (e.g., Treisman & Gelade, 1980; Wolfe, 1994).

Development of Selective Attention

The ability to filter extraneous information is challenging to examine in infancy, and studies of selective attention in this age group tend to involve preferential looking paradigms (Fantz, 1964; Reynolds, 2015; Tafreshi et al., 2014). On these types of tasks, two stimuli are generally pitted against one another, and infants' increased looking time at one of these is interpreted as reflecting selective attention (e.g., Frank et al., 2009; Reynolds, 2015; Teller, 1979; Wattam-Bell, 1996). Generally, the ability to filter efficiently improves with age, such that between 4 years of age and adulthood, filtering becomes faster and more accurate (e.g., Enns & Cameron, 1987; Enns & Girgus, 1985; Pastò & Burack, 1997; Rayner et al., 1980). However, visual search and its development are slightly more complex.

Search tasks generally involve both reaction time and accuracy as measures of search efficiency. Reaction times and accuracy for both feature (single feature) and conjunctive (more than one feature) searches generally improve with age from 6 to 22 years (Trick & Enns, 1998), suggesting an overall increase of search and selective attention efficiency with development. In addition to standard reaction time and accuracy, studies of reaction times in relation to the number of distractors present provide important clues as to *how* participants search and select targets. In *feature*-based search tasks, participants across the lifespan generally perform similarly regardless of how many distractors are present (Gerhardstein & Rovee-Collier, 2002; Woods et al., 2013), suggesting, that as for adults, the addition of more distracting items for children does not impede the search for stimuli that pop out (Trick & Enns, 1998). In contrast, as for adults, the reaction times for *conjunctive* search tasks increase with the number of distractors. Further, younger children show the biggest slow-down compared to older children and adults in their search times with more distractors, indicating that the ability to use selective attention for conjunctive search tasks develops with age (Hommel et al., 2004; Thompson & Massaro, 1989). These findings are consistent with well-established evidence of typical developmental trajectories of visual search across the lifespan when tested in the lab (although see Brennan et al. 2017 for some unique developmental differences for visual search conducted in natural settings).

In sum, developmental studies of selective attention, including filtering and search, suggest that children develop better control over their ability to select what they are attending to, and exhibit greater flexibility in filtering distracting, extraneous perceptual information in service of their goals over the preschool and early elementary years (e.g., Enns & Akhtar, 1989; Tipper & McLaren, 1990). While filtering and searching are two aspects of selective attention that can be studied separately, isolating these processes is more difficult once researchers move away from the standard versions of the Eriksen filtering tasks and featural and conjunctive search tasks and toward more naturalistic tasks, as several DS researchers have done. This is a positive development and is commensurate with the direction of basic science but makes it more difficult to cleanly dissociate these two processes in our analysis, which is why the section below is referred to as selective attention. Wherever possible we distinguish which aspects of selective attention are most prevalent in each task.

Selective Attention Among Individuals With Down Syndrome

Selective Attention in Early Childhood

We found only one empirical investigation of selective attention abilities of individuals with DS in early childhood in which developmental matching strategies were used. Cornish et al. (2007) investigated visual selective attention in young children with DS (mean CA = 63 months; mean MA = 36 months), WS (mean CA = 46 months; mean MA = 29 months), and Fragile X syndrome (FXS; mean CA = 43 months; mean MA = 29 months) compared to TD individuals (mean CA = 35 months; MA range = not reported) matched by MA based on the Bayley Scales of Infant Development (BSID-II;

Bayley, 1993). The participants were required to select 10 large black target circles on a 15-inch computer touchscreen, which, when touched, would reveal a funny face. Targets were surrounded by small black distractor circles of varying amounts (between 6 and 24), depending on the trial. Because their targets and distractors differed on a key feature (size), this task requires a simple feature-based visual search. The young children with DS performed similarly to the TD children at the same developmental level in terms of search speed (mean search time between each identified target), search path (mean distance between successive touches), and different types of errors (touching distractors or re-touching already identified targets). The individuals with DS also showed a significantly faster search speed than the individuals with WS, significantly fewer distractor errors than the individuals with WS, and significantly less re-touching of already identified targets errors than the individuals with FXS. These results suggest that the selective attention mechanisms requiring visual serial search abilities of young children with DS are similar to those of TD children of the same developmental level. Moreover, selective attention may be a relative strength of young children with DS as compared to young children with other genetic syndromes such as WS and FXS. However, conclusions are tentative as they are based on a single experiment conducted with a very small sample (eight participants per clinical group).

Selective Attention in Middle Childhood and Adolescence

All of the studies of selective attention among older children and adolescents with DS have been in the visual domain. For example, Breckenridge, Braddick, & Atkinson (2013) used a simplified visual search task as a part of their Early Childhood Attention Battery (ECAB; Breckenridge, Braddick, & Atkinson, 2013). In this task, the participants were required to point out red apples (targets) among white apples and red strawberries (distractors) on a large, laminated sheet. Because the targets share features with both distractor types and are unique from those distractors only because of the conjunction of color and shape, this search task can be considered a more complex conjunctive features search task. However, it differs slightly from the classic task (e.g., Fig. 11.1d) as multiple targets were presented on each sheet (e.g., 18 targets and 162 distractors). The researchers measured search efficiency by counting how many red apples each child correctly pointed out within 1 minute and how many errors they made. The children with DS and WS whose mental ages were around 4.5, and whose chronological ages were around 9 years of age performed similarly to one another but less well than TD norms based on their mental age.

Munir et al. (2000) used a fairly naturalistic visual filtering and search task to assess the selective attention abilities of children with DS, children with FXS, and two groups of TD children characterized as having either having either "good" attention or "poor" attention on the basis of teacher ratings on the Attention Deficit Disorder with Hyperactivity Comprehensive Teacher Rating Scale (Ullmann et al., 1984). The participants were required to visually search a forest scene containing various distractors (e.g., trees) and to select targets (e.g., egg-shaped ovals) to uncover hidden "monsters" on the screen. For each trial, the time spent to find the target, the number of correct targets identified, the number of errors, and the mean distance moved between the detected targets were recorded. Significant differences between individuals with DS and both groups of TD participants were found on all of these measures, as the participants with DS spent more time on each trial, made more errors, and correctly identified fewer targets (Munir et al., 2000). Compared to the FXS group, the individuals with DS made fewer errors and identified more targets correctly, although the two groups were similar in time spent on each trial and distance moved between each identified target.

In a follow-up, Cornish et al. (2007) reported on an additional visual search task known as the map search task from the Tests of Everyday Attention for Children (TEA-Ch; Manly et al., 2001) that had been completed by these same participant groups. The map search task is very similar to the visual search task used by Munir et al. (2000) in that it is a naturalistic design that requires both filtering and search abilities. The participants are allowed 1 minute to search for and circle pairs of knives and forks on a map of Philadelphia among distractor symbols. The children and adolescents with DS correctly circled fewer target pairings than both the MA-matched TD participants and the participants with FXS, again indicating that visual selective attention abilities appear to be negatively impacted in individuals with DS. In addition, a positive correlation between CA and task performance was found for all groups, and between MA and task performance for all groups except those with DS.

Costanzo et al. (2013) used the sky search task of the TEA-Ch (Manly et al., 2001) and tested adolescents with DS (mean CA = 14.5 years; mean MA = 6.2 years), WS (mean CA = 17.6 years; mean MA = 6.7 years), and MA-matched TD participants (mean CA = 7.4 years; mean MA = 6.9 years). The sky search task is a brief, timed visual search task where participants find as many target spaceships (pairs of identical spaceships) as possible on a sheet filled with distractor spaceship pairs that share the same features as the targets but are not identical to one another. The participants with DS and WS performed similarly to one another but used significantly more time to detect and select each target than the MA-matched TD participants.

Selective Attention in Adulthood

In their study of reflexive covert orienting, Randolph and Burack (2000) also included conditions in which participants needed to ignore distractors in order to index attentional filtering. They found that reaction times were slowed when distractors were present, with no group differences in the impact of distractors on reaction times, suggesting developmentally commensurate filtering abilities. Cornish et al. (2001) assessed selective attention abilities in a more complex task that combined filtering and searching. They tested adults with DS (mean CA = 24 years) and compared them to groups of adults with FXS (mean CA = 23 years), and verbal MA-matched TD participants (mean CA = 13 years);

Cornish et al. reported no significant difference between the groups in term of verbal MA, but they do no report group means. On the map search task of the Test of Everyday Attention (TEA; Robertson et al., 1994), adults with DS found significantly fewer targets than either the persons with FXS or the TD comparison groups.

In sum, simple serial search and filtering appear to be commensurate with developmental expectations in toddlerhood. However, performance deficits are noted for more complex tasks that require participants to filter and search for conjunctive visual targets simultaneously. These challenges are noted across childhood and adolescence and persist in adulthood. Together, these findings suggest that the development of complex selective attention may plateau earlier in persons with DS than in persons with FXS or typical development, at least in the visual domain.

Sustained Attention

Sustained attention involves continued alertness or awareness and is often operationalized as the ability to detect unpredictably and rarely occurring signals over an extended period of time (Robbins, 1998). As such, sustained attentions includes aspects of vigilance, or a state of readiness for infrequent or irregular events (Parasuraman et al., 1998). From this perspective, sustained attention arises from a combination of initial awareness of environmental input and maintenance of awareness regarding the input. This facet of attention is likely familiar to clinicians, and it maps most directly onto the aspect of attention that is at the core of the ADHD diagnosis. In early childhood, the construct is assessed in play-based tasks, whereas studies of later childhood and adolescence frequently rely on vigilance tasks, in which individuals are presented with distractors while they focus on a specific area in space or look for a specific target (Burack, Dawkins, et al., 2012). This is most often accomplished using a continuous performance task (CPT; Rosvold et al., 1956; see Fig. 11.1c), for which participants are asked to respond when an infrequent target appears in a series of nontargets (Ballard, 1996; Eliason & Richman, 1987; Rosvold et al., 1956). Although most CPT paradigms present information in the visual modality, sustained attention can be further delineated into different sensory modalities, such as visual, auditory, or visual-auditory/dual. Because attentional abilities can vary according to the mode of presentation (Baddeley et al., 1986; Smith & Jonides, 1997), sustained attention should be assessed across multiple sensory modalities.

Development of Sustained Attention

Sustained attention skills improve with age in typical development. Infants' attention is fleeting but they soon learn to focus their attention on a particular person or object and can do so for longer periods of time fairly early in development, though early developmental studies are lacking. For older, school-aged children, improvement on CPT tasks, which are the most frequent measure of sustained attention, are noted between ages 5 and 18 years (Aylward et al., 2002). The ability to sustain attention in early childhood is a foundational skill that is built upon in many practical and academic settings, such as expecting young children to sustain their attention over longer and longer instructional times; thus, enhancing our understanding of whether there are sustained attention deficits beyond the global cognitive delays of children with DS is an important first step in developing interventions to support their learning. Many of the studies presented here overlap with those described in the selective attention section, as researchers often have participants complete multiple experiments that are published in different papers.

Sustained Attention Among Individuals With Down Syndrome

Sustained Attention in Early Childhood

Our understanding of sustained attention in the early years of individuals with DS is limited. Extrapolating meaning from the two available studies of sustained attention in toddlers DS is precarious, particularly given the contrasting results of the studies described below; however, this empirical gap emphasizes the importance of careful methodological considerations while investigating attention (or any other aspect of functioning) among persons with DS.

In a study of sustained attention, Krakow and Kopp (1982) found that TD toddlers (mean CA = 15 months; mean MA = 17 months) and toddlers with DS (mean CA = 29 months; mean MA = 17 months) matched on developmental level performed similarly with regards to how long they engaged with available toys. However, qualitative differences were noted between the groups: for example, the group of children with DS exhibited a more limited range of play (e.g., using the same objects in the same sequence). In contrast, Brown et al. (2003) examined sustained attention abilities in toddlers with DS (mean CA = 29 months; mean BSID-II raw score = 100.89) and WS (mean CA = 29 months; mean BSID-II raw score = 101.43) as well as TD infants and toddlers matched on developmental level (mean CA = 15 months; mean BSID-II raw score = 99.44) and CA (mean CA = 30 months; mean BSID-II raw score = 146.76). They found that the children with DS displayed significantly shorter periods of sustained attention and the fewest number of periods of sustained attention as compared to the other groups.

The findings reported by Brown et al. (2003) seem to run counter to those of Krakow and Kopp (1982), although the experimental procedures of these two studies differs noticeably. Krakow and Kopp (1982) coded play sessions for both total duration of on-task play as well as object-social orientation or social interactions with the parent, whereas Brown et al. (2003) instructed parents not to speak to their children and coded only the duration and number of periods of sustained attention. This leaves open the possibility that the engagement with, or level of interest in the toys by children with DS might have been differentially impacted by a lack of social feedback from either the caregiver or the experimenter. This is consistent with evidence from studies of joint attention and infant toy exploration that infants with DS are less likely to manipulate toys in general, but that mothers of 6-month-old infants with DS were able to enhance their infants' ability to attend to toys by directing the child's attention (Landry & Chapieski, 1989). Parents and caregivers may scaffold the performance of the infant and improve the way that infants deploy their attention (Bakeman & Adamson, 1984; Lawson et al., 1992; Mendive et al., 2013).

As with all aspects of attention, future research examining sustained attention in young children with DS should consider the role of external motivating factors, particularly social factors, that may impact the performance of children with DS (e.g., Zigler & Balla, 1977). Thus, differences in sustained attention during infancy may be attenuated by the use of naturalistic or ecologically relevant experimental procedures. If shown to be influential, increasing opportunities for parental maintenance of their children's attention may provide an important avenue for intervention that could have cascading effects on attention, exploration, and ultimately cognitive and social function of infants and toddlers with DS.

Sustained Attention in Middle Childhood and Adolescence–Visual

In contrast to early childhood, sustained attention in individuals with DS in middle childhood and adolescence is well studied and has yielded consistent findings. In the visual modality, across multiple studies and paradigms, children and young adolescents with DS perform similarly to their MA-matched peers on measures of visual sustained attention. For example, Breckenridge, Braddick, Anker, et al. (2013) used a CPT-type paradigm to examine visual sustained attention in a group of children with DS (mean CA = 9.76 years; mean MA = 4.51 years) and WS (mean CA = 8.45 years; mean MA = 4.89 years). The participants were presented with a continuous stream of pictures and were asked to verbally report when any of five target animals appeared. As a group, the children with DS achieved scores on this task that were comparable to those of the WS group and were consistent with developmental level expectations from available norms, providing evidence that visual sustained attention abilities are developmentally on par among individuals with DS. These findings are supported by other studies (e.g., Cornish et al., 2007; Munir et al., 2000) with slightly older individuals.

Employing a spatially focused sustained attention task, Brodeur et al. (2013) investigated the ability of children and adolescents with DS to maintain their attention as they identified targets among distractors on a single image. When the targets were hidden among distractors in a single spatial array, the group of children and adolescents with DS (mean CA = 15.12 years; mean MA = 5.4 years) performed similarly to a group of MA-matched TD children (mean CA = 5.21 years; mean MA = 5.54 years). The groups performed comparably when they were required to identify targets immediately after being shown their locations as well as after a 10-second delay; however, when the task became more complicated and relied on additional cognitive mechanisms that include working memory and executive functioning (both of which have been shown to be an area of relative weakness among individuals with DS relative to their developmental level), the performance of those with DS was poorer than that of the TD children. Thus, the findings from the baseline task, which is a more direct measure of sustained attention than the complex task, provides further evidence of typical visual sustained attention development in DS.

Costanzo et al. (2013) also examined the visual sustained attention abilities in children and adolescents with DS (mean CA = 14.5 years; mean MA = 6.2 years) by comparing their performance to groups of participants with WS (mean CA = 17.6 years; mean MA = 6.7 years) and TD participants (mean CA = 7.4 years; mean MA = 6.9 years) matched on mental age. Visual sustained attention was assessed using the Bells Test (BELLS; Gauthier et al., 1989), which consists of an array of seven columns each containing 5 targets and 40 distractors. The participants were required to sustain their attention on the array while they crossed out each target bell and ignored all other shapes. The group of adolescents with DS scored significantly lower than the group of adolescents with WS but both groups performed similarly to the TD group on this task (i.e., DS < WS; DS = TD; TD = WS). Although this pattern of performance leaves open questions related to differences between those with DS and those with WS, the comparable performance of the DS group to the MA-matched TD participants supports the conclusion of developmentally appropriate visual sustained attention abilities among individuals with DS.

Using a standard CPT task, Shalev et al. (2019) measured sensitivity (which considers both hit rates and false alarms together; Stanislaw & Todorov, 1999) as well as the time course of attentional vigilance by examining how performance changed during the task. Matching was based on verbal mental age (VMA) and performance mental age (PMA). They tested 18 children with DS (mean CA = 7.1 years, mean VMA = 3.5 years; mean PMA = 3.3 years) and compared their performance to 25 children with WS (mean CA = 6.6, mean VMA = 5.25; mean PMA = 3.2 years) of the same PMA and 31 TD children matched on the basis of VMA and PMA. The authors found that individuals with DS performed similarly to MA-matched TD children in their sensitivity to the task and that their pattern of performance over time was similar to the TD group (improved performance over the second half of the task) and better than the participants with WS.

Sustained Attention in Middle Childhood and Adolescence—Auditory

In addition to studying visual sustained attention, Costanzo et al. (2013) also evaluated the auditory sustained attention abilities of the same groups of participants. Auditory sustained attention was assessed using the Score! task of the TEA-Ch (Manly et al., 2001). The Score! task is a 10-trial tone-counting measure in which between 9 and 15 identical tones are presented and participants are asked to silently count the tones and report the total at the end. In contrast to the comparable visual sustained attention task, the children with DS scored significantly lower than the TD children on the Score! task of auditory sustained attention, suggesting that auditory sustained attention skills were weaker than what would be expected given their MA.

In contrast, on the auditory sustained attention subtest on the ECAB, Breckenridge, Braddick, & Atkinson (2013) found that children with DS performed better than what would be expected given their developmental level as well as higher than the children with WS. The auditory sustained attention subtest of the ECAB required participants to listen to a stream of words and identify target words (animals) amongst distractors (familiar items). The discrepant findings between the Costanzo et al. (2013) and Breckenridge, Braddick, Anker, et al. (2013) studies are likely due to the differing nature of their experimental tasks. Costanzo et al. (2013) required participants both to sustain their attention and to remember and update information at the same time. In contrast, the auditory sustained attention task of the ECAB did not require additional cognitive mechanisms such as working memory and executive functioning.

Sustained Attention in Adulthood

We found only one study on the sustained attention abilities among adults with DS. In that study, Cornish et al. (2001) used the elevator counting task to compare auditory sustained attention between groups of adults with FXS (mean CA = 23 years), adults with DS (mean CA = 24 years), and verbal MA-matched TD participants (mean CA = 13 years). No significant differences were found between the groups in term of verbal MA but no group means were reported. In the elevator counting task, the participants were asked to imagine that they were riding up an elevator and silently count a series of monotones to determine what floor they are on (Robertson et al., 1996). The adults with DS and FXS both exhibited performance significantly below that of the MA-matched comparison group (Cornish et al., 2001). However, similar to Costanzo et al. (2013), the elevator counting task requires additional working memory skills above and beyond sustained attention abilities.

In sum, across a range of researchers and paradigms, the body of evidence suggests that visual sustained attention skills in individuals with DS are typical in the context of their general cognitive development. However, sustaining one's attention in the auditory domain appears to be more challenging among persons with DS, as it is in TD, especially when additional cognitive components such as working memory are necessary for successful task completion.

Conclusion

The literature on the development of attention in individuals with DS reflects both the heterogeneity of attention abilities within the population as well as the heterogeneity in the methods, procedures, and participants in the studies. Though the nature of the experimental tasks are disparate, and despite the challenges described above, some general conclusions about the development of attention among persons with DS may be gleaned from the extant literature. One, individuals with DS appear to orient to visual stimuli in their environment similarly to their TD counterparts. Two, selective visual attention appears to be impacted in individuals with DS relative to their cognitive developmental level. Evidence from studies of children, adolescents, and adults indicates that, as compared to MA-matched comparison groups, individuals with DS show deficits in visual selective attention. Three, visual sustained attention in individuals with DS is comparable to MA-matched comparison participants on several tasks, but auditory sustained attention may be more challenging. Four, while performance on simple tasks appears to be commensurate with developmental expectations across multiple facets of attention, performance challenges arise with the addition of complexity or the need for coordination between attention and other cognitive processes such as working memory or executive function.

Reviewing the literature on the development of attention among individuals with DS reveals many avenues for future research to pursue. A quick glance at Tables 11.1 and 11.2 makes it strikingly clear that much of the research to date has focused on the attentional abilities of older children and adolescents with DS, and there is significantly less research on attentional functioning in early childhood and adulthood. Further, the majority of studies have been primarily focused on visual attention, with far fewer studies examining attentional functioning in the auditory domain.

Though more research may be helpful, simply *more* research is not a viable solution for understanding the real-world implications of attention development among individuals with DS. Rather, researchers should continue to strive toward developing paradigms that inform and guide practical solutions to support individuals with DS in achieving their goals. For example, the knowledge that young children with DS appear to demonstrate significantly better sustained attention skills when they are provided with social scaffolding can directly inform and motivate the need for increased one-on-one assistance for young students with DS. In the future, researchers should explore how long these social supports continue to benefit individuals with DS over the lifespan and whether they are more helpful in some facets of attention than others (e.g., more helpful in increasing sustained attention than in improving selective attention).

Research with individuals with DS that is based in more contemporary conceptualizations of attention, and in which the complexity and dynamic nature of attention are addressed, will help to capture more nuanced and comprehensive understanding of the development of attention among persons with DS. For example, researchers examining visual attention among individuals with DS may benefit from the use of naturalistic paradigms such as detecting stop signs in a driving simulation or finding price tag labels on a crowded grocery store shelf. These efforts may both reveal moderators of visual attention abilities in individuals with DS (e.g., Clark et al., 2021) and more directly inform interventions which target real-world adaptive skills. In addition to embracing the complexity of attention per se, future research endeavors should consider embracing the complexity of cognition. Attention is rarely used in isolation and needs to be coordinated with higher-order processes that include memory and executive function for adaptation. Understanding the coordination and interaction of these different components is critical to moving beyond an understanding of not only how attention develops in DS, but also how individuals with DS use their attention in service of their daily life.

Finally, the evidence highlights the importance of considering developmental level when assessing attentional functioning. This consideration is becoming increasingly standard in the domains of cognitive development research (through the use of MA matching and developmental growth curves), and it will continue to be relevant for the clinical understanding of the profile of attentional strengths and weaknesses in individuals with DS, particularly with regards to education, ADHD diagnoses, and medication considerations. Based on the literature reviewed here, sustained attention among persons with DS develops at a pace commensurate with their global development. This suggests that interventions should not necessarily target sustained attention abilities of individuals with DS, though individual differences can and should dictate individualized intervention plans. In contrast to sustained attention, selective attention is the facet of attention that most consistently functions below developmental-level expectations for individuals with DS. This highlights a clear direction for future intervention work that can be tailored uniquely for individuals with DS. Thus, clinical intervention work that seeks to make meaningful impacts to support skill development among individuals with DS will benefit from specifically targeting skills including filtering, searching, and selecting relevant stimuli in the environment (e.g., Tullo et al., 2018).

References

American Psychiatric Association. (2013). *Diagnostic and statistical manual of mental disorders* (5th ed.). https://doi.org/10.1176/appi.books.9780890425596.744053

Ansari, D., Lyons, I. M., Van Eimeren, L., & Xu, F. (2007). Linking visual attention and number processing in the brain: The role of the temporo-parietal junction in small and large symbolic and nonsymbolic number comparison. *Journal of Cognitive Neuroscience, 19*(11), 1845–1853. https://doi.org/10.1162/jocn.2007.19.11.1845

Aylward, G. P., Brager, P., & Harper, D. C. (2002). Relations between visual and auditory continuous performance tests in a clinical population: A descriptive study. *Developmental Neuropsychology, 21*(3), 285–303. https://doi.org/10.1207/S15326942DN2103_5

Baddeley, A., Logie, R., Bressi, S., Sala, S. Della, & Spinnler, H. (1986). Dementia and working memory. *Quarterly Journal of Experimental Psychology Section A, 38*(4), 603–618. https://doi.org/10.1080/14640748608401616

Bakeman, R., & Adamson, L. B. (1984). Coordinating attention to people and objects in mother-infant and peer-infant interaction. *Child Development, 55*(4), 1278–1289. https://doi.org/10.2307/1129997

Ballard, J. C. (1996). Computerized assessment of sustained attention: A review of factors affecting vigilance performance. *Journal of Clinical and Experimental Neuropsychology, 18*(6), 843–863. https://doi.org/10.1080/01688639608408307

Bayley, N. (1993). *Bayley scales of infant development* (2nd ed.). Pearson Education, Inc.

Beck, D. M., & Kastner, S. (2009). Top-down and bottom-up mechanisms in biasing competition in the human brain. *Vision Research, 49*(10), 1154–1165. https://doi.org/10.1016/j.visres.2008.07.012

Birmingham, E., & Kingstone, A. (2009). Human social attention. *Progress in Brain Research, 176*, 309–320. https://doi.org/10.1016/S0079-6123(09)17618-5

Breckenridge, K., Braddick, O., Anker, S., Woodhouse, M., & Atkinson, J. (2013). Attention in Williams syndrome and Down's syndrome: Performance on the new early childhood attention battery. *British Journal of Developmental Psychology, 31*(2), 257–269. https://doi.org/10.1111/bjdp.12003

Breckenridge, K., Braddick, O., & Atkinson, J. (2013). The organization of attention in typical development: A new preschool attention test battery. *British Journal of Developmental Psychology, 31*(3), 271–288. https://doi.org/10.1111/bjdp.12004

Brennan, A. A., Bruderer, A. J., Liu-Ambrose, T., Handy, T. C., & Enns, J. T. (2017). Lifespan changes in attention revisited: Everyday visual search. *Canadian Journal of Experimental Psychology/Revue Canadienne de Psychologie Expérimentale, 71*(2), 160. https://doi.org/10.1037/cep0000130

Brodeur, D. A., Trick, L. M., Flores, H., Marr, C., & Burack, J. A. (2013). Multiple-object tracking among individuals with Down syndrome and typically developing children. *Development and Psychopathology, 25*(2), 545–553. https://doi.org/10.1017/S095457941200123X

Brown, J. H., Johnson, M. H., Paterson, S. J., Gilmore, R., Longhi, E., & Karmiloff-Smith, A. (2003). Spatial representation and attention in toddlers with Williams syndrome and Down syndrome. *Neuropsychologia, 41*, 1037–1046. https://doi.org/10.1016/S0028-3932(02)00299-3

Burack, J. A., Dawkins, T., Stewart, J., Iarocci, G., & Russo, N. (2012). "The mysterious myth of attention deficit . . ." revisited: A discussion of how the developmental approach is transforming the understanding of intellectual disability. *International Review of Research in Developmental Disabilities, 42*, 147–177. https://doi.org/10.1016/B978-0-12-394284-5.00006-1

Burack, J. A., Iarocci, G., Flanagan, T. D., & Bowler, D. M. (2004). On mosaics and melting pots: Conceptual considerations of comparison and matching strategies. *Journal of Autism and Developmental Disorders, 34*(1), 65–73. https://doi.org/10.1023/b:jadd.0000018076.90715.00

Burack, J. A., Jefferies, L. N., Ringo, J., & Landry, O. (2017). Attention. In B. Hopkins, E. Geangu, & S. Linkenauger (Eds.), *The Cambridge encyclopedia of child development* (pp. 259–265). Cambridge University Press. https://doi.org/https://doi.org/10.1017/9781316216491.045

Burack, J. A., Russo, N., Flores, H., Iarocci, G., & Zigler, E. (2012). The more you know the less you know, but that's OK: Developments in the developmental approach to intellectual disability. In J. A. Burack, R. M. Hodapp, G. Iarocci, & E. Zigler (Eds.), *The Oxford handbook of intellectual disability and development* (pp. 1–15). Oxford University Press. https://doi.org/10.1093/oxfordhb/9780195305012.013.0001

Burack, J. A., Russo, N., Green, C. G., Landry, O., & Iarocci, G. (2016). Developments in the developmental approach to intellectual disability. In D. Cicchetti (Ed.), *Developmental psychopathology* (pp. 1–67). Wiley. https://doi.org/10.1002/9781119125556.devpsy301

Burack, J. (2016). How the developmental approach transformed the study of cognition and the science of intellectual disability. *Journal of Intellectual Disability Research, 60*(7–8), 784–791.

Burack, J. A., Evans, D. W., Russo, N., Napoleon, J. S., Goldman, K. J., & Iarocci, G. (2021). Developmental perspectives on the study of persons with intellectual disability. *Annual Review of Clinical Psychology, 17*, 339–363.

Buschman, T. J., & Kastner, S. (2015). From behavior to neural dynamics: An integrated theory of attention. *Neuron, 88*(1), 127–144. https://doi.org/10.1016/j.neuron.2015.09.017

Capone, G., Goyal, P., Ares, W., & Lannigan, E. (2006). Neurobehavioral disorders in children, adolescents, and young adults with Down syndrome. *American Journal of Medical Genetics. Part C, Seminars in Medical Genetics, 142C*, 158–172. https://doi.org/10.1002/ajmg.c

Channell, M. M., Thurman, A. J., Kover, S. T., & Abbeduto, L. (2014). Patterns of change in nonverbal cognition in adolescents with Down syndrome. *Research in Developmental Disabilities, 35*(11), 2933–2941. https://doi.org/10.1016/j.ridd.2014.07.014

Cicchetti, D, Pogge-Hesse, P., Zigler, E., & Balla, D. (1982). *Mental retardation: The developmental-difference controversy*. Routledge.

Cicchetti, Dante. (1984). The emergence of developmental psychopathology. *Child Development, 44*(1), 1–7. https://doi.org/10.2307/1129830

Clark, E., Tullo, D., & Bertone, A. (2021). Perceptual reasoning skills mediate the relationship between attention and math proficiency in individuals with a neurodevelopmental condition. *Research in Developmental Disabilities, 111*, 103880. https://doi.org/10.1016/j.ridd.2021.103880

Corbetta, M., & Shulman, G. L. (2002). Control of goal-directed and stimulus-driven attention in the brain. *Nature Reviews Neuroscience, 3*(3), 201–215. https://doi.org/10.1038/nrn755

Cornish, K. M., Munir, F., & Cross, G. (2001). Differential impact of the FMR-1 full mutation on memory and attention functioning: A neuropsychological perspective. *Journal of Cognitive Neuroscience, 13*(1), 144–150. https://doi.org/10.1162/089892901564126

Cornish, K., Scerif, G., & Karmiloff-Smith, A. (2007). Tracing syndrome-specific trajectories of attention across the lifespan. *Cortex, 43*, 672–685. https://doi.org/10.1016/S0010-9452(08)70497-0

Costanzo, F., Varuzza, C., Menghini, D., Addona, F., Gianesini, T., & Vicari, S. (2013). Executive functions in intellectual disabilities: A comparison between Williams syndrome and Down syndrome. *Research in Developmental Disabilities, 34*(5), 1770–1780. https://doi.org/10.1016/j.ridd.2013.01.024

Dayan, P., Kakade, S., & Montague, P. R. (2000). Learning and selective attention. *Nature Neuroscience, 3*, 1218–1223. https://doi.org/10.1038/81504

DeCasper, A. J., & Fifer, W. P. (1980). Of human bonding: Newborns prefer their mothers' voices. *Science, 208*(4448), 1174–1176. https://doi.org/10.1126/science.7375928

del Hoyo Soriano, L., Rosser, T., Hamilton, D., Wood, T., Abbeduto, L., & Sherman, S. (2020). Gestational age is related to symptoms of attention-deficit/hyperactivity disorder in late-preterm to full-term children and adolescents with Down syndrome. *Scientific Reports, 10*(1), 1–10. https://doi.org/10.1038/s41598-020-77392-5

Duncan, S., & Barrett, L. F. (2007). Affect is a form of cognition: A neurobiological analysis. *Cognition and Emotion, 21*(6), 1184–1211. https://doi.org/10.1080/02699930701437931

Ekstein, S., Glick, B., Weill, M., Kay, B., & Berger, I. (2011). Down syndrome and attention-deficit/hyperactivity disorder (ADHD). *Journal of Child Neurology, 26*(10), 1290–1295. https://doi.org/10.1177/0883073811405201

Eliason, M. J., & Richman, L. C. (1987). The Continuous Performance Test in learning disabled and nondisabled children. *Journal of Learning Disabilities, 20*(10), 614–619. https://doi.org/10.1177/002221948702001007

Enns, J. T. (1993). What can be learned about attention from studying its development? *Canadian Psychology, 34*(3), 271–281. https://doi.org/10.1037/h0078830

Enns, J. T., & Akhtar, N. (1989). A developmental study of filtering in visual attention. *Child Development*, 1188–1199. https://doi.org/10.2307/1130792

Enns, J. T., & Brodeur, D. A. (1989). A developmental study of covert orienting to peripheral visual cues. *Journal of Experimental Child Psychology, 48*(2), 171–189.

Enns, J. T., & Cameron, S. (1987). Selective attention in young children: The relations between visual search, filtering, and priming. *Journal of Experimental Child Psychology, 44*(1), 38–63. https://doi.org/10.1016/0022-0965(87)90021-x

Enns, J. T., & Girgus, J. S. (1985). Developmental changes in selective and integrative visual attention. *Journal of Experimental Child Psychology, 40*(2), 319–337. https://doi.org/10.1016/0022-0965(85)90093-1

Eriksen, B. A., & Eriksen, C. W. (1974). Effects of noise letters upon the identification of a target letter in a nonsearch task. *Perception & Psychophysics, 16*(1), 143–149. https://doi.org/10.3758/bf03203267

Fairhall, S. L., Indovina, I., Driver, J., & Macaluso, E. (2009). The brain network underlying serial visual search: Comparing overt and covert spatial orienting, for activations and for effective connectivity. *Cerebral Cortex, 19*(12), 2946–2958. https://doi.org/10.1093/cercor/bhp064

Fantz, R. L. (1964). Visual experience in infants: Decreased attention to familiar patterns relative to novel ones. *Science, 146*(3644), 668–670. https://doi.org/10.1126/science.146.3644.668

Farroni, T., Johnson, M. H., Brockbank, M., & Simion, F. (2000). Infants' use of gaze direction to cue attention: The importance of perceived motion. *Visual Cognition, 7*(6), 705–718. https://doi.org/10.1080/135062800501443 99

Fiebelkorn, I. C., & Kastner, S. (2020). Functional specialization in the attention network. *Annual Review of Psychology, 71*, 221–249. https://doi.org/10.1146/annurev-psych-010418-103429

Fiebelkorn, I. C., Pinsk, M. A., & Kastner, S. (2018). A dynamic interplay within the frontoparietal network underlies rhythmic spatial attention. *Neuron, 99*(4), 842–853. https://doi.org/10.1016/j.neuron.2018.07.038

Fiebelkorn, I. C., Saalmann, Y. B., & Kastner, S. (2013). Rhythmic sampling within and between objects despite sustained attention at a cued location. *Current Biology, 23*(24), 2553–2558. https://doi.org/10.1016/j.cub.2013.10.063

Fiebelkorn, I. C., Snyder, A. C., Mercier, M. R., Butler, J. S., Molholm, S., & Foxe, J. J. (2013). Cortical cross-frequency coupling predicts perceptual outcomes. *Neuroimage, 69*, 126–137. https://doi.org/10.1016/j.neuroimage.2012.11.021

Flanagan, T., Russo, N., Flores, H., & Burack, J. A. (2008). The developmental approach to the study of down syndrome: Contemporary issues in historical perspective. *Down Syndrome Research and Practice, 12*, 96–100.

Frank, M. C., Vul, E., & Johnson, S. P. (2009). Development of infants' attention to faces during the first year. *Cognition, 110*(2), 160–170. https://doi.org/10.1016/j.cognition.2008.11.010

Fulcher, E. P., Mathews, A., & Hammerl, M. (2008). Rapid acquisition of emotional information and attentional bias in anxious children. *Journal of Behavior Therapy and Experimental Psychiatry, 39*(3), 321–339. https://doi.org/10.1016/j.jbtep.2007.08.003

Gath, A., & Gumley, D. (1986). Behaviour problems in retarded children with special reference to Down's syndrome. *British Journal of Psychiatry, 149*, 156–161. https://doi.org/10.1192/bjp.149.2.156

Gauthier, L., Dehaut, F., & Joanette, Y. (1989). The Bells Test: A quantitative and qualitative test for visual neglect. *International Journal of Clinical Neuropsychology, 11*, 49–54.

Gavrilov, Y., Rotem, S., Ofek, R., & Geva, R. (2012). Socio-cultural effects on children's initiation of joint attention. *Frontiers in Human Neuroscience, 6*, 286. https://doi.org/10.3389/fnhum.2012.00286

Gerhardstein, P., & Rovee-Collier, C. (2002). The development of visual search in infants and very young children. *Journal of Experimental Child Psychology, 81*(2), 194–215. https://doi.org/10.1006/jecp.2001.2649

Goldman, K. J., Flanagan, T., Shulman, C., Enns, J. T., & Burack, J. A. (2005). Voluntary orienting among children and adolescents with Down syndrome and MA-matched typically developing children. *American Journal on Mental Retardation, 110*(3), 157–163. https://doi.org/10.1352/0895-8017(2005)110<157:VOACAA>2.0.CO;2

Grieco, J., Pulsifer, M., Seligsohn, K., Skotko, B., & Schwartz, A. (2015). Down syndrome: Cognitive and behavioral functioning across the lifespan. *American Journal of Medical Genetics. Part C, Seminars in Medical Genetics, 169*(2), 135–149. https://doi.org/10.1002/ajmg.c.31439

Hodapp, R. M., Burack, J. A., & Zigler, E. F. (1990). *The developmental perspective in the field of mental retardation.* Cambridge University Press. https://doi.org/10.1017/cbo9780511582325.002

Hodapp, R. M., & Zigler, E. (1995). Past, present, and future issues in the developmental approach to mental retardation and developmental disabilities. *Developmental Psychopathology, 2*, 299–331.

Hoehl, S., Wiese, L., & Striano, T. (2008). Young infants' neural processing of objects is affected by eye gaze direction and emotional expression. *PLoS One, 3*(6), e2389. https://doi.org/10.1371/journal.pone.0002389

Hommel, B., Li, K. Z. H., & Li, S.-C. (2004). Visual search across the life span. *Developmental Psychology, 40*(4), 545. https://doi.org/10.1037/0012-1649.40.4.545

Hood, B. M., Willen, J. D., & Driver, J. (1998b). Adult's eyes trigger shifts of visual attention in human infants. *Psychological Science, 9*(2), 131–134. https://doi.org/10.1016/s0163-6383(98)91679-4

James, W. (1890) *Principles of Psychology*. Henry Holt and Company.

Jaswal, V. K., Akhtar, N., & Burack, J. A. (2016). *Building bridges: Cognitive development in typical and atypical populations*. Taylor & Francis. https://doi.org/10.1080/15248372.2016.1199633

Johnson, M. H., Posner, M. I., & Rothbart, M. K. (1991). Components of visual orienting in early infancy: Contingency learning, anticipatory looking, and disengaging. *Journal of Cognitive Neuroscience, 3*(4), 335–344. https://doi.org/10.1162/jocn.1991.3.4.335

Kisilevsky, B. S., Hains, S. M. J., Lee, K., Xie, X., Huang, H., Ye, H. H., Zhang, K., & Wang, Z. (2003). Effects of experience on fetal voice recognition. *Psychological Science, 14*(3), 220–224. https://doi.org/10.1111/1467-9280.02435

Krakow, J. B., & Kopp, C. B. (1982). Sustained attention in young Down syndrome children. *Topics in Early Childhood Special Education, 2*(2), 32–42. https://doi.org/10.1177/027112148200200208

Lanfranchi, S., Jerman, O., Dal Pont, E., Alberti, A., & Vianello, R. (2010). Executive function in adolescents with Down syndrome. *Journal of Intellectual Disability Research, 54*(4), 308–319.

Landry, S. H., & Chapieski, M. L. (1989). Joint attention and infant toy exploration: Effects of Down syndrome and prematurity. *Child Development, 60*(1), 103–118. https://doi.org/10.2307/1131076

Lane, K., Stewart, J., Fernandes, T., Russo, N., Enns, J. T., & Burack, J. A. (2014). Complexities in understanding attentional functioning among children with fetal alcohol spectrum disorder. *Frontiers in Human Neuroscience, 8*, 119. https://doi.org/10.3389/fnhum.2014.00119

Lawson, K. R., Parrinello, R., & Ruff, H. A. (1992). Maternal behavior and infant attention. *Infant Behavior and Development, 15*(2), 209–229. https://doi.org/10.1016/0163-6383(92)80024-O

Leclercq, V., & Siéroff, E. (2013). Development of endogenous orienting of attention in school-age children. *Child Neuropsychology, 19*(4), 400–419. https://doi.org/10.1080/09297049.2012.682568

LoBue, V. (2009). More than just another face in the crowd: Superior detection of threatening facial expressions in children and adults. *Developmental Science, 12*(2), 305–313. https://doi.org/10.1111/j.1467-7687.2008.00767.x

Määttä, T., Tervo-Määttä, T., Taanila, A., Kaski, M., & Iivanainen, M. (2006). Mental health, behaviour and intellectual abilities of people with Down syndrome. *Down Syndrome Research and Practice, 11*(1), 37–43. https://doi.org/10.3104/reports.313

Manly, T., Anderson, V., Nimmo-Smith, I., Turner, A., Watson, P., & Robertson, I. H. (2001). The differential assessment of children's attention: The Test of Everyday Attention for Children (TEA-Ch), normative sample and ADHD performance. *Journal of Child Psychology and Psychiatry, 42*(8), 1065–1081. https://doi.org/10.1111/1469-7610.00806

McDonald, J. J., Teder-SaÈlejaÈrvi, W. A., & Hillyard, S. A. (2000). Involuntary orienting to sound improves visual perception. *Nature, 407*(6806), 906–908. https://doi.org/10.1038/35038085

Mendive, S., Bornstein, M. H., & Sebastián, C. (2013). The role of maternal attention-directing strategies in 9-month-old infants attaining joint engagement. *Infant Behavior and Development, 36*(1), 115–123. https://doi.org/10.1016/j.infbeh.2012.10.002

Mervis, C. B., Robinson, B. F., Bertrand, J., Morris, C. A., Klein-Tasman, B. P., & Armstrong, S. C. (2000). The Williams syndrome cognitive profile. *Brain and Cognition, 44*(3), 604–628. https://doi.org/10.1006/brcg.2000.1232

Mirsky, A. F., Anthony, B. J., Duncan, C. C., Ahearn, M. B., & Kellam, S. G. (1991). Analysis of the elements of attention: A neuropsychological approach. *Neuropsychology Review, 2*(2), 109–145. https://doi.org/10.1007/bf01109051

Munir, F., Cornish, K. M., & Wilding, J. (2000). A neuropsychological profile of attention deficits in young males with fragile X syndrome. *Neuropsychologia, 38*(9), 1261–1270. https://doi.org/10.1016/S0028-3932(00)00036-1

Myers, B. A., & Pueschel, S. M. (1991). Psychiatric disorders in persons with Down syndrome. *Journal of Nervous and Mental Disease, 179*(10), 609–613. https://doi.org/10.1097/00005053-199110000-00004

Oxelgren, U. W., Myrelid, Å., Annerén, G., Ekstam, B., Göransson, C., Holmbom, A., Isaksson, A., Åberg, M., Gustafsson, J., & Fernell, E. (2017). Prevalence of autism and attention-deficit–hyperactivity disorder in Down syndrome: A population-based study. *Developmental Medicine & Child Neurology, 59*(3), 276–283. https://doi.org/10.1111/dmcn.13217

Parasuraman, R., Warm, J. S., & See, J. E. (1998). Brain systems of vigilance. In R. Parasuraman (Ed.), *The attentive brain* (pp. 221–256). MIT Press.

Pastò, L., & Burack, J. A. (1997). A developmental study of visual attention: Issues of filtering efficiency and focus. *Cognitive Development, 12*(4), 523–535. https://doi.org/10.1016/S0885-2014(97)90021-6

Petersen, S. E., & Posner, M. I. (2012). The attention system of the human brain: 20 years after. *Annual Review of Neuroscience, 35*, 73–89. https://doi.org/10.1146/annurev-neuro-062111-150525

Plebanek, D. J., & Sloutsky, V. M. (2019). Selective attention, filtering, and the development of working memory. *Developmental Science, 22*(1), e12727. https://doi.org/10.1111/desc.12727

Porter, R., & Winberg, J. (1999). Unique salience of maternal breast odors for newborn infants. *Neuroscience & Biobehavioral Reviews, 23*(3), 439–449. https://doi.org/10.1016/S0149-7634(98)00044-X

Posner, M. I., & Petersen, S. E. (1990). The attention system of the human brain. *Annual Review of Neuroscience, 13*, 25–42. https://doi.org/10.1146/annurev.ne.13.030190.000325

Posner, M. I., Petersen, S. E., Fox, P. T., & Raichle, M. E. (1988). Localization of operations in the human brain. *Science, 240*(4859), 1627–1631.

Randolph, B., & Burack, J. A. (2000). Visual filtering and covert orienting in persons with Down syndrome. *International Journal of Behavioral Development, 24*(2), 167–172. https://doi.org/10.1080/016502500383287

Rayner, K., Well, A. D., & Pollatsek, A. (1980). Asymmetry of the effective visual field in reading. *Perception & Psychophysics, 27*(6), 537–544. https://doi.org/10.3758/bf03198682

Reece, C., Ebstein, R., Cheng, X., Ng, T., & Schirmer, A. (2016). Maternal touch predicts social orienting in young children. *Cognitive Development, 39*, 128–140. https://doi.org/10.1016/j.cogdev.2016.05.001

Reynolds, G. D. (2015). Infant visual attention and object recognition. *Behavioural Brain Research, 285*, 34–43. https://doi.org/10.1016/j.bbr.2015.01.015

Reynolds, J. H., & Desimone, R. (2003). Interacting roles of attention and visual salience in V4. *Neuron, 37*(5), 853–863. https://doi.org/10.1016/S0896-6273(03)00097-7

Richards, J. E. (2001). Attention in young infants: A developmental psychophysiological perspective. *Handbook of Developmental Cognitive Neuroscience, 2*, 479–497. https://doi.org/10.7551/mitpress/7437.003.0036

Ristic, J., & Enns, J. T. (2015). The changing face of attentional development. *Current Directions in Psychological Science, 24*(1), 24–31. https://doi.org/10.1177/0963721414551165

Ristic, J., & Kingstone, A. (2009). Rethinking attentional development: Reflexive and volitional orienting in children and adults. *Developmental Science, 12*(2), 289–296. https://doi.org/10.1111/j.1467-7687.2008.00756.x

Robbins, T. W. (1998). Arousal and attention: Psychopharmacological and neuropsychological studies in experimental animals. In R. Parasuraman (Ed.), *The attentive brain* (pp. 189–220). MIT Press.

Robertson, I. H., Ward, T., Ridgeway, V., & Nimmo-Smith, I. (1996). The structure of normal human attention: The Test of Everyday Attention. *Journal of the International Neuropsychological Society, 2*(6), 525–534. https://doi.org/10.1017/S1355617700001697

Robertson, I. H., Ward, T., Ridgeway, V., Nimmo-Smith, I., & Company, T. V. T. (1994). *The test of everyday attention.* Pearson Assessment.

Roid, G. H., & Miller, L. J. (1997). Leiter international performance scale–revised (Leiter-R). Stoelting.

Rosvold, H. E., Mirsky, A. F., Sarason, I., Bransome, Jr., E. D., & Beck, L. H. (1956). A continuous performance test of brain damage. *Journal of Consulting Psychology, 20*(5), 343. https://doi.org/10.1037/h0043220

Russo, N., Kaplan-Kahn, E. A., Wilson, J., Criss, A., & Burack, J. A. (2021). Choices, challenges, and constraints: a pragmatic examination of the limits of mental age matching in empirical research. *Development and Psychopathology, 33*(2), 727–738.

Shalev, N., Steele, A., Nobre, A. C., Karmiloff-Smith, A., Cornish, K., & Scerif, G. (2019). Dynamic sustained attention markers differentiate atypical development: The case of Williams syndrome and Down's syndrome. *Neuropsychologia, 132*, 107–148.

Shaywitz, B. A., Shaywitz, S. E., Pugh, K. R., Fulbright, R. K., Skudlarski, P., Mencl, W. E., Constable, R. T., Marchione, K. E., Fletcher, J. M., Klorman, R., Lacadie, C., & Gore, J. C. (2001). The functional neural architecture of components of attention in language-processing tasks. *Neuroimage, 13*(4), 601–612. https://doi.org/10.1006/nimg.2000.0726

Smith, E. E., & Jonides, J. (1997). Working memory: A view from neuroimaging. *Cognitive Psychology, 33*(1), 5–42. https://doi.org/10.1006/cogp.1997.0658

Spence, C., Nicholls, M. E. R., Gillespie, N., & Driver, J. (1998). Cross-modal links in exogenous covert spatial orienting between touch, audition, and vision. *Perception & Psychophysics, 60*(4), 544–557. https://doi.org/10.3758/bf03206045

Stanislaw, H., & Todorov, N. (1999). Calculation of signal detection theory measures. *Behavior Research Methods, Instruments, & Computers, 31*(1), 137–149. https://doi.org/10.3758/bf03207704

Steele, A., Karmiloff-Smith, A., Cornish, K., & Scerif, G. (2012). The multiple subfunctions of attention: Differential developmental gateways to literacy and numeracy. *Child Development, 83*(6), 2028–2041. https://doi.org/10.1111/j.1467-8624.2012.01809.x

Tafreshi, D., Thompson, J. J., & Racine, T. P. (2014). An analysis of the conceptual foundations of the infant preferential looking paradigm. *Human Development, 57*(4), 222–240. https://doi.org/10.1159/000363487

Teller, D. Y. (1979). The forced-choice preferential looking procedure: A psychophysical technique for use with human infants. *Infant Behavior and Development, 2*, 135–153. https://doi.org/10.1016/S0163-6383(79)80016-8

Thompson, L. A., & Massaro, D. W. (1989). Before you see it, you see its parts: Evidence for feature encoding and integration in preschool children and adults. *Cognitive Psychology, 21*(3), 334–362. https://doi.org/10.1016/0010-0285(89)90012-1

Tipper, S. P., & McLaren, J. (1990). Evidence for efficient visual selectivity in children. In J. T. Enns (Ed.), *Advances in psychology* (Vol. 69, pp. 197–210). Elsevier. https://doi.org/10.1016/S0166-4115(08)60457-4

Treisman, A. (1998). Feature binding, attention, and object perception. *Philosophical Transactions of the Royal Society of London B: Biological Sciences, 353*(1373), 1295–1306. https://doi.org/10.1016/j.ejpn.2004.03.003

Treisman, A. M., & Gelade, G. (1980). A feature integration theory of attention. *Cognitive Psychology, 12*(1), 97–136. https://doi.org/10.1016/0010-0285(80)90005-5

Trick, L. M., & Enns, J. T. (1998). Lifespan changes in attention: The visual search task. *Cognitive Development, 13*(3), 369–386. https://doi.org/10.1016/s0885-2014(98)90016-8

Tullo, D., Guy, J., Faubert, J., & Bertone, A. (2018). Training with a three-dimensional multiple object-tracking (3D-MOT) paradigm improves attention in students with a neurodevelopmental condition: A randomized controlled trial. *Developmental Science, 21*(6), e12670. https://doi.org/10.1111/desc.12670

Tummeltshammer, K., & Amso, D. (2018). Top-down contextual knowledge guides visual attention in infancy. *Developmental Science, 21*(4), e12599. https://doi.org/10.1111/desc.12599

Ullmann, R. K., Sleator, E. K., & Sprague, R. L. (1984). A new rating scale for diagnosis and monitoring of ADD children. *Psychopharmacology Bulletin, 20*(1), 160–164.

Wainwright, A., & Bryson, S. E. (2002). The development of exogenous orienting: Mechanisms of control. *Journal of Experimental Child Psychology, 82*(2), 141–155.

Wattam-Bell, J. (1996). Visual motion processing in one-month-old infants: Preferential looking experiments. *Vision Research, 36*(11), 1671–1677. https://doi.org/10.1016/0042-6989(95)00236-7

Wolfe, J. M. (1994). Guided search 2.0 a revised model of visual search. *Psychonomic Bulletin & Review, 1*(2), 202–238. https://doi.org/10.3758/BF03200774

Woods, A. J., Göksun, T., Chatterjee, A., Zelonis, S., Mehta, A., & Smith, S. E. (2013). The development of organized visual search. *Acta Psychologica, 143*(2), 191–199. https://doi.org/10.1016/j.actpsy.2013.03.008

Yantis, S. (2005). How visual salience wins the battle for awareness. *Nature Neuroscience, 8*(8), 975–977. https://doi.org/10.1038/nn0805-975

Zigler, E., & Balla, D. (1977). Personality factors in the performance of the retarded: Implications for clinical assessment. *Journal of the American Academy of Child Psychiatry, 16*(1), 19–37. https://doi.org/10.1016/S0002-7138(09)61578-8

CHAPTER

12 Working Memory and Down Syndrome

Elizabeth A. Smith *and* Christopher Jarrold

Abstract

A considerable body of research has explored working memory function in individuals with Down syndrome, given the fact that working memory is a strong predictor of numerous cognitive abilities over the course of development. Understanding working memory among individuals with Down syndrome is therefore key to providing a full picture of their overall cognitive profile. A pattern of poorer verbal working memory relative to less impaired visuospatial working memory has been well documented among individuals with Down syndrome, typically in the context of the Baddeley and Hitch (1974) working memory model. Here the review is extended to explore the nature of working memory capacity in terms of the maintenance of item versus order information in working memory. Deficits in both storage and control are explored, and explanations from different models of memory are considered. The relationship between long-term memory and working memory among persons with Down syndrome is subsequently outlined, and the role of working memory is considered in relation to learning among individuals Down syndrome.

Key Words: Down syndrome, working memory, verbal storage, visuospatial storage, executive control, cognitive profile, development, memory models

Introduction

Working memory refers to the cognitive mechanism for storing and processing the information to which an individual is currently attending (Baddeley, 2003; Cowan, 2008). Only a limited amount of information can be actively maintained in working memory at any given moment, and this information, be it verbal or visual, is held only temporarily. Various cognitive tasks require working memory, such as holding onto numbers while carrying out arithmetic, processing phonemes and words in sequence, and developing ideas and plans (Baddeley, Gathercole, & Papagno, 1998; Daneman & Carpenter, 1980; Kyllonen & Christal, 1990; Logie, Gilhooly, & Wynn, 1994; Page & Norris, 2009). Working memory is ultimately the holding in mind of information in order to do things, that is, to control our actions and responses. We can thus define working memory in terms of two components: "storage" and "control." The term "short-term memory" is sometimes used synonymously with working memory; however, typically short-term memory is used to refer to only the storage component of working memory (Jarrold & Towse, 2006). In this chapter we will instead use the broader term "working memory" throughout. We first provide a general introduction to working memory performance among individuals with Down syndrome and then structure the remainder of the chapter to discuss storage and then control processes in this population specifically.

We further divide storage into the holding in mind of (a) item information and (b) order information in working memory. Explanations underlying particular patterns of difficulty in working memory storage of item versus order information are then explored, with consideration given to different working memory models so as to best interpret dissociations in working memory performance among individuals with Down syndrome. We review executive functions and control in working memory to provide an understanding of the patterns observed among persons with Down syndrome (see also Fidler, Daunhauer, Will, & Schworer, this volume). We also discuss the concept of procedural working memory as it applies to persons with Down syndrome in the context of control. As working memory storage and control are also influenced by long-term memory and other cognitive systems, we address the relationship between the components of working memory and long-term memory among individuals with Down syndrome.

We additionally consider working memory in relation to learning and development among individuals with Down syndrome. In this section, we draw comparisons between other groups of individuals with developmental disabilities, with a focus on both the influence of working memory on vocabulary and the influence of implicit and explicit learning in relation to working memory. Comparing findings in different groups of individuals with developmental disabilities allows us to gain a better understanding of the nature of learning and development in persons with Down syndrome, where similarities and dissociations across groups can provide insight into the antecedents of behavioral outcomes. We end the chapter by considering educational implications.

Working Memory in Down Syndrome

Working memory is a strong predictor of various academic abilities across development (Alloway & Alloway, 2010; Bull, Espy, & Wiebe, 2008; Gathercole, Pickering, Knight, & Stegmann, 2004). Alloway (2009) also reported that working memory was a better predictor of later learning than IQ was in children with learning disability. Because of the cognitive difficulties generally associated with Down syndrome, a degree of difficulty on working memory tasks is to be expected in this population. However, under some circumstances, performance on working memory tasks among individuals with Down syndrome is in fact poorer than would be expected relative to their other cognitive abilities, and this has been observed among both children and adults with Down syndrome (Jarrold & Baddeley, 1997; Jarrold, Baddeley, & Hewes, 1999; Lanfranchi, Cornoldi, & Vianello, 2004; Marcell & Weeks, 1988). A particular pattern of difficulty is observed in persons with Down syndrome, with specific impairment in tasks that involve verbal information; this is relative to performance in comparable visuospatial tasks (Chapman & Hesketh, 2001; Jarrold & Baddeley, 1997) and relative to comparison groups of mental age–matched typically developing children (Brock & Jarrold, 2005; Jarrold & Baddeley, 1997; Jarrold, Baddeley, & Hewes, 2000; Kay-Raining Bird, & Chapman, 1994; Lee, Pennington, & Keenan, 2010; Vicari, Marotta, & Carlesimo, 2004), and groups of mental age–matched children with other learning difficulties (Jarrold, Baddeley, & Hewes, 1999; Jarrold, Cowan, Hewes, & Riby, 2004; Laws & Bishop, 2003; see Godfrey & Lee, 2018, for a recent, comprehensive, review). Additionally, impairments in working memory tasks of either verbal or visuospatial nature have been observed among individuals with Down syndrome as a result of increased demands on control processes. For instance, when participants are asked to process items simultaneously, rather than sequentially, in working memory tasks, a significantly greater impairment in performance is observed among the participants with Down syndrome relative to typically developing comparison groups matched for vocabulary or nonverbal mental age (Lanfranchi et al., 2004; Lanfranchi, Jerman, & Vianello, 2009; Vicari, Carlesimo, & Caltagirone, 1995). However, the impairment on verbal working memory tasks remains for individuals with Down syndrome even on assessments with low task demands, such as a simple verbal span task (immediately repeating back a list of verbal items). Particular patterns of working memory difficulty are therefore related to both storage and control among individuals with Down syndrome.

Working memory models are necessary to provide a framework within which to meaningfully interpret the patterns of working memory performance among individuals with Down syndrome, and we can consider how different models can explain the patterns observed in this population. The nature of storage and control is viewed somewhat differently in different working memory models, and we will touch on these models in the following sections when interpreting the patterns of performance among individuals with Down syndrome. One key difference between models is the way that storage is conceptualized in working memory. According to the Baddeley (1986) model of working memory, which follows directly from the Baddeley and Hitch (1974) model, items are held in separate and distinct stores. In other models, items that are retained in working memory are viewed as reflecting activated long-term memory representations: those items are held in an individual's "focus of attention," rather than a distinct store (Cowan, 1995, 2005; Oberauer, 2002). Whether short-term memory is meaningfully distinct from long-term memory is still a subject of ongoing debate (e.g., Norris, 2017). The pattern of performance among individuals with Down syndrome also contributes to this debate, as the dissociation in verbal versus visuospatial working memory performance among individuals with Down syndrome appears to fit well with the notion of separate and distinct stores, as posited in the Baddeley model (1986).

Storage

Poor Verbal Working Memory in the Context of the Baddeley (1986) Model

While not necessarily observed in every individual with Down syndrome (Vallar & Papagno, 1993), the tendency toward specific difficulties in tasks involving verbal working memory is very common in this population. Overviews of the specific verbal working memory impairment associated with Down syndrome have been published previously (e.g., Baddeley & Jarrold, 2007; Jarrold & Baddeley, 2001; Jarrold, Baddeley, & Phillips, 1999). These overviews consider specific verbal working memory difficulties among individuals with Down syndrome in the context of the Baddeley (1986) working memory model, as much of the research on working memory in Down syndrome has been carried out within this framework. Therefore, we provide only a somewhat brief overview here in the context of this model.

In the Baddeley (1986) model, working memory was proposed to consist of multiple components—separate stores for visual and verbal information, referred to as the visuospatial sketchpad and the phonological loop respectively, and a central executive. The central executive reflects the control component of working memory, as shown in Figure 12.1. Baddeley (2000) later added an "episodic buffer" to address the interaction between long-term memory and working memory. Here we focus on the 1986 model because there has been limited work on the episodic buffer among individuals with Down syndrome. However, we do pick up on the interaction between working memory and long-term memory further on in the chapter.

The notion of separate verbal/visual stores is supported by modality-specific interference findings, as well as by clinical dissociations in neuropsychological patients (Baddeley,

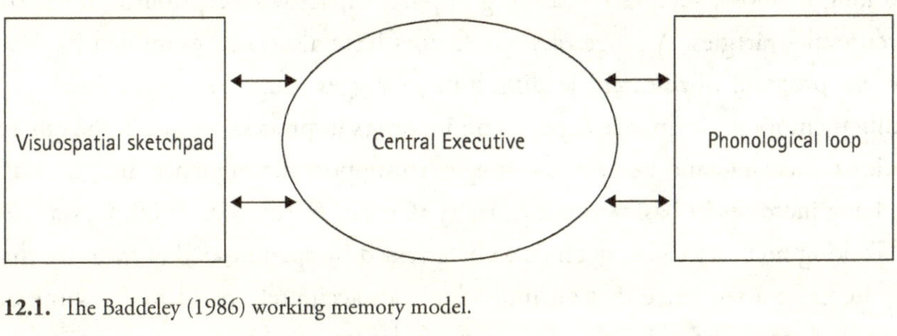

Figure 12.1. The Baddeley (1986) working memory model.

Grant, Wight, & Thomson, 1975; Hale, Myerson, Rhee, Weiss, & Abrams, 1996; Jarrold, Tam, Baddeley, & Harvey, 2011; Toms, Morris, & Foley, 1994; Vallar & Baddeley, 1984). The specific deficit in verbal as opposed to visual working memory performance that has been consistently observed among persons with Down syndrome (Brock & Jarrold, 2005; Jarrold & Baddeley, 1997; Lanfranchi et al., 2004; Marcell & Weeks, 1988; Vicari et al., 2004) can be readily framed as an impairment to the phonological loop component of the Baddeley (1986) working memory model, as this particular system specifically stores and maintains verbal input.

A number of potential other explanations for impaired performance on tasks of verbal working memory among persons with Down syndrome have been explored, including hearing difficulties, lack of verbal rehearsal, and slower speech rates. However, when controlling for such variables, for instance by removing the need for verbal responses or by matching children with Down syndrome with other groups on variables such as rehearsal or speech rate, the impairment is still evident. Hence, none of these areas account fully for the extent of the verbal working memory impairment in persons with Down syndrome (Jarrold et al., 2000; Marcell & Armstrong, 1982; Seung & Chapman, 2000; see Jarrold & Baddeley, 2001; Jarrold, Baddeley, & Phillips, 1999, for detailed reviews). Rather, poor verbal working memory among individuals with Down syndrome may best be explained by a limited phonological storage capacity as we now discuss.

Limited Phonological Storage Capacity Among Individuals With Down Syndrome?

In typical populations, adult working memory capacity is traditionally considered to be around seven items (Miller, 1956), and it has been more recently suggested that this reflects around three to five "chunks" or meaningful units of information (Cowan, 2010). Chen and Cowan (2009) found that when participants were prevented from verbally rehearsing memoranda, they were able to remember approximately three units, regardless of whether the units were single items or learned pairs, supporting the notion of a limit in the number of chunks, rather than single items, that can be stored. However, children's working memory capacity is less than that of adults (Dempster, 1981). Dempster (1981) identified a number of possible factors that might contribute to developmental differences in working memory, such as rehearsal, grouping, capacity, susceptibility to interference, and retrieval strategies. A range of these factors have also been examined by Cowan in his recent program of research, leading him to suggest that the typical development of working memory performance depends on increases in processing speed, the efficiency of attentional focusing, and the use of strategies to support maintenance, but, crucially, also underlying increases in basic storage capacity (Cowan & Alloway, 2009; Cowan, 2010).

Working memory capacity tends to be assessed by span tasks that measure the number of items in a sequence that an individual can accurately recall in the same order as presented. Among individuals with Down syndrome, working memory span for verbal material tends to be much lower than that seen among typically developing comparison groups of children matched for nonverbal ability or vocabulary, indicating that their capacity is significantly impaired relative to their mental age, and even relative to their other verbal abilities. In studies of working memory span among individuals with Down syndrome, the range of span performance tends to fall between two and four items (or one to two chunks), and this remains relatively consistent across late childhood and adulthood. For example, Frenkel and Bourdin (2009) found that a group of individuals with Down syndrome between the ages of 6 and 17 years had a mean verbal span of 2.28 items, ranging from 2–4, while a typically developing comparison group matched for mental age via the Kaufman Intelligence test (Kaufman & Kaufman, 1993) and age 3–7 years had a mean span of 3.02 items (range: 2–5). Frenkel and Bourdin (2009) also found that the verbal span of mental age–matched typically developing comparison children was subject to a much greater increase with age relative to individuals with Down syndrome. Stavroussi, Andreou and Karagiannopoulou (2016) assessed verbal digit span in a group of adults with Down syndrome age 26–38 years, in comparison to a group of adults with intellectual disability of unspecified origin aged 25–39 years matched on receptive vocabulary. Stavroussi et al. report a mean verbal span of 3.25 items for the group with Down syndrome, and a mean verbal span of 4.08 for the comparison group of persons with intellectual disability of unspecified origin (see also Jarrold & Baddeley, 1997; Kay-Raining Bird & Chapman, 1994; Smith & Jarrold, 2014b, for additional comparisons of verbal span among individuals with or without Down syndrome).

Simple verbal span tasks require repeating back a list of verbal items in correct order, and are used as a measure of verbal short-term storage capacity. However, simple span performance might involve more than just short-term memory storage capacity; individuals can use long-term knowledge of the items to improve their serial recall performance (Poirier, Dhir, Saint-Aubin, Tehan, & Hampton, 2011; Roodenrys, Hulme, Lethbridge, Hinton, & Nimmo, 2002). Hence, in order to obtain an estimate of "pure" verbal working memory storage capacity, long-term memory contributions can be distinguished from pure phonological storage in verbal serial recall tasks. This can be done by reducing the extent to which semantic long-term memory knowledge can support working memory, so that performance depends on phonological representation of the information alone. Conversely, stimuli that are phonologically confusable but semantically rich will be difficult to maintain in verbal working memory but could benefit considerably from long-term memory support.

Following this logic, Purser and Jarrold (2005) used phonological confusion as an index of short-term storage and semantic confusion as an index of long-term memory storage in a short-term recognition task. Persons with Down syndrome, with an average vocabulary mental age of 8 years, only showed evidence of phonological confusion for the most recent item in the list, indicating a pure phonological capacity limited to just one item. In contrast, in a typically developing comparison group of children (age 5–6 years) of similar nonverbal ability (measured via Raven's colored progressive matrices; Raven,

Raven, & Court, 1998) but with a lower vocabulary mental age, Purser and Jarrold found evidence of phonological storage across all four list positions. In contrast to phonological storage, the typically developing comparison children showed evidence of semantic confusion effects only at early list positions, indicating the influence of long-term memory knowledge in recalling these items. However, the individuals with Down syndrome did not show evidence of semantic confusion effects for any list positions, indicating that they were not using long-term memory to support their performance in this particular task to the same extent.

However, individuals with Down syndrome have shown evidence of contributions from their long-term memory knowledge to verbal working memory performance in other studies (Brock & Jarrold, 2004; Lee et al., 2010; Smith & Jarrold, 2014a, 2014b) indicating that they are able to benefit from their knowledge of items for some verbal working memory tasks. For example, Lee et al. (2010) measured the extent to which adults with Down syndrome employed either phonological or semantic strategies to support verbal working memory performance by, amongst other manipulations, varying either the phonological or semantic similarity of the to-be-remembered lists. They found a reduced sensitivity to the phonological manipulation among persons with Down syndrome relative to a typically developing comparison group, but a (nonsignificantly) larger effect of the semantic manipulation than seen in the typically developing group. Thus, evidence of the use of long-term knowledge to support recall among individuals with Down syndrome may depend on the nature of the to-be-remembered material. Individuals with Down syndrome show "frequency" and "lexicality" effects, recalling common words more easily than infrequent ones and known words more readily than nonwords (Brock & Jarrold, 2004; Smith & Jarrold, 2014a), However, these effects reflect familiarity with individual words in long-term memory. In contrast, semantic similarity effects upon verbal short-term memory recall depend on knowledge of semantic relations among items. Thus, limitations in relational knowledge (see Laws et al., 2015) could limit the extent of semantic similarity effects seen among persons with Down syndrome.

Storage Capacity: Remembering Items and Remembering the Correct Order of the Items

If individuals with Down syndrome have a severely limited verbal working memory capacity, then this could reflect a limited storage capacity for the items themselves, but also a potential capacity limit on their memory for the order of these items. The amount an individual can recall in working memory tasks depends on both working memory for item information and working memory for order information. If an individual were to mix up the order of phonemes in a word, or mix up the order of the digits in a phone number, this would alter the meaning of that information. Working memory serves as a mental workspace, thus the accurate representation of the correct information in its correct order is vital for correct subsequent learning in many domains.

In classic working memory tasks, working memory for item information and for order information tend not to be distinguished. For instance, an individual's digit span reflects the number of items recalled correctly in order. However, under this criterion, incorrect recall may be due to the failure to recall either the items, the order of items, or both. When verbal item and verbal order working memory are explored separately in typically developing persons, these two aspects of memory are differentially affected by certain variables, indicating that memory for item and order are potentially separable (Baddeley, 1966; Burns, 1996; Conrad & Hull, 1964; DeLosh & McDaniel, 1996; Nairne & Kelley, 2004; Poirier & Saint-Aubin, 1996; Wickelgren, 1965). For example, phonological similarity of to-be-recalled items has been found to result in impaired order memory, relative to phonologically dissimilar lists. In contrast, phonological similarity leads to unimpaired, or sometimes greater, item memory. There are also neuroimaging data (Giraud et al., 2000; Majerus, Poncelet, Van der Linden, et al., 2006) indicating a separation between item and order information in working memory.

Capacity for Item Versus Order Information in Working Memory in Individuals With Down Syndrome

Individuals with Down syndrome may have specific difficulties regarding verbal working memory for item information or for order information, leading to their greater impairment on tasks involving verbal working memory relative to visuospatial working memory tasks. There are different ways in which tasks can be designed to tap item and order memory respectively. Free recall tasks require the participant to recall items irrelevant of order. In contrast, in serial reconstruction tasks the participants have the memory items returned to them and are required only to put these items back into the order that they were first presented. Following this distinction, Brock and Jarrold (2005) compared performance on a free recall and a serial reconstruction task among individuals with Down syndrome with an average vocabulary age of 7 years and found that the participants experienced relatively greater problems reconstructing order than item information. Such a difficulty could have secondary consequences, as Majerus, Poncelet, Greff, and Van der Linden (2006) suggest that serial order memory plays an important role in vocabulary development (see also Ordonez Magro, Attout, Majerus, & Szmalec, 2018). Similarly, Rosin, Swift, Bless, and Vetter (1988) suggest that difficulties in the language domain among persons with Down syndrome may be reflective of broader impairment involving the processing of serial order. Given that individuals with Down syndrome experience some specific problems in the language domain (see Abbeduto, Arias-Trejo, & Thurman, this volume; Chapman & Hesketh, 2000; Chapman & Kay-Raining Bird, 2012, for reviews), particular difficulties regarding memory for order information may play a key role in their impaired language abilities. A comparison can also be drawn here to children with specific language impairment, for whom difficulty remembering the order of items, or sequential information more generally, may play a role in the language difficulties they experience (Hsu & Bishop, 2014).

Evidence of an additional impairment recalling item information in verbal working memory tasks is also seen among individuals with Down syndrome (Brock & Jarrold, 2004; Marcell, Harvey, & Cothran, 1988; Smith & Jarrold, 2014a). For instance, Brock and Jarrold (2004) found that participants with Down syndrome performed more poorly on both an order and an item working memory task, relative to typically developing comparison children of a similar nonverbal ability (assessed via the Raven's colored progressive matrices). However, they also reported that performance on the item task was particularly impaired with the Down syndrome group showing an atypically large lexicality effect, which refers to an advantage for recalling words relative to recalling nonwords. As this is thus thought to reflect the top-down influence of vocabulary knowledge upon short-term memory performance, the significantly larger lexicality effect for the participants with Down syndrome relative to typically developing participants may therefore imply that they rely more heavily on their vocabulary knowledge during verbal short-term memory tasks. However, Brock and Jarrold noted that the individuals with Down syndrome showed poor item memory in general relative to the typically developing comparison group, but had a particular difficulty in recalling item information for nonword stimuli. They therefore interpreted the large lexicality effect as reflecting poor phonological discrimination, and hence particular difficulties in identifying nonwords (see also Lee et al., 2010). These findings suggest that the verbal working memory deficit observed in persons with Down syndrome is the result of difficulties in retaining both order information and item information, both of which are required for successful sequential recall.

The finding of poor item and order memory in individuals with Down syndrome may, however, be influenced by the measures that have been used to assess short-term item memory and short-term order memory. The studies of item and order memory separately among individuals with Down syndrome have tended to involve measures that are not entirely free from interference from item or order respectively. Although free recall tasks are assumed to reflect item memory, since they do not *require* participants to recall items in correct order, participants (including children) very often choose to recall the items in such tasks in the same order as they were presented (Bhatarah, Ward, Smith, & Hayes, 2009; Jarrold et al., 2014; Ward, Tan, & Grenfell-Essam, 2010; see also Farrell, 2012). This means that order memory may still contribute to participants' performance in free recall tasks. The same issue is true for reconstruction tasks, whereby performance reconstructing order has been shown to be influenced by the extent to which the item characteristics are concrete versus abstract (Neath, 1997). This indicates that reconstruction tasks can be affected by item-level factors and so may not provide a very pure measure of order memory.

The use of process dissociation is a more recent approach to the item/order distinction in serial recall that seeks to circumvent such problems (Nairne & Kelley, 2004; Smith & Jarrold, 2014a; Wang, Xuan, & Jarrold, 2016). Originally introduced by Jacoby (1991) as a way to dissociate conscious versus unconscious processes, this method is based on an inclusion condition, whereby two processes contribute to performance, and an exclusion condition, whereby one process contributes to and the other process opposes performance. Nairne and Kelley (2004) adapted the process dissociation method to separate item and order memory, providing purer measures of each. They found the expected effects of given variables on item memory and order memory respectively in typically developing adults. In our own work using this approach, Smith and Jarrold (2014a) also found expected effects of given variables upon working memory for item versus order information among individuals with Down syndrome with a mean verbal mental age of 7.4 years. For instance, phonologically similar lists of items led to poorer order memory, but stronger item memory, among individuals with and without Down syndrome. Using this method, we also found that persons with Down syndrome are significantly impaired relative to vocabulary-matched typically developing comparison groups when recalling both item and order information. This, along with previous findings, indicates that both item and order memory problems contribute to the poorer verbal working memory seen in this population. If capacity is impaired in terms of the ability to remember both item and order information, the nature of a capacity limitation for verbal working memory among individuals with Down syndrome then depends on how we theoretically view item memory and memory for order, an issue which we will now discuss in some detail.

Domain Specificity and Domain Generality in Working Memory for Order Versus Items

According to domain-specific theories, different systems represent verbal and visuospatial information, whereas according to domain-general theories, multiple domains are processed within the same system. The Baddeley (1986) model is a domain-specific account of working memory that readily accommodates the relative difference in verbal versus visuospatial working memory performance in Down syndrome via the suggestion of a specific deficit in the short-term maintenance of verbal item information. However, the mechanism underlying the encoding and maintenance of serial order in either domain is not defined in detail in the model (Hurlstone, Hitch, & Baddeley, 2014). This leaves open the question of whether the serial ordering of verbal as opposed to visual information still rests on a common process or not. Some authors argue for two separate and domain-specific ordering mechanisms on the basis of dual task studies. For example, Saito, Logie, Morita, and Law (2008) explored the extent to which repeating an irrelevant sound or word (articulatory suppression task), which is thought to selectively block verbal rehearsal, moderated typically developing adults' visual or phonological similarity confusions when attempting to recall lists of items in the correct order. Saito et al. (2008) found that the visual similarity effect remained whereas the phonological similarity effect did not. Therefore, order errors that would usually be caused by phonological similarity of items in a list were reduced as a result of the suppression task. The enduring visual similarity effect, in the presence of articulatory suppression, implies that visual order information is stored via a separate mechanism, suggesting a domain-specific order retention (see also Logie, Saito, Morita, Varma, & Norris, 2016; Soemer & Saito, 2016).

In contrast to the above evidence, several other researchers have suggested that serial ordering within working memory rests on a common sequencing mechanism for both verbal and visual memoranda (e.g., Depoorter & Vandierendonck, 2009; Farrell & Oberauer, 2014; Jones, Farrand, Stuart, & Morris, 1995; Morey & Mall, 2012; Vandierendonck, 2016). Studies that have investigated working memory for mixed domain sequences (verbal and visual items within the same list) can also shed light on the nature of memory for order. Domain-specific theories would predict poorer recall of order for items when they are in mixed-domain sequences, due to the additional demands of switching attention between domains. However, a domain-general view, as suggested by Farrell and Oberauer (2014), predicts that memory for the order of items from different domains will be enhanced. This is because a common mechanism underlies memory for the order of all items, and items from different domains are more distinguishable from each other, reducing the degree of inter-item confusion caused from the application of a common ordering system. Farrell and Oberaurer found support for this latter view in an experiment with typically developing adults in which mixed-domain lists led to greater serial recall than lists of items all from the same domain.

Other evidence in support of the notion of a domain-general mechanism for serial order comes from an embedded task approach. Depoorter and Vandierendonck (2009) presented typical adult participants with a primary working memory task and embedded a second working memory task in between presentation and recall of the first task. The embedded task was either an item or an order recall task, and the modality of the embedded task was also manipulated (verbal versus visuospatial items). Presenting an embedded order memory task caused impaired performance on the primary task regardless of the modality of the embedded task. This interference across domains again fits with the notion of a domain-general ordering mechanism.

In a similar vein, Morey and Mall (2012) found evidence for cross-domain interference on serial order reconstruction performance among typical adults. However, the interference effects were not symmetrical. Participants' ability to recall the order of spatial items was disrupted by verbal interference to a large extent. In the other direction, the effect of spatial interference on recall of order of verbal items was weaker. Likewise, in a study of cross-modal interference, Vandierendonck (2016) observed less visuospatial interference on recall of order in a verbal task relative to greater interference of a verbal task upon visuospatial task performance. Morey and Mall as well as Vandierendonck note that the evidence appears to point toward a potential separate resource that specifically supports verbal order information in working memory, *in addition* to a mechanism for processing order information across domains in working memory more generally. An additional verbal resource for maintaining order information may thereby allow for a degree of compensation in one's ability to remember the order of verbal items in the face of spatial interference during working memory tasks. Along similar lines, Camos, Lagner, and Barrouillet (2009) have suggested that the articulatory loop may be available in addition to activated long-term memory for verbal items. This articulatory loop was originally proposed by Baddeley (1986), alongside the phonological store, functioning as a mechanism for verbal rehearsal.

In contrast, a domain-general mechanism for processing order information in working memory, as outlined above, could have something of a spatial aspect to it, which could still support recall of both verbal and visual information. Individuals may rely upon spatial attention when processing order information, with some researchers having suggested that even verbal order information in working memory tasks can be represented both spatially and temporally (Fischer-Baum & Benjamin, 2014; van Dijck, Abrahamse, Majerus, & Fias, 2013; van Dijck & Fias, 2011). For example, van Dijck et al. (2013) and van Dijck & Fias (2011) suggest that typically developing individuals process order information spatially during working memory tasks, even when the items are verbal. Van Dijck and Fias (2011) observed faster responses to early items on the list when they are subsequently presented on the left-hand side of a screen, and faster responses to later items when they are presented on the right side of the screen. Likewise, Fischer-Baum and Benjamin (2014) found presenting items spatially from left to right was beneficial for forward recall among typically developing adults, whereas spatial presentation from right to left was more beneficial for backward recall. These spatial influences on ordered recall led Fischer-Baum and Benjamin to suggest that verbal order information can be represented both spatially *and* temporally.

In sum, one reading of the body of work on how order information is maintained in working memory among typically developing adults is that the phonological loop serves as a domain-specific system for ordering verbal material, which supplements a more general ordering mechanism, which though applicable to all short-term memory tasks may have a spatial aspect to it. Although not accepted by all (e.g., Logie et al., 2016), this reading is well placed to explain the pattern of findings on ordered recall from working memory among individuals with Down syndrome. Poor performance on tasks involving working memory for verbal order information, relative to mental age–matched comparison groups, could reflect an impairment to maintenance of verbal order within the phonological loop. In contrast, a domain-general mechanism for processing order in working memory tasks may be relatively unimpaired among individuals with Down syndrome given their mental age, allowing individuals to perform in line with their mental age–matched peers during visuospatial working memory tasks. Indeed, spatial presentation of verbal items has been found to improve the serial recall performance of children and adolescents with Down syndrome (Duarte, Covre, Braga, & de Macedo, 2011), as they were able to perform in line with a typically developing comparison group. The comparison group had a matched mental age of 6.8 years as measured by the Wechsler Intelligence scale III (Wechsler, 2002). The individuals with Down syndrome also performed in line with a typically developing comparison group matched on vocabulary, with average raw scores of 51.1 (Down syndrome) and 49.3 (typically developing) respectively, as measured by the Peabody picture vocabulary test (Dunn & Dunn, 1981). On other word span tasks that involved verbal only presentation or verbal plus visual presentation but without spatial support, Duarte et al. found that the group of individuals with Down syndrome were significantly poorer than the mental age–matched comparison group.

Working Memory for Item Information

Working memory for items has an inherently domain-specific nature: verbal items are verbal in nature while visual/spatial items are visual/spatial in nature. However, researchers debate exactly how item information is stored and maintained during working memory tasks. The notion of a specialized, distinct phonological store and a distinct visuospatial store is indicative of complete domain specificity at the item level. In contrast, there is an element of domain generality in models in which items in working memory are activated long-term memory representations of the objects in some "focus of attention" (Cowan, 1995, 2005; Oberauer, 2002, 2009; see the first section of this chapter). In these models, items from different domains can be simultaneously attended to as attentional resources are shared across domains. Morey and Cowan (2005) argue for a central storage resource of a domain-general nature in addition to domain-specific "codes." In this scenario, domain-general central storage follows from the deployment of an attentional resource such as a focus of attention or an episodic buffer, depending on the model within which it is framed, while the domain-specific codes are the representations of the memoranda, either held in domain-specific stores or reflecting activated long-term memory representations. If it is assumed that there is not a distinct phonological store, but rather that working memory comprises activated long-term memory representations within an individual's focus of attention, then the poor working memory for verbal item information among individuals with Down syndrome may be thought to directly reflect impoverished verbal codes in memory. However, long-term memory for verbal memoranda does not appear to be prone to the same difficulties as verbal working memory among persons with Down syndrome (Jarrold, Baddeley, & Phillips, 2007). Furthermore, individuals with Down syndrome perform more poorly in verbal working memory tasks than typically developing comparison groups matched on verbal measures such as vocabulary (e.g., Brock & Jarrold, 2005; Jarrold et al., 2000). Verbal working memory therefore appears to be poorer than other verbal abilities among persons with Down syndrome.

One possibility is that the ability to attend to or process verbal information during working memory tasks specifically is subject to impairment among individuals with Down syndrome. Consistent with this, Smith and Jarrold (2014b) found that the ability to temporally group items during verbal working memory tasks was compromised in children and young adults with Down syndrome relative to comparison participants matched on verbal ability via the British Picture Vocabulary Scale (Dunn, Dunn, Whetton, &

Burley, 1997). Temporal grouping refers to the ability to group items together when they are presented in grouped intervals (with longer pauses between groups of items relative to within groups), and thereby improve serial recall performance. Difficulty attending to the temporal context of incoming verbal memoranda may contribute to difficulties processing order, but also to the processing of items, as successfully binding items to a context may allow for chunking and thereby increase capacity for items. Brock and Jarrold (2004) suggest that a temporal context model (e.g., Brown, Preece, & Hulme, 2000) could provide a potential explanation for concurrent order and item impairments. This is because in such models the temporal context signal is used to mark serial positions, and so provides a means of ordering recall of information. However, the temporal context associated with any given item is also used as a cue for retrieval of that item, therefore noise in such a signal could result in item as well as order errors. Poor phonological discrimination and hearing difficulties could further compound performance, and may contribute to noise in the temporal context signal. Vandierendonck (2016) notes that among typically developing individuals rehearsal and temporal grouping may be more effective for verbal, as opposed to visuospatial memoranda, potentially due to an additional compensatory articulatory (phonological) loop-type mechanism. It may be that this type of mechanism involves a temporal context signal specific to verbal items; impairment of this mechanism among individuals with Down syndrome could therefore explain their tendency for a verbal working memory deficit.

To summarize the findings on storage among individuals with Down syndrome, evidence points to a limited capacity for storing verbal memoranda. Poorer working memory for verbal items as well as for the order of these verbal items both contribute to the overall impairment in verbal working memory storage in the Down syndrome population; this pattern is found among both children and young adults with Down syndrome (Brock & Jarrold, 2004, 2005; Smith & Jarrold, 2014a). A specific difficulty involving processing of temporal context could impair both storage of item and order in working memory for the verbal domain specifically. The tendency for a specific verbal working memory deficit remains among individuals with Down syndrome over the course of development and does not appear to vary based on mental age (Hick, Botting, & Conti-Ramsden, 2005; Jarrold, Baddeley, & Phillips, 2002; Jarrold, Thorn, & Stephens, 2009; Marcell & Weeks, 1988). Early intervention is crucial to address both the verbal item and order short-term storage difficulties, as this may have potential for positive secondary effects over the course of development.

Control Component of Working Memory

In addition to storage systems, working memory requires control—the processing or "doing" components of working memory, such as maintaining, inhibiting, and dual processing. There is evidence for deficits in control in addition to specific verbal problems among individuals with Down syndrome (Lanfranchi et al., 2004; Lanfranchi, Jerman,

& Vianello, 2009; Vicari et al., 1995). Compared to two typically developing comparison groups, one matched to the group with Down syndrome on vocabulary and the other group matched on nonverbal mental age, Lanfranchi, Jerman et al. (2009) found that children with Down syndrome (mean age: 13.10; mean nonverbal mental age: 4.10; mean vocabulary age: 4.10) were impaired on tests of verbal working memory. Hence, the impairment was beyond what would be expected simply as a result of individuals' verbal abilities. In the studies carried out by Lanfranchi et al. (2004) and Lanfranchi, Carretti, Spanò and Cornoldi (2009) the level of control was manipulated, where the higher control demands involved simultaneous processing (a double task condition) relative to the lower control demands (a single task condition). The verbal working memory impairment was seen regardless of the degree of control required. In contrast, for visuospatial working memory, the group of individuals with Down syndrome were only impaired relative to the matched comparison groups when the task had higher control demands. Hence, poor executive control among individuals with Down syndrome appears to affect working memory performance across both the verbal and visuospatial domain.

Lanfranchi, Jerman et al. (2009) also found a stronger relationship between performance on high control tasks and a logical thinking intelligence test among participants with Down syndrome than in the typically developing comparison groups. This finding led them to suggest that tasks involving high control may be more automatized among typically developing individuals, placing less demand on general working memory capacity relative to individuals with Down syndrome. To better understand difficulties involving working memory control among individuals with Down syndrome, researchers have investigated whether specific components of control are subject to lesser or greater impairment. Control processes are also referred to as executive functions (i.e., the frontal functions of the brain), and these can be broken down into various different abilities. In the Baddeley (1986) working memory model it is the central executive system that exercises "control" on working memory systems, therefore difficulties involving working memory control processes can be interpreted as reflecting an impaired central executive system. However, different working memory models provide alternative frameworks to understand the nature of impairment to control processes among individuals with Down syndrome.

Procedural Versus Declarative Working Memory

Oberauer (2009) distinguishes between working memory for the to-be-remembered content itself, referred to as declarative working memory, and memory for what to do with that content, such as a particular (cognitive or motor) action, referred to as procedural working memory. The above separation of storage versus executive control or processing somewhat parallels Oberauer's distinction between declarative and procedural working memory. The model proposed by Oberauer can also be considered in relation to the highly influential account of executive functions proposed by Miyake et al. (2000) whose framework of executive functions consists of three key components of memory: updating, inhibition, and shifting. Memory updating could be considered analogous to the control process of replacing or updating representations in declarative memory. In contrast, Oberauer (2009) relates the two other key executive functions highlighted by Miyake and colleagues—inhibition and shifting (or switching)—to procedural working memory. Both inhibition and shifting involve establishing a new task set that is in competition with a previous habitual response.

In terms of applying the above framework to the patterns observed among individuals with Down syndrome, an impairment in procedural working memory might be expected to play out in terms of individuals with Down syndrome showing impairment on working memory tasks that involve greater switching and inhibition demands. A particular difficulty on switching tasks would be indicative of problems updating procedural working memory in that it represents a failure to retrieve the new task set, whereas difficulty inhibiting and thus high error costs on inhibition tasks would represent a failure to prevent the execution of a habitually driven competing action in procedural working memory. As there are often time pressures inherent in working memory tasks, individuals with slower processing speed may be slower to retrieve the new task set in procedural working memory and may thus be more likely to neglect the task goals.

An impairment in terms of the declarative system would be expected to result in difficulties maintaining memory representations (temporary content to context binding), and thus low working memory capacity. Difficulty on memory updating tasks could also be argued to reflect an impairment in the declarative working memory system. However, Oberauer (2009) notes that performance on memory updating tasks may not be particularly helped by high working memory capacity, in that individuals with high capacity have to overcome stronger bindings during updating tasks. Therefore, while individuals with Down syndrome perform poorly on verbal working memory tasks, they may not necessarily be expected to have a specific impairment in working memory updating tasks.

Breaking these areas down to explore which aspects of executive control are impaired among individuals with Down syndrome may help to pinpoint the nature of a deficit in control and how this impacts working memory performance. However, the findings in this area are somewhat mixed as several researchers have reported impaired executive functioning among individuals with Down syndrome (Borella, Carretti, & Lanfranchi, 2013; Lanfranchi, Jerman, Dal Pont, Alberti, & Vianello, 2010; Lee et al., 2015; Rowe, Lavender, & Turk, 2006), but both Smith, Hedge and Jarrold (2019) and Pennington, Mood, Edgin, Stedron, and Nadel (2003) did not find significant differences in executive control between persons with Down syndrome and typically developing children matched on mental age. The matching measure used by Pennington et al. (2003) was the Differential Ability Scales (DAS; Elliott, 1990). The DAS includes both verbal and visual components, indicating that executive function was in line with mental age in the Pennington et al. study; indeed this was the case for all six of the executive function tasks.

The six tasks used to assess prefrontal functions were planning, verbal fluency, nonverbal fluency, inhibition (a "stopping" task), spatial working memory, and a verbal working memory task, thus covering a wide range of prefrontal (executive) functions. Lanfranchi et al. (2010) also covered a wide range of prefrontal functions in their study comparing adolescents with Down syndrome to a typically developing group, with the groups matched on mental age via a logical thinking measure. However, they found significant impairment across all abilities; a working memory task (verbal and visuospatial), an inhibition task (a Stroop type task), a set shifting task, a conceptual shifting task, a planning task, a verbal fluency task, and a sustained attention task. The studies by Lanfranchi et al. (2010) and Pennington et al. both involved adolescents with Down syndrome and included various tasks, but the types of executive function tasks used in these studies were different. Different tasks are often assumed to measure the same underlying component of executive function, but it is not clear that this assumption is always warranted (for reviews, see Karr et al., 2018; Packwood, Hodgett, & Tremblay, 2011). The performance of individuals with Down syndrome may vary depending on the different components of executive function measured. However, apparently inconsistent findings may also reflect the different types of tasks used to tap executive function. A Stroop task (saying "night" when presented with a sun image and saying "day" when presented with a moon and stars) was used to measure inhibitory control in the Lanfranchi et al. (2010) study described above, whereas a stopping task (stopping an automated button press response upon hearing a tone) was used for the same purpose in the Pennington et al. study above. Measures of inhibitory control such as Stroop type tasks involve greater verbal demands (Hamilton & Martin, 2005; Nee, Wager, & Jonides, 2007). Any executive functioning task that involves updating verbal memoranda in working memory may be harder for individuals with Down syndrome because of difficulties involving verbal storage outlined previously.

The characteristics of the comparison group may also lead to different results. Pennington et al. matched adolescents with Down syndrome to a group of younger typically developing children on mental ability, via the DAS. In the Lanfranchi et al. (2010) study the individuals were also adolescents, but the groups were matched via the Logical Operations Test (Vianello & Marin, 1997); this test is thought to place very little demand on verbal abilities. The DAS matching measure involves tests of verbal working memory and phonological processing, among other abilities. Due to poor verbal working memory among individuals with Down syndrome, they may be expected to be matched to a comparison group of higher functioning when matched on measures that place less demand on their verbal abilities, relative to when matched on tasks that place greater demands on verbal abilities.

Differences in the age of participants in studies of executive function may also influence the study findings. For example, Rowe et al. (2006) observed impairment in executive functions among adults with Down syndrome across a variety of executive functioning tasks. In this study the mean age of the participants with Down syndrome was 33 years, with a receptive vocabulary raw score of 14.50 (British Picture Vocabulary Scale; mental age equivalent not reported). The older age of participants may play a role in the difference in findings to that observed in the Pennington et al. study, involving young adolescents (mean age 14 years). The adults in the Rowe et al. study were matched to a comparison group of other individuals with learning difficulty, meaning that the groups were similar in terms of chronological age (mean age of Down syndrome group: 33 years, range: 23.8–40; non-Down syndrome group: 33 years, range: 19–55), in addition to mental age. As the mental age equivalents for the vocabulary raw scores are not reported in the Rowe et al. study, it is not possible to determine if the mental age of participants in this study differs to that in other studies with different executive function findings. Nonetheless, differences in matching measures and the nature of the comparison group, in addition to the types of executive function tasks used, could all influence study outcomes.

Costanzo et al. (2013) compared executive control abilities among a group of children, adolescents, and adults with Down syndrome; a group of individuals with Williams syndrome; and a typically developing comparison group of children (age 7.4), with all groups matched on the Leiter International Performance Scale—Revised, brief version (Leiter—R, Roid & Miller, 1997). The mean mental age of the groups was 6.2 (Down syndrome), 6.7 (Williams syndrome), and 7.4 (typically developing). They found a specific profile among persons with Down syndrome. Both the group with Down syndrome and the group with Williams syndrome were impaired on working memory tasks with a high load, with further impairment on the verbal task among the group of individuals with Down syndrome. Planning ability was less impaired among individuals with Down syndrome relative to individuals with Williams syndrome, such that the accuracy of the participants with Down syndrome was comparable to the typically developing comparison group, although the participants with Down syndrome took longer to execute the plans. Particularly poor performance in terms of shifting ability was observed among the participants with Down syndrome relative to both the participants with Williams syndrome and the typically developing comparison group. However, inhibitory deficits were only observed in a verbal task, not in a visual task among the participants with Down syndrome. It may be that difficulties in verbal storage increase control demands for individuals with Down syndrome. However, some components of executive control appear to be particularly impaired among individuals with Down syndrome, such that performance across domains is affected. Other domains appear less impaired overall, with a pattern of strengths and weaknesses; evidence for a characteristic profile among young children with Down syndrome was reported by Lee et al. (2015), with inhibition emerging as a relative strength.

Age-related changes in the profile of executive function were also investigated by Lee et al. (2015) by examining caregiver reports in a cross-sectional sample of children and young adults with Down syndrome. The same pattern of relative strengths and weaknesses in executive function among individuals with Down syndrome appeared to remain over time from early childhood to early adulthood. Inhibition remained the least impaired, and was also the one component for which the *rate* at which difficulties decreased over time for the sample with Down syndrome was in line with that seen in a typically developing group of children of the same chronological age; it is possible that these difficulties could continue to decrease into later adulthood. However, there is a lack of longitudinal research investigating potential changes in executive function in Down syndrome over the course of development. A considerable body of literature has focused specifically on changes in executive function among older adults with Down syndrome, as declines in executive function have been found to be a common early sign of Alzheimer's Disease in this population (see Lautarescu, Holland, & Zaman, 2017; for a review, see also Strydom, Zaman, & Startin, this volume). Edgin, Clark, Massand, and Karmiloff-Smith (2015) note the possibility that early improvements in executive function, which may occur through interventions/training, may mitigate potential declines in later life.

The profile of relative strengths and weaknesses in executive function among young children with Down syndrome may also have important consequence for their academic achievement. Will, Fidler, Daunhauer, and Gerlach-McDonald (2017) recently reported that executive function was linked to academic achievement in preschoolers with Down syndrome, as it is in typically developing children. Their participants completed a number of executive function tasks including a shifting task and a working memory/inhibition task. The shifting task consisted of sorting cards based on either color or shape. The working memory/inhibition task involved receiving instructions (such as "touch your nose") from a bad puppet and a good puppet character. The preschoolers were told to follow the instructions from the good puppet and to inhibit the instructions from the bad puppet. The task was considered to be a working memory task because the participants had to hold in mind the rules of the game at the same time as receiving and responding to the puppet's instructions. Whereas shifting was the strongest predictor of academic achievement in a typically developing comparison group (matched on nonverbal mental age via the Leiter-R; Roid & Miller, 1997), the task combining demands on working memory and inhibition was the strongest predictor of academic achievement among the children with Down syndrome.

These findings highlight that individuals with Down syndrome experience specific patterns of impairment involving particular aspects of both storage and control in working memory. As touched on previously, working memory is further influenced by long-term memory. In a revision to the Baddeley (1986) model, Baddeley (2000) added the "episodic buffer" to account for the interaction between working memory and long-term memory. While different models of working memory frame the interaction in different ways, researchers ultimately agree that long-term memory knowledge has an influence upon working memory, and that working memory has a key role in long-term learning. Hence, in the following section we consider the reciprocal relationship between long-term memory and working memory among individuals with Down syndrome.

Influence of Long-Term Memory Upon Working Memory Performance Among Individuals With Down Syndrome

Long-term memory knowledge contributes to performance on working memory tasks in typically developing populations. Individuals show superior recall of words relative to nonwords (Hulme, Maughan, & Brown, 1991), concrete words relative to abstract words (Paivio, Clark, & Khan, 1988), and higher frequency relative to lower frequency words (Roodenrys et al., 2002). Individuals with Down syndrome have also been shown to benefit from long-term memory knowledge during working memory tasks (Brock & Jarrold, 2005; Lee, Pennington, & Keenan, 2010; Smith & Jarrold, 2014a, 2014b). However, the degree to which individuals with Down syndrome benefit from their long-term memory knowledge may be reduced relative to their peers. For instance, although individuals with Down syndrome have been shown to benefit from semantic relations among items in a list, they appear to benefit to a lesser extent than vocabulary matched typically developing peers (Smith & Jarrold, 2014b). Purser and Jarrold (2005) found no evidence of a semantic similarity effect among participants with Down syndrome, also indicating that long-term memory may not support working memory to the same extent among individuals with Down syndrome as compared to typically developing individuals matched on nonverbal mental ability (Raven's colored progressive matrices; Raven et al. 1998). Another possibility is that individuals with Down syndrome have a shallower understanding of semantics, as suggested by Laws et al. (2015) who found that vocabulary depth may be poorer than vocabulary breadth among individuals with Down syndrome. Benefiting from semantic similarity during working memory tasks may require vocabulary depth: an individual not only has to recognize the items, but also has to understand how the items are related. This could potentially explain why the benefit of semantic similarity of items in working memory tasks is sometimes reduced among persons with Down syndrome relative to comparison groups. Long-term knowledge therefore provides some compensation for poor verbal working memory, but potentially to a lesser extent than comparison groups.

Working memory for nonwords presents a particular challenge for individuals with Down syndrome, with individuals showing a more pronounced impairment relative to typically developing individuals when recalling lists of nonwords relative to their degree of impairment recalling real words (Brock & Jarrold, 2005). When recalling nonwords, individuals clearly cannot rely on the kinds of semantic representations that would be available for known words, although there is evidence that typically developing children's memory for nonwords is affected by the extent to which items conform to the typical phonological properties of their language (Munson, Edwards, & Beckman, 2005). As with nonword recall, performance in nonword repetition tasks has also been shown to be impaired among individuals with Down syndrome (e.g., Laws, 1998). Holding novel phonological forms in verbal working memory has been suggested as a key route to learning language (Baddeley et al., 1998; Gathercole, Service, Hitch, Adams, & Martin, 1999), thus raising the question of how individuals with Down syndrome are able to develop vocabulary abilities beyond that of their verbal working memory ability.

Laws and Gunn (2004) reported a relationship between phonological working memory and later language among individuals with Down syndrome, including later grammar abilities (see also Jarrold et al., 2009). Hence, phonological working memory appears to play at least some role in language development for individuals with Down syndrome. However, Mosse and Jarrold (2010, 2011) suggested that phonological working memory is not the only route for vocabulary acquisition; individuals with Down syndrome appear to be able to acquire long-term verbal knowledge via implicit long-term learning, relying to a lesser extent on the phonological working memory route than their peers (see also Majerus & Barisnikov, 2018). Mosse and Jarrold (2010) found an intact Hebb repetition learning effect among individuals with Down syndrome, which refers to the long-term learning of sequence repetitions across the trials of a short-term memory task (Hebb, 1961). This potentially indicates intact implicit long-term learning of information, and offers a potential explanation for the discrepancy between relatively strong vocabulary and relatively weaker verbal working memory abilities in this population.

Comparisons can also be drawn between individuals with Down syndrome and those with other developmental disabilities, with similarities and differences between groups providing an insight into the nature of working memory in these populations. More specifically, a number of comparisons with other groups highlight the way in which working memory may be related to learning among persons with Down syndrome.

The Influence of Working Memory on Learning and Development Among Individuals With Down Syndrome and Other Groups With Developmental Disabilities

Developmental disabilities are often associated with particular cognitive profiles. The specific patterns of relative strengths and weaknesses among different groups can be compared, and we can consider whether instances in which we see similar patterns of performance may be driven by the same or different underlying causes (Karmiloff-Smith 2013). As previously noted, individuals with Down syndrome develop vocabulary abilities that are stronger than one might expect given their deficit in verbal working memory; they have a profile of relative strengths and weaknesses in the language domain, with receptive vocabulary tending to be a strength relative to much poorer expressive vocabulary and syntax (Chapman, Kay-Raining Bird, & Schwartz, 1990; Laws, 1998; Næss, Lyster, Hulme, & Melby-Lervåg, 2011).

Individuals with specific language impairment (SLI) are often reported to show similar patterns to individuals with Down syndrome in terms of their language profile, with both groups experiencing grammatical difficulties and expressive language difficulties (Laws & Bishop, 2004; Rice, Warren, & Betz, 2005). Individuals with SLI have also been found to experience difficulties in tasks involving verbal working memory (Archibald & Gathercole, 2006; Bishop, North, & Donlan, 1996; Conti-Ramsden & Hesketh 2003; Gathercole & Baddeley, 1990). Such similarities between individuals with SLI and individuals with Down syndrome are indicative of a potential link between poor verbal working memory and language development. Indeed, Archibald and Gathercole (2006) suggest that problems in verbal working memory could play a causal role in some of the language learning difficulties associated with SLI; the same may also be the case among individuals with Down syndrome.

While there are similarities among individuals with Down syndrome and individuals with SLI, it is also important to consider differences that may point to distinct underlying causes of the apparently similar verbal working memory and language impairments. The pattern of difficulties experienced among individuals with SLI may also be associated with a procedural learning deficit. Ullman and Pierpont (2005) suggested that the brain structures underlying procedural memory may be impaired among individuals with SLI, and this results in an impairment in implicit sequence learning and the learning of grammar rules. Additionally, a procedural learning deficit is argued to account for poorer working memory across both the verbal and visuospatial domains (Hick et al., 2005), given the sequential nature of working memory storage and recall. Impaired learning of implicit sequences among individuals with SLI has been observed in numerous studies (Evans, Saffran, & Robe-Torres, 2009; Hsu & Bishop, 2014; Lum, Gelgic, & Conti-Ramsden, 2010; Tomblin, Mainela-Arnold, & Zhang, 2007). Impaired Hebb repetition learning has also been observed among individuals with dyslexia (Szmalec, Loncke, Page, & Duyck, 2011), another group that has also been found to have impaired verbal working memory (e.g., Smith-Spark & Fisk, 2007). Research also highlights that SLI and dyslexia often co-occur (Bishop & Snowling, 2004).

In contrast, as outlined previously, individuals with Down syndrome show evidence of implicit long-term learning of sequences (e.g., intact Hebb repetition effects) that do not appear reduced relative to typically developing comparison groups matched on vocabulary (Mosse & Jarrold, 2010). Thus, while a procedural or sequential processing impairment may arguably explain some of the language and working memory difficulties associated with SLI and dyslexia, it does not provide a feasible explanation for all the difficulties in verbal working memory or language among individuals with Down syndrome.

To sum up these findings: among individuals with Down syndrome, verbal working memory appears to be an underlying impairment, which may play a part in explaining difficulties in poor expressive language. An implicit learning route may be supporting receptive vocabulary among individuals with Down syndrome, where implicit learning leads to long-term recognition. Concordantly, Hulme and MacKenzie (1992) found a weaker correlation between phonological memory and receptive vocabulary among individuals with Down syndrome relative to what is observed in typical development (see also Jarrold et al., 2009; Laws, 1998). Among individuals with SLI and dyslexia, evidence is less supportive of a direct link between verbal working memory and expressive vocabulary, but may instead reflect poor processing of sequential information more generally (e.g., Hsu & Bishop, 2014; though see also Majerus et al., 2009 and Guiraud et al., 2018, for an alternative account).

Patterns of working memory performance across other groups with developmental disability also indicate that separate components of the working memory system can be impaired in different populations. A comparison is often drawn between individuals with Down syndrome and individuals with Williams syndrome, who, in contrast to the specific verbal working memory deficit associated with the Down syndrome population, show a specific deficit in visuospatial working memory, relative to less-impaired verbal working memory (Wang & Bellugi, 1994; Jarrold, Baddeley, & Hewes, 1999). The comparison between Down syndrome and Williams syndrome highlights that both verbal and visuospatial memory can be selectively impaired. Other developmental disabilities are rather associated with a general working memory deficit across domains; children and adolescents with fragile X syndrome (mean mental age: 5 years) have been found to experience both visuospatial and verbal working memory deficits (Lanfranchi, Cornoldi, Drigo, & Vianello, 2009). However, the working memory deficit among individuals with fragile X syndrome only appears to be present when the working memory task demands a high level of control, thus indicating an impairment in the control component of working memory. Additionally, Munir, Cornish, and Wilding (2000) found that children and adolescents with fragile X syndrome may have a limited attentional capacity relative to typically developing comparison children matched on verbal mental age (British Picture Vocabulary scale; Dunn et al., 1997). This deficit was also relative to individuals with Down syndrome at a similar chronological age as well as verbal mental age (mean mental age of 6.77 in fragile X group and 6.09 in Down syndrome group), indicating that greater impairments in attentional capacity and executive control are observed across domains among individuals with fragile X syndrome.

Thus, across different groups with developmental disability, impairment in working memory can occur at the level of specific domains (verbal or visual) or instead reflect a domain-general impairment in working memory control. Additionally, domain-general impairments potentially outside of the working memory system can lead to impaired working memory performance, where poor working memory is an indirect consequence of broader processing or attentional difficulties. These different levels of working memory impairment will all have effects on learning; however, understanding the underlying cause is key to targeting interventions appropriately. Among individuals with Down syndrome, the pattern of difficulties on working memory tasks appear to be driven by specific impairments within the working memory system itself, at the level of both storage and control. Thus, whereas interventions for groups such as SLI and dyslexia might be best focused on sequence learning or discrimination of input, and interventions for individuals with fragile X might be best focused on attention skills, interventions for individuals with Down syndrome need to be focused on directly addressing both verbal working memory storage difficulties and domain-general control difficulties.

Educational Implications and Future Directions

The pattern of difficulties in working memory among individuals with Down syndrome has been observed in groups consisting of children, adolescents, and adults (e.g., Carney et al. 2013; Frenkel & Bourdin, 2009; Jarrold et al., 2009; see also Godfrey & Lee, 2018, for a review). As difficulties in working memory do not appear to resolve over the course of development, early intervention is essential to support individuals as early as possible and maximize their learning potential. In their recent review, Godfrey and Lee (2018) note that there are no cognitive studies on working memory reported in preschool children and infants with Down syndrome because of a difficulty designing tasks that can capture working memory in these younger individuals. However, neurological research suggests that early differences in the brains of individuals with Down syndrome may be precursors for the emergent profile of working memory impairment seen in later childhood and adulthood (Edgin et al., 2015). In particular, Down syndrome appears to be associated with compromised development of the hippocampus, prefrontal cortex, and cerebellum, with some differences even observed in the brain prenatally (Edgin, 2013; see also Fidler, Daunhauer, Will, & Schworer, this volume). It has been suggested that early compromised hippocampal development may play a role in later patterns of memory impairment among groups with Down syndrome (Gomez & Edgin, 2016). Providing intervention as early as possible has the potential to alter brain development and to allow for possible cascading benefits. Routes such as minimizing sleeping difficulties early in development have been suggested to have the potential to alter brain development for individuals with Down syndrome. It is also essential to provide effective behavioral interventions as early as possible to allow young children to develop strategies in areas of difficulty such as verbal working memory. Supporting verbal working memory early in development may in turn improve expressive vocabulary and subsequent academic attainment more generally. One route may be to improve individuals' ability to attend to the temporal context of incoming verbal memoranda; this could involve techniques to increase attention to phonology and rhythm. Early intervention to target executive control among children with Down syndrome may also be very valuable given the evidence for subsequent links to academic development (see also Fidler, Daunhauer, Will, & Schworer, this volume).

Summary and Conclusion

In summary, individuals with Down syndrome tend to experience a specific pattern of impairment in working memory, which is not simply a reflection of their general cognitive ability. A specific deficit in verbal working memory is now a long-standing and consistent finding among the Down syndrome population, and this deficit appears to reflect limited memory for both item and order information. A domain-specific temporal processing deficit may offer a potential explanation for the limitations in storage for both item and order information in verbal working memory among individuals with Down syndrome. Other issues experienced by individuals with Down syndrome, such as poor hearing and phonological discrimination difficulties, may further compound individuals' verbal working memory performance.

Recent evidence points to the possibility of a domain-general ordering mechanism that, in addition to a verbal-specific temporal mechanism, supports serial recall in typically developing individuals. This proposed domain-general ordering mechanism appears to be in line with mental age among individuals with Down syndrome, in turn allowing for visuospatial serial recall performance that is in line with mental age.

In addition to a pattern of impaired working memory storage, individuals with Down syndrome also experience impaired control in working memory tasks. Different degrees of impairment across various components of executive control have been observed among persons with Down syndrome; this may, in part, reflect different measures and comparison groups being used across studies. It may also reflect differences in the nature of the tasks being used to compare different components of executive function within studies. Some aspects of executive control appear to be relatively less impaired than other areas among individuals with Down syndrome. Inhibition may be more in line with mental age in both childhood and adulthood than other executive functions, such as task switching. Future research is needed to determine the exact nature of executive control difficulties among individuals with Down syndrome over development and how this affects performance across working memory tasks.

Long-term memory knowledge appears to support working memory performance for individuals with Down syndrome, but the benefit is not as large as that seen among their typically developing peers. This may contribute to poorer working memory performance in individuals with Down syndrome relative to their peers. Verbal working memory is related to later vocabulary knowledge among individuals with Down syndrome. However, implicit learning may also be relied upon as an alternative route for obtaining long-term vocabulary knowledge where possible in this population.

These findings among individuals with Down syndrome inform us about working memory more generally. For example, separate components of the working memory system can be specifically impaired. While domain-general mechanisms may be in place for processing order information, verbal memoranda may be additionally supported by a domain-specific temporal processing mechanism. Likewise, the evidence from individuals with Down syndrome indicates that executive control may not necessarily be entirely constrained by general mental age, but rather that different components of control can be relatively stronger or weaker. Findings among individuals with Down syndrome also suggest that an implicit learning route for verbal information exists and that this may allow compensation in some areas of language learning (e.g., implicit learning of phoneme sequences may support receptive vocabulary) but perhaps not others; verbal working memory may be essential for effective phonological awareness and expressive language skills. This kind of analysis, informed by current theoretical approaches in the broader literature, helps us to be more specific about strengths and weaknesses in functioning and areas for future research; this is important given the crucial role of working memory in academic achievement and various day to day skills. Thus, understanding the underlying causes of working memory impairment among individuals with Down syndrome is essential and may indicate how best to support these individuals throughout their development.

References

Alloway, T. P. (2009). Working memory, but not IQ, predicts subsequent learning in children with learning difficulties. *European Journal of Psychological Assessment, 25*(2), 92–98.

Alloway, T. P., & Alloway, R. G. (2010). Investigating the predictive roles of working memory and IQ in academic attainment. *Journal of Experimental Child Psychology, 106*(1), 20–29.

Archibald, L. M., & Gathercole, S. E. (2006). Short-term and working memory in specific language impairment. *International Journal of Language & Communication Disorders, 41*(6), 675–693.

Baddeley, A. D. (1966). Short-term memory for word sequences as a function of acoustic, semantic and formal similarity. *Quarterly Journal of Experimental Psychology, 18*(4), 362–365.

Baddeley, A. D. (1986). *Working memory.* Oxford: Clarendon Press.

Baddeley, A. (2000). The episodic buffer: A new component of working memory? *Trends in Cognitive Science, 4*(11), 417–423.

Baddeley, A. (2003). Working memory and language: An overview. *Journal of Communication Disorders, 36*(3), 189–208.

Baddeley, A., Gathercole, S., & Papagno, C. (1998). The phonological loop as a language learning device. *Psychological Review, 105*(1), 158–173.

Baddeley, A. D., Grant, W., Wight, E., & Thomson, N. (1975). Imagery and visual working memory. *Attention and Performance, V,* 205–217.

Baddeley, A. D., & Hitch, G. (1974). Working memory. *Psychology of Learning and Motivation, 8,* 47–89.

Baddeley, A., & Jarrold, C. (2007). Working memory and Down syndrome. *Journal of Intellectual Disability Research, 51*(12), 925–931.

Bhatarah, P., Ward, G., Smith, J., & Hayes, L. (2009). Examining the relationship between free recall and immediate serial recall: Similar patterns of rehearsal and similar effects of word length, presentation rate, and articulatory suppression. *Memory & Cognition, 37*(5), 689–713.

Bishop, D. V., North, T., & Donlan, C. (1996). Nonword repetition as a behavioural marker for inherited language impairment: Evidence from a twin study. *Journal of child Psychology and Psychiatry, 37*(4), 391–403.

Bishop, D. V., & Snowling, M. J. (2004). Developmental dyslexia and specific language impairment: Same or different? *Psychological Bulletin, 130*(6), 858.

Borella, E., Carretti, B., & Lanfranchi, S. (2013). Inhibitory mechanisms in Down syndrome: Is there a specific or general deficit? *Research in Developmental Disabilities, 34*(1), 65–71.

Brock, J., & Jarrold, C. (2004). Language influences on verbal short-term memory performance in Down syndrome: Item and order recognition. *Journal of Speech Language and Hearing Research, 47*(6), 1334–1346.

Brock, J., & Jarrold, C. (2005). Serial order reconstruction in Down syndrome: Evidence for a selective deficit in verbal short-term memory. *Journal of Child Psychology and Psychiatry, 46*(3), 304–316.

Brown, G. D. A., Preece, T., & Hulme, C. (2000). Oscillator-based memory for serial order. *Psychological Review, 107*(1), 127–181.

Bull, R., Espy, K. A., & Wiebe, S. A. (2008). Short-term memory, working memory, and executive functioning in preschoolers: Longitudinal predictors of mathematical achievement at age 7 years. *Developmental Neuropsychology, 33*(3), 205–228.

Burns, D. J. (1996). The item-order distinction and the generation effect: The importance of order information in long-term memory. *American Journal of Psychology, 109*(4), 567–580.

Camos, V., Lagner, P., & Barrouillet, P. (2009). Two maintenance mechanisms of verbal information in working memory. *Journal of Memory and Language, 61*(3), 457–469.

Carney, D. P., Henry, L. A., Messer, D. J., Danielsson, H., Brown, J. H., & Rönnberg, J. (2013). Using developmental trajectories to examine verbal and visuospatial short-term memory development in children and adolescents with Williams and Down syndromes. *Research in Developmental Disabilities, 34*(10), 3421–3432.

Chapman, R. S., & Hesketh, L. J. (2000). Behavioral phenotype of individuals with Down syndrome. *Developmental Disabilities Research Reviews, 6*(2), 84–95.

Chapman, R. S., & Hesketh, L. J. (2001). Language, cognition, and short-term memory in individuals with Down syndrome. *Downs Syndrome Research and Practice, 7*(1), 1–7.

Chapman, R. S., & Kay-Raining Bird, E. (2012). Language development in childhood, adolescence, and young adulthood in persons with Down syndrome. In J. A. Burack, R. M. Hodapp, G. Iarocci, & E. Zigler (Eds.), *The Oxford Handbook of Intellectual Disability and Development* (pp. 167–183). New York, NY: Oxford University Press.

Chapman, R. S., Kay-Raining Bird, E., & Schwartz, S. E. (1990). Fast mapping of words in event contexts by children with Down syndrome. *Journal of Speech and Hearing Disorders, 55*(4), 761–770.

Chen, Z., & Cowan, N. (2009). Core verbal working memory capacity: The limit in words retained without covert articulation. *The Quarterly Journal of Experimental Psychology, 62*(7), 1420–1429.

Conrad, R., & Hull, A. J. (1964). Information, acoustic confusion and memory span. *British Journal of Psychology, 55*(4), 429–432.

Conti-Ramsden, G., & Hesketh, A. (2003). Risk markers for SLI: A study of young language-learning children. *International Journal of Language & Communication Disorders, 38*(3), 251–263.

Costanzo, F., Varuzza, C., Menghini, D., Addona, F., Gianesini, T., & Vicari, S. (2013). Executive functions in intellectual disabilities: A comparison between Williams syndrome and Down syndrome. *Research in Developmental Disabilities, 34*(5), 1770–1780.

Cowan, N. (1995). Attention and memory: An integrated framework. Oxford, UK: Oxford University Press.

Cowan, N. (2005). Working memory capacity. Hove, UK: Psychology Press.

Cowan, N. (2008). What are the differences between long-term, short-term, and working memory? *Progress in Brain Research, 169*, 323–338.

Cowan, N. (2010). The magical mystery four: How is working memory capacity limited, and why? *Current Directions in Psychological Science, 19*(1), 51–57.

Cowan, N., & Alloway, T. P. (2009). Development of working memory in childhood. In M. Courage & N. Cowan (Eds.), The development of memory in infancy and childhood (pp. 303–342). London: Psychology Press.

Daneman, M., & Carpenter, P. A. (1980). Individual differences in working memory and reading. *Journal of Verbal Learning and Verbal Behavior, 19*(4), 450–466.

DeLosh, E. L., & McDaniel, M. A. (1996). The role of order information in free recall: Application to the word-frequency effect. *Journal of Experimental Psychology-Learning Memory and Cognition, 22*(5), 1136–1146.

Dempster, F. N. (1981). Memory span: Sources of individual and developmental differences. *Psychological Bulletin, 89*, 63–100.

Depoorter, A., & Vandierendonck, A. (2009). Evidence for modality-independent order coding in working memory. *The Quarterly Journal of Experimental Psychology, 62*(3), 531–549.

Duarte, C. P., Covre, P., Braga, A. C., & de Macedo, E. C. (2011). Visuospatial support for verbal short-term memory in individuals with Down syndrome. *Research in Developmental Disabilities, 32*(5), 1918–1923.

Dunn, L. M., & Dunn, L. M. (1981). *Peabody Picture Vocabulary Test: Revised.* Circle Pines, MN: American Guidance Service.

Dunn, L. M., Dunn, L. M., Whetton, C., & Burley, J. (1997). *British Picture Vocabulary Scale Second Edition.* Windsor, England: NFER-Nelson.

Edgin, J. O. (2013). Cognition in Down syndrome: A developmental cognitive neuroscience perspective. *Wiley Interdisciplinary Reviews: Cognitive Science, 4*(3), 307–317.

Edgin, J. O., Clark, C. A. C., Massand, E., & Karmiloff-Smith, A. D. (2015). Building an adaptive brain across development: Targets for neurorehabilitation must begin in infancy. *Frontiers in Behavioral Neuroscience, 9*, 232.

Elliott, C. D. (1990). *Differential Ability Scales*. San Diego, CA: Harcourt, Brace, Jovanovich.

Evans, J. L., Saffran, J. R., & Robe-Torres, K. (2009). Statistical learning in children with specific language impairment. *Journal of Speech, Language, and Hearing Research, 52*(2), 321–335.

Farrell, S. (2012). Temporal clustering and sequencing in short-term memory and episodic memory. *Psychological Review, 119*(2), 223–271.

Farrell, S., & Oberauer, K. (2014). Working memory for cross-domain sequences. *The Quarterly Journal of Experimental Psychology, 67*(1), 33–44.

Fischer-Baum, S., & Benjamin, A. S. (2014). Time, space, and memory for order. *Psychonomic Bulletin & Review, 21*(5), 1263–1271.

Frenkel, S., & Bourdin, B. (2009). Verbal, visual, and spatio-sequential short-term memory: Assessment of the storage capacities of children and teenagers with Down's syndrome. *Journal of Intellectual Disability Research, 53*(2), 152–160.

Gathercole, S. E., & Baddeley, A. D. (1990). Phonological memory deficits in language disordered children: Is there a causal connection? *Journal of Memory and Language, 29*(3), 336–360.

Gathercole, S. E., Pickering, S. J., Knight, C., & Stegmann, Z. (2004). Working memory skills and educational attainment: Evidence from national curriculum assessments at 7 and 14 years of age. *Applied Cognitive Psychology, 18*(1), 1–16.

Gathercole, S. E., Service, E., Hitch, G. J., Adams, A.-M., & Martin, A. J. (1999). Phonological short-term memory and vocabulary development: Further evidence on the nature of the relationship. *Applied Cognitive Psychology, 13*(1), 65–77.

Giraud, A. L., Lorenzi, C., Ashburner, J., Wable, J., Johnsrude, I., Frackowiak, R., & Kleinschmidt, A. (2000). Representation of the temporal envelope of sounds in the human brain. *Journal of Neurophysiology, 84*(3), 1588–1598.

Godfrey, M., & Lee, N. R. (2018). Memory profiles in Down syndrome across development: A review of memory abilities through the lifespan. *Journal of Neurodevelopmental Disorders, 10*, 5.

Gómez, R. L., & Edgin, J. O. (2016). The extended trajectory of hippocampal development: Implications for early memory development and disorder. *Developmental Cognitive Neuroscience, 18*, 57–69.

Guiraud, H., Bedoin, N., Krifi-Papoz, S., Herbillon, V., Caillot-Bascoul, A., Gonzalez-Monge, S., & Boulenger, V. (2018). Don't speak too fast! Processing of fast rate speech in children with specific language impairment. *PloS one, 13*(1).

Hale, S., Myerson, J., Rhee, S. H., Weiss, C. S., & Abrams, R. A. (1996). Selective interference with the maintenance of location information in working memory. *Neuropsychology, 10*(2), 228–240.

Hamilton, A. C., & Martin, R. C. (2005). Dissociations among tasks involving inhibition: A single-case study. *Cognitive, Affective, & Behavioral Neuroscience, 5*(1), 1–13.

Hebb, D. O. (1961). Brain mechanisms and learning. In J. F. Delafresnaye (Ed.), *Distinctive features of learning in the higher animal* (pp. 37–46). New York, NY: Oxford University Press.

Hick, R. F., Botting, N., & Conti-Ramsden, G. (2005). Short-term memory and vocabulary development in children with Down syndrome and children with specific language impairment. *Developmental Medicine & Child Neurology, 47*(8), 532–538.

Hsu, H. J., & Bishop, D. V. (2014). Sequence-specific procedural learning deficits in children with specific language impairment. *Developmental Science, 17*(3), 352–365.

Hulme, C., & Mackenzie, S. (1992). *Working memory and severe learning difficulties*. Hillsdale, NJ: Lawrence Erlbaum.

Hulme, C., Maughan, S., & Brown, G. D. A. (1991). Memory for familiar and unfamiliar words: Evidence for a long-term memory contribution to short-term memory span. *Journal of Memory and Language, 30*(6), 685–701.

Hurlstone, M. J., Hitch, G. J., & Baddeley, A. D. (2014). Memory for serial order across domains: An overview of the literature and directions for future research. *Psychological Bulletin, 140*(2), 339.

Jacoby, L. L. (1991). A process dissociation framework—separating automatic from intentional uses of memory. *Journal of Memory and Language, 30*(5), 513–541.

Jarrold, C., & Baddeley, A. D. (1997). Short-term memory for verbal and visuospatial information in Down's syndrome. *Cognitive Neuropsychiatry, 2*(2), 101–122.

Jarrold, C., & Baddeley, A. (2001). Short-term memory in Down syndrome: Applying the working memory model. *Down Syndrome Research and Practice, 7*(1), 17–23.

Jarrold, C., Baddeley, A. D., & Hewes, A. K. (1999). Genetically dissociated components of working memory: Evidence from Down's and Williams syndrome. *Neuropsychologia, 37*, 637–651. doi:10.1016/S0028-3932(98)00128-6

Jarrold, C., Baddeley, A. D., & Hewes, A. K. (2000). Verbal short-term memory deficits in Down syndrome: A consequence of problems in rehearsal? *Journal of Child Psychology and Psychiatry and Allied Disciplines, 41*(2), 233–244.

Jarrold, C., Baddeley, A., & Phillips, C. (1999). Down syndrome and the phonological loop: The evidence for, and importance of, a specific verbal short-term memory deficit. *Down Syndrome Research and Practice, 6*(2), 61–75.

Jarrold, C., Baddeley, A. D., & Phillips, C. E. (2002). Verbal short-term memory in Down syndrome: A problem of memory, audition, or speech? *Journal of Speech, Language, and Hearing Research, 45*(3), 531–544.

Jarrold, C., Baddeley, A. D., & Phillips, C. (2007). Long-term memory for verbal and visual information in Down syndrome and Williams syndrome: Performance on the Doors and People Test. *Cortex, 43*(2), 233–247.

Jarrold, C., Cowan, N., Hewes, A. K., & Riby, D. M. (2004). Speech timing and verbal short-term memory: Evidence for contrasting deficits in Down syndrome and Williams syndrome. *Journal of Memory and Language, 51*(3), 365–380.

Jarrold, C., Hall, D., Harvey, C. E., Tam, H., Towse, J. N., & Zarandi, A. L. (2014). What can we learn about immediate memory from the development of children's free recall? *The Quarterly Journal of Experimental Psychology, 68*, 1871–1894.

Jarrold, C., Tam, H., Baddeley, A. D., & Harvey, C. E. (2011). How does processing affect storage in working memory tasks? Evidence for both domain-general and domain-specific effects. *Journal of Experimental Psychology: Learning, Memory, and Cognition, 37*(3), 688–705.

Jarrold, C., Thorn, A. S., & Stephens, E. (2009). The relationships among verbal short-term memory, phonological awareness, and new word learning: Evidence from typical development and Down syndrome. *Journal of Experimental Child psychology, 102*(2), 196–218.

Jarrold, C., & Towse, J. N. (2006). Individual differences in working memory. *Neuroscience, 139*(1), 39–50.

Jones, D., Farrand, P., Stuart, G., & Morris, N. (1995). Functional equivalence of verbal and spatial information in serial short-term memory. *Journal of Experimental Psychology: Learning, Memory, and Cognition, 21*(4), 1008.

Karmiloff-Smith, A. (2013). Challenging the use of adult neuropsychological models for explaining neurodevelopmental disorders: Developed versus developing brains. *The Quarterly Journal of Experimental Psychology, 66*, 1–14. doi:10.1080/17470218.2012.744424

Karr, J. E., Areshenkoff, C. N., Rast, P., Hofer, S. M., Iverson, G. L., & Garcia-Barrera, M. A. (2018). The unity and diversity of executive functions: A systematic review and re-analysis of latent variable studies. *Psychological Bulletin, 144*(11), 1147–1185.

Kaufman, A. S., & Kaufman, N. L. (1993). *Kaufman Adolescent and Adult Intelligence Test (KAIT)*. Circle Pines, MN: American Guidance Service.

Kay-Raining Bird, E., & Chapman, R. S. (1994). Sequential recall in individuals with Down syndrome. *Journal of Speech, Language, and Hearing Research, 37*(6), 1369–1380.

Kyllonen, P. C., & Christal, R. E. (1990). Reasoning ability is (little more than) working memory capacity?! *Intelligence, 14*(4), 389–433.

Lanfranchi, S., Carretti, B., Spanò, G., & Cornoldi, C. (2009). A specific deficit in visuospatial simultaneous working memory in Down syndrome. *Journal of Intellectual Disability Research, 53*(5), 474–483.

Lanfranchi, S., Cornoldi, C., Drigo, S., & Vianello, R. (2009). Working memory in individuals with fragile X syndrome. *Child Neuropsychology, 15*(2), 105–119.

Lanfranchi, S., Cornoldi, C., & Vianello, R. (2004). Verbal and visuospatial working memory deficits in children with Down syndrome. *American Journal on Mental Retardation, 109*(6), 456–466.

Lanfranchi, S., Jerman, O., Dal Pont, E., Alberti, A., & Vianello, R. (2010). Executive function in adolescents with Down syndrome. *Journal of Intellectual Disability Research, 54*(4), 308–319.

Lanfranchi, S., Jerman, O., & Vianello, R. (2009). Working memory and cognitive skills in individuals with Down syndrome. *Child Neuropsychology, 15*(4), 397–416.

Lautarescu, B. A., Holland, A. J., & Zaman, S. H. (2017). The early presentation of dementia in people with down syndrome: A systematic review of longitudinal studies. *Neuropsychology Review, 27*(1), 31–45.

Laws, G. (1998). The use of nonword repetition as a test of phonological memory in children with Down syndrome. *Journal of Child Psychology and Psychiatry, 39*, 1119–1130.

Laws, G., & Bishop, D. V. M. (2003). A comparison of language abilities in adolescents with Down syndrome and children with specific language impairment. *Journal of Speech Language and Hearing Research, 46*(6), 1324–1339.

Laws, G., & Bishop, D. V. (2004). Verbal deficits in Down's syndrome and specific language impairment: A comparison. *International Journal of Language & Communication Disorders, 39*(4), 423–451.

Laws, G., Briscoe, J., Ang, S.-Y., Brown, H., Hermena, E., & Kapikian, A. (2015). Receptive vocabulary and semantic knowledge in children with SLI and children with Down syndrome. *Child Neuropsychology, 21*(4), 490–508.

Laws, G., & Gunn, D. (2004). Phonological memory as a predictor of language comprehension in Down syndrome: a five-year follow-up study. *Journal of Child Psychology and Psychiatry, 45*(2), 326–337.

Lee, N. R., Anand, P., Will, E., Adeyemi, E. I., Clasen, L. S., Blumenthal, J. D., . . . & Edgin, J. O. (2015). Everyday executive functions in Down syndrome from early childhood to young adulthood: evidence for both unique and shared characteristics compared to youth with sex chromosome trisomy (XXX and XXY). *Frontiers in Behavioral Neuroscience, 9*.

Lee, N. R., Pennington, B. F., & Keenan, J. M. (2010). Verbal short-term memory deficits in Down syndrome: Phonological, semantic, or both? *Journal of Neurodevelopmental Disorders, 2*(1), 9–25.

Logie, R. H., Gilhooly, K. J., & Wynn, V. (1994). Counting on working memory in arithmetic problem solving. *Memory & Cognition, 22*(4), 395–410.

Logie, R. H., Saito, S., Morita, A., Varma, S., & Norris, D. (2016). Recalling visual serial order for verbal sequences. *Memory & Cognition, 44*, 590.

Lum, J. A., Gelgic, C., & Conti-Ramsden, G. (2010). Procedural and declarative memory in children with and without specific language impairment. *International Journal of Language & Communication Disorders, 45*(1), 96–107.

Majerus, S., & Barisnikov, K. (2018). Verbal short-term memory shows a specific association with receptive but not productive vocabulary measures in Down syndrome. *Journal of Intellectual Disability Research, 62*, 10–20. doi:10.1111/jir.12443

Majerus, S., Leclercq, A. L., Grossmann, A., Billard, C., Touzin, M., Van der Linden, M., & Poncelet, M. (2009). Serial order short-term memory capacities and specific language impairment: No evidence for a causal association. *Cortex, 45*(6), 708–720.

Majerus, S., Poncelet, M., Greffe, C., & Van der Linden, M. (2006). Relations between vocabulary development and verbal short-term memory: The relative importance of short-term memory for serial order and item information. *Journal of Experimental Child Psychology, 93*(2), 95–119.

Majerus, S., Poncelet, M., Van der Linden, M., Albouy, G., Salmon, E., Sterpenich, V., . . . Maquet, P. (2006). The left intraparietal sulcus and verbal short-term memory: Focus of attention or serial order? *Neuroimage, 32*(2), 880–891.

Marcell, M. M., & Armstrong, V. (1982). Auditory and visual sequential memory of Down syndrome and nonretarded children. *American Journal of Mental Deficiency, 87*(1), 86–95.

Marcell, M. M., Harvey, C. F., & Cothran, L. P. (1988). An attempt to improve auditory short-term memory in Down's syndrome individuals through reducing distractions. *Research in Developmental Disabilities, 9*(4), 405–417.

Marcell, M. M. & Weeks, S. L. (1988). Short-term memory difficulties and Down's syndrome. *Journal of Mental Deficiency Research*, 32, 153–162.

Miller, G. A. (1956). The magical number seven, plus or minus two: Some limits on our capacity for processing information. *Psychological Review, 63*(2), 81–97.

Miyake, A., Friedman, N. P., Emerson, M. J., Witzki, A. H., Howerter, A., & Wager, T. D. (2000). The unity and diversity of executive functions and their contributions to complex "frontal lobe" tasks: A latent variable analysis. *Cognitive Psychology, 41*(1), 49–100.

Morey, C. C., & Cowan, N. (2005). When do visual and verbal memories conflict? The importance of working memory load and retrieval. *Journal of Experimental Psychology: Learning, Memory, and Cognition, 31*(4), 703.

Morey, C. C., & Mall, J. T. (2012). Cross-domain interference costs during concurrent verbal and spatial serial memory tasks are asymmetric. *The Quarterly Journal of Experimental Psychology, 65*(9), 1777–1797.

Mosse, E. K., & Jarrold, C. (2010). Searching for the Hebb effect in Down syndrome: Evidence for a dissociation between verbal short-term memory and domain-general learning of serial order. *Journal of Intellectual Disability Research, 54*(4), 295–307.

Mosse, E. K., & Jarrold, C. (2011). Evidence for preserved novel word learning in Down syndrome suggests multiple routes to vocabulary acquisition. *Journal of Speech, Language, and Hearing Research, 54*(4), 1137–1152.

Munir, F., Cornish, K. M., & Wilding, J. (2000). Nature of the working memory deficit in fragile-X syndrome. *Brain and Cognition, 44*(3), 387–401.

Munson, B., Edwards, J., & Beckman, M. E. (2005). Relationships between nonword repetition accuracy and other measures of linguistic development in children with phonological disorders. *Journal of Speech, Language and Hearing Research, 48*, 61–78.

Næss, K. A. B., Lyster, S. A. H., Hulme, C., & Melby-Lervåg, M. (2011). Language and verbal short-term memory skills in children with Down syndrome: A meta-analytic review. *Research in Developmental Disabilities, 32*(6), 2225–2234.

Nairne, J. S., & Kelley, M. R. (2004). Separating item and order information through process dissociation. *Journal of Memory and Language, 50*(2), 113–133.

Neath, I. (1997). Modality, concreteness, and set-size effects in a free reconstruction of order task. *Memory & Cognition, 25*(2), 256–263.

Nee, D. E., Wager, T. D., & Jonides, J. (2007). Interference resolution: Insights from a meta-analysis of neuroimaging tasks. *Cognitive, Affective, & Behavioral Neuroscience, 7*(1), 1–17.

Norris, D. (2017). Short-term memory and long-term memory are still different. *Psychological Bulletin, 143*, 992–1009.

Oberauer, K. (2002). Access to information in working memory: Exploring the focus of attention. *Journal of Experimental Psychology: Learning, Memory, and Cognition, 28*(3), 411.

Oberauer, K. (2009). Design for a working memory. *Psychology of Learning and Motivation, 51*, 45–100.

Ordonez Magro, L., Attout, L., Majerus, S., & Szmalec, A. (2018). Short-and long-term memory determinants of novel word form learning. *Cognitive Development, 47*, 146–157. doi:10.1016/j.cogdev.2018.06.002

Packwood, S., Hodgetts, H. M., & Tremblay, S. (2011). A multiperspective approach to the conceptualization of executive functions. *Journal of Clinical and Experimental Neuropsychology, 33*(4), 456–470.

Page, M. P. A., & Norris, D. (2009). A model linking immediate serial recall, the Hebb repetition effect and the learning of phonological word forms. *Philosophical Transactions of the Royal Society of London B: Biological Sciences, 364*(1536), 3737–3753.

Paivio, A., Clark, J., & Khan, M. (1988). Effects of concreteness and semantic relatedness on composite imagery ratings and cued recall. *Memory & Cognition, 16*(5), 422–430.

Pennington, B. F., Moon, J., Edgin, J., Stedron, J., & Nadel, L. (2003). The neuropsychology of Down syndrome: Evidence for hippocampal dysfunction. *Child development, 74*(1), 75–93.

Poirier, M., Dhir, P., Saint-Aubin, J., Tehan, G., & Hampton, J. (2011). The Influence of Semantic Memory on Verbal Short-term Memory. In B. Kokinov, A. Karmiloff-Smith, & N. J. Nersessian (Eds.), *European Perspectives on Cognitive Science*. Sofia, Bulgaria: New Bulgarian University Press.

Poirier, M., & Saint-Aubin, J. (1996). Immediate serial recall, word frequency, item identity and item position. *Canadian Journal of Experimental Psychology, 50*(4), 408–412.

Purser, H. R. M., & Jarrold, C. (2005). Impaired verbal short-term memory in Down syndrome reflects a capacity limitation rather than atypically rapid forgetting. *Journal of Experimental Child Psychology, 91*(1), 1–23.

Raven, J., Raven, J. C., & Court, J. H. (1998). Coloured progressive matrices. Oxford, UK: Oxford University Press.

Rice, M. L., Warren, S. F., & Betz, S. K. (2005). Language symptoms of developmental language disorders: An overview of autism, Down syndrome, fragile X, specific language impairment, and Williams syndrome. *Applied Psycholinguistics, 26*(1), 7–27.

Roid, G. H., & Miller, L. J. (1997). *Leiter International Performance Scale—Revised: Examiner's manual.* Wood Dale, IL: Stoelting.

Roodenrys, S., Hulme, C., Lethbridge, A., Hinton, M., & Nimmo, L. M. (2002). Word-frequency and phonological-neighborhood effects on verbal short-term memory. *Journal of Experimental Psychology: Learning, Memory, and Cognition, 28*(6), 1019–1034.

Rosin, M. M., Swift, E., Bless, D., & Kluppel Vetter, D. (1988). Communication profiles of adolescents with Down syndrome. *Journal of Childhood Communication Disorders, 12*(1), 49–64.

Rowe, J., Lavender, A., & Turk, V. (2006). Cognitive executive function in Down's syndrome. *British Journal of Clinical Psychology, 45*(1), 5–17.

Saito, S., Logie, R. H., Morita, A., & Law, A. (2008). Visual and phonological similarity effects in verbal immediate serial recall: A test with kanji materials. *Journal of Memory and Language, 59*(1), 1–17.

Seung, H. K., & Chapman, R. (2000). Digit span in individuals with Down syndrome and in typically developing children: Temporal aspects. *Journal of Speech Language and Hearing Research, 43*(3), 609–620.

Soemer, A., & Saito, S. (2016). Domain-specific processing in short-term serial order memory. *Journal of Memory and Language, 88*, 1–17.

Smith, E., Hedge, C., & Jarrold, C. (2019). A novel framework to measure executive function in Down syndrome, with applications for early clinical diagnosis of dementia. *American Journal on Intellectual and Developmental Disabilities, 124*(4), 354–373. https://doi.org/10.1352/1944-7558-124.4.354

Smith, E., & Jarrold, C. (2014a). Demonstrating the effects of phonological similarity and frequency on item and order memory in Down syndrome using process dissociation. *Journal of Experimental Child Psychology, 128*, 69–87.

Smith, E., & Jarrold, C. (2014b). Grouping, semantic relation and imagery effects in individuals with Down syndrome. *Research in Developmental Disabilities, 35*(11), 3162–3174.

Smith-Spark, J. H., & Fisk, J. E. (2007). Working memory functioning in developmental dyslexia. *Memory, 15*(1), 34–56.

Stavroussi, P., Andreou, G., & Karagiannopoulou, D. (2016). Verbal Fluency and Verbal Short-Term Memory in Adults with Down Syndrome and Unspecified Intellectual Disability. *International Journal of Disability, Development and Education, 63*(1), 122–139.

Szmalec, A., Loncke, M., Page, M., & Duyck, W. (2011). Order or disorder? Impaired Hebb learning in dyslexia. *Journal of Experimental Psychology: Learning, Memory, and Cognition, 37*(5), 1270.

Tomblin, J. B., Mainela-Arnold, E., & Zhang, X. (2007). Procedural learning in adolescents with and without specific language impairment. *Language Learning and Development, 3*, 269–293.

Toms, M., Morris, N., & Foley, P. (1994). Characteristics of visual interference with visuospatial working memory. *British Journal of Psychology, 85*(1), 131–144.

Ullman, M. T., & Pierpont, E. I. (2005). Specific language impairment is not specific to language: The procedural deficit hypothesis. *Cortex, 41*(3), 399–433.

Vallar, G., & Baddeley, A. D. (1984). Phonological short-term store, phonological processing and sentence comprehension: A neuropsychological case study. *Cognitive Neuropsychology, 1*(2), 121–141.

Vallar, G., & Papagno, C. (1993). Preserved vocabulary acquisition in Down's syndrome: The role of phonological short-term memory. *Cortex, 29*(3), 467–483.

Vandierendonck, A. (2016). Modality independence of order coding in working memory: Evidence from cross-modal order interference at recall. *The Quarterly Journal of Experimental Psychology, 69*(1), 161–179.

van Dijck, J.-P., Abrahamse, E. L., Majerus, S., & Fias, W. (2013). Spatial attention interacts with serial-order retrieval from verbal working memory. *Psychological Science, 24*(9), 1854–1859.

van Dijck, J.-P., & Fias, W. (2011). A working memory account for spatial–numerical associations. *Cognition, 119*(1), 114–119.

Vianello R. & Marin M. L. (1997). OLC: Operazioni Logiche e Conservazione. Progetto MS. Junior, Bergamo.

Vicari, S., Carlesimo, A., & Caltagirone, C. (1995). Short-term memory in persons with intellectual disabilities and Down's syndrome. *Journal of Intellectual Disability Research, 39*(6), 532–537.

Vicari, S., Marotta, L., & Carlesimo, G. A. (2004). Verbal short-term memory in Down's syndrome: An articulatory loop deficit? *Journal of Intellectual Disability Research, 48*, 80–92.

Wang, P. P., & Bellugi, U. (1994). Evidence from two genetic syndromes for a dissociation between verbal and visual-spatial short-term memory. *Journal of Clinical and Experimental Neuropsychology, 16*, 317–322. doi:10.1080/01688639408402641

Wang, X., Xuan, Y., & Jarrold, C. (2016). Using a process dissociation approach to assess verbal short-term memory for item and order information in a sample of individuals with a self-reported diagnosis of dyslexia. *Frontiers in Psychology, 7*.

Ward, G., Tan, L., & Grenfell-Essam, R. (2010). Examining the relationship between free recall and immediate serial recall: The effects of list length and output order. *Journal of Experimental Psychology: Learning, Memory, and Cognition, 36*(5), 1207.

Wechsler, D. (2002). Escalas de Inteligência Wechsler para Crianças: Manual (3rd ed.|V. L. Marques de Figueiredo, Adaptação e padronização brasileira). São Paulo, SP: Casa do Psicólogo.

Wickelgren, W. A. (1965). Short-Term-Memory for Phonemically Similar Lists. *American Journal of Psychology, 78*(4), 567–574.

Will, E., Fidler, D. J., Daunhauer, L., & Gerlach-McDonald, B. (2017). Executive function and academic achievement in primary–grade students with Down syndrome. *Journal of Intellectual Disability Research, 61*(2), 181–195.

CHAPTER

13 Executive Function in Down Syndrome: Links to Adaptation and Treatment Implications

Deborah J. Fidler, Lisa A. Daunhauer, Emily Schworer, *and* Lina Patel

Abstract

This chapter presents a review of existing research on the presentation of executive function in persons with Down syndrome. Contemporary scientific work regarding the development of executive function in persons with Down syndrome is reviewed, with an emphasis on profiles associated with childhood, adolescence, and adulthood. The valid assessment of executive function and methodological considerations are also discussed, including the importance of developing phenotype-sensitive and reliable measures of executive function that account for the broader profile of strengths and challenges associated with Down syndrome. Future areas of research are identified that can inform intervention approaches to target the development of goal-directed behavior and adaptation in this population.

Key Words: executive function, cognitive phenotype, Down syndrome, assessment, intervention

Executive Function in Down Syndrome: Links to Adaptation and Treatment Implications

While global cognitive delays have been a hallmark feature of Down syndrome (DS) since early characterizations of the condition in the scientific literature, advances in the study of neurodevelopmental pathways in DS have led to a more refined understanding of critical aspects of the DS cognitive phenotype. Neuropathology studies of humans with DS and mouse models of DS have characterized the pronounced impact of DS on particular neural structures, including the prefrontal cortex (Edgin, Pennington, & Mervis, 2010; Nadel, 2003; Reeves & Garner, 2007). This aspect of the neuroanatomical phenotype in DS is implicated in the cognitive challenges associated with DS, particularly in the area of executive function.

Executive function (EF) refers to a set of cognitive processes that facilitate purposeful, regulated behavior. Throughout the lifespan, EF is increasingly used across settings to reach goals that vary in complexity—from packing a lunch to solving a math problem. While the scientific discussion continues regarding the specific architecture of EF, most frameworks include the constructs of working memory (see Smith & Jarrold, this volume), cognitive flexibility, inhibitory control, and planning, among other cognitive functions. It is the interplay between EF component processes that make it possible for individuals to organize their behavior in ongoing ways to reach goals throughout their day. Amid the continuing theoretical conversations regarding EF, there is converging evidence for the practical importance of EF as a set of skills that emerges early in development. To date, EF has been linked to academic achievement (Best, Miller, & Naglieri, 2011; Blair & Razza, 2007), health behaviors (Riggs, Huh, Chou, Spruijt-Metz, & Pentz, 2012), and adaptive behavior (Gilotty, Kenworthy, Sirian, Black, & Wagner, 2002; Pugliese et al., 2016; Ware et al., 2012), and these associations have also been demonstrated in studies of individuals with DS (Daunhauer, Gerlach-McDonald, Will, & Fidler, 2017; Tomaszewski, Fidler, Talapatra, & Riley, 2018; Will, Fidler, Daunhauer, & Gerlach-McDonald, 2017).

In the broader field of lifespan development, there is clear evidence for the influential role of EF development during childhood, with a recognition of EF as an important construct impacting outcomes in clinical populations such as autism spectrum disorder (ASD) and attention deficit and hyperactivity disorder (ADHD; Biederman et al., 2004; Lawson et al., 2015; Rosenthal et al., 2013). Growth in this area of research has generated insights regarding a DS-specific profile of strengths and challenges in EF in childhood and throughout the lifespan that has shed new light on our basic understanding of the DS cognitive phenotype. There is also recent evidence relating EF to critical adaptation outcomes among persons with DS (Daunhauer, Fidler, & Will, 2014; Tomaszewski et al., 2018; Will et al., 2017), as has been reported in children without DS, suggesting that effective EF intervention in DS will have an important impact on quality of life in this population. However, despite these findings, researchers have faced methodological issues and other challenges related to the study of EF in DS that must be addressed for a richer understanding of this construct to emerge in this population.

In this chapter, we review the current conceptualizations of the construct of EF, highlighting specific topics of relevance for persons with DS. We will then present a review of the current state of knowledge regarding the development of EF from childhood to adulthood in persons with DS, its implications for outcomes of interest and intervention, and methodological issues to be addressed in future research.

Overview of Recent Conceptualizations of Executive Function

While the majority of individuals with DS experience global developmental delays, the study of EF among persons with DS has begun to offer an important window into the link between cognitive delays and everyday functioning in this group. Researchers in developmental science and allied disciplines have continued to refine our understanding of EF and have continued to pose new questions. With the understanding that much of this work continues to evolve, our most recent understanding of EF converges on the following ideas.

1. EF involves higher-order regulation of lower-level processes. A defining feature of EF and its component processes is that they involve top-down control of other cognitive, emotional, and behavioral processes (Müller & Kerns, 2015). This type of higher-order regulation is necessary for an individual to exert control over their behavior—to refrain from automatic responses, to keep track of the status of a task to see it through to completion, and to flexibly try different strategies to reach a goal. While the prefrontal cortex is widely understood to be a critical region for EF, different aspects of regulatory control are thought to be associated with different neuroanatomical subregions. The dorsolateral prefrontal cortex plays an active role in supporting working memory and cognitive flexibility, while the orbitofrontal cortex is thought to play a more active role in impulse control (Müller & Kerns, 2015).

2. EF component processes appear to be dissociable but related to one another (Miyake et al., 2000). Numerous component processes contribute to the top-down control exerted by EF, including working memory, inhibition, cognitive flexibility, and planning. Additional constructs that are included in various models of EF include aspects of attention regulation, verbal and visual-design fluency, and task monitoring, among others (Friedman & Miyake, 2017). While these processes are recruited in concert with one another during goal-directed behavior, component EF processes appear to develop somewhat independently of one another. Within current models of EF, low correlations are observed between performances on various EF tasks in which specific component processes are emphasized, suggesting dissociability between these different domains. Friedman and Miyake (2017) note that several possible factors contribute to this lack of association beyond dissociability, including issues related to measurement. For example, certain EF measures may lack psychometric validity/reliability, leading to diverging, unassociated performances across tasks. The perpetual challenges presented by task impurity also likely account for the lack of association observed on different types of EF tasks, in that an assessment of EF component processes are likely to include additional cognitive elements (temporal processing, visual processing) or other EF component processes.

Despite the evidence of dissociability of EF processes, Miyake et al. (2000) have reported that latent factors can be observed across tasks and that these factors show evidence of a more unified EF architecture. Using latent variable modeling, a methodological approach used to identify the common variance among different measures, Miyake et al. observed latent variables that corresponded to underlying EF constructs. They also reported that EF component latent variables were more strongly correlated with one another than performances on individual tasks, suggesting that EF components are more integrated than would be suggested by simple examinations of inter-task association (Miyake et al., 2000). Moreover, there appears to be a developmental component to the architecture of EF, in that EF performance patterns are more unified during early childhood, but dissociability among EF component processes becomes more pronounced during middle childhood (Brydges, Fox, Reid, & Anderson, 2014; Wiebe et al., 2011).

3. EF emerges during early childhood and continues to develop throughout adolescence and early adulthood. While EF is a construct of interest across the lifespan, developmental researchers have closely examined the specific sequence of acquired EF capabilities during the preschool years. Findings from this extensive work indicate that most typically developing (TD) children develop the ability to use rules flexibly, resist prepotent behaviors, and plan/sequence actions for goal-directed purposes between the ages of 3 and 5 years (Carlson, 2005). Also, the presentation of EF during early childhood tends to predict aspects of adaptation, with individual differences in EF often showing continuity over time (Carlson, Mandell, & Williams, 2004). Only recently, however, have researchers begun to inquire about the foundational cognitive abilities that precede these developmental changes in EF during the preschool years (Hendry et al., 2016). In particular, early attention regulation, processing speed, rudimentary cognitive flexibility, and early self-regulation have been identified as early precursors that may be important foundations for the emergence of EF competences during the first 5 years (Hendry et al., 2016). More comprehensive accounts of continuity from early infant neuropsychological processing into EF performance in preschool and beyond will likely be an active area of future research.

4. Impairments in EF occur in numerous neurodevelopmental conditions, often with specific patterns of relative competences and pronounced impairments (Russo, Dawkins, Huizinga, & Burack, 2012). Because numerous dissociable EF constructs work in concert with one another, the atypical presentation of EF is prone to vary in accordance with different neurodevelopmental presentations. It follows, then, that the phenotypic presentation of EF profiles can differ in both subtle and pronounced ways across individuals with different types of diagnostic conditions. As Ozonoff and Jensen (1999) described, based on patterns of task performance, individuals with ASD can be characterized as demonstrating predominating difficulty in the EF domain of cognitive flexibility. In contrast, EF inhibition challenges are more likely observed in individuals with ADHD (Ozonoff & Jensen, 1999), and difficulties have been linked to specific patterns of atypical activation in the prefrontal cortex and cingulate gyrus during tasks that involve inhibitory control and error detection in this population (Rubia, Smith, Brammer, Toone, & Taylor, 2005). As will be described in greater depth below, DS predisposes individuals to global delays in the development of EF as well as to more pronounced difficulties with working memory and planning than would be expected based on developmental status (Daunhauer, Fidler, Hahn, et al., 2014; Lee et al., 2011; Smith & Jarrold, this volume).

5. EF can be measured in laboratory settings or via self/proxy report, but these approaches may assess different aspects of EF. Just as the scientific conceptualization of EF has evolved, approaches to EF assessment have undergone extensive examination and discussion. The two general approaches to the assessment of EF carry with them different sets of advantages and disadvantages. The direct assessment approach, which is conducted using either standardized assessments or laboratory measures, has the advantage of carefully controlling numerous factors, including the isolation of specific EF components through the selection of complementary tasks, and the objectivity of independent raters of performance. However, direct assessment in laboratory conditions can be considered "too controlled," and lacking in ecological validity (Chaytor, Schmitter-Edgecombe, & Burr, 2006), raising issues regarding the generalizability and utility of performances observed. In addition, even when conducted under a carefully controlled set of conditions, laboratory assessment may be confounded by performance anxiety with an unknown examiner, or task impurity wherein EF tasks may be influenced by other cognitive domains, such as visuospatial processing (Müller & Kerns, 2015).

In contrast to laboratory-based assessment of EF, standardized self- and proxy-report measures have been developed to probe for performance on EF-related tasks in everyday situations (Chan, Shum, Toulopoulou, & Chen, 2008). These measures, such as the Behavior Rating Inventory of Executive Function (BRIEF; Gioia, Espy, & Isquith, 2003; Gioia, Isquith, Guy, & Kenworthy, 2000), are focused on contextual EF performance based on the developmental level of those being assessed, such that preschool-aged children are administered questions regarding the use of EF skills during play and preschool learning, and adults are asked about EF performance in work and leisure time activities. While self- and proxy-report measures have the advantage of ecological validity, they face concerns regarding reporter bias. Specifically, reporter perceptions of normative functioning on a given task may vary, and the expectations that a reporter has regarding what is an acceptable performance in a specific area may differ (e.g., Daunhauer, Fidler, Hahn, et al., 2014; Mares, McLuckie, Schwartz, & Saini, 2007). Thus, while self- and proxy-report measures and direct assessment approaches both capture EF skills, they are increasingly thought to measure different aspects of EF (efficiency of processing versus successful goal-pursuit; Toplak, West, & Stanovitch, 2013) as scores on similar domains of functioning have been found to be only modestly or minimally correlated with one another (e.g., Daunhauer et al., 2017; Toplak et al., 2013).

Cognitive Phenotype Associated with Down Syndrome

While DS predisposes individuals to global developmental delays, the neurocognitive phenotype associated with DS involves a complex pattern of areas of relative strength and challenge across numerous domains of information processing (as reviewed in several chapters in this volume). Some aspects of this phenotypic profile have been well-studied over the past several decades, including the contrast between visual and verbal processing, implicit versus explicit memory, and short-term memory difficulties (Carlesimo, Marotta, & Vicari, 1997; Jarrold & Baddeley, 1997; Vicari, Bellucci & Carlesimo, 2000; for reviews, see Jarrold & Brock, 2012; Vicari, 2012). Similarly, EF (Russo et al., 2012) is becoming better understood with new research generated in the past decade.

Despite the recent nature of interest in EF in persons with DS, the broader topic of goal-directed behavior has been a focus of the DS literature for several decades. Some of the earliest work examined this issue from a temperament perspective, with evidence from parent report studies indicating that children with DS are less persistent and more distractible than other children (Gunn & Berry, 1985; Gunn & Cuskelly, 1991). Other researchers have addressed aspects of this issue from a sensory processing perspective, with converging reports of "low registration," "low energy/weak," or "underresponsive/seeks sensation" in school-aged children with DS (Bruni, Cameron, Dua, & Noy, 2010; Wuang & Su, 2011). When this issue has been examined through the lens of behavioral presentations in persons with DS, the findings have indicated increased levels of noncompliance associated with less adaptive outcomes (Patti & Tsiouris, 2006; Will et al., 2017).

While temperament, behavioral compliance, and sensory issues each address important related constructs, the issue of goal-directed behavior in persons with DS has been examined most directly from a motivation-orientation perspective (Fidler, 2006; Gunn & Berry, 1985; Wishart, 2001). Studies in this area were rooted in the foundational personality-motivation work that was focused on individuals with intellectual disability (then "mental retardation") more broadly, as research on individuals with intellectual disability moved beyond the simple study of cognitive impairments (Zigler & Burack, 1989; Zigler & Hodapp, 1986). DS specific work from this perspective is primarily focused on mastery-motivation, or the degree to which an individual is internally driven to engage with their environment in effective ways (Morgan, Harmon, & Maslin-Cole., 1990). Studies within this framework were initially focused on decreased levels of mastery motivation in persons with DS. For toddlers with DS, Ruskin, Mundy, Kasari, and Sigman (1994) described a profile of less engagement in goal-directed object play, shorter sequences of goal-directed behavior, and a greater likelihood of rejecting toys than developmentally matched TD children.

On standardized measures of mastery motivation, 5-year-old children with DS were found to have lower scores relative to norms, with some within-group variability predicting outcomes in adaptive behavior (Niccols, Atkinson, & Pepler, 2003). In laboratory contexts, young children with DS were shown to opt for more social rather than instrumental strategies, with off-task social behavior described as a strategy to distract from more challenging tasks at hand (Fidler, 2006; Pitcairn & Wishart, 1994). However, these findings have come into question, as between-group differences involving persons with DS and developmentally matched TD children have not consistently been found on this dimension when experimental tasks have been used (Gilmore & Cuskelly, 2011).

Thus, while questions regarding the nature of goal-directed behavior in persons with DS have been examined from numerous perspectives, including temperament, sensory, behavioral, and motivation-orientation frameworks, the examination of goal-directed behavior from a cognitive perspective has much to contribute to this ongoing conversation. Adopting an EF framework for understanding issues related to goal-directed behavior makes it possible to understand this issue from a cognitive perspective, and as an important aspect of the cognitive phenotype in persons with DS. In the following section, we provide an overview of research on the cognitive underpinnings of goal-directed behavior in DS, in the form of EF.

Executive Function in Down Syndrome: Current Progress

The investigation into EF performance in persons with DS has grown at a steady pace in recent years, leading to some overarching preliminary findings (see Table 13.1 for a review of existing work). Across both laboratory and informant reported methodologies, individuals with DS are at elevated risk for relative challenges in working memory (see Smith & Jarrold, this volume), with greater uncertainty about risk for challenges in other areas such as cognitive flexibility/shifting, inhibition, and planning (Daunhauer, Fidler, Hahn, et al., 2014; Daunhauer et al., 2017; Loveall, Conners, Tungate, Hahn, & Osso, 2017; Pennington, Moon, Edgin, Stedron, & Nadel, 2003; Rowe, Lavender, & Turk, 2006; Zelazo, Burack, Benedetto, & Frye, 1996). Most researchers report global EF challenges (Camp, Karmiloff-Smith, Thomas, & Farran, 2016; Lanfranchi, Jerman, Dal Pont, Alberti, & Vianello, 2010; Lee et al., 2011; Loveall et al., 2017), whereas others specify areas of competence, even when using MA-matched TD comparison groups (Carney, Brown, & Henry, 2013; Pennington et al., 2003). Another approach to reporting findings is to account for overall EF challenges, and then work to identify the severity of those challenges in DS when compared to other genetic syndromes or disorders (Costanzo et al., 2013; Edgin, 2003; Kogan et al., 2009; Rowe et al., 2006; Wilde & Oliver, 2017). In addition, links between important biomedical factors, such as sleep apnea, to compromised EF outcomes in DS have also been identified (Breslin et al., 2014; Chen, Spanò, & Edgin, 2013). Each method of inquiry adds to the larger, rapidly growing field of research on EF among persons with DS across the lifespan.

Laboratory Measure Findings

Laboratory-based studies have contributed to the current understanding of EF in persons with DS across various age groups, with a trend toward more research on adolescents and adults. Lanfranchi et al. (2010) identified global EF challenges in adolescents with DS when compared to an MA-matched TD group, with individuals with DS demonstrating impairments in working memory, response inhibition, shifting, and planning. However, challenges only in the areas of working memory and response inhibition were reported by Pennington et al. (2003). When teens and adults have been studied together in laboratory-based work, cognitive flexibility has also been reported as an area of relative challenge in comparison both to MA-matched persons with WS and to MA-matched TD groups (Campbell et al., 2013; Costanzo et al., 2013; Zelazo et al., 1996).

The overwhelming majority of laboratory-based EF research in persons with DS has focused on challenges in the component process of working memory. Within the significant working-memory challenges in persons with DS, there is a general trend toward better performance on visual-spatial working memory compared to verbal working memory

Table 13.1. Research Studies on Executive Function in Down Syndrome

Citation	Task	Comparison Group/s	Matching Strategy	CA for DS group: *M* (range)	DS Findings
Kopp, Krakow, & Johnson, 1983	Inhibition (delayed reward)	TD	MA and language age using Gesell developmental exam	4 y (2–5)	Deficits in inhibitory control, decreased latency to touch reward.
Vicari, Carlesimo, & Caltagirone, 1995	Working memory (verbal & spatial backward span)	TD, DD	CA matched to DD group, MA matched to TD group using Leiter	17 y	Deficits in backward span for both verbal and spatial measures.
Zelazo, Burack, Benedetto, & Frye, 1996	Cognitive flexibility (card sort)	TD	MA using PPVT-R	23 y (16–30)	Deficits in card sort using more than one rule.
Dawson, Meltzoff, Osterling, Rinaldi, & Brown, 1998	Cognitive flexibility (visual orientation to stimuli)	TD, ASD	MA using VABS communication and PLS	5 y	Performed better than children with ASD and similarly to TD group when orienting to social and nonsocial stimuli.
Kasari & Freeman, 2001	Planning (solvable and unsolvable puzzles)	TD, DD	MA using Stanford-Binet-IV and Reynell Developmental Language Scales	8 y (6–11)	Requested more help and exhibited less task persistence, taking longer than TD and DD to complete the puzzles.
Edgin, 2003	EF battery (backward digit & Corsi span, verbal & spatial problem solving, card sort)	WS	CA	18 y (13–23)	Performed better on spatial problem solving than WS group, but poorer on verbal problem solving and cognitive flexibility.
Pennington, Moon, Edgin, Stedron, & Nadel, 2003	EF battery (stop task, stockings of Cambridge)	TD	MA using DAS	15 y (11–19)	Deficits in working memory and response inhibition, but not planning.
Lanfranchi, Cornoldi, & Vianello, 2004	Working memory (verbal & spatial tasks)	TD	MA using Logical Operations test	12 y (7–18)	Deficits in working memory, with more pronounced differences in verbal tasks.

Fidler, Hepburn, Mankin, & Rogers, 2005	Planning (object retrieval)	TD, DD	CA matched to DD group, MA matched to TD group using MSEL	3 y (2–4)	Requested more help and deficits in on praxis task battery.
Rowe, Lavender, & Turk, 2006	EF battery (digit/spatial span, finger tapping, Tower of London, Weigl color form sort test, verbal fluency)	DD	CA	33 y (23–40)	Deficits in working memory, fluency, shifting, planning and inhibition, with less pronounced differences on spatial span task.
Kogan et al., 2009	Working memory and inhibition (modified version of Wisconsin General Test Apparatus)	2 TD groups, FXS	CA matched to one TD group, MA matched to second TD group and FXS group using PPVT-III	17 y (11–36)	Deficits on visual-spatial working memory task, and strengths on egocentric spatial learning and object discrimination.
Edgin, Pennington, & Mervis, 2010	Working memory (verbal & spatial backward span)	WS	CA	18 y (13–23)	No significant difference between groups on verbal or spatial working memory tasks.
Lanfranchi, Jerman, Dal Pont, Alberti, & Vianello, 2010	EF battery (modified Stroop, Tower of London, modified card sort, verbal-visuospatial dual tasks)	TD	MA using Logical Operations test	15 y (11–18)	Global EF deficits (working memory, response inhibition, shifting, and planning/problem-solving).
Lee et al., 2011	BRIEF-P	-	-	6 y (4–10)	Deficits in global EF composite. Specific challenges in working memory and plan/organize with relative strengths in emotional control.
Lanfranchi, Baddeley, Gathercole, & Vianello, 2012	Working memory (verbal & spatial tasks)	TD	Receptive language using PPVT-R	13 y (8–23)	Deficits in working memory, with more pronounced differences in verbal tasks.

(*continued*)

Table 13.1. *Continued*

Citation	Task	Comparison Group/s	Matching Strategy	CA for DS group: *M* (range)	DS Findings
Borella, Carretti, Lanfranchi, 2013	Inhibitory control (animal Stroop, proactive interference task, directed forgetting task) and working memory (verbal & spatial)	TD	Receptive language using PPVT-R	14 y (10–19)	Deficits in verbal working memory and ability to suppress irrelevant information.
Campbell et al., 2013	Cognitive flexibility (Flexible Item Selection Task)	-	-	15 y (9–23)	Deficits in cognitive flexibility strongly associated with verbal mental age.
Carney, Brown, Henry, 2013	EF battery (Listening Span task, Odd-One-Out test, Verbal Inhibition Motor Inhibition, Word Generation, Design Fluency, Category Switching)	TD, WS	no specific matching technique, ages and IQ using Stanford-Binet broadly similar	13 y (10–19)	Deficits in both verbal and spatial working memory tasks and verbal domain of cognitive flexibility task. Inhibition and fluency performance did not differ from TD group.
Costanzo et al., 2013	EF battery (digit span, nonword repetition, Corsi span, Tower of London, Category Fluency test, Weigl color form sort test, alternative category fluency task, trail making test, forma/forma task, Stroop task, go-nogo task)	TD, WS	MA using Leiter-R	15 y (8–21)	Both group deficits in auditory sustained and visual selective attention, visual categorization, and working memory. DS-specific deficits include shifting, and verbal memory, along with relative strength in planning.
Daunhauer et al., 2014	BRIEF-P	TD	MA using Leiter-R	8 y (5–11)	Deficits in working memory and planning as reported by both parents and teachers. Deficits in inhibition reported by parents.
Fidler, Will, Daunhauer, Gerlach-McDonald, & Visootsak, 2014	Planning (object-related generativity task)	TD, DD	MA using Leiter-R	8 y	Deficits in initiating actions on new objects and producing novel functional acts.

Lee et al., 2015	BRIEF	TD, sex chromosome trisomy	CA and maternal education level	11 y (7–17)	Deficits in working memory and monitoring. Relative strengths in emotional control and organization of materials.
Pritchard, Kalback, McCurdy, & Capone, 2015	BRIEF-P	DS+ASDDS+ DBD	CA	7 y (3–13)	Strongest EF deficits in DS groups with a co-occurring disorder.
Roberts & Richmond 2015	A-not-B	TD	Receptive language using MSEL	4 y (3–5)	No group differences on A-not-B performance.
Camp, Karmiloff-Smith, Thomas, & Farran, 2016	BRIEF and problem-solving questionnaire	TD, WS	CA and RCPM match to WS group	18 y (12–24)	Deficits in problem-solving and global EF performance in DS and WS groups, but more severe in WS group.
Daunhauer et al. 2017	EF battery (Pony gator working memory/inhibition task, snack delay, card sort, planning-generativity, BRIEF-P)	TD	MA using Leiter-R	7 y (5–11)	Deficits in working memory/ inhibition and planning.
Loveall, Conners, Tungate, Hahn, & Osso, 2017	BRIEF & BRIEF-P	-	-	13 (2–35)	Deficits in global EF and specifically working memory across lifespan, coupled with relative strength in emotional control.
Wilde & Oliver, 2017	BRIEF-P	SMS	MA using VABS II- SF	8 y (3–15)	Deficits in global EF in both groups, with pronounced working memory challenges and strengths in emotional control in DS group.
Tomaszewski et al. 2018	BRIEF-A	-	-	26 y (18–43)	Deficits in shifting, working memory, plan/organizing, and task monitoring. Relative strengths in inhibition, emotional control, self-monitoring, and organization of materials.

(Borella, Carretti, Lanfranchi, 2013; Lanfranchi, Baddeley, Gathercole, & Vianello, 2012; Lanfranchi, Cornoldi, & Vianello, 2004; Rowe et al., 2006). This pattern has been found in immediate short-term memory, but not working memory (Edgin, Pennington, et al., 2010). This type of granular examination of EF profiles using laboratory approaches has identified even more subtle dissociations among persons with DS. Within the visual-spatial working-memory strength, for example, sequential visual-spatial working memory is reportedly stronger than simultaneous visual-spatial working memory in persons with DS when compared to TD children at similar verbal mental ages (Lanfranchi, Carretti, Spanò, & Cornoldi, 2009).

Additional laboratory-based studies have indicated that inhibitory control is an area of challenge among adolescents with DS relative to MA-matched TD groups, as they experience difficulties with the ability to suppress irrelevant information during task completion (Borella et al., 2013). However, others (Carney et al., 2013) have reported inhibition performances in persons with DS that were comparable to TD individuals with a similar MA. A potential explanation of conflicting findings in this area could be that the operationalization of inhibition is variable and sometimes includes several types of functions, such as behavioral inhibition or disregarding interference (Borella et al., 2013). In other cases, elements of inhibitory control are integrated with other tasks involving executive functions (Zelazo & Müller, 2011). Despite these issues, research on adolescents and adults has worked to characterize the EF profile in persons with DS, and while questions remain, much progress had been made in examining syndrome specific strengths and challenges in EF among persons with DS.

Early Development of Executive Function

To understand the developmental origins of EF outcomes in persons with DS, researchers have also utilized laboratory-based approaches to examine performances at younger ages. Preschoolers ages 3–5 years with DS have been shown to perform similarly to receptive language-matched TD children on specific EF tasks, including object location retention, deferred imitation, and A-not-B tasks (Roberts & Richmond, 2015). However, early challenges in planning have been identified in young children with DS (Fidler, Hepburn, Mankin, & Rogers, 2005). Difficulties with planning are also evident on laboratory measures administered to individuals with DS during middle childhood, including puzzle (Kasari & Freeman, 2001) and generativity tasks (Fidler, Will, Daunhauer, Gerlach-McDonald, & Visootsak, 2014).

Regarding the early presentation of other EF processes, difficulties with inhibition have been reported in preschoolers with DS, as measured by the time and ability to delay touching a reward (Kopp, Krakow, & Johnson, 1983). In addition, by middle childhood, students with DS exhibit specific deficits in working memory/inhibition and planning on laboratory-based measures, and a nonsignificant trend for challenges in shifting as well, when compared to MA-matched TD children (Daunhauer et al., 2017). However, shifting has been shown to be stronger in young children with DS than in children with ASD, highlighting the importance of considering comparison groups when interpreting EF findings from persons with DS (Dawson, Meltzoff, Osterling, Rinaldi, & Brown, 1998). These findings provide evidence for some degree of disruption in the early developmental foundations of EF in persons with DS using laboratory-based measures. However, more scientific work in this area is needed to inform targeted early intervention related to EF and adaptation.

Questionnaire Findings

Another predominating approach to EF measurement involves using proxy-report measures, usually in the form of questionnaires. Questionnaire ratings are thought by some to be potentially more clinically meaningful than laboratory-based assessments because they approximate EF performance in real-world contexts (Toplak et al., 2013). In addition, though laboratory-based approaches to EF assessment in persons with DS have led to some discrepant outcomes, questionnaire-based approaches have generated more consistent findings.

Across two different proxy-report studies utilizing Behavior Rating Inventory of EF-Preschool (BRIEF-P) with different cohorts of children, similar global EF challenges have been reported in young children with DS, with more pronounced limitations reported in the areas of working memory and planning/organization (Lee et al., 2011; Daunhauer, Fidler, Hahn, et al., 2014). Evidence from other studies has confirmed the global EF and working-memory deficits in school-aged children and adolescents using the BRIEF (Camp et al., 2016; Loveall et al., 2017). Relative strengths in emotional control (emotion modulation and corresponding behavioral responses) for persons with DS between ages 2 and 18 years have been identified and replicated across multiple studies using the BRIEF (Lee et al., 2011; Loveall et al., 2017; Wilde & Oliver, 2017).

The BRIEF and BRIEF-P have also been administered in studies in which persons with DS were compared to individuals with other clinical diagnoses, including sex chromosome trisomy, DS with comorbid ASD, and Smith-Magenis syndrome (SMS; Lee et al., 2015; Pritchard, Kalback, McCurdy, & Capone, 2015; Wilde & Oliver, 2017). The findings are consistent with evidence related to deficits in working memory and strengths in emotional control (Lee et al., 2015; Wilde & Oliver, 2017) and also reveal that the strongest EF challenges are in groups of persons with both DS and a co-occurring disorder (Pritchard et al., 2015). Thus, while laboratory-based work on EF in persons with DS can shed light on issues related to the efficiency of processing in this population, additional useful EF-related information has also been generated via proxy/self-report approaches, with an emphasis on EF in the context of everyday goal-directed behavior.

Methodological Considerations in Assessing Executive Function for Individuals with Down Syndrome

With the increased focus on EF processes in persons with DS, the need for methodological sophistication and consideration has become more pronounced. In the broader context of translational science, researchers and clinicians in the United States have been charged with better aligning intervention with an individual's specific needs; this approach is referred to as the Precision Medicine Initiative (National Institutes of Health, 2015). Precision, or personalized, medicine is pertinent to selecting optimal assessments in addition to intervention for individuals with DS (Lemons et al., 2018). To better account for individual variability within DS, it is critical to assess relevant domains, such as EF, accurately (e.g., Daunhauer, Fidler, Hahn, et al., 2014). Furthermore, the precise assessment of individuals with DS, particularly for assessment related to cognition, must also account for relative competencies and weaknesses associated with the phenotypic profile, which includes relative challenges in assessment-relevant areas such as verbal processing and motor skills. At present, the valid assessment of EF in DS has posed particular challenges to researchers. For example, Edgin et al. (2017) found that EF assessments demonstrated the weakest test-retest reliability in the psychometrically evaluated Arizona Cognitive Test Battery for individuals with DS.

Moreover, to better understand EF performance in individuals with DS when using standardized assessments, the development of scores based on an individuals' MA, rather than their chronological age, would be useful (e.g., Daunhauer, Fidler, Hahn, et al., 2014). Because nearly all individuals with DS have intellectual disability (Tsao & Kindelberger, 2009), utilizing chronological age norms may provide very little information to researchers and clinicians. However, comparing individuals with DS to MA norms affords the advantage of understanding executive performance while controlling for overall levels of developmental delay (Burack, Iarocci, Flanagan, & Bowler, 2004; Burack, Russo, Flores, Iarocci, & Zigler, 2011; Dykens & Hodapp, 2007; Fidler, Daunhauer, Will, Gerlach-McDonald, & Schworer, 2016; Mervis & Klein-Tasman, 2004; Seltzer, Abbeduto, Wyngaarden Krauss, Greenberg, & Swe, 2004).

Beyond phenotypic considerations, the accurate measurement of EF in early development has been a lively topic in the developmental science literature (Willoughby & Blair, 2016; Willoughby, Blair, Wirth, & Greenberg, 2010). Over the past decade, researchers have adapted traditional neuropsychological tasks for use in developmentally young children (e.g., Carlson, 2005; Diamond, 1991; Espy, 1997; Rose, Feldman, & Jankowski, 2009; Rose, Feldman, Jankowski, & Van Rossem, 2007; Willoughby et al., 2010; Yerys & Munakata, 2006; Zelazo et al., 2003). Adaptations include shortening or simplifying task demands and presenting tasks as play (e.g., Carlson, 2005; Yerys, Hepburn, Pennington, & Rogers, 2007). While these modifications have become increasingly common, some researchers have acknowledged the need for standards regarding this approach (Willoughby et al., 2010). For example, Willoughby et al. (2010) recommended avoiding the use of pass/fail or other dichotomous measures, unclear or lack of explicit administration procedures, and underpowered sample sizes in laboratory studies of EF.

Another methodological consideration regarding the selection and use of tasks to assess EF in DS, as well as other populations, is the issue of task impurity (Friedman &

Miyake, 2017). Though EF tasks are designed to target specific component processes of EF, such as inhibition or working memory, in most cases, tasks often recruit additional cognitive processing skills, or even other EF component processes. Executive function tasks developed to assess individuals with young MAs are particularly prone to this methodological concern. For example, a classic snack delay task that is designed to assess behavioral inhibition requires a child to hear a rule and wait to retrieve a snack from under a clear glass when a bell is rung (Carlson, 2005). This task has multiple components in addition to inhibitory control, including verbal comprehension and memory, that may influence whether or not the child will activate the inhibitory control to resist taking the snack immediately. The classic Dimensional Change Card Sort (Zelazo, 2006) cognitive flexibility task, as another example, also makes demands on multiple domains. In addition to flexibly shifting from the use of different rules, the task requires visual perception of different shapes and colors on cards and then memory of the rules for successful task completion (Zelazo, 2006). Although this issue is impossible to avoid entirely, Friedman and Miyake (2017) suggest that using multiple EF tasks to assess each domain can help minimize measurement distortion due to task impurity.

Assessment Throughout the Lifespan

To date, most EF assessment work has been focused on older children, adolescents, and adults. However, EF foundations begin to emerge during infancy and toddlerhood (Hendry et al., 2016) and can be operationalized during these early stages. In very young children with DS, the assessment of EF may help researchers to identify challenges before they can have far-reaching impacts in areas such as adaptive behavior and academic achievement (Edgin, Clark, Massand, & Karmiloff-Smith, 2015; Stagni, Giacomini, Guidi, Ciani, & Bartesaghi, 2015). To date, however, there has been very little emphasis on the validation of EF assessment in early childhood in DS. On the other end of the lifespan, developmentally sensitive and accurate EF evaluation may predict later life adaptive outcomes, such as employment status (Tomaszewski et al., 2018), and maladaptive outcomes, such as early-onset Alzheimer's disease (Lautarescu, Holland, & Zaman, 2017). To advance the development of reliable and valid measures of EF across the lifespan, researchers will need to consider features of the DS phenotype at different life stages. These lifespan issues may include motor delays in early development (Daunhauer & Fidler, 2011), as well as behavioral and psychological changes in later development (Lautarescu et al., 2017).

In summary, there are numerous methodological considerations that researchers will need to address in future work on EF in persons with DS, including establishing consensus regarding phenotype-sensitive adaptations, appropriate task structure, comparison group selection, and task impurity issues. Furthermore, there is still work to be done to develop phenotype-sensitive and reliable measures of EF in later childhood and adulthood for individuals with DS (e.g., Edgin et al., 2017). Without psychometrically sound evaluation of EF skills, there is the potential to misunderstand targets for intervention and to misinterpret the effects of potentially beneficial interventions, whether they are pharmaceutical, medical, educational, or behavioral. Therefore, continued research on the assessment of EF in DS is critical for future intervention development and outcomes for this population.

Executive Function and Adaptation in Down Syndrome

Down syndrome predisposes individuals to a complex pattern of EF challenges and competencies throughout the lifespan. The EF difficulties are observable during early childhood, and as such, the influence of EF on various outcomes in home, school, and community settings has the potential to demonstrate far-reaching effects (Daunhauer, Fidler, Hahn, et al., 2014; Daunhauer et al., 2017; Lee et al., 2011). These difficulties may primarily be implicated in the behavioral presentation of individuals with DS. Children and young adults with Down syndrome demonstrate increased behavioral challenges (25–35 percent) as compared to TD (5–25 percent) through childhood and adolescence (Brauner & Stephens, 2006; van Gameren-Oosterom et al., 2013). Consistent with this clinical presentation, Daunhauer, Fidler, and Will (2014) found that in school settings, individuals with DS exhibit challenges with compliance to adult directives and school rules, task behavior-completion, positive interactions, safety, and behavior regulation.

Executive functions may play a critical role in aspects of the clinical presentation in DS. For example, difficulties with working memory may contribute to struggles with task completion, necessitating 1:1 support during educational activities. Although Daunhauer, Fidler, and Will (2014) found that teacher-reported global EF was linked to school function, they did not examine associations between specific EF components and school adaptation. Different EF processes are implicated in the range of behavioral challenges described above. While challenges in working memory for individuals with DS may result in difficulty with task completion, difficulties with transitioning from one activity to another may be consistent with identified challenges in cognitive flexibility or shifting. Similarly, poor boundaries, aggression, and safety concerns (wandering or running away from adults) may reflect underlying difficulties with response inhibition, an aspect of inhibitory control.

In the context of academic performance, there is mounting evidence that components of EF predict early literacy and math achievement in primary school-aged children with DS (Will, Gerlach-McDonald, Fidler, & Daunhauer, 2016). In addition, teacher ratings of EF predict school function (the adaptive behaviors that support learning in the school context) more powerfully than either nonverbal IQ or language ability in primary grade students with DS (Daunhauer, Fidler, & Will, 2014). Executive function difficulties may also contribute to difficulties with functioning in the home and community settings. For examples, in an analysis of 274 questionnaires completed by parents of individuals with

DS between the ages of 2 and 22, Patel, Wolter-Warmerdam, Leifer, & Hickey,(2018) found that the majority of respondents (n = 187; 68 percent) reported concerns regarding impulsivity, 183 (67 percent) indicated concerns regarding poor boundaries, and 206 (75 percent) indicated concerns regarding running or wandering away from adults. Compensatory strategies with environmental supports can be implemented to help, but without improvement in working memory, planning, and other EF components, individuals with DS may continue to show difficulties with purposeful, goal-directed behavior, resulting in decreased independence.

Interventions for Executive Function for Individuals With Down Syndrome

With mounting evidence for the role of EF in critical educational and functional outcomes in DS, there is a growing understanding of the critical need for effective intervention in this area. Childhood EF intervention research is promising, with data suggesting that EF and related outcomes can change positively in response to behavioral intervention in TD children (Riggs, Jahromi, Razza, Dillworth, & Mueller, 2006) and those at-risk for delays (e.g., Bierman, Nix, Greenberg, Blair, & Domitrovich, 2008). While many EF interventions have been focused on other diagnostic populations such as ASD (Kenworthy et al., 2014) and ADHD (Rabiner, Murray, Skinner, & Malone, 2010), comprehensive EF intervention has yet to be researched in individuals with DS.

Working-Memory Training

To date, the primary focus of EF intervention work with persons with DS has been in the area of working-memory training. This work grew out of foundational studies on the effectiveness of auditory working-memory rehearsal in children with DS (e.g., Conners, Rosenquist, Arnett, Moore, & Hume, 2008; Conners, Rosenquist, & Taylor, 2001). In other diagnostic groups, such as individuals with acquired brain injuries or children with ADHD, computerized training has been widely applied to improve working memory (e.g., Klingberg, 2010). This approach utilizes distributed practice coupled with an adaptive or scaled component, such that practice is adjusted to be less or more challenging based on prior performance (Klingberg, 2010).

In recent years, researchers have begun to examine the impact of computerized working-memory training on school-aged children and adolescents with DS. Bennett, Holmes, and Buckley (2013) tested a computerized training program, Junior Cogmed Working Memory Training, with school-aged children with DS (n = 21) using a waitlist control design. Following approximately 13 weeks of intervention, the participants in the treatment group showed statistically significant advances in trained tasks (those tasks that were more similar to the tasks in the computer program, e.g., assessing visuospatial short-term memory). An important outcome to note about this study was that the amount of training completed by each participant was positively associated with performance on both trained and untrained tasks. These findings indicate the possibility of a dose-response effect for working-memory training in school-age children with DS. While this study is promising, further research is needed with larger samples and with additional directly measured, nontrained tasks (such as those related to performance in academics and adaptation) to determine whether training can be transferred.

In another working-memory training study, Pulina, Carretti, Lanfranchi, and Mammarella,(2015) targeted the spatial-simultaneous components of visual-spatial working memory in individuals with DS. The intervention involved an adaptation of a computerized working-memory training program and incorporated phenotypically informed adaptations based on their team's previous iterations of this intervention. These adaptations included minimizing language processing and abstract reasoning aspects of the intervention program (for details see Lanfranchi, Mammarella, Carretti, & Pulina, 2014). Using this adapted working-memory training program, Pulina et al., (2015) targeted both child and adolescent participants with DS (n = 39) to engage in the computer program twice a week for 4 weeks. Additionally, the participants were randomized into one of two groups. In one group, an expert led the participant computer sessions, and in the other group, the participants' parents led the sessions. The results of this study indicated that all of the participants benefitted, whether they were assigned to the expert-led or parent-led conditions. However, the expert-led group participants performed slightly better on average on most measures. Overall, following the intervention, both groups of participants showed stronger performances on trained tasks with a large magnitude of effect. Additionally, both groups performed nontrained near-transfer and far-transfer tasks more competently, but with small effects. Thus, in addition to demonstrating the effects of the intervention itself, this study provides evidence that a parent-led approach is feasible, which is important from an implementation perspective.

Lanfranchi, Pulina, Carretti, and Mammarella (2017) further examined additional children and adolescents with DS (n = 61) using the same computerized program described above. However, the participants were randomly assigned to a training program, an active control group (vocabulary activities), or a passive control group (waitlist). Following the intervention period, the participants who completed the computerized training program showed stronger performances on most measures of working memory than the participants in either of the two control groups, providing further evidence that a phenotype-specific computerized training program for working memory elicits greater competencies in working memory when compared to alternative or nontreatment control conditions.

Collectively, the working-memory training studies reviewed here demonstrate that children and adolescents with DS can engage in working-memory training and benefit from it (Lanfranchi et al., 2017), even when it is completed in their everyday environments (Bennett et al., 2013) or led by a parent (Pulina et al., 2015). However, much more information is needed to make informed intervention choices for this population. Future research should aim to clarify whether an investment of time in working-memory training will have benefits that translate into everyday lives, such as improvements in academic achievement or adaptive behavior. Areas for future working-memory training research include identifying the "active" ingredients of working-memory training for this population, individual variability associated with treatment response, long-term effects, and optimal dosage, frequency, and timing for intervention.

Additional Executive Function Treatment Approaches

In addition to working-memory training, current approaches to EF treatment in DS have begun to include more biomedical approaches, such as sleep apnea intervention (Breslin, Edgin, Bootzin, & Goodwin, & Nadel, 2011) and the development of pharmaceutical treatments (de la Torre et al., 2016; Hart et al., 2017). Below we summarize the major research findings in these areas.

The incidence of sleep apnea in individuals with DS is high (Breslin et al., 2011), which is relevant for the treatment of EF because sleep disturbance has shown positive associations with the EF component process of cognitive flexibility in individuals with DS (Breslin et al., 2014). Co-occurring health issues are not always accounted for when studying development in children with neurodevelopmental disabilities such as DS, yet these research findings highlight that health issues such as sleep apnea are very likely a critical source of variability in cognitive trajectories. Between 40 and 60 percent of preschoolers with DS have obstructive sleep apnea (OSA), and the origins of these difficulties are observable even in infancy, as at least 30 percent of infants older than 6 months have demonstrated OSA through polysomnography assessment (Goffinski et al., 2015; Shott et al., 2006). Parent report and actigraphy data suggest that school-age children with DS exhibit fragmented sleep (sleep punctuated by periods of frequent awakenings and restlessness; Ashworth, Hill, Karmiloff-Smith, & Dimitriou, 2013). Currently, clinicaltrials.gov (National Institutes of Health—U.S. National Library of Medicine, 2018) reports two active treatment trials for OSA in DS. Given the statistical associations between sleep and cognitive flexibility, such studies may demonstrate downstream effects onto cognition and EF outcomes; however, no findings have yet been published in this area.

Another means of treating cognitive challenges, including EF, for individuals with DS may be the use of pharmaceuticals and dietary supplements. At present, pharmaceuticals treatments are thought to have the potential to rescue cognitive function, including EF, by targeting aspects of the brain and neurofunction affected by trisomy 21. Some human pharmaceutical treatments trials have targeted cognition in DS (Hart et al., 2017) guided by findings from earlier DS mouse model research (for a review see Gardiner, 2015; Hart et al., 2017; Stagni et al., 2015). To date, researchers have reported limited or no significant changes in cognitive function in pharmaceutical trials for individuals with DS (e.g., Boada et al., 2012), with one notable exception in a recent study of green tea extract (epigallocatechin-3-gallate, EGCG). In this study using a double-blind placebo-controlled trial, 16- to 34-year-olds with DS (n = 87) participated in either a group that received

EGCG plus 12 months of cognitive training or a group that received a placebo and 12 months of cognitive training (de la Torre et al., 2016). The group that received the EGCG plus cognitive training had significantly enhanced outcomes, including improved inhibitory control, though the effects were small to medium ($d = 0.27$ for total score; $d = 0.28$ for response time).

With the exception of de la Torre et al.'s (2016) findings, this work is still in early stages, with an initial track record of primarily null results. The reasons for this early lack of observed effects in pharmaceutical trials may be attributable to factors beyond the effects of the potential treatments. In addition to questions regarding the impact of a candidate pharmaceutical agent on neural function, researchers have hypothesized that outcome measures used in clinical trials for individuals with DS may not be adequately sensitive to detect growth and change (Hart et al., 2017). This potential issue arises from the challenges of using assessments that have not been psychometrically validated for individuals with DS. Many assessments that have been used in previous treatment studies with persons with DS were standardized on neurotypical populations and do not account for known relative challenges in the phenotypic profile associated with DS (Daunhauer et al., 2017; Hart et al., 2017; Keeling et al., 2017).

Future innovations in intervention research will be critical for our understanding of how cognition in general, and EF in particular, may be enhanced for individuals with DS. In addition, from an implementation perspective, the low-incidence of DS will necessitate the use of creative approaches to provide behavioral/educational intervention trials to groups who do not live in urban areas near major medical clinics. There is some promising evidence for the utility of a "train the trainer" approach (e.g., Bennett et al. 2013; Pulina et al., 2015) using teaching assistants and parents. This approach also could be optimized with the addition of secure video-conferencing for coaching and questions.

An additional issue that researchers have begun to face relates to the role of social media and its influence on intervention research. Today, social media groups often offer support to diagnostic groups such as individuals with DS and their families, and in this context, families participating in treatments may share their experiences. While such support networks may offer invaluable resources to individuals with DS and their families, social media sharing may also influence research findings by skewing participant recruitment, knowledge about the intervention conditions, informant reports, and expectations for change. There are both benefits and additional methodological complexities that will need to be accounted for in treatment research within the context of social media. Despite these new issues, the open spirit of social media encourages important advances for individuals with DS and their families, including increased advocacy; access and influence; and the prioritization of their opinions, needs, and goals.

Conclusion

The growing scientific knowledge based regarding EF in DS offers much promise for improving our understanding of cognitive outcomes in DS and their relation to adaptation in naturalistic environments throughout the lifespan. Over the past decade, methodological approaches have become increasingly more refined, revealing the nuances of the EF profile in DS during different phases of the lifespan and across different EF subdomains. The groundwork for translational work is firmly in place, and the next generation of work in this area will require the application of this work to improve intervention and education planning in childhood, and supports and services in adolescence and adulthood. As is observed in the general population, EF has been linked to a range of important outcomes that impact quality of life among persons with DS. Therefore, the translation of this work into practice has the potential to support the development of purposeful, goal-directed behavior in persons with DS, which has important implications for independence and self-determination at all ages.

References

Ashworth, A., Hill, C. M., Karmiloff-Smith, A., & Dimitriou, D. (2013). Cross syndrome comparison of sleep problems in children with Down syndrome and Williams syndrome. *Research in Developmental Disabilities, 34*, 1572–1580. doi:10.1016/j.ridd.2013.01.031

Bennett, S. J., Holmes, J., & Buckley, S. (2013). Computerized memory training leads to sustained improvement in visuospatial short-term memory skills in children with Down syndrome. *American Journal on Intellectual and Developmental Disabilities, 118*(3), 179–192. doi:10.1352/1944-7558-118.3.179

Best, J. R., Miller, P. H., & Naglieri, J. A. (2011). Relations between EF and academic achievement from ages 5 to 17 in a large, representative national sample. *Learning and Individual Differences, 21*(4), 327–336. doi:10.1016/j.lindif.2011.01.007

Biederman, J., Monuteaux, M. C., Doyle, A. E., Seidman, L. J., Wilens, T. E., Ferrero, F., . . . & Faraone, S. V. (2004). Impact of executive function deficits and attention-deficit/hyperactivity disorder (ADHD) on academic outcomes in children. *Journal of Consulting and Clinical Psychology, 72*(5), 757. doi:10.1037/0022-006X.72.5.757

Bierman, K. L., Nix, R. L., Greenberg, M. T., Blair, C. & Domitrovich, C. E. (2008). Executive functions and school readiness intervention: Impact, moderation, and mediation in the Head Start REDI program. *Development and Psychopathology, 20*, 821–843. doi:10.1017/S0954579408000394

Blair, C., & Razza, R. P. (2007). Relating effortful control, executive function, and false belief understanding to emerging math and literacy ability in kindergarten. *Child Development, 78*(2), 647–663. doi:10.1111/j.1467-8624.2007.01019.x

Boada, R., Hutaff-Lee, C., Schrader, A., Weitzenkamp, D., Benke, T. A., Goldson, E. J., & Costa, A. C. (2012). Antagonism of NMDA receptors as a potential treatment for Down syndrome: A pilot randomized controlled trial. *Translational Psychiatry, 2*, e141.

Borella, E., Carretti, B., & Lanfranchi, S. (2013). Inhibitory mechanisms in Down syndrome: Is there a specific or general deficit? *Research in Developmental Disabilities, 34*, 65–71. doi:10.1016/j.ridd.2012.07.017

Brauner, C. B., & Stephens, C. B. (2006). Estimating the prevalence of early childhood serious emotional/behavioral disorders: Challenges and recommendations. *Public Health Rep, 121*(3), 303–310.

Breslin, J., Spanò, G., Bootzin, R., Anand, P., Nadel, L. & Edgin, J. O. (2014). Obstructive sleep apnea and cognition in Down syndrome, Developmental Medicine and Child Neurology, 56 (7), 657–664.

Breslin, J. H., Edgin, J. O., Bootzin, R. R., Goodwin, J. L. & Nadel, L. (2011). Parental report of sleep problems in Down syndrome. *Journal of Intellectual Disability Research, 55*(11), 1086–1091.

Bruni, M., Cameron, D., Dua, S., & Noy, S. (2010). Reported sensory processing of children with Down syndrome. *Physical & Occupational Therapy in Pediatrics, 30*(4), 280–293. doi:10.3109/01942638.2010.486962

Brydges, C. R., Fox, A. M., Reid, C. L., & Anderson, M. (2014). The differentiation of executive functions in middle and late childhood: A longitudinal latent-variable analysis. *Intelligence, 47*, 34–43. doi:10.1016/j.intell.2014.08.010

Burack, J. A., Iarocci, G., Flanagan, T., & Bowler, D. M. (2004). On melting pots and mosaics: Conceptual considerations for matching strategies. *Journal of Autism and Developmental Disorders, 34*, 65–73.

Burack, J. A., Russo, N., Flores, H., Iarocci, G., & Zigler, E. (2011). The more we know, the less we know, but that's OK: Developmental implications for theory, methodology, and interpretation. In J. A. Burack, R. M. Hodapp, G. Iarocci, & E. Zigler (Eds.), *The Oxford handbook of intellectual disability and development*, pp. 1–12 (2nd ed.). New York: Oxford University Press. doi:10.1093/oxfordhb/9780195305012.001.0001

Camp, J. S., Karmiloff-Smith, A., Thomas, M. S. C., & Farran, E. K. (2016). Cross-syndrome comparison of real-world executive functioning and problem solving using a new problem-solving questionnaire. *Research in Developmental Disabilities, 59*, 80–92. doi:10.1016/j.ridd.2016.07.006

Campbell, C., Landry, O., Russo, N., Flores, H., Jacques, S., & Burack, J. A. (2013). Cognitive flexibility among individuals with Down syndrome: Assessing the influence of verbal and nonverbal abilities. *American Journal on Intellectual and Developmental Disabilities, 118*, 193–200. doi:10.1352/1944-7558-118.3.193

Carlesimo, G. A., Marotta, L., & Vicari, S. (1997). Long-term memory in mental retardation: Evidence for a specific impairment in subjects with Down's syndrome. *Neuropsychologia*, 35, 71–79.

Carlson, S. M. (2005). Developmentally sensitive measures of executive function in preschool children. *Developmental Neuropsychology, 28*, 595–616. doi:10.1207/s15326942dn2802_3

Carlson, S. M., Mandell, D. J., & Williams, L. (2004). Executive function and theory of mind: Stability and prediction from ages 2 to 3. *Developmental Psychology, 40*(6), 1105–1122. doi:10.1037/0012-1649.40.6.1105

Carney, D. P. J., Brown, J. H., & Henry, L. A. (2013). Executive function in Williams and Down syndromes. *Research in Developmental Disabilities, 34*, 46–55. doi:10.1016/j.ridd.2012.07.013

Chan, R. C., Shum, D., Toulopoulou, T., & Chen, E. Y. (2008). Assessment of executive functions: Review of instruments and identification of critical issues. *Archives of Clinical Neuropsychology, 23*(2), 201–216. doi:10.1016/j.acn.2007.08.010

Chaytor, N., Schmitter-Edgecombe, M., & Burr, R. (2006). Improving the ecological validity of executive functioning assessment. *Archives of Clinical Neuropsychology, 21*(3), 217–227. doi:10.1016/j.acn.2005.12.002

Chen, C. C. J., Spanò, G., & Edgin, J. O. (2013). The impact of sleep disruption on executive function in Down syndrome. *Research in Developmental Disabilities, 34*(6), 2033–2039.

Conners, F. A., Rosenquist, C. J., Arnett, L., Moore, M. S., & Hume, L. E. (2008). Improving memory span in children with Down syndrome. *Journal of Intellectual Disability Research, 52*(3), 244–255. doi:0.1111/j.1365-2788.2007.01015.x

Conners, F. A., Rosenquist, C. J., & Taylor, L. A. (2001). Memory training for children with Down syndrome. *Down Syndrome Research and Practice, 7*, 25–33.

Costanzo, F., Varuzza, C., Menghini, D., Addona, F., Gianesini, T., & Vicari, S. (2013). Executive functions in intellectual disabilities: A comparison between Williams syndrome and Down syndrome. *Research in Developmental Disabilities, 34*, 1770–1780. doi:10.1016/j.ridd.2013.01.024

Daunhauer, L. A., & Fidler, D. J. (2011). The Down syndrome behavioral phenotype: Implications for practice and research in occupational therapy. *Occupational Therapy in Healthcare, 25*, 7–25. doi:10.3109/07380577.2010.535601

Daunhauer, L. A., Fidler, D. J., Hahn, L., Will, E., Lee, N. R., & Hepburn, S. (2014). Profiles of everyday executive functioning in young children with Down syndrome. *American Journal on Intellectual and Developmental Disabilities, 119*, 303–318. doi:10.1352/1944-7558-119.4.303

Daunhauer, L. A., Fidler, D. J., & Will, E. (2014). School function in students with Down syndrome. *American Journal of Occupational Therapy*, 68, 167–176. doi:10.5014/ajot.2014.009274

Daunhauer, L. A., Gerlach-McDonald, B., Will, E., & Fidler, D. (2017). Performance and ratings based measures of executive function in school-aged children with Down syndrome. *Developmental Neuropsychology, 42*(6), 351–368. doi:10.1080/87565641.2017.1360303

Dawson, G., Meltzoff, A. N., Osterling, J., Rinaldi, J., & Brown, E. (1998). Children with autism fail to orient to naturally occurring social stimuli. *Journal of Autism and Developmental Disorders, 28*, 479–485.

de la Torre, R., de Sola, S., Hernandez, G., Farre, M., Pujol, J., Rodriguez, J., . . . TESDAD study group. (2016). Safety and efficacy of cognitive training plus epigallocatechin 3 gallate in young adults with

Down's syndrome (TESDAD): A double-blind, randomised, placebo-controlled, phase 2 trial. *Lancet Neurol, 15(8),* 801–810.

Diamond, A. (1991). Neuropsychological insights into the meaning of object concept development. In S. Carey, & R. Gelman (Eds.), *The epigenesis of mind: Essays on biology and cognition* (pp. 67–110). Hillsdale, NJ: Erlbaum.

Dykens, E. N., & Hodapp, R. M. (2007). Three steps toward improving the measurement of behavior in behavioral phenotype research. *Child and Adolescent Psychiatric Clinics of North America, 16,* 617–630. doi:10.1016/j.chc.2007.02.001

Edgin, J. O. (2003). A neuropsychological model for the development of the cognitive profiles in mental retardation syndromes: Evidence from Down syndrome and Williams syndrome [proquest information & learning]. In *Dissertation Abstracts International: Section B: The Sciences and Engineering* (Vol. 64, Issue 3–B, p. 1522).

Edgin, J. O., Anand, P., Rosser, T., Pierpont, E. I., Figueroa, C., Hamilton, D., . . . Sherman, S. (2017). The Arizona Cognitive Test Battery for Down Syndrome: Test-retest reliability and practice effects. *American Journal on Intellectual and Developmental Disabilities, 122,* 215–234. doi:10.1352/1944-7558-122.3.215

Edgin, J. O., Clark, C. C., Massand, E., & Karmiloff-Smith, A. (2015). Building an adaptive brain across development: Targets for neurorehabilitation must begin in infancy. *Frontiers in Behavioral Neuroscience, 9,* 232. doi:10.3389/fnbeh.2015.00232

Edgin, J. O., Mason, G. M., Allman, M. J., Capone, G. T., De Leon, I., Maslen, C., Reeves, R. H., Sherman, S. L., & Nadel, L. (2010). Development and validation of the Arizona cognitive test battery for Down syndrome. *Journal of Neurodevelopmental Disorders, 2,* 149–164. doi:10.1007/s11689-010-9054-3

Edgin, J. O., Pennington, B. F., & Mervis, C. B. (2010). Neuropsychological components of intellectual disability: The contributions of immediate, working, and associative memory. *Journal of Intellectual Disability Research, 54,* 406–417. doi:10.1111/j.1365-2788.2010.01278.x

Espy, K. A. (1997). The Shape School: Assessing executive function in preschool children. *Developmental Neuropsychology, 13*(4), 495–499. doi:10.1080/87565649709540690

Fidler, D. J. (2006). The emergence of a syndrome-specific personality profile in young children with Down syndrome. *Down Syndrome: Neurobehavioural Specificity,* 139–152.

Fidler, D. J., Daunhauer, L. A., Will, E., Gerlach-McDonald, B., & Schworer, E. (2016). The central role of etiology in science and service in intellectual disability. *International Review of Research in Developmental Disabilities, 52,* 35–69.

Fidler, D. J., Hepburn, S. L., Mankin, G., & Rogers, S. J. (2005). Praxis skills in young children with Down syndrome, other developmental disabilities, and typically developing children. *The American Journal of Occupational Therapy, 59,* 129–138.

Fidler, D. J., Will, E., Daunhauer, L. A., Gerlach-McDonald, B., & Visootsak, J. (2014). Object–related generativity in children with Down syndrome. *Research in Developmental Disabilities, 35,* 3379–3385. doi:10.1016/j.ridd.2014.07.024

Friedman, N., & Miyake, N. (2017). Unity and diversity of executive functions: Individual differences as a window on cognitive structure. *Cortex: A Journal Devoted to the Study of the Nervous System and Behavior, 86,* 186–204. doi:10.1016/j.cortex.2016.04.023

Gardiner, K. J. (2015). Pharmacological approaches to improving cognitive function in Down syndrome: current status and considerations. *Drug Design, Development and Therapy, 9,* 103–125. doi:10.2147/DDDT.S51476

Gilmore, L., & Cuskelly, M. (2011). Observational assessment and maternal reports of motivation in children and adolescents with Down syndrome. *American Journal on Intellectual and Developmental Disabilities, 116*(2), 153–164.

Gilotty, L., Kenworthy, L., Sirian, L., Black, D. O., & Wagner, A. E. (2002). Adaptive skills and executive function in autism spectrum disorders. *Child Neuropsychology, 8*(4), 241–248. doi:10.1076/chin.8.4.241.13504

Gioia, G. A., Espy, K. A., & Isquith, P. K. (2003). Behavior rating inventory of executive function preschool version. Lutz, FL: Psychological Assessment Resources, Inc.

Gioia, G. A., Isquith, P. K., Guy, S. C., & Kenworthy, L. (2000). Test review behavior rating inventory of executive function. *Child Neuropsychology, 6*(3), 235–238. doi:10.1076/chin.6.3.235.3152

Goffinski, A., Stanley, M. A., Shepherd, N., Duvall, N., Jenkinson, S. B., Davis, C., . . . Roper, R. J. (2015). Obstructive sleep apnea in young infants with Down syndrome evaluated in a Down syndrome specialty clinic. *American Journal of Medical Genetics Part A, 167*(2), 324–330.

Gunn, P., & Berry, P. (1985). The temperament of Down's syndrome toddlers and their siblings. *Journal of Child Psychology and Psychiatry*, *26*(6), 973–979. doi:10.1111/j.1469-7610.1985.tb00610.x

Gunn, P., & Cuskelly, M. (1991). Down syndrome temperament: The stereotype at middle childhood and adolescence. *International Journal of Disability, Development and Education*, *38*, 59–70. doi:10.1080/0156655910380106

Handbook of Child Psychology and Developmental Science (pp. 571–623). John Wiley & Sons: New York.

Hart, S., Visootsak, S., Tamburri, J., Phuong, P., Baumer, P., Hernandez, N., . . . Spiridigliozzi, P. (2017). Pharmacological interventions to improve cognition and adaptive functioning in Down syndrome: Strides to date. Americ*an Journal of Medical Genetics*, *173*(11), 3029–3041.

Hendry, A., Jones, E. J., & Charman, T. (2016). Executive function in the first three years of life: Precursors, predictors and patterns. *Developmental Review*, *42,* 1–33. doi:10.1016/j.dr.2016.06.005

Jarrold, C., & Baddeley, A. D. (1997). Short-term memory for verbal and visuospatial information in Down's syndrome. *Cognitive Neuropsychiatry*, *2*(2), 101–122. doi:10.1080/135468097396351

Jarrold, C., & Brock, J. (2012). Short-term memory and working memory in mental retardation. In J. A. Burack, R. M. Hodapp, G. Iarocci, & E. Zigler (Eds.), Oxford library of psychology. The Oxford handbook of intellectual disability and development (pp. 109–124). Oxford: Oxford University Press.

Kasari, C., & Freeman, S. F. N. (2001). Task-related social behavior in children with Down syndrome. *American Journal on Mental Retardation*, *106*, 253–264.

Keeling, L., Spiridigliozzi, L., Hart, G., Baker, S., Jones, J., & Kishnani, H. (2017). Challenges in measuring the effects of pharmacological interventions on cognitive and adaptive functioning in individuals with Down syndrome: A systematic review. *American Journal of Medical Genetics*, *173*(11), 3058–3066.

Kenworthy, L., Anthony, L. G., Naiman, D. Q., Cannon, L., Wills, M. C., Luong-Tran, C., . . . Wallace, G.L. (2014). Randomized controlled effectiveness trial of executive function intervention for children on the autism spectrum. *Journal of Child Psychology and Psychiatry*, *55*, 374–383. doi:10.1111/jcpp.12161

Klingberg, T. (2010). Training and plasticity of working memory. *Trends in Cognitive Sciences*, *14*(7), 317–324. doi:10.1016/j.tics.2010.05.002

Kogan, C. S., Boutet, I., Cornish, K., Graham, G. E., Berry-Kravis, E., Drouin, A., & Milgram, N. W. (2009). A comparative neuropsychological test battery differentiates cognitive signatures of Fragile X and Down syndrome. *Journal of Intellectual Disability Research*, *53*, 125–142.

Kopp, C. B., Krakow, J. B., & Johnson, K. L. (1983). Strategy production by young Down syndrome children. *American Journal of Mental Deficiency*, *88*, 164–169.

Lanfranchi, S., Baddeley, A., Gathercole, S., & Vianello, R. (2012). Working memory in Down syndrome: Is there a dual task deficit? *Journal of Intellectual Disability Research*, *56*, 157–166. doi:10.1111/j.1365-2788.2011.01444.x

Lanfranchi, S., Carretti, B., Spanò, G., & Cornoldi, C. (2009). A specific deficit in visuospatial simultaneous working memory in Down syndrome. *Journal of Intellectual Disability Research*, *53*(5), 474–483. doi:10.1111/j.1365-2788.2009.01165.x

Lanfranchi, S., Cornoldi, C., & Vianello, R. (2004). Verbal and visuospatial working memory deficits in children with Down syndrome. *American Journal on Mental Retardation*, *109*, 456–466. doi:10.1352/0895-8017(2004)109<456:VAVWMD>2.0.CO;2

Lanfranchi, S., Jerman, O., Dal Pont, E., Alberti, A., & Vianello, R. (2010). Executive function in adolescents with Down syndrome. *Journal of Intellectual Disability Research*, *54*, 308–319. doi:10.1111/j.1365-2788.2010.01262.x

Lanfranchi, S., Mammarella, I., Carretti, B., & Pulina, F. (2014). How to improve spatial-simultaneous working memory in Down syndrome: A computerized training. Symposium: Intervention programs for individuals with Down syndrome. Sweden: ECIDD.

Lanfranchi, S., Pulina, F., Carretti, B., & Mammarella, I. C. (2017). Training spatial-simultaneous working memory in individuals with Down syndrome. *Research in Developmental Disabilities*, *64*, 118–129. doi:10.1016/j.ridd.2017.03.012

Lautarescu, B. A., Holland, A. J., & Zaman, S. (2017). The early presentation of dementia in people with Down syndrome: A systematic review. *Neuropsychological Review*, *27*, 31–45. doi:10.1007/s11065-017-9341-9

Lawson, R. A., Papadakis, A. A., Higginson, C. I., Barnett, J. E., Wills, M. C., Strang, J. F., . . . & Kenworthy, L. (2015). Everyday executive function impairments predict comorbid psychopathology in autism spectrum and attention deficit hyperactivity disorders. *Neuropsychology*, *29*(3), 445. doi:10.1037/neu0000145

Lee, N. R., Anand, P., Will, E., Adeyemi, E. I., Clasen, L. S., Blumenthal, J. D., . . . Edgin, J. O. (2015). Everyday executive functions in Down syndrome from early childhood to young adulthood: Evidence for both unique and shared characteristics compared to youth with sex chromosome trisomy (XXX and XXY). *Frontiers in Behavioral Neuroscience, 9*(264), 1–15. doi:10.3389/fnbeh.2015.00264

Lee, N. R., Fidler, D. J., Blakeley-Smith, A., Daunhauer, L., Robinson, C., & Hepburn, S. L. (2011). Caregiver report of executive functioning in a population-based sample of young children with Down syndrome. *American Journal on Intellectual and Developmental Disabilities, 116*, 290–304. doi:10.1352/1944-7558-116.4.290

Lemons, C. J., King, S. A, Davidson, K. A., Puranik, C. S., Al Otaiba, S., & Fidler, D. J. (2018). Personalized reading intervention for children with Down syndrome. *Journal of School Psychology, 66*, 67–84. doi.org/10.1016/j.jsp.2017.07.006

Loveall, S. J., Conners, F. A., Tungate, A. S., Hahn, L. J., & Osso, T. D. (2017). A cross-sectional analysis of executive function in Down syndrome from 2 to 35 years. *Journal of Intellectual Disability Research, 61*, 877–887. doi:10.1111/jjr.12396

Mares, D., McLuckie, A., Schwartz, M., & Saini, M. (2007). Executive function impairments in children with attention-deficit hyperactivity disorder: Do they differ between school and home environments? *The Canadian Journal of Psychiatry, 52*(8), 527–534. doi:10.1177/070674370705200811

Mervis, C. & Klein-Tasman, B. P. (2004). Methodological issues in group-matching designs alpha levels for control variable comparisons and measurement characteristics of control and target variables. *Journal of Autism and Developmental Disabilities, 34*, 7–17.

Miyake, A., Friedman, N. P., Emerson, M. J., Witzki, A. H., Howerter, A., & Wager, T. D. (2000). The unity and diversity of executive functions and their contributions to complex "frontal lobe" tasks: A latent variable analysis. *Cognitive Psychology, 41*, 49–100. doi:10.1006/cogp.1999.0734

Morgan, G. A., Harmon, R. J., & Maslin-Cole, C. A. (1990). Mastery motivation: Definition and measurement. *Early Education and Development, 1*(5), 318–339.

Müller, U., & Kerns, K. (2015). The development of executive function. In R. Lerner (Ed).

Nadel, L. (2003). Down's syndrome: A genetic disorder in biobehavioral perspective. *Genes, Brain & Behavior, 2*(3), 156–166. doi:10.1034/j.1601-183X.2003.00026.x

National Institutes of Health. (2015). NIH precision medicine initiative. *NIH MedlinePlus*, 10(3), 19–21.

National Institutes of Health—U.S. National Library of Medicine. (2018). ClinicalTrials.gov [Database] Retrieved from https://clinicaltrials.gov.

Niccols, A., Atkinson, L., & Pepler, D. (2003). Mastery motivation in young children with Down's syndrome: Relations with cognitive and adaptive competence. *Journal of Intellectual Disability Research, 47*(2), 121–133.

Ozonoff, S., & Jensen, J. (1999). Brief report: Specific executive function profiles in three neurodevelopmental disorders. *Journal of Autism and Developmental Disorders, 29*(2), 171–177.

Patel, L., Wolter-Warmerdam, K., Leifer, N., & Hickey, F. (2018). Behavioral characteristics of individuals with Down syndrome. *Journal of Mental Health Research in Intellectual Disabilities, 11*(3), 221–246.

Patti, P. J., & Tsiouris, J. A. (2006). Psychopathology in adults with Down syndrome: Clinical findings from an outpatient clinic. *International Journal on Disability and Human Development, 5*(4), 357–364.

Pennington, B. F., Moon, J., Edgin, J., Stedron, J., & Nadel, L. (2003). The neuropsychology of Down syndrome: Evidence for hippocampal dysfunction. *Child Development, 74*, 75–93.

Pitcairn, T. K., & Wishart, J. G. (1994). Reactions of young children with Down's syndrome to an impossible task. *British Journal of Developmental Psychology, 12*(4), 485–489. doi:10.1111/j.2044-835X.1994.tb00649.x

Pritchard, A. E., Kalback, S., McCurdy, M., & Capone, G. T. (2015). Executive functions among youth with Down syndrome and co-existing neurobehavioral disorders. *Journal of Intellectual Disability Research, 59*, 1130–1141. doi:10.1111/jir.12217

Pugliese, C. E., Anthony, L. G., Strang, J. F., Dudley, K., Wallace, G. L., Naiman, D. Q., & Kenworthy, L. (2016). Longitudinal examination of adaptive behavior in autism spectrum disorders: Influence of executive function. *Journal of Autism and Developmental Disorders, 46*(2), 467–477. doi:10.1007/s10803-015-2584-5

Pulina, F., Carretti, B., Lanfranchi, S., & Mammarella, I. (2015). Improving spatial-simultaneous working memory in Down syndrome: Effect of a training program led by parents instead of an expert. *Frontiers in Psychology, 6*, 1–9.

Rabiner, D. L., Murray, D. W., Skinner, A. T., & Malone, P. S. (2010). A randomized trial of two promising computer-based interventions for students with attention difficulties. *Journal of Abnormal Child Psychology, 38*, 131–142. doi:10.1007/s10802-009-9353-x

Reeves, R. H., & Garner, C. C. (2007). Year of unprecedented progress in Down syndrome basic research. *Mental Retardation and Developmental Disabilities Research Reviews, 13*(3), 215–220. doi:10.1002/mrdd.20165

Riggs, N. R., Huh, J., Chou, C. P., Spruijt-Metz, D., & Pentz, M. A. (2012). Executive function and latent classes of childhood obesity risk. *Journal of Behavioral Medicine, 35*(6), 642–650. doi:10.1007/s10865-011-9395-8

Riggs, N., R., Jahromi, L. B., Razza, R. P., Dillworth-Bart, J. E., & Mueller, U. (2006). Executive function and the promotion of social-emotional competence. *Journal of Applied Developmental Psychology, 27*, 300–309. doi:10.1016/j.appdev.2006.04.002

Roberts, L. V., & Richmond, J. L. (2015). Preschoolers with Down syndrome do not yet show the learning and memory impairments seen in adults with Down syndrome. *Developmental Science, 18*, 404–419. doi:10.1111/desc.12225

Rose, S. A., Feldman, J. F., & Jankowski, J. J. (2009). A cognitive approach to the development of early language. *Child Development, 80*, 13.4–150. doi:10.1111/j.1467-8624.2008.01250.x

Rose, S. A., Feldman, J. F., Jankowski, J. J., & Van Rossem, R. (2007). A cognitive cascade in infancy: Pathways from prematurity to later mental development. *Intelligence, 36*, 367–378. doi:10.1016/j.intell.2007.07.003

Rosenthal, M., Wallace, G. L., Lawson, R., Wills, M. C., Dixon, E., Yerys, B. E., & Kenworthy, L. (2013). Impairments in real-world executive function increase from childhood to adolescence in autism spectrum disorders. *Neuropsychology, 27*, 13. doi:10.1037/a0031299

Rowe, J., Lavender, A., & Turk, V. (2006). Cognitive executive function in Down's syndrome. *British Journal of Clinical Psychology, 45*, 5–17. doi:10.1348/014466505X29594

Rubia, K., Smith, A. B., Brammer, M. J., Toone, B., & Taylor, E. (2005). Abnormal brain activation during inhibition and error detection in medication-naive adolescents with ADHD. *American Journal of Psychiatry, 162*(6), 1067–1075. doi:10.1176/appi.ajp.162.6.1067

Ruskin, E. M., Mundy, P., Kasari, C., & Sigman, M. (1994). Object mastery motivation of children with Down syndrome. *American Journal on Mental Retardation, 98* (4), 499–509.

Russo, N., Dawkins, T., Huizinga, M., Burack, J. A. (2012). Executive function across syndromes associated with intellectual disabilities: A developmental perspective. *The Oxford Handbook of Intellectual Disability and Development*, 2, 125–137.

Seltzer, M. M., Abbeduto, L., Wyngaarden Krauss, M., Greenberg, J., & Swe, A. (2004). Comparison groups in autism family research: Down syndrome, fragile X syndrome and schizophrenia. *Journal of Autism and Developmental Disorders, 34*, 41–417.

Shott, S. R., Amin, R., Chini, B., Heubi, C., Hotze, S., & Akers, R. (2006). Obstructive sleep apnea: should all children with Down syndrome be tested?. *Archives of Otolaryngology–Head & Neck Surgery, 132*(4), 432–436.

Stagni, F., Giacomini, A., Guidi, S., Ciani, E., & Bartesaghi, R. (2015). Timing of therapies for Down syndrome: The sooner, the better. *Frontiers in Behavioral Neuroscience, 9*, 265. doi:10.3389/fnbeh.2015.00265

Tomaszewski, B., Fidler, D., Talapatra, D., & Riley, K. (2018). Adaptive behavior, executive function and employment in adults with Down syndrome. *Journal of Intellectual Disability Research, 62*, 41–52. doi:10.1111/jir.12450

Toplak, M. E., West, R. F., & Stanovich, K. E. (2013). Practitioner review: Do performance-based measures and ratings of executive function assess the same construct? *Journal of Child Psychology and Psychiatry, 54*(2), 131–143. doi:10.1111/jcpp.12001

Tsao, R., & Kindelberger, R. (2009). Variability of cognitive development in children with Down syndrome: Relevance of good reasons for using the cluster procedure. *Research in Developmental Disabilities, 30*(3), 426–432.

van Gameren-Oosterom, H. B., Fekkes, M., van Wouwe, J. P., Detmar, S. B., Oudesluys-Murphy, A. M., & Verkerk, P. H. (2013). Problem behavior of individuals with Down syndrome in a nationwide cohort assessed in late adolescence. *Journal of Pediatrics, 163*(5), 1396–1401. doi:10.1016/j.jpeds.2013.06.054

Vicari, S., Bellucci, S., & Carlesimo, G. A. (2000). Implicit and explicit memory: A functional dissociation in persons with Down syndrome. *Neuropsychologia, 38*(3), 240–251.

Vicari, S., Carlesimo, A., & Caltagirone, C. (1995). Short-term memory in persons with intellectual disabilities and Down's syndrome. *Journal of Intellectual Disability Research, 39*, 532–537.

Vicari, S. (2012). Memory and learning in intellectual. J. A. Burack, R. M. Hodapp, G. Iarocci, & E. Zigle (Eds.). *The Oxford handbook of intellectual disability and development* (p. 97), New York: Oxford University Press.

Ware, A. L., Crocker, N., O'Brien, J. W., Deweese, B. N., Roesch, S. C., Coles, C. D., . . . & Jones, K. L. (2012). Executive function predicts adaptive behavior in children with histories of heavy prenatal alcohol exposure and attention-deficit/hyperactivity disorder. *Alcoholism: Clinical and Experimental Research, 36*(8), 1431–1441. doi:10.1111/j.1530-0277.2011.01718.x

Wiebe, S. A., Sheffield, T., Nelson, J. M., Clark, C. A., Chevalier, N., & Espy, K. A. (2011). The structure of executive function in 3-year-olds. *Journal of experimental child psychology, 108*(3), 436–452.

Wilde, L., & Oliver, C. (2017). Brief report: Contrasting profiles of everyday executive functioning in Smith-Magenis syndrome and Down syndrome. *Journal of Autism and Developmental Disorders, 47*, 2602–2609. doi:10.1007/s10803-017-3140-2

Will, E., Fidler, D. J., Daunhauer, L., & Gerlach-McDonald, B. (2017). Executive function and academic achievement in primary—Grade students with Down syndrome. *Journal of Intellectual Disability Research, 61*(2), 181–195. doi:10.1111/jir.12313

Will, E. A., Gerlach-McDonald, B., Fidler, D. J., & Daunhauer, L. A. (2016). Impact of maladaptive behavior on school function in Down syndrome. *Research in Developmental Disabilities, 59*, 328–337. doi:10.1016/j.ridd.2016.08.018

Willoughby, M. T., & Blair, C. B. (2016). Measuring executive function in early childhood: A case for formative measurement. *Psychological assessment, 28*(3), 319.

Willoughby, M. T., Blair, C. B., Wirth, R. J., & Greenberg, M. (2010). The measurement of executive function at age 3 years: Psychometric properties and criterion validity of a new battery of tasks. *Psychological Assessment, 22*(2), 306–317. doi:10.1037/a0018708

Wishart, J. (2001). Motivation and learning styles in young children with Down syndrome. *Down Syndrome Research and Practice, 7*(2), 47–51.

Wuang, Y. P., & Su, C. Y. (2011). Correlations of sensory processing and visual organization ability with participation in school-aged children with Down syndrome. *Research in Developmental Disabilities, 32*(6), 2398–2407. doi:10.1016/j.ridd.2011.07.020

Yerys, B. E., Hepburn, S. L., Pennington, B. F., & Rogers, S. J. (2007). Executive function in preschoolers with autism: Evidence consistent with a secondary deficit. *Journal of Autism Developmental Disorders, 37*, 1068–1079. doi:10.1007/s10803-006-0250-7

Yerys, B. E., & Munakata, Y. (2006). When labels hurt but novelty helps: children's perseveration and flexibility in a card-sorting task. *Child Development, 77*(6), 1589–1607. doi:10.1111/j.1467-8624.2006.00961.x

Zelazo P. D. (2006). The dimensional change card sort (DCCS): A method of assessing executive function in children. *Nature Protocols, 1*, 297–301. doi:10.1038/nprot.2006.46

Zelazo, P. D., Burack, J. A., Benedetto, E., & Frye, D. (1996). Theory of mind and rule use in individuals with Down's syndrome: A test of the uniqueness and specificity claims. *Journal of Child Psychology and Psychiatry and Allied Disciplines, 37*, 479–484.

Zelazo, P. D., & Müller, U. (2011). Executive function in typical and atypical development. In U. Goswami (Ed.), *The Wiley-Blackwell handbook of childhood cognitive development* (pp. 574–603). Wiley-Blackwell.

Zelazo, P. D., Müller, U., Frye, D., Marcovitch, S., Argitis, G., Boseovski, J., . . . Sutherland, A. (2003). The development of executive function in early childhood. *Monographs of the Society for Research in Child Development, 68*, vii–137.doi:10.1111/j.1540-5834.2003.06803001.x

Zigler, E., & Burack, J. A. (1989). Personality development and the dually diagnosed person. *Research in Developmental Disabilities, 10*(3), 225–240.

Zigler, E., & Hodapp, R. M. (1986). Understanding mental retardation. New York: Cambridge University Press.

CHAPTER

14 Language Development in Down Syndrome

Leonard Abbeduto, Natalia Arias-Trejo, Angela John Thurman, Jessica Ramos-Sanchez, *and* Laura del Hoyo Soriano

Abstract

This chapter is a review of research on language development in individuals with Down syndrome. The development of various aspects of language is described from infancy to adulthood, with a focus on gestures and prelinguistic communication, speech, vocabulary, syntax, and pragmatics. In each area, the profile of relative strengths and weaknesses is described, as well as the trajectory of development, differences relative to other disorders, and the influence of other aspects of the phenotype of individuals with Down syndrome (e.g., memory impairments). Research is briefly reviewed on possible influences of the social and linguistic environments of individuals with Down syndrome on their language development. The chapter focuses on research on the learning of English as a first language; however, where possible, data from other languages and cultures is considered. Directions for future research are outlined.

Key Words: Down syndrome, language, communication, speech, phonology, gestures, vocabulary, syntax, pragmatics, maternal language, auditory memory, hearing

Introduction

Studies of language development in syndromes with identifiable genetic causes such as Down syndrome (DS) are essential for developing treatments that can optimize outcomes in language, cognition, and adaptive functioning in affected individuals. Such studies are also relevant to understanding language development more generally (Abbeduto, McDuffie, Thurman, & Kover, 2016). By examining relationships between various aspects of language ability and other domains of psychological and behavioral functioning (e.g., memory) within a syndrome, we can learn about the prerequisites for, and contributors to, language development in all children, as well as the functional consequences of particular genes and genetic variations. In addition, by making cross-syndrome comparisons, it should be possible to distinguish between language impairments that are the consequence of general cognitive delay (e.g., intellectual disability) and those that are syndrome specific, resulting from the unique genotypes, characteristics, and experiences of individuals with specific syndromes (del Hoyo Soriano, Thurman, & Abbeduto, 2018).

In this chapter, we summarize the literature on the language impairments and course of language development in persons with DS. We examine the relationships of language to other dimensions of the DS phenotype and highlight similarities and differences between persons with DS and those with other commonly occurring genetic syndromes associated with intellectual disability. We also review the ways in which caregiver behavior shapes, and is shaped by, the individual with DS. Finally, we briefly consider general issues in the assessment and treatment of language impairments in individuals with DS.

Brief Overview of Typical Language Development

Research on language development in individuals with DS has been shaped by the changing theoretical perspectives on language and its development emerging in work on typical populations (Abbeduto, Keller-Bell, Richmond, & Murphy, 2006). Beginning in the 1960s and into the 1980s, nativism was the dominant perspective, as espoused by the linguist Noam Chomsky (1975, 1988) and others (e.g., Fodor, 1983; Pinker, 1996). This perspective includes four interrelated claims:

(1) The human brain is specifically designed to learn language and, thus, every child has an innate capacity to learn language.
(2) The capacity to learn language is defined by mechanisms that are specifically linguistic and operate in modular fashion (i.e., with little input from, or dependency on, other cognitive systems or skills).
(3) Children need only limited exposure to language to learn it. They need to hear only a few key examples to know which of all possible human languages he/she is learning.
(4) The goal of language development is mastery of a set of abstract, deterministic, tacitly known rules that guide speaking and listening, but whose application is often distorted by "trivial" performance factors, such as memory, attention, or motivation.

These assumptions have largely been shown to be incorrect or, at best, overly simplistic. There are now various theoretical models, along with compelling empirical data, documenting the following characteristics of typical language development (Abbeduto, Keller-Bell, et al., 2006):

(1) Although the child may well be innately prepared to learn language, the mechanisms are not specifically linguistic; instead, learning language depends on largely the same mechanisms as do other types of learning. For example, children construct linguistic categories and rules by tracking recurring patterns in the language they hear and the situations in which language occurs, and they use all sources of information available to them, from the acoustic

properties of language to the nature of the objects to which language refers, to the social intentions of speakers (Saffran & Kirkham, 2018). In terms of understanding language development in individuals with DS, the implication is that language, like all learning, will be negatively impacted, although the extent of the impact remains to be determined.

(2) Learning language draws on the entire cognitive system and, thus, individual differences in cognitive ability affect language learning in fundamental and potentially dramatic ways. For example, the ability to parse, store, and access auditory information is essential for learning vocabulary and syntax, such that individuals with stronger auditory memory skills show better progress in language learning (Baddeley, 2001). Moreover, because the cognitive system itself develops with age and experience, developments in cognition can set the stage for new linguistic achievements. For example, the onset of intentionality in the behavior of the infant near 9 months of age changes the nature of social interaction in ways that facilitate recognition of the mappings between objects and events in the world and the words heard (Bates, Bretherton, Beeghly-Smith, & McNew, 1982; Mundy & Newell, 2007). In terms of understanding language development in individuals with DS, the implication is that the profile of behavioral relative strengths and weaknesses that defines the phenotype of affected individuals will shape their language development and that the relationships between language and cognition may change over the course of development.

(3) Learning language depends on extensive exposure to language (Hart & Risley, 1995) and a supportive learning environment, which can be conceptualized as a series of interacting contexts or systems of influence, such as the family, school, and peer group (Bronfenbrenner & Ceci, 1994; Cross, 2017; Vandell, Pierce, & Dadisman, 2005). Moreover, the nature and role in development of these settings change over the course of development (Cross, 2017). Adult caregivers play an especially important role throughout all phases of language development. Indeed, variations in the amount of language heard and the nature of the interactions that parents and other caregivers have with children have a substantial influence on the rate of language learning. In areas such as vocabulary, this input is an important source of individual differences (Bornstein, Tamis-LeMonda, & Haynes, 1999; Hoff & Naigles, 2002; Landry, Smith, & Swank, 2006; Smith, Adamson, & Bakeman, 1988). In terms of understanding language development in individuals with DS, the implication is that environmental influences will play a role in shaping the trajectory of language. It has even been suggested that suboptimal learning environments may be even more influential for individuals with DS than is the case for otherwise typically developing (TD) children because the former

have less capacity to "rise above" such environments because of their cognitive impairments (Abbeduto et al., 2016). Moreover, the behavioral phenotype of individuals with DS may actually challenge caregivers and others to provide optimal experiences for language development.

(4) Performance factors, such as memory and attention, are not trivial factors obscuring true linguistic competence, but rather critical determinants of how language is learned and used (Chapman et al., 1992). Moreover, variability in performance should be expected and is a function of the "state" of the information processing system at any given point in time. In terms of understanding language development in individuals with DS, the implication is that the profile of relative strengths and weaknesses that defines the behavioral phenotype of affected individuals can lead to asynchronies in performance across different language tasks or modalities.

In this chapter, we have organized our review in ways that reflect more recent alternatives to the nativist approach. We begin by considering aspects of the behavioral phenotype of individuals with DS that are likely to shape their language development. We carry this interest in the broader behavioral phenotype in which language learning is embedded throughout the chapter, considering relationships among linguistic and nonlinguistic skills and the ways in which their unique phenotype may lead to different profiles of language development in individuals with DS relative to those with either typical development or intellectual disability of different etiology. We also review the prelinguistic achievements that set the stage for language development in individuals with DS. In considering language development in individuals with DS, we organize the review around major components (i.e., speech and phonology, vocabulary, syntax, and pragmatics) because each component depends on different skills and experiences and so poses differential challenges for individuals with DS. In each section, we also consider performance factors, especially distinguishing the problems that individuals with DS experience with the expressive (i.e., speaking) and receptive (i.e., listening) modalities. We close the review by a consideration of research on environmental influences, focusing on parental influences on language development in individuals with DS.

Down Syndrome Phenotype and Its Implications for Language Development

Language is among the most affected domains of neurocognitive functioning in persons with DS and is arguably the greatest barrier to independent living and meaningful inclusion in the community (Abbeduto, Warren, & Conners, 2007). Moreover, treating the language impairments of individuals with DS will require identifying the ways in which the DS phenotype promotes and hinders language development (Abbeduto et al., 2007). Thus, we briefly consider those aspects of the behavioral phenotype of DS that help to shape language development. Further, more detailed information is available in other chapters in this volume.

The cognitive challenges experienced by individuals with DS are likely to shape many aspects of their language development. Problems in visual and verbal attention and memory formation can be detected before the end of the first year of life and may impact language development (Delabar et al., 2016; D'Souza et al., 2015; Karmiloff-Smith et al., 2016). Individuals with DS also have especially severe impairments in the phonological loop component of working memory (i.e., the ability to encode, process, and retrieve auditory information), which have been hypothesized to contribute to the speech and language difficulties associated with a number of disorders (Pierpont, Richmond, Abbeduto, Kover, & Brown, 2011), including DS (Buckley & Bird, 2001; Conners, Moore, Loveall, & Merrill, 2011; Jarrold & Baddeley, 2001; Jarrold, Baddeley, & Phillips, 2002). Hearing loss and oral motor difficulties are also common in DS (Chapman, Seung, Schwartz, & Bird, 1998) and are likely to interact with impairments in the phonological loop to impact language development and speech articulation (Martin, Klusek, Estigarribia, & Roberts, 2009; Stoel-Gammon, 2001). Other aspects of the memory system are also impaired in DS, including the intentional processing involved in resource allocation, as reflected in, for example, tasks involving the backward recall of both verbal and visual information (Vicari, Carlesimo, & Caltagirone, 1995).

Other challenges associated with DS may also contribute to the language impairments of affected individuals. Congenital heart disease is related to poorer receptive and expressive language in DS toddlers (Alsaied et al., 2016). Sleep disturbance, resulting in part from obstructive sleep apnea, also is related to reduced expressive language in preschoolers with DS, probably by disrupting the memory consolidation that typically occurs during sleep (Edgin et al., 2015). In addition, infantile spasm history is linked to greater difficulties in receptive and expressive language (Tapp, Anderson, & Visootsak, 2015). Other comorbidities, such as hypothyroidism and autism spectrum disorder (ASD), also are associated with greater language difficulties in this population (Hepburn, Philofsky, Fidler, & Rogers, 2008; Lavigne et al., 2017; Naerland, Bakke, Storvik, Warner, & Howlin, 2017; Warner, Howlin, Salomone, Moss, & Charman, 2017). For example, congenital hypothyroidism is 28 times more prevalent in infants with DS than in the general population (Fort et al., 1984) and ASD has been found to occur in as many as 40 percent of individuals with DS in one study (Warner, Moss, Smith, & Howlin, 2014). These comorbid conditions may exert their influence on language either directly or indirectly (i.e., through other aspects of neurocognition).

As the DS phenotype changes rather dramatically with chronological age (CA), many individuals with DS often experience a cognitive decline in adulthood reflecting neuropathology associated with Alzheimer's disease (see Helman, Van Pelt, Schmitt, & Head, this volume; Startin, Zaman, & Strydom, this volume). In fact, DS confers a virtually 100 percent risk of developing the neuropathology associated with Alzheimer's disease, often as early as the fourth decade of life (Hartley et al., 2017). The neuropathology leads to a high incidence of early onset of dementia in individuals with DS (Lott, 2012). It is likely, of course, that language will be impacted by this cognitive decline, although which aspects of language and to what degree are not well understood. In this chapter, we focus on development into adulthood, touching only briefly on the linguistic indicators of early cognitive decline.

Language Development in Individuals With Down Syndrome

Although language is a tightly integrated system of knowledge and procedures for speaking and listening, it is useful to dissect it into components when examining the profile of development and impairments. Among individuals with DS, all stages of development and components of language show some degree of impairment, from mastery of the sounds of language to the use of language for social ends. Nevertheless, the profile of impairments, and of relative strengths and weaknesses, differ across language components and processes.

Prelinguistic Foundations

Relative to other neurodevelopmental disorders, there is a substantial body of research considering the early developmental period for children with DS. This is likely due to the relatively high incidence of DS, as well as the fact that awareness and technological advancements allow for the early diagnosis of DS in contrast to, for example, fragile X syndrome (FXS), which is not typically diagnosed until age 3 years on average (Bailey, Raspa, Bishop, & Holiday, 2009).

Prelinguistic vocalizations. Despite problems with oral-motor development (Kumin & Bahr, 1999), similarities have been observed between infants with DS and TD infants with regard to the frequency of vocalizations produced and in the developmental sequence of their vocalizations, including the onset of canonical babbling (i.e., production of consonant/vowel speech-like productions, such as "ba;" e.g., Dodd, 1972; Oller, Eilers, Neal, & Cobo-Lewis, 1998; Smith & Oller, 1981; Smith & Stoel-Gammon, 1996). Nevertheless, there is evidence that early communicative difficulties may emerge within late infancy for children with DS (e.g., Adamson, Bakeman, Deckner, & Romski, 2009; Mervis & Robinson, 2000). For example, Legerstee, Bowman, and Fels (1992) found that the CA at which infants with DS begin to alter their vocalizations according to the context (e.g., when looking at people versus objects) was approximately two months later than has been reported for TD infants, although consistent with mental age (MA) expectations. Furthermore, the integration of findings across studies suggests that infants with DS may produce fewer speech-like (melodic) vocalizations and more non-speech-like (vocalic) vocalizations than do TD infants (e.g., Legerstee, 1991; Legerstee et al., 1992). In addition, Lynch et al. (1995) found that the onset of canonical babbling for their group of infants with DS was delayed by approximately two months relative to the age reported in TD infants. The production of canonical babbling was also less stable for the infants with DS.

Due to the relatively small numbers of participants and considerable heterogeneity among the participants in studies of prelinguistic vocalizations in infants with DS, the extent to which data from these studies can be generalized to the larger population of individuals with DS is unclear. Furthermore, the lack of comparisons to appropriately matched children with other neurodevelopmental disorders or developmental delays in these studies limits our understanding of the syndrome specificity of the developmental patterns described. In addition, longitudinal studies are needed to understand the extent to which these early patterns of development predict long-term language development.

Gestures/nonverbal communication. Young children with DS demonstrate a relative strength in the use of gestures. Franco and Wishart (1995) demonstrated that the frequency and variety of gestures produced is comparable if not higher in DS relative to younger TD children with similar overall communicative ability. Such findings have led some researchers to argue that children with DS may compensate for their often protracted periods of oral speech development with their gestural productions (Singer-Harris, Bellugi, Bates, Jones, & Rossen, 1997). This relative strength in the gestural domain also distinguishes children with DS from those with other conditions such as Williams syndrome (WS), for whom gesturing is an area of particular weakness (John & Mervis, 2010; Rowe, Peregrine, & Mervis, 2005).

There is also evidence suggesting that the communicative functions of gestures used by children with DS may differ from other groups. For example, there is evidence of difficulties with components of joint attention (the ability to coordinate attention between people and objects), such as reciprocal eye contact (e.g., Berger, 1990; Berger & Cunningham, 1983), which may result in part from a low level of visual exploration by children with DS (Kasari, Mundy, Yirmiya, & Sigman, 1990). Despite delays relative to CA expectations, children with DS are as likely to initiate and respond to the joint attention initiations of others as are their MA-matched TD peers (Sigman et al., 1999). In contrast, nonverbal requesting appears to be an area of challenge for children with DS. Indeed, several investigators have found that children with DS make fewer nonverbal requests than MA-matched TD peers (e.g., Beeghly, Weiss-Perry, & Cicchetti, 1990; Fidler, Philofsky, Hepburn, & Rogers, 2005; Mundy, Kasari, Sigman, & Ruskin, 1995; Sigman et al., 1999). Commenting and requesting gestures are often associated with better linguistic communication and therefore delays in these nonverbal communication skills may also contribute to the well-documented language deficits in DS (e.g., Chan & Iacono, 2001; Mundy et al., 1995; Yoder & Warren, 2004; Zampini & D'Odorico, 2009, 2011a).

Individuals with DS also integrate gestures and language differently than TD children. Children with DS seem to primarily use "equivalent" combinations, such as waving goodbye and saying "bye," whereas TD children are more likely to use "complementary" combinations, such as pointing at a bird and saying "bird," and "supplementary" combinations, such as signing "more" and saying "cookie" (Zampini & D'Odorico, 2011a). Furthermore, the ability to pair gestures with words has been associated with the onset of two-word verbal utterances in children with DS, although "supplementary" and "complementary" combinations are generally believed to be the best predictors of the emergence of word combinations (e.g., Bates & Dick, 2002; Capirci, Iverson, Pizzuto, & Volterra, 1996; Iverson & Goldin-Meadow, 2005). These differences in how words and gestures are combined occur even though the frequency with which gestures are paired with words is similar for children with DS and TD children matched on language age, MA, and expressive vocabulary size (e.g., Iverson, Longobardi, & Caselli, 2003; Zampini & D'Odorico, 2011a).

Speech Development

From the first years of life, children with DS, like their TD peers, must learn about the sound system, or phonology, of their native language. Moreover, in typical development, phonological development is essential for building a broader, stable lexicon, as well as other aspects of language (Curtin & Zamuner, 2014). Unfortunately, there are significant gaps in our knowledge of the phonological development of children with DS, especially the understanding of how they perceive speech during infancy and the toddler years.

Etiological factors. Children with DS have distinct biological characteristics that impact their phonological development. A high incidence of chronic ear disease has been widely reported in children with DS as compared to their TD peers and to children with other neurodevelopmental disorders (Dahle & McCollister, 1986; Downs, 1980; Kanamori, Witter, Brown, & Williams-Smith, 2000; Shott, 2006). Chronic ear disease (such as otitis media) accounts for a high incidence in the DS population of conductive, mixed, and sensorineural hearing loss, and a greater severity and extended periods of untreated ear disease and associated hearing loss negatively affect speech and language development (see Roberts et al., 2004).

Differences in the skeletal and muscular systems of individuals with DS (particularly those pertaining to orofacial features) also may impose some limitations on their articulatory performance and therefore their phonological development. Problems such as a mild degree of dysphonia, a smaller middle and lower facial skeleton that reduces upper airway size, poorly differentiated mid-face muscles, and a relatively large tongue are implicated in the speech difficulties of individuals with DS (Bersu & Opitz, 1980; Guimaraes, Donnelly, Short, Amin, & Kalra, 2008; Uong et al., 2001).

Speech production. There is ongoing debate in the field as to whether the phonological development of children with DS is delayed or qualitatively distinct from that of TD children. A comprehensive review of the literature suggests a combination of both developmental (Barnes et al., 2009; Bleile & Schwarz, 1984; Borsel, 1996; Smith & Stoel-Gammon, 1983; Stoel-Gammon, 1980) and atypical patterns (Cleland, Wood, Hardcastle, Wishart & Timmins, 2010; Sommers, Patterson, & Wildgen, 1988). For instance, a delayed emergence of phonemes has been reported in children with DS, although the pattern of emergence is similar to that of their TD counterparts (Dodd, Leahy, & Hambly, 1989; Kumin, Councill, & Goodman, 1994). A delayed suppression of phonological processes, which leads to simplified and immature productions of TD children (e.g., final stop devoicing, final stop deletion, initial stop cluster reduction, and final consonant de-aspiration), has also been found in children with DS. For example, Smith and Stoel-Gammon (1983) examined the rates of suppression of phonological processes over 3 years in a longitudinal study of 3-year-old children with DS and 18–24 month-old TD children. These investigators noted smaller rates of suppression of phonological processes per year for the children with DS (6 percent) than for TD children (38 percent), thereby indicating slower developmental progress for the children with DS. Moreover, phonological processes (such as final consonant deletion of voiced stops and cluster reduction of nasals) tend to persist even at older ages in individuals with DS rather than being replaced with accurate speech reductions as in TD children, suggesting ongoing delay and impairment in DS (Shriberg & Widder, 1990; Sommers et al., 1988).

Many aspects of the speech impairments of individuals with DS can be seen as reflecting particularly serious delays relative to typical development. Stoel-Gammon (1980, 2001) documented the most frequently occurring patterns of phonological acquisition in children with DS (CAs 3:10–6:3). They are (1) consonant clusters produced as singleton consonants, (2) omission of word-final consonants, (3) target fricatives and affricates produced as stops, (4) de-aspiration of aspirated voiceless stops in initial positions, (5) word-initial liquids produced as glides, (6) word-final liquids produced as vowels or omitted altogether, and (7) devoicing of word-final obstruents. These patterns are like those found among younger TD toddlers and preschoolers as they develop, suggesting an extensive delay rather than an atypical developmental process.

The phonological development of children with DS, however, is also characterized by unique patterns rather than simply delays relative to TD children. In an articulation test, children with DS were found to make more consonant errors and reduced word shapes due to omitted syllables, reduced consonant clusters, and deletion of consonant singletons (Roberts et al., 2005). Further, although Cleland et al. (2010) reported that 15 children and adolescents with DS (9.83–18.75 CA) showed a high percentage (66.23 percent) of the phonological processes reported in younger TD children (2.0–5.11 CA) by Dodd, Zhu, Crosbie, Holm, and Ozanne (2002), all of the individuals with DS had at least one atypical phonological error (e.g., initial consonant deletion).

Speech impairments also distinguish individuals with DS from those with other neurodevelopmental disorders, such as FXS. In particular, Barnes et al. (2009) found greater delays in measures of phonological accuracy and phonological process occurrence than in matched individuals with FXS and TD children, although these investigators studied only males.

Speech perception. Few studies have been focused on the speech perception abilities of children with DS due largely to the challenges of working with very young children with DS and the difficulty of creating tasks sensitive to the phenotypic characteristics of the syndrome (e.g., greater hearing loss and reduced attention spans). However, research with adolescents and adults with DS suggests that the ability to form stable, long-term phonological representations of words might be hampered because of problems in verbal short-term memory (Brock & Jarrold, 2004; Jarrold, Thorn, & Stephens, 2009; Laws, 2002). Jarrold et al. (2009) examined the learning of new words in 22 adolescents and adults with DS (14–29 CA) and found impairments both in their verbal short-term memory (measured in tasks of serial recall, item recognition, and order recognition) and their ability to learn the phonological form (sound units) of novel words but not their physical referents, as compared to 5- to 8-year-old TD children. These investigators found that their participants with DS were unsuccessful at learning the phonological forms of new words because of their inability to maintain an accurate phonological representation of the novel items in memory. Jarrold et al. also found that verbal working memory problems were associated with poor performance on the phonological awareness tasks of alliteration detection, deletion, and rhyme detection. Similar results have been found in the measurement of the phonological awareness abilities of children with DS, who show notably poor performance in tasks that require making judgments of the rhyme units of words (Cardoso-Martins, Michalick, & Pollo, 2002; Snowling, Hulme, & Mercer, 2002).

Researchers have linked some of the speech perception problems of individuals with DS to their neurobiological substrates, such as anomalous cerebral lateralization. For example, evidence from studies of dichotic listening have indicated greater left ear advantages, which suggests that individuals with DS use their right hemispheres to process speech input to a greater extent than TD individuals (Bunn, Roy, & Elliott, 2007; Elliott & Weeks, 1993; Elliott, Weeks, & Chua, 1994; Welsh & Elliott, 2001).

Summary. There is still much we do not know about the abilities of children with DS to learn and process the sound structure and characteristics of their language. Further research on their sensitivity to phonological cues in language input, their use of phonological information to cluster their early vocabularies, as well as their development of phonotactical knowledge, is needed to further our understanding of the phonological development of individuals with DS.

Lexical Development

Although delayed relative to typical CA expectations, lexical development in DS tends to be less impaired, on average, than other linguistic abilities. The appearance of the first words spoken by children with DS can occur between 12 and 24 months of age (Berglund, Eriksson, & Johansson, 2001), which is not drastically different from TD children; however, the subsequent acquisition of words occurs at a slower pace and with greater variability.

Milestones, trajectories, and profiles. Oliver and Buckley (1994) indicated that individuals with DS learn the same vocabulary as their TD peers, but with a delay of 18 months that becomes more evident with development. More evidence is needed to assess whether the DS phenotype is characterized by simply a delay in lexical development, but with a trajectory like that of TD children, or by a different trajectory.

Even after they begin to produce words, there is evidence suggesting a preference in young children with DS to use gestures rather than spoken words (Kaat-van den Os, Jongmans, Volman, & Lauteslager, 2015; Stefanini, Caselli, & Volterra, 2007). This preference for gestures, however, changes with development. For example, Kaat-van den Os, Volman, Jongmans, and Lauteslager (2017) reported that in a period of 18 months, only 10 percent of the children included in their study progressed from using only gestures to using gestures plus spoken words, and another 10 percent progressed from using gestures plus spoken words to using mainly spoken words.

The MacArthur-Bates Communicative Development Inventory (CDI; Fenson et al., 1993), in which a caregiver informant marks the words the child understands or says, has been widely used to measure early vocabularies in children with TD as well as in children with DS. In studies in which the CDI has been used, the productive vocabularies of young children with DS have been found to be smaller than those of their MA-matched TD peers (Miller, 1992, 1999). In a longitudinal study with DS children with a MA between 12 and 17 months, Miller (1999) demonstrated that TD children matched on MA had larger vocabularies, both in comprehension and production, throughout development, although the difference became larger as MA increased.

Use of the CDI has also documented delays in vocabulary in children with DS learning languages other than English. Zampini and D'Odorico (2013) administered the Italian version of the CDI at 6-month intervals to study word production. These investigators found lower productive vocabulary sizes for children with DS that were well below CA expectations for TD children based on the Italian CDI normative data in Caselli, Pasqualetti, and Stefanini (2007). Instead, the scores for the children with DS were more similar to those for younger TD children who were analogous in their developmental levels. Similarly, Caselli et al. (1998) found vocabulary scores in Italian children with DS (CA 10–49 months) were alike those of younger TD children matched on lexical comprehension scores. Using an adaptation of the Spanish CDI for DS individuals (Galeote, Soto, Checa, Gómez, & Lamela, 2008), Galeote, Sebastian, Checa, Rey, and Soto (2011) found that oral production and oral plus gestural production were similar for MA-matched children with DS and TD children (MA 9–27 months).

Although individuals with DS display CDI profiles that are generally consistent with their levels of cognitive functioning, studies using the CDI have also shown some aspects of their vocabulary development do not match expectations relative to other aspects of their cognition and language. For example, using an adaptation of the Spanish CDI for DS individuals (Galeote et al., 2008), Galeote et al. (2011) found, among other things, that children with DS (MA 9–27 months) had higher CDI scores than MA-matched TD children in both lexical comprehension and gestural production. Galeote et al. (2011) argued that the additional life experience of children with DS associated with their greater CA was the main factor contributing to this difference. In a study of Italian children with DS (mean MA 30.7 months) as compared to a group of TD children matched by

MA and socioeconomic status, Vicari, Caselli, and Tonucci (2000) found similar scores in production for individual words on the Italian version of the CDI, although the DS group produced simpler and more telegraphic sentences. The DS group also scored lower on receptive grammar on a verbal comprehension test than did their TD counterparts (Vicari et al., 2000). We expand on these problems in syntax in a subsequent section of this chapter.

A common milestone in lexical development is the vocabulary spurt/naming explosion, a period of rapid increase in vocabulary acquisition, which occurs in many TD children between the ages of 18 and 24 months (Ganger & Brent, 2004; Goldfield & Reznick, 1990). This vocabulary spurt/naming explosion is observed in some children with DS, although it is delayed (Berglund, Eriksson, & Johansson, 2001; Miller, 1999; Oliver & Buckley, 1994). In a longitudinal study of recordings of children with DS (ages 12–28 months) that was focused on vocabulary growth from the periods of first words to the consolidation of two-word phrases, Oliver and Buckley (1994) reported that only 5 of the 12 children (CA 28–38 months) exhibited a clear vocabulary spurt. For the remaining seven children, evidence of a rapid surge in language acquisition was less obvious. In another longitudinal study, Zampini and D'Odorico (2013) found that none of the children in their sample displayed vocabularies of fifty words or more at 30 months of age. In fact, Zampini and D'Odorico found that increases in vocabulary size did not occur until 36 months of age, on average, for their sample of children with DS, 18 in a longitudinal study and 27 in a cross-sectional study. In some children with DS, however, the vocabulary spurt in children with DS can occur as late as 5 years of age (Caselli, Marchetti, & Vicari, 1994). For example, Berglund et al. (2001) reported that in a sample of Swedish children with DS, the fifty-word milestone was most often achieved at age 5 (75 percent), with the rest of the children reaching that milestone at age 3 or 4 years.

As described in the next section on syntax, individuals with DS produce shorter, less complex utterances than expected for their CA, as reflected in, for example, lower mean length of utterance in morphemes (MLUs). In terms of vocabulary, this reduction in utterance length is systematic, with certain categories or types of words more likely to be omitted than others. Relative to TD children, individuals with DS include fewer functional words, such as articles, prepositions, and pronouns (Chapman et al., 1998; Vicari, Caselli, Gagliardi, Tonucci, & Volterra, 2002; Zampini & D'Odorico, 2011b). In narrative and conversational recordings of adolescents with DS, Chapman (1997) found that children and adolescents with DS tended to omit words from closed-class grammatical categories. Similarly, in a free-play session with their parents, Italian children with DS (mean MA 30 months) were again found to have particular deficits in producing closed-class words (Zampini & D'Odorico, 2011b) as compared with a control group of TD children of the same MA and vocabulary size, although the two groups produced equal numbers of nouns. In contrast, using the adapted version of the Spanish CDI, Checa, Galeote, and Soto (2016) found no difference in the number of nouns, predicates (verbs and adjectives), social words, or closed-class words produced by children with DS and their TD peers matched by sex, MA (9–29 months), and vocabulary size. The extent to which these differences across studies arise from language and cultural differences, other characteristics of the participants, or the measures used to assess language is not clear.

Qualitative aspects of the expressive vocabulary profiles of individuals with DS have also been examined and have generally indicated that verbs pose a special challenge for them. For example, Nash and Snowling (2008) examined narrative production and found that young adults with DS (mean MA 5.62 years) tended to omit verbs for their descriptions of story episodes relative to TD children matched by MLU. In a similar vein, Loveall, Channell, Abbeduto, and Conners (2019) found that when producing narratives, adolescents and young adults with DS used fewer verbs than nonverbal cognitive-level matched TD children and used a less diverse set of verbs than individuals with intellectual disabilities of other etiologies.

Arias-Trejo, Angulo-Chavira, and Barrón-Martínez (2019) used an eye-tracking paradigm to illuminate the reasons for these difficulties individuals DS have with verbs. These investigators found that children with DS (mean MA 5.48 years) were capable of employing the semantic information embedded in a verb (e.g., "read") to anticipate a target ("book" versus "chair"). Arias-Trejo et al. also found that the both children with DS and TD children demonstrated a visual preference for a target semantically related to a heard informative verb and a lack of preference for a visual target preceded by a noninformative verb (e.g., "see"). Thus, omission of verbs may reflect syntactic rather than lexical-semantic problems, an issue to which we return in the next section.

More generally, expressive vocabulary deficits may be the result of insufficient short-term memory (Nadel, 1999), specifically phonological short-term memory problems or difficulties in accessing word knowledge for the purposes of oral production, as well as verbal short-term memory itself (Næss, Lyster, Hulme, & Melby-Lervag, 2011). Chapman and Hesketh (2001) demonstrated that auditory short-term memory and CA are predictors of early vocabulary scores, and Laws (1998) found a correlation of word and nonword repetition tasks with phonological memory and receptive vocabulary in a group of children with DS. Difficulties in lexical development also have been explained by different factors such as the cognitive delay itself, recurrent auditory problems, access to education, and sleep efficiency, among others. For example, Anand, Misra, Demara, Clark, and Edgin (2017) reported that sleep efficiency correlates positively with the number of words produced by 12- to 18-month-olds in a 5-minute recording of their utterances (see Anand & Edgin, this volume, on sleep disorder and its correlates in children with DS).

As is true for TD children, the lexical development of children with DS is shaped by developments in other cognitive domains. For example, Abreu-Mendoza and Arias-Trejo (2017) found that children with DS who have larger receptive vocabularies also know the meaning of more words that express numerical concepts. These investigators evaluated the understanding of number words using the give-a-number task (Wynn, 1990) and their receptive vocabulary using the task for that purpose from the Mexican adaptation of the WPPSI-III (Wechsler, 2011). After controlling for CA, Abreu-Mendoza and Arias-Trejo found that receptive vocabulary scores explained 15 percent of the variance in number word knowledge. These findings, along with a previous study (Porter, 1999), suggest a strong link between lexical and numerical development in children with DS.

Syndrome specificity. Comparison with other neurodevelopmental disorders has allowed for a better understanding of the linguistic profile of people with DS and the association of specific linguistic problems with particular cognitive deficits. These comparisons have mainly been made with Specific Language Impairment (SLI) and WS (see Ypsilanti & Grouios, 2008 for a review). Broadly speaking, individuals with SLI experience difficulties in phonology and grammar production, but have typical range IQ scores (Laws & Bishop, 2003). Children with SLI also have strengths in comprehension over production (Montgomery, 2000). Using the Test for Reception of Grammar (Bishop, 2003), Laws and Bishop (2003) found that a group of individuals with DS and another with SLI had similar abilities in receptive vocabulary when compared to a group of TD children matched for nonverbal MA. However, the TD children were better with syntax than were the children with either DS or SLI. The two experimental groups also had more errors in expressive language (as opposed to receptive language) than the comparison group. The similarities between DS and SLI individuals may be due to similar deficits in short-term memory, particularly in the phonological domain, or they may be modulated by different mechanisms.

Early studies comparing individuals with DS and those with WS were motivated largely by an interest in the seemingly intact language abilities of individuals with WS despite their intellectual disability, with DS being seen as a convenient comparison (Bellugi, Wang, & Jernigan, 1994). More recent studies have clarified that individuals with WS have milder cognitive impairments than do those with DS, on average, which makes the comparison of language skills in the two groups more complicated (e.g., Mervis & John, 2010). Nonetheless, these studies have yielded insights into the language phenotype associated with DS.

Studies in which the CDI has been used indicate differences in expressive vocabulary between individuals with DS and those with WS. Singer-Harris et al. (1997) studied samples of children with a mean age of 34 months and found that the number of words expressed as gestures on the Words and Gestures form of the CDI was greater for children with DS than for children with WS. Using the Words and Sentences form for children with a mean age of 45 months, Singer-Harris et al. also found, however, that the children with WS outperformed the children with DS on expressive vocabulary. Also using the Words and Sentences form, Mervis and Robinson (2000) found better expressive vocabulary in children with WS than in those with DS (mean age 30 months). Similar differences were reported by Bellugi et al. (1994).

Using a direct assessment (i.e., the Peabody Picture Vocabulary Test; Dunn, Dunn, Whetton, & Burley, 1997) rather than parent report, Klein and Mervis (1999) did not find significant differences in receptive vocabulary between 9- and 10-year-old children with WS or DS. This pattern is consistent with those studies that have reported that receptive vocabulary in DS children is a strength relative to other aspects of cognitive functioning, including expressive vocabulary (Glenn & Cunningham, 2005; Iverson, Longobardi, & Caselli, 2003).

In addition to examining which words are learned and at what rate, researchers have been interested in the ways in which individuals with DS process lexical information and use that information to speak and listen. For example, Ypsilanti, Grouios, Zikouli, and Hatzinikolaou (2006) compared naming speed for colors, pictures, numbers, letters, and single words, and found no differences between children with DS and those with WS matched on MA (as measured by the Wechsler Intelligence Scale for Children-III; WISC-III). The children with DS, however, produced more errors in naming pictures and words than did those with WS and TD. Such findings suggest that individuals with DS may represent and/or access lexical information in less complete or organized ways than TD children or even those with other neurodevelopmental disorders.

Summary. The lexical development of individuals with DS is characterized by substantial delays relative to CA, but there are asynchronies across modalities and word types, and there are commonalities and differences relative to other neurodevelopmental disorders. These asynchronies and cross-disorder differences reflect, at least in part, the unique cognitive profile of DS.

Syntactic Development

Learning a language requires more than learning sounds and words. Every language has its own grammatical rules that impose constraints on the ways in which words are combined into phrases and sentences to express complex meanings. Thus, learning syntax requires mastering conventions about word order, morphological inflections (e.g., past tense markings), and the formal categories of different words (e.g., to distinguish nouns from verbs), as well as the capacity to create and understand the complex semantic structures that map on to grammatical combinations. The task of learning syntax is one of the most challenging aspects of language development for persons with DS (Abbeduto et al., 2016; Chapman, Schwartz, & Bird, 1991; Fowler, 1990; Martin et al., 2009). In this section, we consider expressive syntax, or the ability when speaking to combine words in ways that conform to the rules of the language, separately from receptive syntax, or the ability to determine the meaning of multiword phrases and sentences, because they show different patterns of impairment in individuals with DS.

Expressive syntax. Expressive syntax is typically more delayed than receptive syntax in persons with DS (Abbeduto et al., 2001; Chapman, Hesketh, & Kistler, 2002; Eadie, Fey, Douglas, & Parsons, 2002) and is an area of particular weakness, with expressive syntax less well developed than that of nonverbal MA-matched TD peers on average (Chapman et al., 1998). These problems with expressive syntax may have their roots in the problems in prelinguistic requesting observed in persons with DS (Mundy et al., 1995), although other cognitive impairments and hearing loss, as well as the level of receptive language, also play a role (Chapman et al., 1991; Chapman et al., 2002). The severity of impairments in expressive syntax distinguishes DS from other neurodevelopmental disorders, including FXS (Finestack, Sterling, Abbeduto, 2013; Martin, Losh, Estigarribia, Sideris, & Roberts, 2013; but see del Hoyo et al., 2018 for an exception).

However, not all aspects of expressive syntax are equally impaired. For example, Hesketh and Chapman (1998) found that children with DS produced significantly fewer grammatical verbs (e.g., forms of *do*, *be*, or *have*) and main verbs per utterance relative to TD children matched on MLU. In addition, those individuals with DS who had MLUs in excess of 3.5 used a significantly higher number of different main, but not grammatical, verbs as compared to TD children matched on MLU. Thus, in individuals with DS, longer MLU does not necessary imply the appropriate use of verbs as it does in the course of typical development. Limited verb use relative to nonverbal MA-matched TD children has also been observed for adolescents and young adults with DS (Loveall et al., 2019). Although this deficit in verb use may reflect in part a failure to understand their semantic content (Loveall, Channell, Phillips, Abbeduto, & Conners, 2016), the omission of verbs is in large measure a failure to understand their syntactic potentialities and constraints. Verb use is also impaired partly because of the well-documented challenges that individuals with DS have in auditory short-term memory (Chapman et al., 2002). Moreover, this impairment in verb use is not observed in individuals with intellectual disability due to other causes and therefore may be unique to DS (Loveall et al., 2019).

Individuals with DS also have especially serious challenges using grammatical morphemes, including copula verbs (e.g., *is* in *Bill is kind*), auxiliary verbs (e.g., *is* in *Jane is running*), articles, and the use of grammatical function words such as prepositions, tense and nontense bound morphemes (e.g., *ed* to mark past tense), and third person singular "s" (e.g., *s* in *The boy runs*; Chapman et al. 1998; Roberts, Price, et al., 2007). In terms of the use of functional morphemes, children with DS have difficulty with binding reflexive pronouns (e.g., understanding that the pronoun refers to *John* in *John dressed himself* but not in *John dressed him*), with their performance in this regard being poorer than that of same-aged children with SLI (Fortunato-Tavares et al., 2015). However, not all languages use these stronger types of personal pronouns (him/her); instead, using syntactically weaker personal pronouns, such as pronominal clitics (e.g., Spanish: Baauw Escobar, & Philip, 1997; Italian: McKee, 1992; Greek: Varlokosta, 2000). Thus, the patterns of impairment associated with DS may be somewhat different across languages.

Individuals with DS also produce utterances that are often poorly formed relative to the syntactic conventions of their language (Finestack & Abbeduto, 2010). For example, in a study involving the use of a wordless picture book to elicit narratives (Keller-Bell &

Abbeduto, 2007), adolescents and adults with DS produced more grammatically incorrect utterances than did same-aged individuals with FXS matched for nonverbal MA. This difference emerged although the former used several types of narrative devices (e.g., exclamations and onomatopoeia) more frequently, thereby producing somewhat richer narratives. These findings are consistent with those of Boudreau and Chapman (2000) and Miles and Chapman (2002) that individuals with DS produce narratives that are more sophisticated than expected for their levels of expressive syntactic skill. In part, the grammatical errors observed by Keller-Bell and Abbeduto (2007) may reflect the problems with verbs and grammatical morphemes already described.

Although expressive syntax is generally an area of substantial weakness, there are some areas of relative strength within expressive syntax in persons with DS, as documented by Thordardottir, Chapman, and Wagner (2002) in a study of the specific syntactic structures used by adolescents with DS. The utterances produced by these adolescents were examined for ten specific syntactic constructions in a narrative context (e.g., conjoined sentences, full propositional complements, simple noninfinitive wh-clauses, among others). The findings indicated that when compared to a comparison group of TD preschoolers matched on MLU, the adolescents with DS did not differ as regards the types and frequency of complex syntactic forms used. In fact, the adolescents with DS actually had a slightly higher mean than did MLU-matched peers with regard to complex syntax (i.e., multi-clause utterance) use.

Although cross-sectional comparisons between individuals with DS and variously matched groups of TD children or individuals with other neurodevelopmental disorders have been common, longitudinal studies of syntactic development have been relatively infrequent. This is true despite the fact that nativist claims about strong biological constraints on language learning, including the assumption of a CA-related critical period, had led to the claim that little progress in syntactic skills was possible for individuals with DS after early adolescence (Chapman et al., 1998). However, this assumption of a DS plateau has not been supported by longitudinal data. In fact, the picture emerging from research on expressive syntax thus far shows that individuals with DS can continue to learn syntax beyond adolescence, through at least 20 years of age. In particular, in a longitudinal study, Chapman et al. (2002) found that MLU continued to increase, on average, during adolescence in a large cohort of individuals with DS. This evidence must be considered tentative, however, because MLU is only a gross indicator of syntactic ability and increases in MLU can be driven by a number of other factors, including lexical advances. Accordingly, more nuanced analytical frameworks may be useful in understanding the nature of the advances comprising increases in MLU among individuals with DS.

In assessing the findings about expressive syntax, the method of assessment must be considered, as even in the case of expressive language sampling, different sampling contexts can influence expressive syntax and other dimensions of the language produced (Abbeduto, Benson, Short, & Dolish, 1995; Berry-Kravis et al., 2013; Chapman et al., 1998; Kover

& Abbeduto, 2010; Kover, McDuffie, Abbeduto, & Brown, 2012). Moreover, context effects may vary as a function of age, developmental level, and neurodevelopmental disorder. Therefore, the range of methods should be expanded in assessing expressive syntax in individuals with DS to provide a more comprehensive picture of their development and suggest hypotheses about the factors that shape their expressive syntactic performance.

Receptive syntax. Although delayed relative to CA expectations, receptive syntax is, on average, less problematic than verbal expression of syntax in DS (Chapman et al., 1991; Miller, 1999; Miolo, Chapman, & Sindberg, 2005). By adolescence, however, receptive syntax begins to lag behind nonverbal cognition as well as other aspects of language, such as receptive vocabulary (Chapman et al., 1991; Finestack & Abbeduto, 2010; Finestack et al., 2013; Phillips, Loveall, Channell, & Conners, 2014; Rosin, Swift, Bless, & Vetter, 1988). The extent of impairment observed for receptive syntax is dependent on the nature of the listening task, with sentences or tasks that place greater demands on auditory memory (e.g., by presenting longer verbal stimuli), being especially challenging for individuals with DS (Miolo et al., 2005; Oakes Kover, & Abbeduto, 2013; Witecy & Penke, 2017). Moreover, measures of auditory memory, such as digit recall and nonword repetition, predict variation in receptive syntax in DS (Miolo et al., 2005; Witecy & Penke, 2017), as they do in other neurodevelopmental disorders, such as FXS (Pierpont, Richmond, Abbeduto, Kover, & Brown, 2011). Moreover, individuals with DS appear to have worse auditory than visual skills (D'Souza, D'Souza, Johnson, & Karmiloff-Smith, 2016), and exhibit especially severe impairments in short-term memory and working memory (Jarrold et al., 2002), which may contribute to receptive syntax problems more generally (Witecy & Penke, 2017).

Comparisons with other neurodevelopmental disorders also have suggested a receptive syntax profile that may be specific to children with DS. For example, in contrast to those with DS, individuals with FXS do not display an asynchrony between receptive syntax and vocabulary, at least in adolescence and young adulthood. The receptive syntax and vocabulary of the latter, although delayed relative to CA expectations, is largely consistent with nonverbal cognitive expectations even in adolescence (Abbeduto et al., 2003).

Individuals with DS may also bring a unique set of processes to bear on the task of understanding syntax. Oakes et al. (2013) conducted a detailed analysis of error patterns on the Test for Reception of Grammar-2 (Bishop, 2003) for cognitively matched children and adolescents with DS or FXS as well as younger TD children. They found that the participants with DS were more likely to make syntactic errors (e.g., selecting a foil that violated word-order constraints) than either of the other participant groups. Using the German version of the TROG (Fox, 2006), Witecy and Penke (2017) also found a preponderance of syntactic rather than lexical errors in German-speaking individuals with DS. These findings raise the possibility that individuals with DS not only have syntactic problems, but also might try to leverage their lexical knowledge to solve syntactic problems, reflecting perhaps an atypical developmental course.

The developmental course of receptive syntax in adolescence and into adulthood for DS also contrasts with the optimistic picture that has emerged of continued growth for expressive syntax. In a 6-year longitudinal study of the trajectories of syntax comprehension in 31 participants with DS, between the ages of 5 and 20 years old at baseline, Chapman et al. (2002) found that CA at the first measurement was a predictor of the change in slope for growth in receptive syntax (Chapman et al., 2002). Based on hierarchical linear modeling, younger participants showed a positive slope, whereas the slope was actually negative for those who entered the study near a CA of 17 years, indicating that the trajectory into young adulthood was one of loss of receptive syntactic skills. If replicated in a larger sample and with different measures of receptive syntax, this trend could reflect an early stage of Alzheimer's disease-related decline (Menéndez, 2005).

The picture of adult development is complicated by Witecy and Penke's (2017) finding that German-speaking individuals with DS showed a positive correlation between performance on a standardized test of receptive syntax and CA in children and adolescents. In contrast to Chapman et al., these investigators found no CA-related loss (or growth) among adults 20 to 40 years old. However, this was a cross-sectional study, whereas Chapman et al.'s (2002) was longitudinal. In addition, Chapman et al.'s participants were learning English, whereas Witecy and Penke's participants were learning German. Longitudinal replications of the trajectory of receptive syntax, preferably using a comprehensive multi-method approach to assessment to ensure that the findings are not specific to a single measure would be useful, as would replications across languages to understand the interaction between the language being learned and CA-related brain changes. Moreover, more fine-grained analyses of performance across different types of syntactic structures and elements, which may be associated with different developmental trajectories (Oakes et al., 2013; Witecy & Penke, 2017), are needed to illuminate what aspects of receptive syntax are most subject to decline, which in turn would provide insight into the factors contributing to those declines.

Summary. Syntax is an area of special challenge, with expressive syntax more impaired than receptive syntax, but the latter possibly more sensitive to Alzheimer's disease-related factors and decline. DS is distinguished by the severity and profile of syntactic impairments from other neurodevelopmental disorders, including FXS, WS, and SLI. Memory impairments and other aspects of the phenotype of individuals with DS play a role in shaping syntactic development.

Pragmatic Development

Pragmatics refers to the use of language for social interaction (Bryant, 2009; Landa, 2005). Pragmatic abilities enable speakers to express their thoughts and listeners to determine the meanings intended by other people's utterances. These abilities require knowledge of the mechanics of communication (e.g., that speakers take turns) as well as various supporting competencies, such as the ability to make inferences, to appreciate differences in people's knowledge, and to recall previous interactions with particular social partners.

The delays in nonverbal intentional communication during the prelinguistic period described previously fall within the realm of pragmatics.

Early difficulties with social referencing, an iterative situation in which one person uses another person's interpretation of an event to inform their own understanding of that event, have also been documented in children with DS. In a series of studies, Thurman and Mervis (2013) addressed how children with DS between 42 and 71 months of age, as compared to children with WS, navigate this social situation. These investigators found that the children with DS evidenced difficulty using an adult's expression of fear to regulate their own behavior, a skill that typically emerges around 12 months of age. Overall, the children with DS evidenced more social competence on the component skills theorized to support the social referencing process, although difficulties recognizing the communicative significance of fearful expressions was observed in the DS group. Not surprisingly, pragmatic delays continue after the onset of language in individuals with DS.

Children with DS use their earliest verbalizations to express the same social, or pragmatic, functions (e.g., requesting, commenting, answering), and with the same relative frequencies, as do younger TD children at a similar level of linguistic sophistication (Coggins, Carpenter, & Owings, 1983; Owens & MacDonald, 1982). Such findings suggest that individuals with DS eventually come to understand, albeit more slowly, that language is a tool to be used for the same set of communicative goals as do TD children. Children with DS also are able to maintain a topic, formulating utterances that contribute new semantic information to previous utterances in the conversation, both their own utterances and those produced by other people, at least in a manner consistent with MA expectations (Roberts, Martin, et al., 2007; Tannock, 1988).

Individuals with DS also display areas of relative pragmatic strength, including in managing some facets of the narrative genre. When retelling the story depicted in a wordless picture book or wordless film, children and adolescents with DS include more story elements, inferential relationships, and plot components than do TD children with similar expressive syntax skills, suggesting that the former can compensate for their syntactic limitations (Boudreau & Chapman, 2000; Miles & Chapman, 2002; Miles, Chapman, & Bridge, 2006). In contrast, children with DS display lower gist and verbatim recall than MA-matched TD children when recalling verbally presented stories with minimal visual support (Bird & Chapman, 1994; Bird, Chapman, & Schwartz, 2004). Thus, the ability of individuals with DS to compensate for their expressive syntax limitations is modest (Abbeduto et al., 2007) and highly dependent on access to visual supports (Miles et al., 2006).

Despite having a basic ability to use language to perform essential pragmatic functions and in managing some genres of talk, older children and adolescents with DS also have especially serious problems in crafting verbalizations that effectively convey their intended meanings. Abbeduto, Murphy et al. (2006) used a non-face-to-face referential task that required the participant to describe a novel shape so that it could be selected by a listener from among other novel shapes. They found that the adolescents and young adults with

DS produced more ambiguous (i.e., non-discriminating) descriptions of their intended referents than did the younger TD children matched on nonverbal MA. The individuals with DS also were less likely to scaffold their listener's understanding of the description by saying, for example, "it looks sort of like a boat" rather than simply "it's a boat." Abbeduto, Murphy et al. suggested that individuals with DS may not understand what constitutes a referentially adequate message from the perspective of a listener and that this problem is not solely a reflection of their limited vocabulary and syntax. Abbeduto, Murphy et al. found no evidence that this failure of the youth with DS was related to performance on measure of theory of mind (i.e., an ability to represent other people's mental states); however, the pattern of correlations suggested that the failing was more closely related to managing the linguistic rather than the social-cognitive dimensions of the task.

The ability to recognize and signal comprehension problems also appears to be a relative pragmatic weakness for individuals with DS. In a simple direction-following task, Abbeduto et al. (2008) found that school-age children and adolescents with DS were less likely to signal noncomprehension of inadequate messages (e.g., by saying, "Which one?") than were TD children matched on nonverbal MA. Moreover, these deficits were most pronounced as the task became more complex in terms of the number of possible referents to which the message could refer or the obviousness of the inadequacy (e.g., messages with multiple potential referents were less likely to elicit a signal of noncomprehension than were messages with no referent).

Little is known about the specificity of the pragmatic profile of DS because there have been so few comparisons of individuals with DS to those with other neurodevelopmental disorders under the same task conditions. In many domains of pragmatics, individuals with DS appear to be less impaired, on average, than those with other conditions (Martin et al., 2009). For example, individuals with DS are less likely to be verbally perseverative or to produce utterances that are unrelated or tangential to the topic at hand than are individuals with FXS (Belser & Sudhalter, 2001; Ferrier, Bashir, Meryash, Johnston, Wolff, 1991; Roberts, Martin, et al., 2007; Sudhalter, Cohen, Silverman, & Wolf-Schein, 1990). They are also less likely than CA-matched individuals with WS to use stereotyped language or inappropriate means of initiating a conversation (Laws & Bishop, 2004). However, individuals with DS also display both areas of weakness relative to those with other neurodevelopmental disorders and areas of common impairment. In the Abbeduto, Murphy et al. (2006) study of non-face-to-face referential communication, the participants with DS were as likely to produce ambiguous descriptions, but were less likely to include linguistic scaffolding, than were participants with FXS matched on CA and nonverbal IQ. In addition, children and adolescents with DS appear to be less apt to signal noncomprehension under at least some conditions than are individuals with ASD or FXS (without co-occurring ASD) matched on indices of developmental level (Abbeduto et al., 2008; Martin et al., 2017).

Summary. DS is associated with an uneven profile of relative strengths and weaknesses in the domain of pragmatics that is distinct from other neurodevelopmental disorders. The relationship of this profile to other aspects of the DS language and cognitive phenotype has seldom been examined, although, not surprisingly, impairments in other aspects of language (e.g., syntax) appear to correlate with pragmatic impairments (Abbeduto et al., 2008). There is a need for more investigation into pragmatics and DS, particularly using longitudinal designs, with a focus on domains such as turn taking, understanding of nonliteral language, topic initiation and maintenance, and others that have yet to be explored. Such data are critical to developing a comprehensive approach to treating pragmatic problems.

Caregiver Influences

In this section, we consider studies focused on the role of parents in shaping language development in children with DS. A number of dimensions of parental talk and interactional style that are associated with the language and communicative skills of individuals with DS are identified. Although language development is influenced by other people (e.g., peers), contexts (e.g., school), and informational sources (e.g., television), these influences have been less well studied among individuals with DS; hence, our exclusive focus on parents, who no doubt also are the first and strongest influence on language learning in the early years of life.

Numerous studies have documented the ways in which parents support the language development of young children with DS. For example, Legerstee, Varghese, and Van Beek (2002) considered the effects of maternal interaction style on the referential communication of infants with DS (CA 6–20 months) and found that the mothers' maintenance of infant attention was positively associated with the infants' referential communication, although this relationship appeared stronger for more cognitively advanced infants. Additionally, the findings from sequential analyses suggested that the infants with DS often became distracted and disengaged from the interaction unless their mothers worked to redirect their attention. This pattern was primarily observed in children with DS who demonstrated more limited cognitive ability, suggesting that the mothers used redirecting as a strategy for successfully promoting referential communication.

In a study of somewhat older children, Roach, Barratt, Miller, and Leavitt (1998) found that the frequency with which mothers of children with DS (CA 16–30 months) used "supporting" behaviors, such as verbalizations or actions that encouraged the child's object exploration, was positively associated with children's frequency of object play and vocalization. However, this pattern was not observed among mothers of TD children matched on either CA or MA. In addition, mothers of children with DS demonstrated more supporting object behaviors than did mothers of either group of TD children. Supportive object behaviors were defined in this project as the "facilitation of the child's interaction with an object by holding it, moving it close, or otherwise supporting the child in play or by giving, taking, or receiving a toy from the child" (Roach et al., 1998, pg. 80). These findings suggest that mothers of children with DS adapt to the unique characteristics and behaviors of their children with DS, presumably in an effort to engage them in more sustained and satisfying social interaction.

In contrast to the previous studies reviewed, which examined concurrent relationships among maternal and child behaviors, Adamson and colleagues (e.g., Adamson, Deckner, & Bakeman, 2010; Adamson, Bakeman, Deckner, & Nelson, 2012; Adamson et al. 2009) conducted a series of studies to examine the role of joint parent-child engagement in later language acquisition in children with DS (mean CA: approximately 30 months) using a longitudinal design. These investigators used both observational state coding (e.g., time spent in joint engagement state) and observer rating methods. Among other findings, Adamson and colleagues demonstrated that mother-child interactions characterized by high rates of symbol-infused joint engagement (i.e., the dyad was actively engaged with the same referent and responding to the language heard) predicted later receptive and expressive language outcomes over and above the children's initial language capacity. In addition, Adamson et al. (2010) found that individual differences in the children's interest/attention toward people and objects predicted the frequency of coordinated joint engagement states (i.e., child and parent were actively involved with the same referent and the child was actively acknowledging the parent's participation) as well as how quickly the child began to attend to symbols used during this state.

Dimitrova, Ozçalışkan, and Adamson (2016) focused specifically on the ways in which parents of infants with DS responded to their children' gestures, with the hypothesis being that such responses could facilitate the transition from gesture to word. The participants were 23 children with DS who at study initiation had a mean age of 30 months (range: 20–40 months). The findings indicated that the children with DS frequently indicated references uniquely through the use of gestures prior to development of referential labels. Furthermore, the parents of the children with DS were observed to translate, or restate, the majority of these gestures into words. Dimitrova et al. also found that the referents translated into words by parents were more likely to enter into children's subsequent vocabularies relative to referents that were not translated into words by parents, supporting a casual role for these parental translations in the development of language by children with DS.

Summary. Environmental factors, as captured by the concept of *parental responsivity*, reflected in behaviors that support child engagement in social interaction and object exploration while providing rich verbal import matched to the child's focus of attention, play a key role in shaping the communicative development of children with DS. Thus, within these interactions, child and parent both influence, and are influenced by, each other. Indeed, the slowed rate of development of children with DS and their atypical behavioral profile clearly make it more difficult for parents to provide appropriate and supportive verbal input or other types of support. For example, the poor speech intelligibility of individuals with DS may make it more difficult for parents (and others) to know how to expand the immature utterances of a child with DS into more mature, but semantically consistent, utterances. Moreover, the lessened motivation of children with DS to engage and persist in object exploration (Ruskin, Mundy, Kasari, & Sigman, 1994) can result in fewer opportunities for parents to translate child referential gestures into a verbal form.

These complex parent-child interactions are likely to change as children develop and will have different effects at different ages or developmental levels. Thus, longitudinal investigations of this complexity and the dynamic bidirectional influence of both parental and child factors in interactions (Adamson et al., 2009) is vital to advancing our understanding of environmental influences on language learning in children with DS. Although the studies on the associations between parental responsivity and language skills in children with DS have been focused on the early childhood period, parental responsivity continues to facilitate language development well beyond this period in children with neurodevelopmental disorders (Brady, Warren, Fleming, Keller, & Sterling, 2014). From a clinical perspective, the shaping of language learning by the environment suggests that improvements in language in children with DS are possible by systematizing, enriching, and optimizing their environments (see Warren and colleagues, this volume by Warren and colleagues).

Conclusions and Future Directions

The evidence clearly indicates that DS is associated with substantial delays relative to CA expectations in all aspects of language and that these delays are evident early in development and even in the prelinguistic achievements that typically set the stage for language development. At the same time, the delays are greater in some facets of language than in others, with expressive syntax being an area of especially severe impairment (i.e., with a lag relative to nonverbal MA) and receptive vocabulary being an area of relative strength, at least when it comes to concrete vocabulary (with functioning at or in advance relative to nonverbal MA). Pragmatics is on, average, a relative strength, although here too some areas of skill seem more impaired, even relative to level of cognitive functioning (such as signaling noncomprehension of problematic messages during listening). However, there are developmental changes in the linguistic profile of DS, as evidenced, for example, by the increasing lag in the development of receptive syntax relative to nonverbal cognition beginning in adolescence. There also is some evidence of continued improvement in language at least until the young adult years, although some limited evidence indicates that declines in language ability may begin during that same time. The profile of relative strengths and weaknesses in language distinguishes DS from other neurodevelopmental disorders associated with intellectual disability, such as FXS and WS, as well as from individuals with SLI. Importantly, there is little evidence of qualitative differences between DS and TD or other neurodevelopmental disorders; that is, the evidence to date suggests largely differences in degree of impairment, not in developmental sequence or approach to learning, although the data addressing the "delay versus difference" issue to date are limited.

There are areas of language and of the factors shaping language development in individuals with DS in which more research is needed, especially if we are to develop effective interventions to improve language learning and use in this population. In particular, more data are needed regarding the relationships between linguistic achievements and other aspects of the DS phenotype. Thus far, there is evidence for the role of hearing and phonological memory in explaining some of the language-learning problems of people with DS; however, explorations of the contributions of other phenotypic strengths and weaknesses, particularly in social cognition, have seldom been addressed. Moreover, studies of the relationships between language and other aspects of the DS phenotype have largely been focused on concurrent correlations. Long-term longitudinal studies are needed to establish causal relationships and to chart the dynamic relationships among various dimensions of the phenotype over the course of development as well as to identify possible plateaus, or skills that are never acquired.

There also is a need to understand the relationships among different aspects of language over development so that we can develop interventions that might be able to produce generalized gains. For example, do improvements in expressive syntax translate into appropriate uses in social interaction (i.e., pragmatics)? Does teaching vocabulary, especially verbs, lead to improvements in syntax? In examining these relationships, there needs to be a focus on a range of phenotypic domains, including physical health (e.g., thyroid problems, sleep apnea). More data are needed about the ways in which language learning shapes other aspects of the DS phenotype, such as the acquisition of literacy skills, basic numerical skills, and even adaptive function, so that we can target for intervention those linguistic skills that are essential prerequisites to a wider array of life skills and improved quality of life.

There also is a need to develop measures that more precisely isolate difficulties with language from other aspects of the behavioral phenotype characterizing individuals with DS, and that are appropriate for individuals of a wider range of abilities. The use of alternative methodologies, including comprehension tests with low cognitive demands such as preferential-looking paradigms, would allow us to better understand language development in individuals with DS by isolating purely linguistic skills from the motivational, motoric, and cognitive skills that are often required to make even a simple pointing response on a test such as the PPVT or TROG. Indeed, many standardized tests used to assess language require quite complex skills, include hypothetical reasoning and inferencing, to make a response, thereby raising ambiguity whether "failure" should be ascribed to the language skills being targeted or the complex cognitive skills needed to respond. In addition, there is a need to conduct basic psychometric analyses, determining, for example, test-retest reliability and sensitivity to change of the measures used. Understanding the psychometric properties of the measures used in research on DS will allow us to begin to determine the best design for our studies (e.g., the sample size needed to adequately test hypotheses) or the appropriate measures to be used in studies designed to determine treatment efficacy. In addition, most measures and studies continue to be focused on the "products" rather than the "processes" of learning. Instead, we need measures that provide insights into not only what has or has not been learned, but also how the individual goes about trying to learn. The latter measures will provide more useful targets for intervention and more useful outcome measures for studies focused on testing the efficacy of pharmacological or behavioral interventions. The recent advent of research on low demand measures (Arias-Trejo et al., 2019), on the psychometric properties of some language measures

(Esbensen et al., 2017), and on learning processes (Oakes et al., 2013) is a hopeful sign that there will soon be a battery of measures that will accelerate understanding and treatment of language learning difficulties of individuals with DS.

More research is needed on environmental influences on language development in individuals with DS so that we can understand the full array of such influences and thereby the potential paths for changing the trajectory of language in different developmental periods. Research into parental behavior needs to involve a longitudinal approach so that bidirectional causal relationships can be investigated, and researchers need to take a life-course perspective so that the accumulated history of caregiver-child interactions is considered. Information on experiences in other important social contexts is needed as well. Relationships with siblings and peers play important roles in the language development of TD children, but these relationships are largely unexplored from the perspective of language development in the DS literature. Schooling is recognized as an important contributor to development, yet the role of schooling in the language development of individuals with DS has been largely ignored. Language is both shaped by, and shapes, experiences in all of the many contexts in which people with DS live, again necessitating a longitudinal approach with attention to bidirectional relationships.

Cross-cultural studies of development of language abilities of the DS population are also needed as they can allow us to distinguish between problems specific to the characteristics of a group of languages in comparison to those that are language independent. Characteristics of the language learner with DS, the properties of the language being learned, and the patterns of social interaction of the culture are likely to interact to shape language development in individuals with DS. Languages that depend heavily on word order rather than word inflections, for example, may tax the poor phonological memory of individuals with DS, possibly making languages like English more difficult for them to learn than languages such as Portuguese. Understanding these complex relationships will be required to ensure appropriate linguistic and cultural adaptations of intervention approaches for the needs of the individual with DS.

References

Abbeduto, L., Benson, G., Short, K., & Dolish, J. (1995). Effects of sampling context on the expressive language of children and adolescents with mental retardation. *Mental Retardation, 33*(5), 279–288.

Abbeduto, L., Keller-Bell, Y., Richmond, E. K., & Murphy, M. M. (2006). Research on language development and mental retardation: History, theories, findings, and future directions. In L. M. Glidden (Ed.), *International Review of Research in Mental Retardation*. New York: Academic Press.

Abbeduto, L., McDuffie, A., Thurman, A. J., & Kover, S. T. (2016). Language development in individuals with intellectual and developmental disabilities. *International Review of Research in Developmental Disabilities, 50*, 71–118.

Abbeduto, L., Murphy, M. M., Cawthon, S. W., Richmond, E. K., Weissman, M. D., Karadottir, S., & O'Brien, A. (2003). Receptive language skills of adolescents and young adults with Down or fragile X syndrome. *American Journal on Mental Retardation, 149*(3), 149–160.

Abbeduto, L., Murphy, M. M., Kover, S. T., Giles, N. D., Karadottir, S., Amman, A., Nollin, K. A. (2008). Signaling noncomprehension of language: A comparison of fragile X syndrome and Down syndrome. *American Journal on Mental Retardation, 113*(3), 214.

Abbeduto, L., Murphy, M. M., Richmond, E. K., Amman, A., Beth, P., Weissman, M. D., Karadottir, S. (2006). Collaboration in referential communication: Comparison of youth with Down syndrome or fragile X syndrome. *American Journal on Mental Retardation, 111*(3), 170.

Abbeduto, L., Pavetto, M., Kesin, E., Weissman, M. D., Karadottir, S., O'Brien, A., & Cawthon, S. (2001). The linguistic and cognitive profile of Down syndrome: Evidence from a comparison with fragile X syndrome. *Down's Syndrome, Research and Practice: The Journal of the Sarah Duffen Centre/University of Portsmouth, 7*(1), 9–15.

Abbeduto, L., Warren, S. F., & Conners, F. A. (2007). Language development in Down syndrome: From the prelinguistic period to the acquisition of literacy. *Mental Retardation and Developmental Disabilities Research Reviews, 13*(3), 247–261.

Abreu-Mendoza, R. A., & Arias-Trejo, N. (2017). Counting abilities in Down syndrome: The role of the one-to-one correspondence principle and receptive vocabulary. *Neuropsychology, 31*(7), 750–758.

Adamson, L. B., Bakeman, R., Deckner, D. F., & Nelson, P. B. (2012). Rating parent-child interactions: Joint engagement, communication dynamics, and shared topics in autism, Down syndrome, and typical development. *Journal of Autism and Developmental disorders, 42*(12), 2622–2635.

Adamson, L. B., Bakeman, R., Deckner, D. F., & Romski, M. (2009). Joint engagement and the emergence of language in children with autism and Down syndrome. *Journal of Autism and Developmental Disorders, 39*(1), 84–96.

Adamson, L. B., Deckner, D. F., & Bakeman, R. (2010). Early interests and joint engagement in typical development, autism, and Down syndrome. *Journal of Autism and Developmental Disorders, 40*(6), 665–676.

Alsaied, T., Marino, B. S., Esbensen, A. J., Anixt, J. S., Epstein, J. N., & Cnota, J. F. (2016). Does congenital heart disease affect neurodevelopmental outcomes in children with Down syndrome? *Congenital Heart Disease, 11*(1), 26–33.

Anand, P., Misra, S., Demara, B., Clark, C. A. C., & Edgin, J. O. (2017). *The development of sleep and language in infants with Down syndrome.* Paper presented at the Society for Research in Child Development, Austin, TX.

Arias-Trejo, N., Angulo-Chavira, A. Q., & Barrón-Martínez, J. B. (2019). Verb-mediated anticipatory eye movements in people with Down syndrome. *International Journal of Language & Communication Disorders, 54*(5),756–766. doi:10.1111/1460-6984.12473

Baauw, S., Escobar, M. A., & Philip, W. (1997). *A delay of principle b-effect in Spanish speaking children: The role of lexical feature acquisition.* In A. Sorace, C. Heycock, & R. Shillcock (Eds.), *Proceedings of the GALA 97 Conference on Language Acquisition* (pp. 16–21). University of Edinburgh.

Baddeley AD. (2001). Is working memory still working? *American Psychologist, 56*(11), 851–864.

Bailey, D. B., Raspa, M., Bishop, E., & Holiday, D. (2009). No change in the age of diagnosis for fragile X syndrome: Findings from a national parent survey. *Pediatrics, 124*(2), 527–533.

Barnes, E., Roberts, J., Long, S. H., Martin, G. E., Berni, M. C., Mandulak, K. C., & Sideris, J. (2009). Phonological accuracy and intelligibility in connected speech of boys with fragile X syndrome or Down syndrome. *Journal of Speech Language and Hearing Research, 52*(4), 1048.

Bates, E., Bretherton, I., Beeghly-Smith, M., & McNew, S. (1982). Social bases of language development: A reassessment. *Advances in Child Development and Behavior, 16*, 7–75.

Bates, E., & Dick, F. (2002). Language, gesture, and the developing brain. *Developmental Psychobiology, 40*, 293–310.

Beeghly, M., Weiss-Perry, B., & Cicchetti, D. (1990). Beyond sensorimotor functioning: Early communicative and play development of children with Down syndrome: A developmental perspective. Cambridge, UK: Cambridge University Press.

Bellugi, U., Wang, P. P., & Jernigan, T. L. (1994). Williams syndrome: An unusual neuropsychological profile. In S. H. Broman & J. Grafman (Eds.), *Atypical cognitive profile in developmental disorders. Implications for brain function* (pp. 23–56). London: Lawrence Erlbaum.

Belser, R. C., & Sudhalter, V. (2001). Conversational characteristics of children with fragile X syndrome: Repetitive speech. *American Journal on Mental Retardation, 106*(1), 28.

Berger, J. (1990). Interactions between parents and their infants with Down syndrome. In D. Cicchetti & M. Beeghly (Eds.), *Children with Down syndrome* (pp. 101–146). Cambridge, UK: Cambridge University Press.

Berger, J., & Cunningham, C. C. (1983). Development of early vocal behaviors and interactions in Down's syndrome and nonhandicapped infant-mother pairs. *Developmental Psychology, 19*(3), 322–331.

Berglund, E., Eriksson, M., & Johansson, I. (2001). Parental reports of spoken language skills in children with Down syndrome. *Journal of Speech, Language, and Hearing Research, 44*, 179–191.

Berry-Kravis, E., Doll, E., Sterling, A., Kover, S. T., Schroeder, S. M., Mathur, S., & Abbeduto, L. (2013). Development of an expressive language sampling procedure in fragile X syndrome. *Journal of Developmental & Behavioral Pediatrics, 34*(4), 245–251.

Bersu, E. T., & Opitz, J. M. (1980). Anatomical analysis of the developmental effects of aneuploidy in man: The down syndrome. *American Journal of Medical Genetics*, 5(4), 339–420. doi:10.1002/ajmg.1320050411.

Bird, E. K., & Chapman, R. S. (1994). Sequential recall in individuals with Down syndrome. *Journal of Speech and Hearing Research, 37*(6), 1369–1380.

Bird, E. K., Chapman, R. S., & Schwartz, S. E. (2004). Fast mapping of words and story recall by individuals with Down syndrome. *Journal of Speech, Language, and Hearing Research, 47*(6), 1286–1300.

Bishop, D. (2003). *Test for Reception of Grammar, Version 2.* London, UK: Pearson Assessment.

Bleile, K., & Schwarz, I. (1984). Three perspectives on the speech of children with Down's syndrome. *Journal of Communication Disorders, 17*(2), 87–94.

Bornstein, M. H., Tamis-LeMonda, C. S., & Haynes, O. M. (1999). First words in the second year: Continuity, stability, and models of concurrent and predictive correspondence in vocabulary and verbal responsiveness across age and context. *Infant Behavior and Development, 22*(1), 65–85.

Borsel, J. V. (1996). Articulation in Down's syndrome adolescents and adults. *European Journal of Disorders of Communication, 31*(4), 415–444.

Boudreau, D. M., & Chapman, R. S. (2000). The relationship between event representation and linguistic skill in narratives of children and adolescents with Down syndrome. *Journal of Speech, Language, and Hearing Research, 43*(5), 1146–1159.

Brady, N., Warren, S. F., Fleming, K., Keller, J., & Sterling, A. (2014). Effect of sustained maternal responsivity on later vocabulary development in children with fragile X syndrome. *Journal of Speech Language and Hearing Research, 57*(1), 212.

Brock, J., & Jarrold, C. (2004). Language influences on verbal short-term memory performance in Down syndrome: Item and order recognition. *Journal of Speech, Language, and Hearing Research, 47*(6), 1334–1346.

Bronfenbrenner, U., & Ceci, S. J. (1994). Nature-nurture reconceptualized in developmental perspective: A bioecological model. *Psychological Review, 101*(4), 568–586.

Bryant, J. B. (2009). Pragmatic language development. In E. L. Bavin (Ed.), *The Cambridge handbook of child language* (pp. 339–354). New York: Cambridge University Press.

Buckley, S., & Bird, G. (2001). Memory development for individuals with Down syndrome– An overview. *Down Syndrome Issues and Information.*

Bunn, L., Roy, E. A., & Elliott, D. (2007). Speech perception and motor control in children with Down syndrome. *Child Neuropsychology, 13*(3), 262–275.

Capirci, O., Iverson, J. M., Pizzuto, E., & Volterra, V. (1996). Communicative gestures during the transition to two-word speech. *Journal of Child Language, 23*, 645–673.

Cardoso-Martins, C., França Michalick, M., & Cury Pollo, T. (2002). Is sensitivity to rhyme a developmental precursor to sensitivity to phoneme? Evidence from individuals with Down syndrome. *Reading and Writing: An Interdisciplinary Journal, 15*, 439–454.

Caselli, M. C., Marchetti, C., & Vicari, S. (1994). Conoscenze lessicali e primo sviluppo morfosintattico [Lexical knowledge and first morphosyntactic development]. In A. Contardi & S. Vicari (Eds.), *Le persone Down. Aspetti neuropsicologici, educativi e sociali [People with Down syndrome: Neuropsychological, educational and social aspects]* (pp. 28–48). Milan, Italy: Franco.

Caselli, M. C., Pasqualetti, P., & Stefanini, S. (2007). *Parole e frasi nel "primo vocabolario del bambino." Nuovi dati normativi fra 18 e 36 mesi e Forma breve del questionario* [Words and sentences in "children's first words." New normative data between 18 and 36 months and short form of the inventory]. Milan, Italy: Franco Angeli.

Caselli, M. C., Vicari, S., Longobardi, E., Lami, L., Pizzoli, C., & Stella, G. (1998). Gestures and words in early development of children with Down syndrome. *Journal of Speech, Language, and Hearing Research, 41*, 1125–1135.

Chan, J., & Iacono, T. (2001). Gesture and word production in children with down syndrome. *Augmentative and Alternative Communication, 17*(2), 73–87.

Chapman, R. (1997). Language development in children and adolescents with Down syndrome. *Mental Retardation and Developmental Disabilities Research Review, 3*, 307–312.

Chapman, R., & Hesketh, L. (2001). Language, cognition and short-term memory in individuals with Down Syndrome. *Down's Syndrome, Research and Practice: The Journal of the Sarah Duffen Centre/University of Portsmouth, 1*, 1–7.

Chapman, R. S., Hesketh, L. J., & Kistler, D. J. (2002). Predicting longitudinal change in language production and comprehension in individuals with Down syndrome: Hierarchical linear modeling. *Journal of Speech, Language, and Hearing Research, 45*(5), 902–915.

Chapman, R. S., Schwartz, S. E., & Bird, E. K. (1991). Language skills of children and adolescents with Down syndrome: I. Comprehension. *Journal of Speech and Hearing Research, 34*(5), 1106–1120.

Chapman, R. S., Seung, H., Schwartz, S., & Bird, E. K. (1998). Language skills of children and adolescents with Down syndrome: II. Production deficits. *Journal of Speech, Language, and Hearing Research, 41*(4), 861–873.

Chapman, R. S., Sindberg, H., Bridge, C., Gigstead, K., & Hesketh, L. (2006). Effect of memory support and elicited production on fast mapping of new words by adolescents with Down syndrome. *Journal of Speech, Language, and Hearing Research, 49*(1), 3–15.

Chapman, R. S., Streim, N., Crais, E., Salmon, D., Strand, E., & Negri, N. (1992). Child talk. Assumptions of a developmental process model for early language learning. In R. S. Chaamn (Ed.), *Processes in language acquisition and disorders* (pp. 3–19). St. Louis, MO: Mosby.

Checa, E., Galeote, M., & Soto, P. (2016). The composition of early vocabulary in Spanish children with Down syndrome and their peers with typical development. *American Journal of Speech-Language Pathology, 25*, 605–619.

Chomsky, N. (1975). *Reflections on language*. New York: Random House.

Chomsky, N. (1988). *Language and problems of knowledge: The Managua lectures*. Cambridge, MA: MIT Press.

Cleland, J., Wood, S., Hardcastle, W., Wishart, J., & Timmins, C. (2010). Relationship between speech, oromotor, language and cognitive abilities in children with Down's syndrome. *International Journal of Language & Communication Disorders, 45*(1), 83–95.

Coggins T. E., Carpenter R. L., & Owings N. O. (1983). Examining early intentional communication in Down's syndrome and nonretarded children. *British Journal of Disorders of Communication, 18*, 99–107.

Conners, F. A., Moore, M. S., Loveall, S. J., & Merrill, E. C. (2011). Memory profiles of Down, Williams, and fragile X syndromes: Implications for reading development. *Journal of Developmental and Behavioral Pediatrics, 32*(5), 405–417.

Cross, W. E. (2017). Ecological factors in human development. *Child Development, 88*(3), 767–769.

Curtin, S., & Zamuner, T. S. (2014). Understanding the developing sound system: Interactions between sounds and words. *WIREs Cognitive Science, 5*(5), 589–602.

D'Souza, D., D'Souza, H., Johnson, M. H., & Karmiloff-Smith, A. (2016). Audio-visual speech perception in infants and toddlers with Down syndrome, fragile X syndrome, and Williams syndrome. *Infant Behavior and Development, 44*, 249–262.

D'Souza, D., D'Souza, H., Johnson, M. H., Karmiloff-Smith, A., Bates, E., Hartung, J., & Kushnerenko, E. (2015). Concurrent relations between face scanning and language: A cross-syndrome infant study. *PLOS One, 10*(10), e0139319.

Dahle, A. J., & McCollister, F. P. (1986). Hearing and otologic disorders in children with Down syndrome. *American Journal of Mental Deficiency, 90*(6), 636–642.

del Hoyo Soriano, L., Thurman, &, Abbeduto, L. (2018). Specificity: A phenotypic comparison of communication-relevant domains between youth with Down syndrome and fragile X syndrome. *Frontiers in Genetics, 9*, 424.

Delabar, J.-M., Allinquant, B., Bianchi, D., Blumenthal, T., Dekker, A., Edgin, J., & Busciglio, J. (2016). Changing paradigms in Down syndrome: The First International Conference of the Trisomy 21 Research Society. *Molecular Syndromology, 7*(5), 251–261.

Dimitrova, N., Özçalışkan, Ş., & Adamson, L. B. (2016). Parents' translations of child gesture facilitate word learning in children with autism, Down syndrome and typical development. *Journal of Autism and Developmental Disorders, 46*(1), 221–231.

Dodd, B. J. (1972). Comparison of babbling patterns in normal and Down-syndrome infants. *Journal of Mental Deficiency Research, 16*, 35–40.

Dodd, B., Leahy, J., & Hambly, G. (1989). Phonological disorders in children: Underlying cognitive deficits. *British Journal of Developmental Psychology, 7*(1), 55–71.

Dodd, B., Zhu, H., Crosbie, S., Holm, A., & Ozanne, A. (2002). *Diagnostic evaluation of articulation and phonology (DEAP)*. Psychology Corporation.

Downs, M. (1980). The hearing of Down's individuals. *Seminars in Hearing, 1*(1), 25–37.

Dunn, L. M., Dunn, L. M., Whetton, C., & Burley, J. (1997). The British Picture Vocabulary Scale (2nd ed.). Windsor, UK: NFER-Nelson.

Eadie, P. A., Fey, M. E., Douglas, J. M., & Parsons, C. L. (2002). Profiles of grammatical morphology and sentence imitation in children with specific language impairment and Down syndrome. *Journal of Speech, Language, and Hearing Research, 45*(4), 720–732.

Edgin, J. O., Tooley, U., Demara, B., Nyhuis, C., Anand, P., & Spanò, G. (2015). Sleep disturbance and expressive language development in preschool-age children with Down syndrome. *Child Development, 86*(6), 1984–1998.

Elliott, D., & Weeks, D. J. (1993). Cerebral specialization for speech perception and movement organization in adults with Down's syndrome. *Cortex: A Journal Devoted to the Study of the Nervous System and Behavior, 29*(1), 103–113.

Elliott, D., Weeks, D. J., & Chua, R. (1994). Anomalous cerebral lateralization and Down syndrome. *Brain and Cognition, 26*(2), 191–195.

Esbensen, A. J., Hooper, S. R. Fidler, D., Hartley, S., Edgin, J., Liogier d'Ardhuy, X., . . . Outcome Measures Working Group. (2017). Outcome measures for clinical trials in Down syndrome. *American Journal on Intellectual and Developmental Disabilities, 122*, 247–281.

Fenson, L., Dale, P. S., Reznick, J. S., Thal, D., Bates, E., Hartung, J., & Reilly, J. S. (1993). *User's guide and technical manual for the MacArthur Communicative Development Inventories*. San Diego, CA: Singular Press.

Ferrier, L. J., Bashir, A. S., Meryash, D. L., Johnston, J., & Wolff, P. (1991). Conversational skills of individuals with fragile-X syndrome: A comparison with autism and Down syndrome. *Developmental Medicine and Child Neurology, 33*(9), 776–788.

Fidler, D. J., Philofsky, A., Hepburn, S. L., & Rogers, S. J. (2005). Nonverbal requesting and problem-solving by toddlers with Down syndrome. *American Journal on Mental Retardation, 110*(4), 312.

Finestack, L. H., & Abbeduto, L. (2010). Expressive language profiles of verbally expressive adolescents and young adults with Down syndrome or fragile X syndrome. *Journal of Speech, Language, and Hearing Research, 53*, 1334–1348.

Finestack, L. H., Sterling, A. M., & Abbeduto, L. (2013). Discriminating Down syndrome and fragile X syndrome based on language ability. *Journal of Child Language, 40*(1), 244–265.

Fodor, J. A. (1983). *The modularity of mind*. Cambridge, MA: MIT Press.

Fort, P., Lifshitz, F., Bellisario, R., Davis, J., Lanes, R., Pugliese, M., . . . David, R. (1984). Abnormalities of thyroid function in infants with Down syndrome. *Journal of Pediatrics, 104*, 545–549.

Fortunato-Tavares, T., Andrade, C. R. F., Befi-Lopes, D., Limongi, S. O., Fernandes, F. D. M., & Schwartz, R. G. (2015). Syntactic comprehension and working memory in children with specific language impairment, autism or Down syndrome. *Clinical Linguistics & Phonetics, 29*(7), 499–522.

Fowler, A. E. (1990). Language abilities in children with Down syndrome: Evidence for a specific syntactic delay. In D. Cicchetti, &M. Beeghly (Eds.), *Children with Down syndrome: A developmental perspective* (pp. 302–328). New York: Cambridge University Press.

Fox, A. V. (2006). TROG-D. *Test zur Überprüfung des Grammatikverständnisses. Handbuch. Das Gesundheitsforum*. Idstein: Schulz-Kirchner Verlag.

Franco, F., & Wishart, J. G. (1995). Use of pointing and other gestures by young children with Down syndrome. *American Journal of Mental Retardation, 100*(2), 160–182.

Galeote, M., Sebastian, E., Checa, E., Rey, R., & Soto, P. (2011). The development of vocabulary in Spanish children with Down syndrome: Comprehension, production, and gestures. *Intellectual & Developmental Disability, 36*, 184–196.

Galeote, M., Soto, P., Checa, E., Gómez, A., & Lamela, E. (2008). The acquisition of productive vocabulary in Spanish children with Down syndrome. *Journal of Intellectual and Developmental Disability, 33*, 292–302.

Ganger, J., & Brent, M. R. (2004). Reexamining the vocabulary spurt. *Developmental Psychology, 40*, 621–632.

Glenn, S., & Cunningham, C. (2005). Performance of young people with Down syndrome on the Leiter-R and British Picture Vocabulary Scales. *Intellectual and Developmental Disabilities, 4*, 239–244.

Goldfield, B. A., & Reznick, J. S. (1990). Early lexical acquisition: Rate, content, and the vocabulary spurt. *Journal of Child Language, 17*(1), 171–183.

Guimaraes, C. V. A., Donnelly, L. F., Shott, S. R., Amin, R. S., & Kalra, M. (2008). Relative rather than absolute macroglossia in patients with Down syndrome: Implications for treatment of obstructive sleep apnea. *Pediatric Radiology, 38*(10), 1062–1067.

Hart, B., & Risley, T. R. (1995). *Meaningful differences in the everyday experience of young American children.* Baltimore, MD: Brookes.

Hartley, S. L., Handen, B. L., Devenny, D., Mihaila, I., Hardison, R., Lao, P. J., . . . Christian, B. T. (2017). Cognitive decline and brain amyloid-β accumulation across 3 years in adults with Down syndrome. *Neurobiology of Aging, 58*, 68–76.

Hepburn, S., Philofsky, A., Fidler, D. J., & Rogers, S. (2008). Autism symptoms in toddlers with Down syndrome: A descriptive study. *Journal of Applied Research in Intellectual Disabilities, 21*(1), 48–57.

Hesketh, L. J., & Chapman, R. S. (1998). Verb use by individuals with Down syndrome. *American Journal on Mental Retardation, 103*, 288–304.

Hoff, E., & Naigles, L. (2002). How children use input to acquire a lexicon. *Child Development, 73*(2), 418–433.

Iverson, J. M., & Goldin-Meadow, S. (2005). Gesture paves the way for language development. *Psychological Science, 16*(5), 367–371.

Iverson, J. M., Longobardi, E., & Caselli, M. C. (2003). Relationship between gestures and words in children with Down's syndrome and typically developing children in the early stages of communicative development. *International Journal of Language & Communication Disorders, 38*(2), 179–197.

Jarrold, C., & Baddeley, A. (2001). Short-term memory in Down syndrome: Applying the working memory model. *Down's Syndrome, Research and Practice: The Journal of the Sarah Duffen Centre/University of Portsmouth, 7*(1), 17–23.

Jarrold, C., Baddeley, A. D., & Phillips, C. E. (2002). Verbal short-term memory in Down syndrome: A problem of memory, audition, or speech? *Journal of Speech, Language, and Hearing Research, 45*, 531–544.

Jarrold, C., Thorn, A. S. C., & Stephens, E. (2009). The relationships among verbal short-term memory, phonological awareness, and new word learning: Evidence from typical development and Down syndrome. *Journal of Experimental Child Psychology, 102*(2), 196–218.

John, A. E., & Mervis, C. B. (2010). Comprehension of the communicative intent behind pointing and gazing gestures by young children with Williams syndrome or Down syndrome. *Journal of Speech, Language, and Hearing Research, 53*(4), 950–960.

Kaat-van den Os, D. J. A., Jongmans, J. M., Volman, M. J. M., & Lauteslager, P. E. M. (2015). Do gestures pave the way? A systematic review of the transitional role of gesture during the acquisition of early lexical and syntactic milestones in young children with Down syndrome. *Child Language Teaching and Therapy, 31*, 71–84.

Kaat-van den Os, D. t., Volman, C., Jongmans, M., & Lauteslager, P. (2017). Expressive vocabulary development in children with Down syndrome: A longitudinal study. *Journal of Policy and Practice in Intellectual Disabilities, 14*, 311–318. doi:10.1111/jppi.12212

Kanamori, G., Witter, M., Brown, J., & Williams-Smith, L. (2000). Otolaryngologic manifestations of Down syndrome. *Otolaryngologic Clinics of North America, 33*(6), 1285–1292.

Karmiloff-Smith, A., Al-Janabi, T., D'Souza, H., Groet, J., Massand, E., Mok, K., & Strydom, A. (2016). The importance of understanding individual differences in Down syndrome. *F1000Research*, 5.

Kasari, C., Mundy, P., Yirmiya, N., & Sigman, M. (1990). Affect and attention in children with Down syndrome. *American Journal of Mental Retardation, 95*(1), 55–67.

Keller-Bell, Y. D., & Abbeduto, L. (2007). Narrative development in adolescents and young adults with fragile X syndrome. *American Journal on Mental Retardation, 112*(4), 289–299.

Klein, B. P., & Mervis, C. B. (1999). Contrasting patterns of cognitive abilities of 9- and 10-year-olds with Williams syndrome or Down syndrome. *Developmental Neuropsychology, 16*, 177–196.

Kover, S. T., & Abbeduto, L. (2010). Expressive language in male adolescents with fragile X syndrome with and without comorbid autism. *Journal of Intellectual Disability Research, 54*, 246–265.

Kover, S. T., McDuffie, A., Abbeduto, L., & Brown, W. T. (2012). Effects of sampling context on spontaneous expressive language in males with fragile X syndrome or Down syndrome. *Journal of Speech, Language, and Hearing Research, 55*(4), 1022–1038.

Kumin, L., & Bahr, D. C. (1999). Patterns of feeding, eating, and drinking in young children with Down syndrome with oral motor concerns. *Down Syndrome Quarterly, 4*, 1–8.

Kumin, L., Councill, C., & Goodman, M. (1994). A longitudinal study of the emergence of phonemes in children with Down syndrome. *Journal of Communication Disorders, 27*(4), 293–303.

Landa, R. J. (2005). Assessment of social communication skills in preschoolers. *Mental Retardation and Developmental Disabilities Research Reviews, 11*, 247–252.

Landry, S. H., Smith, K. E., & Swank, P. R. (2006). Responsive parenting: Establishing early foundations for social, communication, and independent problem-solving skills. *Developmental Psychology, 42*(4), 627.

Lavigne, J., Sharr, C., Elsharkawi, I., Ozonoff, A., Baumer, N., Brasington, C., . . . Skotko, B. G. (2017). Thyroid dysfunction in patients with Down syndrome: Results from a multi-institutional registry study. *American Journal of Medical Genetics, Part A, 173*(6), 1539–1545.

Laws, G. (1998). The use of nonword repetition as a test of phonological memory in children with Down syndrome. *Journal of Child Psychology and Psychiatry, 39*, 1119–1130.

Laws, G. (2002). Working memory in children and adolescents with Down syndrome: Evidence from a colour memory experiment. *Journal of Child Psychology and Psychiatry, and Allied Disciplines, 43*(3), 353–364.

Laws, G., & Bishop, D. V. M. (2003). A comparison of language abilities in adolescents with Down syndrome and children with specific language impairment. *Journal of Speech, Language, and Hearing Research, 46*, 1324–1339.

Laws, G., & Bishop, D. V. M. (2004). Pragmatic language impairment and social deficits in Williams syndrome: A comparison with Down's syndrome and specific language impairment. *International Journal of Language & Communication Disorders, 39*(1), 45–64.

Legerstee, M. (1991). Changes in the quality of infant sounds as a function of social and nonsocial stimulation. *First Language, 11*(33), 327–343.

Legerstee, M., Bowman, T. G., & Fels, S. (1992). People and objects affect the quality of vocalizations in infants with Down syndrome. *Early Development and Parenting, 1*(3), 149–156.

Legerstee, M., Varghese, J., & Van Beek, Y. (2002). Effects of maintaining and redirecting infant attention on the production of referential communication in infants with and without Down syndrome. *Journal of Child Language, 29*(1), 23–48.

Lott, I. (2012). Neurological phenotypes for Down syndrome across the life span. *Progress in Brain Research, 197*, 101–121.

Loveall, S. J., Channell, M. M., Abbeduto, L., & Conners, F. A. (2019). Verb production by individuals with Down syndrome during narration. *Research in Developmental Disabilities, 85*, 82–91.

Loveall, S. J., Channell, M. M., Phillips, B. A., Abbeduto, L., & Conners, F. A. (2016). Receptive vocabulary analysis in Down syndrome. *Research in Developmental Disabilities, 55*, 161–172.

Lynch, M. P., Oller, D. K., Steffens, M. L., Levine, S. L., Basinger, D. L., & Umbel, V. (1995). Onset of speech-like vocalizations in infants with Down syndrome. *American Journal on Mental Retardation, 100*(1), 68–86.

Martin, G. E., Barstein, J., Hornickel, J., Matherly, S., Durante, G., & Losh, M. (2017). Signaling of noncomprehension in communication breakdowns in fragile X syndrome, Down syndrome, and autism spectrum disorder. *Journal of Communication Disorders, 65*, 22–34.

Martin, G. E., Klusek, J., Estigarribia, B., & Roberts, J. E. (2009). Language characteristics of individuals with Down syndrome. *Topics in Language Disorders, 29*(2), 112–132.

Martin, G. E., Losh, M., Estigarribia, B., Sideris, J., & Roberts, J. (2013). Longitudinal profiles of expressive vocabulary, syntax and pragmatic language in boys with fragile X syndrome or Down syndrome. *International Journal of Language & Communication Disorders, 48*(4), 432–443.

McKee, C. (1992). A comparison of pronouns and anaphors in Italian and English acquisition. *Language Acquisition, 2*(1), 21–54.

Menéndez, M. (2005). Down syndrome, Alzheimer's disease and seizures. *Brain and Development, 27*(4), 246–252.

Mervis, C. B., & John, A. E. (2010). Cognitive and behavioral characteristics of children with Williams syndrome: Implications for intervention approaches. *American Journal of Medical Genetics, Part C, 154C*, 229–248.

Mervis, C. B., & Robinson, B. F. (2000). Expressive vocabulary ability of toddlers with Williams syndrome or Down syndrome: A comparison. *Developmental Neuropsychology, 17*(1), 111–126.

Miles, S., & Chapman, R. S. (2002). Narrative content as described by individuals with Down syndrome and typically developing children. *Journal of Speech Language and Hearing Research, 45*(1), 175–189.

Miles, S., Chapman, R., & Sindberg, H. (2006). Sampling context affects MLU in the language of adolescents with Down syndrome. *Journal of Speech Language and Hearing Research, 49*(2), 325–337.

Miller, J. F. (1992). Development of speech and language in children with Down syndrome. In I. T. Lott & E. E. McCoy (Eds.), *Down syndrome: Advances in medical care* (pp. 39–50). New York: Wiley-Liss.

Miller, J. F. (1999). Profiles of language development in children with Down syndrome. In J. Miller, M. Leddy, & L. Leavitt (Eds.), *Improving the communication of people with Down syndrome* (pp. 11–39). Baltimore. MD: Brookes.

Miolo, G., Chapman, R. S., & Sindberg, H. A. (2005). Sentence comprehension in adolescents with Down syndrome and typically developing children: Role of sentence voice, visual context, and auditory-verbal short-term memory. *Journal of Speech, Language, and Hearing Research, 48*(1), 172–188.

Montgomery, J. W. (2000). Verbal working memory and sentence comprehension in children with specific language impairment. *Journal of Speech, Language and Hearing Research, 43*, 293–308.

Mundy, P., Kasari, C., Sigman, M., & Ruskin, E. (1995). Nonverbal communication and early language acquisition in children with Down syndrome and in normally developing children. *Journal of Speech and Hearing Research, 38*(1), 157–167.

Mundy, P. & Newell, L. (2007). Attention, joint attention and social cognition. *Current Directions in Psychological Science, 16*, 269–274.

Nadel, L. (1999). Down syndrome in cognitive neuroscience perspective. In H. Tager-Flusberg (Ed.) *Neurodevelopmental disorders: Contributions to a new framework from the cognitive neurosciences* (pp. 187–221). Cambridge, MA: MIT Press.

Naerland, T., Bakke, K. A., Storvik, S., Warner, G., & Howlin, P. (2017). Age and gender-related differences in emotional and behavioural problems and autistic features in children and adolescents with Down syndrome: A survey-based study of 674 individuals. *Journal of Intellectual Disabilities Research, 61*(6), 594–603.

Næss, K. A., Lyster, S. A., Hulme, C., & Melby-Lervag, M. (2011). Language and verbal short-term memory skills in children with Down syndrome: A meta-analytic review. *Research in Developmental Disabilities, 32*, 2225–2234.

Nash, H. M., & Snowling, M. J. (2008). Semantic and phonological fluency in children with Down Syndrome: Atypical organization of language or less efficient retrieval strategies? *Cognitive Neuropsychology, 5*, 690–703.

Oakes, A., Kover, S. T., & Abbeduto, L. (2013). Language comprehension profiles of young adolescents with fragile X syndrome. *American Journal of Speech-Language Pathology, 22*(4), 615.

Oliver, B., & Buckley, S. (1994). The language development of children with Down's syndrome: First words to two-word phrases. *Down Syndrome: Research & Practice, 2*, 71–75.

Oller, D. K., Eilers, R. E., Neal, A. R., & Cobo-Lewis, A. B. (1998). Late onset canonical babbling: A possible early marker of abnormal development. *American Journal on Mental Retardation, 103*(3), 249–263.

Owens, R. E., & MacDonald, J. D. (1982). Communicative uses of the early speech of nondelayed and Down syndrome children. *American Journal of Mental Deficiency, 86*(5), 503–510.

Phillips, B. A., Loveall, S. J., Channell, M. M., & Conners, F. A. (2014). Matching variables for research involving youth with Down syndrome: Leiter-R versus PPVT-4. *Research in Developmental Disabilities, 35*(2), 429–438.

Pierpont, E. I., Richmond, E. K., Abbeduto, L., Kover, S. T., & Brown, W. T. (2011). Contributions of phonological and verbal working memory to language development in adolescents with fragile X syndrome. *Journal of Neurodevelopmental Disorders, 3*(4), 335–347.

Pinker, S. (1996). *The language instinct.* New York: Norton.

Porter, J. (1999). Learning to count: A difficult task. *Down's Syndrome, Research and Practice: The Journal of the Sarah Duffen Centre/University of Portsmouth, 6*, 85–94.

Roach, M. A., Barratt, M. S., Miller, J. F., & Leavitt, L. A. (1998). The structure of mother–child play: Young children with Down syndrome and typically developing children. *Developmental Psychology, 34*(1), 77–87.

Roberts, J., Hunter, L., Gravel, J., Rosenfeld, R., Berman, S., Haggard, M., & Wallace, I. (2004). Otitis media, hearing loss, and language learning: Controversies and current research. *Journal of Developmental and Behavioral Pediatrics , 25*(2), 110–122.

Roberts, J., Long, S. H., Malkin, C., Barnes, E., Skinner, M., Hennon, E. A., & Anderson, K. (2005). A comparison of phonological skills of boys with fragile X syndrome and Down syndrome. *Journal of Speech Language and Hearing Research, 48*(5), 980.

Roberts, J., Martin, G. E., Moskowitz, L., Harris, A. A., Foreman, J., & Nelson, L. (2007). Discourse skills of boys with fragile X syndrome in comparison to boys with Down syndrome. *Journal of Speech Language and Hearing Research, 50*(2), 475.

Roberts, J., Price, J., Barnes, E., Nelson, L., Burchinal, M., Hennon, E. A., Hooper, S. R. (2007). Receptive vocabulary, expressive vocabulary, and speech production of boys with fragile X syndrome in comparison to boys with Down syndrome. *American Journal on Intellectual and Developmental Disabilities, 177*(3), 177–193.

Rosin, M. M., Swift, E., Bless, D., & Kluppel Vetter, D. (1988). Communication profiles of adolescents with Down syndrome. *Communication Disorders Quarterly, 12*(1), 49–64.

Rowe, M. L., Peregrine, E., & Mervis, C. B. (2005). *Communicative development in toddlers with Williams syndrome.* Poster Presented at the Meeting of the Society for Research in Child Development, Atlanta, GA.

Ruskin, E. M., Mundy, P., Kasari, C., & Sigman, M. (1994). Object mastery motivation of children with Down syndrome. *American Journal of Mental Retardation, 98*(4), 499–509.

Saffran, J. R., & Kirkham, N. Z. (2018). Infant statistical learning. *Annual Review of Psychology, 69*, 181–203.

Shott, S. R. (2006). Down syndrome: Common otolaryngologic manifestations. *American Journal of Medical Genetics Part C: Seminars in Medical Genetics, 142C*(3), 131–140.

Shriberg, L. D., & Widder, C. J. (1990). Speech and prosody characteristics of adults with mental retardation. *Journal of Speech, Language, and Hearing Research, 33*(4), 627–653.

Sigman, M., Ruskin, E., Arbeile, S., Corona, R., Dissanayake, C., Espinosa, M., & Zierhut, C. (1999). Continuity and change in the social competence of children with autism, Down syndrome, and developmental delays. *Monographs of the Society for Research in Child Development, 64*(1), 1–114.

Singer-Harris, N. G., Bellugi, U., Bates, E., Jones, W., & Rossen, M. (1997). Contrasting profiles of language development in children with Williams and Down syndromes. *Developmental Neuropsychology, 13*(3), 345–370.

Smith, B. L., & Oller, D. K. (1981). A comparative study of pre-meaningful vocalizations produced by normally developing and Down's syndrome infants. *The Journal of Speech and Hearing Disorders, 46*(1), 46–51.

Smith, B. L., & Stoel-Gammon, C. (1983). A longitudinal study of the development of stop consonant production in normal and Down's syndrome children. *The Journal of Speech and Hearing Disorders, 48*(2), 114–118.

Smith, B. L., & Stoel-Gammon, C. (1996). A quantitative analysis of reduplicated and variegated babbling in vocalizations by Down syndrome infants. *Clinical Linguistics & Phonetics, 10*(2), 119–129.

Smith, C. B., Adamson, L. B., & Bakeman, R. (1988). Interactional predictors of early language. *First Language, 8*(23), 143–156.

Snowling, M. J., Hulme, C., & Mercer, R. C. (2002). A deficit in rime awareness in children with Down syndrome. *Reading and Writing, 15*(5/6), 471–495.

Sommers, R. K., Patterson, J. P., & Wildgen, P. L. (1988). Phonology of Down syndrome speakers, ages 13–22. *Journal of Childhood Communication Disorders, 12*(1), 65–91.

Stefanini, S., Caselli, M. C., & Volterra, V. (2007). Spoken and gestural production in a naming task by young children with Down syndrome. *Brain and Language, 3*, 208–221.

Stoel-Gammon, C. (1980). Phonological analysis of four Down's syndrome children. *Applied Psycholinguistics, 1*(1), 31–48.

Stoel-Gammon, C. (2001). Down syndrome phonology: Developmental patterns and intervention strategies. *Down's Syndrome, Research and Practice: The Journal of the Sarah Duffen Centre/University of Portsmouth, 7*(3), 93–100.

Sudhalter, V., Cohen, I. L., Silverman, W., & Wolf-Schein, E. G. (1990). Conversational analyses of males with fragile X, Down syndrome, and autism: Comparison of the emergence of deviant language. *American Journal of Mental Retardation, 94*(4), 431–441.

Tannock, R. (1988). Mothers' directiveness in their interactions with their children with and without Down syndrome. *American Journal of Mental Retardation, 93*(2), 154–165.

Tapp, S., Anderson, T., & Visootsak, J. (2015). Neurodevelopmental outcomes in children with Down syndrome and infantile spasms. *Journal of Pediatric Neurology, 13*(2), 74–77.

Thordardottir, E. T., Chapman, R. S., & Wagner, L. (2002). Complex sentence production by adolescents with Down syndrome. *Applied Psycholinguistics, 23*, 163–183.

Thurman, A. J., & Mervis, C. B. (2013). The regulatory function of social referencing in preschoolers with Down syndrome or Williams syndrome. *Journal of Neurodevelopmental Disorders, 5*(1), 2.

Uong, E. C., Mcdonough, E. M., Tayag-Kier, C. e., Zhao, H., Haselgrove, J., Mahboubi, S., . . . Pack, A. I.> (2001). Magnetic Resonance Imaging of the Upper Airway in Children with Down Syndrome. *American Journal of Respiratory and Critical Care Medicine, 163*(3), 731–736.

Vandell, D. L., Pierce, K. M., & Dadisman, K. (2005). Out-of-school settings as a developmental context for children and youth. *Advances in Child Development and Behavior, 33*, 43–77.

Varlokosta, S. (2000). Lack of clitic-pronoun distinctions in the acquisition of Principle B in Child Greek. In *Proceedings of the 24th annual Boston University Conference on Language Development* (pp. 738–748). Somerville, MA: Cascadilla Press.

Vicari, S., Carlesimo, A., & Caltagirone, C. (1995). Short-term memory in persons with intellectual disabilities and Down's syndrome. *Journal of Intellectual Disability Research, 39*(6), 532–537.

Vicari, S., Caselli, M. C., Gagliardi, C., Tonucci, F., & Volterra, V. (2002). Language acquisition in special populations: A comparison between Down and Williams syndromes. *Neuropsychologia, 40*, 2461–2470.

Vicari, S., Caselli, M. C., & Tonucci, F. (2000). Asynchrony of lexical and morphosyntactic development in children with Down Syndrome. *Neuropsychologia, 38*, 634–644.

Warner, G., Howlin, P., Salomone, E., Moss, J., & Charman, T. (2017). Profiles of children with Down syndrome who meet screening criteria for autism spectrum disorder (ASD): A comparison with children diagnosed with ASD attending specialist schools. *Journal of Intellectual Disability Research, 61*(1), 75–82.

Warner, G., Moss, J., Smith, P., & Howlin, P. (2014). Autism characteristics and behavioural disturbances in ~ 500 children with Down's syndrome in England and Wales. *Autism Research, 7*(4), 433–441.

Wechsler, D. (2011). Escala Wechsler de Inteligencia para los niveles preescolar y primario-III. (M. Moderno Ed.).

Welsh, T. N., & Elliott, D. (2001). The processing speed of visual and verbal movement information by adults with and without Down syndrome. *Adapted Physical Activity Quarterly, 18*(2), 156–167.

Witecy, B., & Penke, M. (2017). Language comprehension in children, adolescents, and adults with Down syndrome. *Research in Developmental Disabilities, 62*, 184–196.

Wynn, K. (1990). Children's understanding of counting. *Cognition, 36*, 155–193.

Yoder, P. J., & Warren, S. F. (2004). Early predictors of language in children with and without Down syndrome. *American Journal on Mental Retardation, 109*(4), 285–300.

Ypsilanti, A., & Grouios, G. (2008). Linguistic profile of individuals with Down syndrome: Comparing the linguistic performance of three developmental disorders. *Child Neuropsychology, 14*, 148–170.

Ypsilanti, A., Grouios, G., Zikouli, A., & Hatzinikolaou, K. (2006). Speed of naming in children with Williams and Down syndromes. *Journal of Intellectual and Developmental Disability, 31*, 87–94.

Zampini, L., & D'Odorico, L. (2009). Communicative gestures and vocabulary development in 36-month-old children with Down's syndrome. *International Journal of Language & Communication Disorders, 44*(6), 1063–1073.

Zampini, L., & D'Odorico, L. (2011a). Gesture production and language development: A longitudinal study of children with Down syndrome. *Gesture, 11*, 174–193.

Zampini, L., & D'Odorico, L. (2011b). Lexical and syntactic development in Italian children with Down's syndrome. *Language & Communication Disorders, 46*, 386–396.

Zampini, L., & D'Odorico, L. (2013). Vocabulary development in children with Down syndrome: Longitudinal and cross-sectional data. *Intellectual & Developmental Disability, 4*, 310–317.

CHAPTER

15 Motor Function in Persons With Down Syndrome

Shannon D. R. Ringenbach, Nathaniel E. Arnold, Kahyun Nam, Simon D. Holzapfel, Chih-Chia Chen, Corinna Lopez, *and* Monica Szeto

Abstract

This chapter reviews fine- and gross-motor function research in persons with Down syndrome (DS) across the lifespan. Fine-motor function consists of movements of the small muscles in the body such as the fingers and hands used to perform many activities of daily living, including writing, using a zipper, tying shoe laces, eating with a spoon, and using scissors. In contrast, gross-motor function consists of movements of the larger muscles of the body such as the leg muscles to perform essential skills such as walking, jumping, climbing, and swimming. In general, both fine- and gross-motor function are slower, more variable, and delayed in persons with DS. Multiple movement interventions are available for individuals with DS, including physical therapy, equine therapy, virtual reality gaming, Assisted Cycling Therapy, walking, and aerobic and strength training. These as well as other exercise interventions and their results on fine- and gross-motor function in persons with DS across the lifespan were reviewed. In general, early research focused more on anatomical differences in persons with DS, whereas more recently the focus has been on differences in neural mechanisms and how they can be altered for the benefit of motor and cognitive improvements in persons with DS. Future research should rethink exercise interventions to require fast movements in young children with DS and to determine the lasting effects on motor and cognitive skills that will ultimately improve longevity and quality of life for persons with DS.

Key Words: intervention, therapy, motor skills, cognitive, Down syndrome, neural, Assisted Cycling Therapy

Persons with Down syndrome (DS) are most often characterized as individuals with cognitive and language deficits. The presence of an extra 21st chromosome, however, also creates significant fine (e.g., writing, dressing, etc.) and gross (e.g., walking, stair climbing, etc.) motor challenges. While infants and young children with DS achieve motor skills in the same order as compared to those with typical development, they are significantly delayed (Winders, 1997). For example, the child with Down syndrome walks approximately 1 year later than the typical child, which also delays the development of social, perceptual, and cognitive development. Furthermore, the movements of individuals with Down syndrome are often slower and less consistent throughout their lifespan. Motor function is crucial for completing activities of daily living (e.g., feeding, grooming, handling money, walking, etc.) for people with DS. Thus, motor function is an extremely important area to understand in persons with DS.

In this chapter, we review research concerning fine- and gross-motor functioning, the connection of motor skills to cognition, and recent alternative and exercise movement therapies. Finally, we conclude with a new way to think of movement therapy for persons with DS.

Review of Motor Functioning

Fine-Motor Function

Fine-motor function consists of movements of the small muscles of the body such as the fingers, wrists, and toes. Movements of the small muscles include using utensils to eat, using zippers and buttons to dress, using writing or typing to communicate, and using money to purchase items. Clearly, fine-motor function is essential for activities of daily living and independence. Among persons with Down syndrome, however, these fine-motor skills are performed more slowly and less consistently, and the skills develop later than in the typical population. For example, a study was conducted of fine-motor and perceptual motor development among 22 children with DS between the ages of 4.5 and 14 years (Spano et al., 1999). The participants completed two standardized assessments: the Movement ABC test, which is used to measure fine- and gross-motor function, and the Developmental Test of Visual Motor Integration, which is used to measure the ability to copy shapes. For both assessments, all of the children scored below the 5th percentile for their chronological age. On the Developmental Test of Visual Motor Integration specifically, all of the participants scored between an age range of 2 to 4 years, which is considerably lower than their chronological age. On the Movement ABC, the fine-motor skills (such as peg insertion, threading beads, and drawing between two lines) were more delayed than gross-motor skills in children with DS. These findings demonstrate that fine- and gross-motor skills in persons with DS develop at a delayed rate and continue to be immature into adolescence.

Because persons with DS have motor skills below that of age-matched peers (Block, 1991), their ability to perform functional tasks of daily living are often limited. In a cross-sectional retrospective chart review of 271 children with DS ranging in age from 4 months to 18 years old, Frank and Esbensen (2015) expanded the fine-motor skills studied to include more activities of daily living such as handwriting, scissor usage, and the self-care skills of feeding and dressing. They found that persons with DS were significantly delayed with these tasks as well and that an increase in the complexity of tasks increased the difference between persons with DS and typical chronological age-matched peers. More recently, Marchal et al. (2016) conducted a large longitudinal study with 181 children with DS and measured mental and motor development using the Bayley Scales of Infant Development (BSID-II) at ages 6, 12, and 24 months and followed up at 10.7 years. At the 10.7 year mark, Marchal et al. administered the Movement Assessment Battery for Children (M-ABC 2) to assess motor skill and found that the participants were delayed compared to the norm in aiming, catching, and manual dexterity. This is consistent with other evidence that catching is an area of weakness in persons with DS, which may be due to the complex timing, spatial calculation, and coordination involved in catching (Savelsbergh, van der Kamp, Ledebt, & Planinsek, 2000).

Research on reaching- and pointing-type tasks in adults with DS has consistently shown slower reaction times (Anson & Mawston, 2000) and slower movement times (for a review refer to Weeks, Chua, & Elliott, 2000). Two decades of research with adults with DS found that motor performance of discrete tasks (e.g., rapid one-time movements) was most effective using visual instructions. Elliott and colleagues (Elliott, Weeks, & Elliott, 1987; Maraj et al., 2002, 2007) proposed a model of atypical cerebral specialization only for verbal perception in persons with DS. According to this model, verbal-motor skills in individuals with Down syndrome are delayed because of the specialization of speech perception in the right hemisphere in these individuals; this is opposite to that found in the typical population and opposite to the motor planning and production areas of the brain. This separation of speech perception and movement centers in the brain creates slower, more variable movements with more errors following verbal instructions. This is why visual instructions are the most effective for rapid, simple fine-motor skills in persons with DS. However, benefits for persons with DS have been reported in unimanual and bimanual coordination in continuous (i.e., lasting for 30 seconds) drawing (Ringenbach, Chen, Mulvey, & Jung, 2012; Ringenbach, Mulvey, Van Gemmert, Stankus, & Maraj, 2009) and continuous drumming tasks (Ringenbach, Beachy, & Mulvey, 2007) with auditory instructions. This suggests that the type of instructions may differ with the type of motor skill being taught (i.e., visual instructions for rapid fine movements and auditory instructions for continuous fine movements) and that this may be due to the different brain organization of persons with DS (i.e., as explained above, verbal perception in the opposite hemisphere as movement planning).

While fine-motor impairments in persons with DS were originally attributed to shorter hands and lax ligaments, evidence from magnetic resonance imaging research indicates that some of the brain structures, such as the cerebellum and brainstem, are smaller in persons with DS (Jernigan & Bellugi, 1990). This supports the foundational explanation by Henderson, Morris, and Frith (1981), who attributed deficits in hand-eye coordination or visual motor function and reaction time to the reduced size of the cerebellum and brainstem (i.e., ~66% of normal weight); reduced myelination in the frontal lobe and cerebellum; and fewer neurons in the temporal, frontal, parietal, and occipital lobes of the cortex. Overall, the evidence indicates that delayed, slower, and more variable fine-motor function is consistently found among persons with DS and may be related to differences in the brain structures controlling fine-motor skills. While direct measurements of cortical structure and function are scarce, recent research is investigating the treatment of DS-related neurocognitive impairment during pregnancy in mice and shows promise for improving aberrant cortical formation and thus abnormal behaviors in mice with DS (Nakano-Kobayashi et al., 2017).

Gross-Motor Function

Gross-motor function consists of movements of the large muscles such as the legs, which are involved in walking, jumping, climbing, swimming, and standing from a chair. Thus, gross-motor function is particularly essential to activities of daily living, independence, and quality of life for persons with DS. Similar to fine-motor function, gross-motor function is delayed, slower, and more variable than typically developing (TD) peers. For example, walking in infants with DS is typically delayed 1 year, which was often thought to be due in part to increased joint laxity and decreased muscle tone (Winders, 1997). Even when infants with DS achieve walking, they demonstrate shorter stride length, slower velocity, and wider step width than peers without DS (Kubo & Ulrich, 2006). As measured by electromyographic electrodes (e.g., measures of muscle activity), toddlers with DS were able to activate their leg muscles by using energy-efficient strategies with less frequent muscle activation, longer muscle duration, and more timing variability than TD peers (Chang, Kubo, & Ulrich, 2009). The longer duration of muscle activity was thought to be needed to stabilize their lax joints. Thus, children with DS accomplished the motor skill of walking by using a different strategy than typical toddlers to overcome their biomechanical limitations. Additionally, only about 50% of children with DS are able to walk up stairs, run, and jump by the age of 5 years, and the development of these skills is generally not complete until 6.2 years of age, whereas among TD children stair climbing occurs around 10–15 months, running occurs around 18–24 months, and jumping around 2–3 years (Palisano et al., 2001).

Research among older children and adults with DS shows continued differences in walking. In one example, Rigoldi, Galli, and Albertini (2011) examined 32 children with DS when they were children (aged 6.7–11.7 years), teenagers (13.5–19.9 years), and adults (31.9–42.7 years) and compared their gait to 10 TD children (5.5–10.7 years), 15 TD teenagers (16.2–19.9 years), and 16 TD adults (33.3–41.9 years) during self-selected walking speed along a 10-meter walkway. Although the gait parameters among the participants with DS improved from childhood to the teenage years, they still displayed shorter step length and larger step width than their age-matched TD peers. This is consistent with findings from analyses of walking on a treadmill in preadolescents with DS, in which researchers found improvements in muscle activity (e.g., reduced stiffness) after walking practice (Smith, Kubo, Black, Holt, & Ulrich, 2007; Ulrich, Haehl, Buzzi, Kubo, & Holt, 2004). Thus, improvement in gait over time suggests that children with DS develop some compensations for their poor balance (e.g., wider step width) and other unique physical characteristics such as low muscle tone and joint laxity.

While walking on the ground is different than treadmill walking, walking around obstacles is important to examine because it is more similar to what we may encounter in daily living. For example, in a study of step length and toe clearance of obstacles in five children with DS (5–6 years old), Virji-Babul and Brown (2004) found that the children with DS were more likely than typical children of the same age to hit the obstacle due to lower toe clearance and to stop before a higher obstacle. These findings suggest that anticipatory adjustments of children with DS were not as effective as typical children, demonstrating that balance and locomotor agility continue to be relative weaknesses during childhood. Subsequently, Vimercati, Galli, Rigoldi, and Albertini (2013) investigated unobstructed walking, walking over an obstacle on the ground, and walking over an obstacle at 10% of the participant's height among young adults with DS (mean age of 22). They also found a lack of anticipatory movement adjustments and that the young adults' lead feet did not go as high or raise as early as that of the typical participants.

In adults with DS, walking has been shown to be less economical, leading to slower walking speeds (Smith & Ulrich, 2008), greater step frequency and step width (Agiovlasitis, McCubbin, Yun, Pavol, & Widrick, 2009), and high levels of muscle co-contraction (Aruin, Almeida, & Latash, 1996). In a study of obstacle avoidance among 12 older adults (35–62 years old) with DS who walked unobstructed on a pressure sensitive walkway (a GAITRrite mat) using standard steps, Smith and Ulrich (2008) found that, compared to typical adults, older adults with DS walked slower with shorter and wider steps and spent more time in the most stable portion of the gait cycle with both legs on the ground (i.e., double support phase). Furthermore, during obstacle avoidance, the older adults with DS again spent more time in double support than typical adults, and two participants were unable to perform the obstacle avoidance stepping task. Thus, this lack of anticipatory movements seen in gait does not appear to improve across development. This finding may be explained by the reduced size of the cerebellum in persons with DS (Frith & Frith, 1974; Guidi, Bonasoni, Ciani, & Bartesaghi, 2010), which may be responsible for hypotonia and coordination deficits seen in gross-motor function.

Relation of Motor Function to Cognitive Function

Historically, motor and cognitive function have been studied separately in the typical population because they were not thought to develop at the same time, with motor development occurring earlier than cognitive development (for a review, see Diamond, 2000). However, neuroimaging research has shown that the cerebellum, which had been traditionally known to aid in motor function, may play a large role in cognitive function. Similarly, the prefrontal cortex, which had been known for its role in cognitive function, has been shown to also have a role in motor function (Berman et al., 1995; Courchesne et al., 1994; Desmond, Gabrieli, Wagner, Ginier, & Glover, 1997). Thus, this led Diamond (2000) to argue that both motor and cognitive development are more related than previously thought. Piek, Dawson, Smith, and Gasson (2008) provided evidence for this in typical children when they examined fine and gross movements (e.g., measured with the McCarron Assessment of Neuromuscular Development; MAND) and cognitive function (e.g., measured with the Wechsler Intelligence Scale for Children; WISC-IV) over time among typical children 0–4 years old and 6–11 years. They found that gross-motor function had a strong positive relationship to working memory and processing speed. A similar relationship was found among children with DS by Marchal et al. (2016), who reported that cognitive and motor milestones among children with DS at 24 months were predictive of motor skills at 10.7 years old.

A similar connection between motor and cognitive function was found among 12 adolescents with DS by Chen, Ringenbach, Albert, and Semken (2014), who measured fine-motor function with the Purdue Pegboard task, which involves putting small dowels in holes with either the dominant hand alone, the nondominant hand alone, or both hands. Cognitive function, specifically working memory, was measured by the Corsi-Block tapping; memory span with the Auditory Memory span test; and cognitive planning with the Tower of London. The findings indicated a positive relationship between motor and cognitive function in adolescents with DS and suggested that the persons with DS with the highest cognitive planning and verbal working memory performance also had the most advanced fine manual dexterity. This finding is consistent with neuroimaging research in the typical population for whom Schall (2003) and Weiss et al. (2003) found positive relationships between motor and cognitive function that were mediated by the co-activation of the prefrontal area and cerebellum. Thus, with similar findings of positive relationships between motor and cognitive function as reported above, it is more convincing that the prefrontal cortex and the cerebellum are both involved during motor and cognitive tasks among persons with DS. This relationship was also found among people with dementia and related cognitive impairment, in which exercise training significantly improved cognitive function and behavior (Heyn, Abreu, & Ottenbacher, 2004). Thus, exercise or therapeutic approaches using movement would be a logical approach for improving motor and cognitive function in persons with DS across their lifespan.

Therapeutic Approaches

Traditional

For over 20 years, physical therapists have provided therapy to improve motor function for persons with DS of all ages. One physical therapist, Patricia Winders, has written several books on gross-motor skills in children with DS as guides for parents and professionals (Winders, 1997). She emphasizes the physical limitations such as hypotonia (i.e., low muscle tone), increased joint flexibility, shorter arms and legs, and decreased strength. Winders also encourages practicing movements when the child is alert, practicing the movements they like first, practicing movements for short periods of time, varying the way that skills are practiced to assess individual preferences, considering each child's temperament, and learning each child's motivator because attention varies. This book is an important resource because Winders provided activities and motor milestone checklists. Around this same time, Maryanne Bruni (1998), an occupational therapist, also wrote a book for parents and professionals on fine-motor skills in children with DS. While physical therapy and occupational therapy are standard approaches to improving motor function in populations with movement deficits, there is an emergence of research on alternative therapeutic approaches to improving movement function specifically in DS.

Alternative

One example of an alternative therapy for improving motor function is horseback/equine therapy, or hippotherapy. Copetti, Mota, Graup, Menezies, and Venturini (2007) investigated the effect of horseback therapy on the kinematics of gait in three children (5.2–9.8 years) with DS. They found that 13 sessions of horseback riding therapy with continuous use of the feet on the stirrups while walking and trotting on sand and asphalt improved stability of the ankle joint in the balance phase of walking. This may be caused by the strengthening of the dorsiflexor muscles during horseback therapy during which the feet are in the stirrups, creating increased movement in the ankle. Thus, this alternative type of therapy can be used to promote improvements in motor function, specifically gross-motor function related to walking in children with DS.

Another alternative therapy involved the Power Pumper, which is a four-wheeled seated riding mobility device. Hauck and Ulrich (2015) investigated 30 minutes of riding two times per week for 2 weeks with 12 children with DS (5–7 years old) and 12 children without DS (5–7 years old) and found an increase in time spent in moderate-to-vigorous physical activity outside of the Power Pumper practice. These findings suggest that participation by persons with DS in a social environment, even with less structured exercise, can lead to engagement in more time in other higher-intensity physical activity.

A more technological alternative therapy that also provides entertainment with exercise are video games (e.g., Wii). In one study, Wuang, Chiang, Su, and Wang (2011) randomized 110, 7–12 year olds with DS into either a Wii Sports group or a standard occupational therapy group. Fifty children with DS (7–12 years old) were in a no-intervention control group. The activity groups participated for 60 minutes twice a week for 24 weeks. The Bruininks-Oseretsky Test of Motor Proficiency, the Developmental Test of Visual Motor Integration, and the Test of Sensory Integration Function were given pre- and post-24 weeks. The findings indicated that the Wii group performed better than the standard occupational therapy group and the no-activity group in fine-motor integration, upper limb coordination, running speed, and agility. In another study using the Wii as an intervention to test the effects of a strength and agility, Lin and Wuang (2012) randomly split 92 adolescents with DS (13–18 years old) into an exercise group (N = 46) and no-exercise group (N = 46). The exercise group participated in a 6-week intervention consisting of three 35-minute sessions per week. The program consisted of a 5-minute treadmill warm-up exercise at a pace of 2.0–3.0 kph, a 10-minute break, then a 20-minute exercise program based in virtual reality (VR). The participants were able to pick from 15 different sport games on the Wii system and reached 50%–60% of max heartrate by the end of the session. Pre- and postintervention measures were taken for both groups using a hand-held dynamometer to measure the grip strength and a BOT-2 test to assess strength and agility performance of hip extensors, hip flexors, knee extensors, knee flexors, hip abductors, and ankle plantar/flexors. The main finding was that the lower extremity muscle strength and agility performance significantly improved in the exercise group after the 6-week intervention as compared to the no-exercise group. The greatest muscle strength gains were seen in the knee flexors and extensors. In general, an exercise training program utilizing fun, virtual-reality style games is capable of improving muscle strength and agility performance in adolescents with DS.

In a study with Wii as a movement therapy in adults with DS, Silva et al. (2017) randomly divided 27 adults (18–60 years old) into 30 minutes of Wii Fit balance board activities (N = 14; e.g., free run, heading, table tilt, snowboard slalom, tightrope tension, hula hoop, balance bubble, etc.), 30 minutes of sports-related games (e.g., Wii sports, Will sports resort) and dancing games (e.g., Just Dance II) completed three times per week for 8 weeks. Thirteen adults with DS were randomized into a control group that did not have any intervention. The findings showed improvements in the shuttle run, sit and reach, standing broad jump, 30 second sit ups, six minute walk test (6MWT), and timed up and go (TUG) in the Wii group over the control group. Thus, playing a virtual reality gaming activity improved many types of gross-motor skills among adults with DS, which is consistent with the evidence that virtual reality gaming can improve motor function among persons with DS all different ages.

Exercise

Another approach to improving motor function across the lifespan in persons with DS is through exercise interventions to improve physical fitness, strength, and overall health. Exercise interventions have been shown to be very valuable among children with DS. Specifically, Ulrich, Ulrich, Angulo-Kinzler, and Yun (2001) showed that infants who trained on a treadmill walked earlier than infants who did not. Furthermore, they were able to better explore and develop their perceptual-motor behavior, which is so important for activities of daily living and independence. Similarly, infants who received high-intensity treadmill training by increasing the speed of the treadmill displayed higher levels of leg activity that were sustained after 1 year (Angulo-Barroso, Burghardt, Lloyd, & Ulrich, 2008). In an early intervention study, Looper and Ulrich (2010) examined 17 infants with DS comparing corrective foot alignment orthoses and treadmill training conducted for 8 minutes a day for 5 days a week with the treadmill training alone. Initially, the infants in both groups showed increased gross-motor function measure (GMFM) scores, although after 1 month of walking experience, the treadmill training alone group showed higher GMFM scores with higher standing, walking, running, and jumping scores than the treadmill and orthoses group. The finding that improvements in gross-motor function in infants with DS last for months post-intervention (Ulrich, Burghardt, Lloyd, Tiernan, and Hornyak, 2001; Ulrich, Lloyd, Tiernan, Looper, & Angulo-Barroso, 2008) is clinically significant for maintaining continued motor function and independence among infants with DS.

Different exercise interventions in older children with DS have also shown positive results on motor function. Ulrich et al. (2011) conducted a bicycle intervention in which children with DS (8–15 years old) were separated into a no-intervention (N = 27) or bicycle intervention (N = 34) group. Ulrich et al. believed that increasing the physical activity and motor skills of children with DS via a culturally normal activity would positively influence patterns of physical activity important for continued motor functioning and health. Their findings supported this hypothesis, as the intervention group spent less sedentary time, as measured by Actical accelerometers, 7 weeks and even 1 year after the intervention.

Strength training is another type of exercise intervention appropriate for adolescents with DS. For example, Shields, Taylor, Wee, Wollersheim, O'Shea, and Fernhall (2013) argued that adequate muscle strength is important for adolescents with DS, especially as they transition to adulthood, because low muscle tone can make daily activities in the work force a challenge. In their study, 34 adolescents with DS (14–22 years old) completed a 10-week progressive resistance training program designed to improve work task performance, muscle strength, and physical activity. The program included seven exercises three for upper body, three for lower body, and one for the trunk. The social program group included 34 adolescents with DS of the same age range who completed a 90-minute social program with a student mentor once a week for 10 weeks. The social program comprised of art activities, watching movies, baking, and listening to music. Measures were taken at baseline, immediately after intervention (11 weeks), and 3 months postintervention (24 weeks). The findings indicated that the progressive resistance training group experienced an increase in upper and lower limb strength at week 11 but maintained only lower limb strength at week 24. Similarly, a significant increase in physical activity levels in the progressive resistance training group was evidenced at week 11 but not at week 24. The findings indicate that this program was effective at increasing muscle strength and physical activity levels, although its effect on work task performance was not examined.

While much research is focused on children with DS, some research has included older adults with DS. This is increasingly important, as the increase in life expectancy for persons with DS has increased from 35 years old in 1982 to 55 years old or older today (Bittles & Glasson, 2004). This has led to many more persons with DS who need to maintain independence and their physical health into later adulthood. Carmeli, Kessel, Coleman, and Ayalon (2002) highlighted that the maintenance of muscle strength and dynamic balance are important for lengthening the life expectancy in elderly adults with

DS. In their study, 16 older adults with DS (57–65 years old) walked on a treadmill three times per week for 25 consecutive weeks, initially for 10–15 minutes, gradually increasing to 45 minutes per session for 6 months. The speed of the treadmill was below the threshold of breathlessness but as fast as the participant could tolerate. The treadmill walking group was compared to 10 older adults in a no-activity control group on measures of leg strength and dynamic balance. After 6 months, knee extension and flexion isokinetic strength and dynamic balance measured by a TUG test were improved in the walking group as compared to the control group.

Other research has examined the effect of exercise interventions on physical fitness in persons with DS, with some findings of improved exercise capacity (Pitetti, Climstein, Campbell, & Barrett, 1992) and improved heart rate recovery (Giagkoudaki, Dimitros, Kouidi, & Deligiannis, 2010; Rimmer, Heller, Wang, & Valerio, 2004; Shields, Taylor, & Dodd, 2008). However, in a meta-analysis of exercise interventions in persons with DS, Andriolo, El Dib, Ramos, Atallah, and da Silva (2010) found insufficient evidence to argue for increased physical outcomes of aerobic exercise in persons with DS. Although the results were promising, only three high-quality research studies were included. In the typical population, voluntary exercise has been shown to improve physical, cognitive, and health outcomes (Penedo & Dahn, 2005). Thus, more research needs to address the influence of exercise on improving motor function in persons with DS across the lifespan.

Cognitive

A trending topic is the relationship between motor and cognitive function, with the underlying question of whether being fit or exercising more can make you smarter. Evidence from children both with and without attention-deficient/hyperactivity disorder (ADHD) suggests that greater physical activity is associated with better grades (Pontifex, Saliba, Raine, Picchietti, & Hillman, 2013). Similarly, among typical older adults, increased activity is associated with increased memory (O'Brien, Ottoboni, Tessari, & Setti, 2017). In healthy adults, functional near-infrared spectroscopy (fNIRS), which combines physiological monitoring and functional neuroimaging, found significant improvement in cognitive function (e.g., the Stroop task) that was related to brain activation in the lateral prefrontal cortices in both hemispheres following an acute bout of moderate intensity exercise (e.g., cycling) (Yanagisawa et al., 2010). Recent research with persons with DS has also shown consistent findings, with typical populations finding a positive relationship between motor and cognitive function among persons with DS following moderate intensity exercise.

Chen and Ringenbach (2019) have found that acute (e.g., one session) treadmill walking exercise improves verbal-fluency performance (e.g., naming things that start with different letters) in adolescents and young adults with DS. Chen, Ringenbach, Crews, Kulinna, and Amazeen (2015) also found improvements in cognitive function (specifically, improved inhibition) in young adults with DS following a single 20-minute bout of moderate-intensity treadmill walking. Chen and Ringenbach (2016) further found that moderate-intensity treadmill walking was more beneficial for improving choice reaction time over high-intensity treadmill walking. In a cycling exercise, Ringenbach, Albert, Chen, and Alberts (2014) found that one session of Assisted Cycle Therapy (fast-rate cycling with the help of a motor) improved cognitive planning and reaction time in adolescents with DS more than voluntary cycling and no cycling.

Longer moderate-intensity exercise programs of cycling three times per week for 8 weeks also found improvements in measures of cognitive function, including reaction time (i.e., speed of processing information) and inhibition (Ringenbach et al., 2016), working memory (Holzapfel et al., 2016), and adaptive behaviors (e.g., cleaning, going to school, preparing a meal, etc.; Ringenbach et al., 2019) in adolescents with DS. Furthermore, when manual dexterity (specifically bimanual coordination) was improved following Assisted Cycling Therapy three times per week for 8 weeks, improvements were also seen in cognitive planning (Holzapfel et al., 2015).

Recent Research

Assisted Cycle Therapy

Alberts, Linder, Penko, Lowe, and Phillips (2011) have proposed a model to explain the improvements in fine-motor function and cognitive function following gross-motor exercise in terms of changes in neural plasticity, neurogenesis, and so forth (see Figure 15.1). This model has recently been modified for persons with DS by the Sensorimotor Development Research Lab at Arizona State University.

Assisted Cycle Therapy (ACT) is an exercise paradigm (see Figure 15.1) in which movement is generated by a mechanical motor at a rapid rate that could not be achieved voluntarily in persons with deficits in movement speed. This rapid rate of movement results in increased intrinsic feedback through receptors that help us move, such as Golgi tendon organs (GTO) and muscles spindles, or cardiovascular responses through changes in heart rate. Information from these receptors have been shown to increase the presence of neurotrophic factors including brain-derived neurotrophic factor (BDNF), dopamine, glial-derived neurotrophic factor (GDNF), and insulin growth factor (IGF_3) in the brain (Alberts et al., 2011) In addition, increases in neurotrophic factors can lead to neurological changes, including neurogenesis, neuroprotection, plasticity, and neural repair (Petzinger et al., 2010), which in turn have led to improvements in cognitive function and motor function in persons with Parkinson's disease (Ridgel, Vitek, & Alberts, 2009) and persons with DS (Ringenbach, Albert, Chen, & Alberts, 2014).

This innovative gross-motor exercise addresses the limitation of some populations, especially persons with DS, who are incapable due to physiological and psychosocial factors of moving at a fast enough rate to gain the benefits of exercise. This is consistent with psychosocial evidence that persons with DS favor solitary and sedentary activities (Jobling &

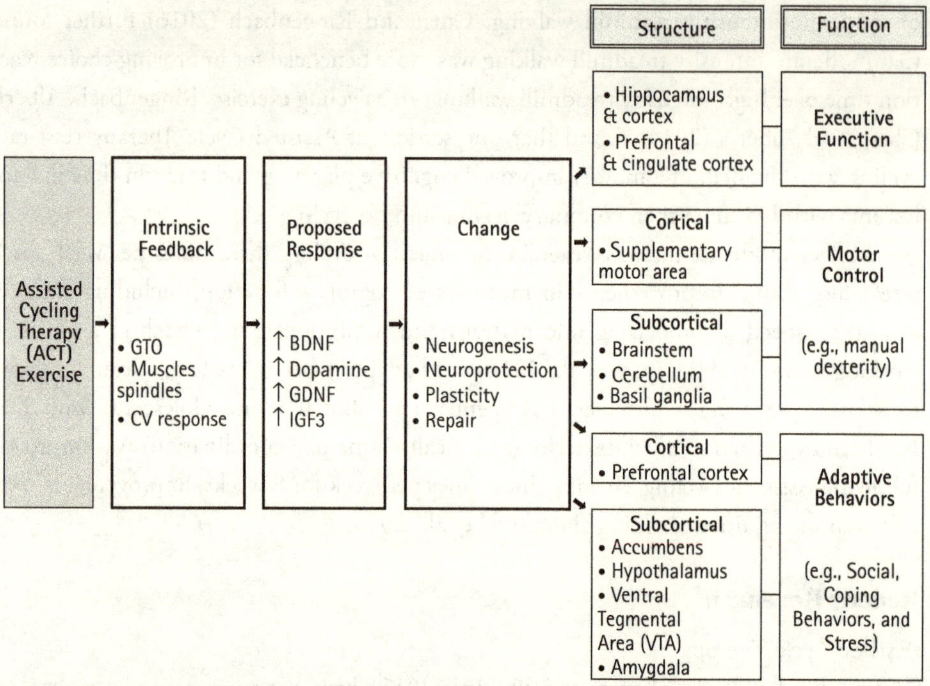

Figure 15.1. Schematic depicting the proposed effect of ACT on central nervous system structure and function. From Ringenbach et al. (2021).

Cuskelly, 2002). Furthermore, approximately 61% persons with DS have been shown to have low exercise tolerance or willingness to exercise, which affects their exercise time and intensity and, as research shows, motor and cognitive benefits (Ringenbach, Chen, Albert, Lichtsinn, & Alberts, 2013). As a result, on average 43% of persons with DS are obese (Pastore et al., 2000), which limits the available muscular strength for persons with DS to produce rapid movement or exercise. Thus, a fundamental limitation of previous rehabilitation and exercise therapy and interventions is that exercise was dependent on voluntary performance, which is affected by reduced muscular strength (i.e., hypotonicity) and negative attitudes toward exercise among persons with DS. Thus, ACT innovates by reducing the muscular requirements of a gross-motor exercise and allows for the increase of movement rate faster than could be achieved on a treadmill or during other exercise interventions.

ACT has been found to improve motor function in other neurological populations that move slowly. Research with persons with Parkinson's disease found that assisted exercise, pedaling on the ACT bicycle at a rate 35% greater than their preferred voluntary rate, improved clinical motor function as assessed by Unified Parkinson's Disease Rating Scale, as well as fine-motor function (e.g., stabilized bimanual dexterity; Ridgel et al., 2009). Initial fMRI data indicated that one session of ACT in adults with Parkinson's disease resulted in greater cortical activation, particularly for the supplementary motor and prefrontal areas that are responsible for fine- and gross-motor function, as well as cognitive function (e.g., motor planning, inhibition, set shifting, etc.). ACT is therefore innovative in that it is proposed to improve motor and cognitive functioning by promoting the formation of new neurons (i.e., neurogenesis) and/or reorganizing a damaged nervous system (i.e., neurorehabilitation).

Thus, persons with DS who move slowly can be assisted (e.g., by a mechanical motor in stationary cycling) in exercising at a rate greater than what they can sustain voluntarily in order to gain the motor and cognitive improvements following exercise. Furthermore, the model and results of ACT may explain the previous nonsignificant therapeutic benefits of voluntary rate exercise among adolescents and adults with DS (Andriolo et al., 2010). Recent data by Chen et al. (2014) using the bicycle pictured in Figure 15.2, support this observation.

After acute bouts of ACT, but not after voluntary cycling or no cycling, improvements were found in manual dexterity as measured by the mean change in total number of pegs moved in adolescents with DS (see Fig. 15.3; Chen et al., 2014). Because improvements in the motor performance of the nonexercised muscles occurred (i.e., improved upper limb

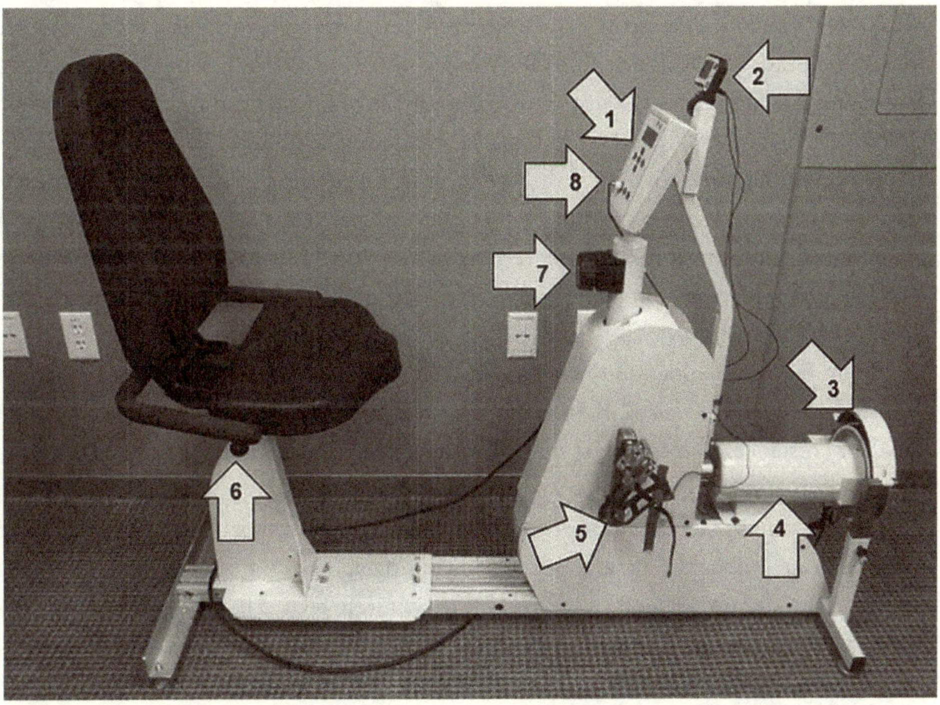

Figure 15.2. Theracycle (Exercycle, Franklin, MA) research model. (1) Time and cadence control panel with time and cadence display, (2) SRM (Schoberer-Rad Messtechnik, Jülich, Germany) Powercontrol V, (3) magnetic resistance belt, (4) electric motor, (5) pedal arm fulcrum (the SRM Powermeter is incorporated in the crank arm located on the other side), (6) lever to adjust seat horizontally, (7) resistance dial, (8) magnetic safety tether. Photograph by Shannon Ringenbach, 2012.

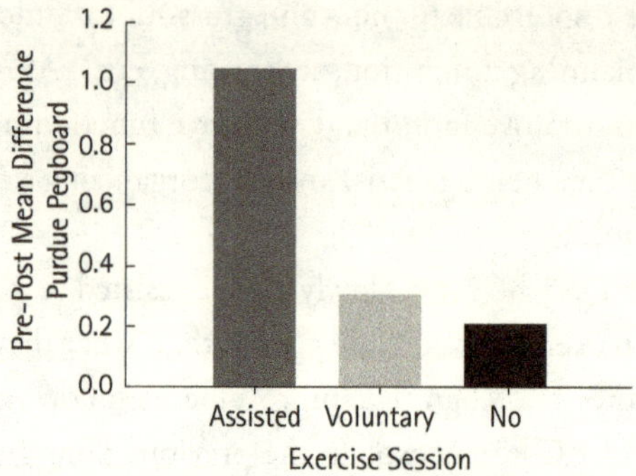

Figure 15.3. Pre-post difference in Purdue Pegboard as a measure of manual dexterity as a function of exercise session in adolescents with DS after acute sessions. From Ringenbach et al. (2014).

fine-motor function following lower extremity gross-motor exercise), one explanation is that ACT leads to changes in neural mechanisms in the brain, which leads to improvements in global motor function. Similarly, after a longer 8-week ACT gross-motor intervention in adolescents with DS, improvements were also found in fine-motor function as measured by the Purdue Pegboard, following ACT but not voluntary cycling or no cycling (Holzapfel et al., 2015). When lower extremity ACT has been found to improve upper extremity motor function, researchers (Ridgel et al., 2009; Ringenbach et al., 2014) reasoned that enhanced fine-motor functioning of the upper extremities following lower extremity exercise would support the hypothesis that ACT is capable of altering central motor processing, as the upper extremities were not exercised. Furthermore, improvements in fine-motor function (i.e., bimanual dexterity) could not be the result of changes in the muscles of the upper extremities or explained by practice effects because both ACT and voluntary cycling groups were exposed to an equal number of practice and test trials. Instead, the improvements may be indicative of biobehavioral/neural changes in the brain.

In an 8-week intervention study with ACT and voluntary cycling with adolescents with DS, Holzapfel et al. (2015) found that improvements in the 6-minute walk test (6MWT) distance, a gross-motor task, correlated positively with improvements in cognitive function, including verbal fluency, short-term memory, and cognitive planning ability. In addition, a positive relationship was found between fine-motor function, as measured by the Purdue Pegboard Test, and cognitive planning ability, as measured by the Tower of London. Thus, improvements in executive function were related to improvements in fine- *and* gross-motor function, suggesting that cognitive function and the execution of motor tasks are closely related in adolescents and adults with DS.

The interrelatedness of motor and cognitive function is also supported by other studies with children with DS. For example Schott and Holfelder (2015) studied 11 boys and 7 girls between the ages of 7 and 11 years old with and without DS on their motor and cognitive abilities. They found that the children with DS demonstrated impaired inhibitory control and set switching as measured by the Trails-P, as well as locomotor and object control skills, as measured by the TGMC-2, compared to age-matched TD children. Furthermore, distraction was found to be significantly related to locomotor and object-control skills. Schott and Holfelder (2015) commented that improvements in both cognitive and motor function may be due to the regions in the brain such as the prefrontal cortex, basal ganglia, and cerebellum that interact and communicate during motor and cognitive functions. This is consistent with the model of improvements in cognitive function following ACT exercise in persons with DS. As can be seen in Figure 15.1, ACT seems to be able to target both motor and cognitive domains simultaneously because the high rate of exercise increases activity in the prefrontal cortex and other brain regions that are important for cognitive function. This was evident in Ringenbach et al.'s (2016) findings of improvements in manual dexterity and 6MWT distance as well as in multiple domains of cognitive function following ACT among adolescents with DS.

Taken together, recent research shows improvements in fine- and gross-motor function in adolescents and older adults with DS following ACT. Furthermore, we suggest that these improvements in motor skills may be a result of rebuilding neural structures in the motor and prefrontal cortex following ACT. The importance of this research is that it is a nonsurgical, nonpharmaceutical approach to improving motor functions in populations who move slowly due to neurological disabilities and has shown promising results in persons with DS.

Rethinking Exercise Interventions

It is abundantly clear from research in infants with DS (Ulrich, Ulrich, Angulo-Kinzler, & Yun, 2001) that early intervention is the most effective strategy for improving fine- and gross-motor function. Furthermore, many traditional, alternative, and exercise therapeutic approaches resulted in improvements in fine- and/or gross-motor function. The connection between motor and cognitive functioning is becoming clear and may be related to specific brain structures in persons with DS. Thus, recent research on the positive influence of motor interventions on cognitive functioning in persons with DS is particularly exciting. While results from exercise interventions are promising in adult populations with neurological conditions, research was previously limited in its scope because the physical characteristics of the exercise equipment/bicycle was built for adults as can be seen in Figure 15.4.

Thus, we believe strongly that, in the future, researchers should rethink how exercise interventions are delivered to persons with DS to examine moderate- to light-intensity exercise interventions at a fast rate in infants and young children with DS. This would provide an early opportunity to rebuild neural connections and gain lifelong motor and

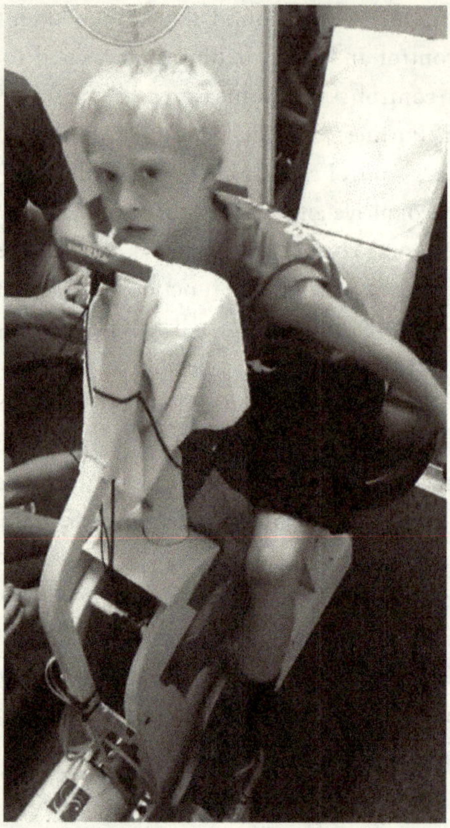

Figure 15.4. Ten-year-old child with DS on Assisted Cycle. Photograph by Shannon Ringenbach, 2012.

cognitive improvements. This is vital because it would ultimately improve their personal and societal functioning, independence, and thus the quality of life throughout their lifespan.

References

Agiovlasitis, S., McCubbin, J. A., Yun, J., Pavol, M. J., & Widrick, J. J. (2009). Economy and preferred speed of walking in adults with and without Down syndrome. *Adapted Physical Activity Quarterly*, *26*(2), 118–130.

Alberts, J. L., Linder, S. M., Penko, A. L., Lowe, M. J., & Phillips, M. (2011). It is not about the bike, it is about the pedaling: Forced exercise and Parkinson's disease. *Exercise and Sport Science Reviews*, *39*(4), 177–186.

Andriolo, R. B., El Dib, R. P., Ramos, L., Atallah, A. N., & da Silva, E. M. (2010). Aerobic exercise training programmes for improving physical and psychosocial health in adults with Down syndrome (Review). *Cochrane Database of Systematic Reviews*, *12*(5), 1–62.

Angulo-Barroso, R., Burghardt, A. R., Lloyd, M., & Ulrich, Dale A. (2008). Physical activity in infants with Down syndrome receiving a treadmill intervention. *Infant Behavior & Development*, *31*(2), 255–269.

Anson, G. J., & Mawston, G. A. (2000). Characteristics of perceptual-motor behavior associated with Down syndrome. In D. Weeks, R. Chua, & D. Elliott (Eds.), *Perceptual-Motor Behavior in Down Syndrome* (pp 1–24). Human Kinetics.

Aruin, A. S., Almedia, G. L., & Latash, M. L. (1996). Organization of a simple two-joint synergy in individuals with Down syndrome. *American Journal of Mental Retardation, 101*, 256–268.

Berman, K. F., Ostrem, J. L., Randoulph, C., Gold, J., Goldberg, T. E., Coppola, R., Carson, R. E., Herscovitch, P., & Weinberger, D. R. (1995). Physiological activation of a cortical network during performance of the Wisconsin Card Sorting Test: A positron emission tomography study. *Neuropsychologia, 33*, 1027–1046.

Bittles, A. H., & Glasson, E. J. (2004). Clinical, social and ethical implications of changing life expectancy in Down syndrome. *Developmental Medicine Child Neurology, 46*, 282–286.

Block, M. E. (1991). Motor development in children with Down syndrome: A review of the literature. *Adapted Physical Activity Quarterly, 8*, 179–209.

Bruni, M. (1998). *Fine motor skills in children with Down syndrome: A guide for parents and professionals.* Woodbine House, Inc.

Carmeli, E., Kessel, S., Coleman, R., & Ayalon, M. (2002). Effects of a treadmill walking program on muscle strength and balance in elderly people with Down syndrome. *Journal of Gerontology, 57*(2), 106–110.

Chang, C.-L., Kubo, M., & Ulrich, B. D. (2009). Emergence of neuromuscular patterns during walking in toddlers with typical development and with Down syndrome. *Human Movement Science, 28*(2), 283–296.

Chen, C.-C., & Ringenbach, S. D. R. (2016). Dose-response relationship between intensity of exercise and cognitive performance in individuals with Down syndrome: A preliminary study. *Journal of Intellectual Disability Research, 60*(6), 606–614.

Chen, C.-C, & Ringenbach, S. D. R. (2019). The effect of acute exercise on the performance of verbal fluency in adolescents and young adults with DS: A pilot study. *Journal of Intellectual Disability Research, 63*(6), 614–623. https://doi.org/10.1111/jir.12603.

Chen, C., Ringenbach, S. D. R., Albert, A., & Semken, K. (2014). Fine motor control is related to cognitive control in adolescents with Down syndrome. *International Journal of Disability, Development and Education, 61*(1), 6–15.

Chen, C.-C., Ringenbach, S. D. R., Crews, D., Kulinna, P. H., & Amazeen, E. L. (2015). The association between a single bout of moderate physical activity and executive function in young adults with Down syndrome: A preliminary study. *Journal of Intellectual Disability Research, 59*, 589–598. https://doi.org/10.1111/jir.12163.

Copetti, F., Mota, C. B., Graup, S., Menezes, K., & Venturini, E. (2007). Angular kinematics of the gait of children with Down's syndrome after intervention with hippotherapy. *Brazilian Journal of Physical Therapy, 11*(6), 503–507.

Courchesne, E., Townsend, J. P., Akshoomoff, N. A., Saitoh, O., Yeung-Courchesne, R., Lincoln, A., James, H., Haas, R. H., Schreibman, L., & Lau, L. (1994). Impairment in shifting attention in autistic and cerebellar patients. *Behavioral Neuroscience, 108*(5), 848–865.

Desmond, J. E., Gabrieli, J. D. E., Wagner, A. D., Ginier, B. I., & Glover, G. H. (1997). Lobular patterns of cerebellar activation in verbal working memory and finger-tapping tasks as revealed by functional MRI. *Journal of Neuroscience, 17*(24), 9675–9685.

Diamond, A. (2000). Close interrelation of motor development and cognitive development and of the cerebellum and prefrontal cortex. *Child Development, 71*(1), 44–56.

Elliott, D., Weeks, D. J., & Elliott, C. L. (1987). Cerebral specialization in individuals with Down syndrome. *American Journal on Mental Retardation, 92*, 263–271.

Frank, K., & Esbensen, A. J. (2015). Fine motor and self-care milestones for individuals with Down syndrome using a retrospective chart review. *Journal of Intellectual Disability Research, 59*(8), 719–729.

Frith, U., & Frith, C. D. (1974). Specific motor disabilities in Downs syndrome. *Journal of Child Psychology and Psychiatry, 15*(4), 293–301.

Giagkoudaki, F., Dimitros, E., Kouidi, E., & Deligiannis, A. (2010). Effects of exercise training on heart rate variability indices in individuals with Down syndrome. *Journal of Sport Rehabilitation, 19*(2), 173–83.

Guidi, S., Bonasoni, P., Ciani, E., & Bartesaghi, R. (2010). Reduced granule cell precursor proliferation in the cerebellum of fetuses with Down syndrome. *International Journal of Developmental Neuroscience, 28*(8), 712.

Hauck, J. L., & Ulrich D. A. (2015). Acute effects of a therapeutic mobility device on physical activity and heart rate in children with Down syndrome. *Research Quarterly for Exercise and Sport, 86*, 260–266.

Henderson, S. E., Morris, J., & Frith, U. (1981). The motor deficit in Down's syndrome children: A problem of timing? *Journal of Child Psychiatry, 22*(3), 233–245.

Heyn, P., Abreu, B. C., & Ottenbacher, K. J. (2004). The effects of exercise training on elderly persons with cognitive impairment and dementia: A meta-analysis. *Archives of Physical Medicine and Rehabilitation, 85*(10), 1694–1704.

Holzapfel, S. D., Ringenbach, S. D. R, Mulvey, G. M., Sandoval-Menendez, A. M., Birchfield, N., & Tahiliani, S. R. (2016). Differential effects of Assisted Cycling Therapy (ACT) on short-term and working memory of adolescents with Down syndrome. *Journal of Cognitive Psychology, 28*(8), 990–1003. https://doi.org/10.1080/20445911.2016.1205592.

Holazpfel, S. D., Ringenbach, S. D. R., Mulvey, G. M., Sandoval-Menendez, A. M., Cook, M. R., Ganger, R. O., & Bennett, K. (2015). Improvements in manual dexterity relate to improvements in cognitive planning after assisted cycling therapy (ACT) in adolescents with Down syndrome. *Research in Developmental Disabilities, 45–46*, 261–270.

Jernigan, T. L., & Bellugi, U. (1990). Anomalous brain morphology on magnetic resonance images in Williams syndrome and Down syndrome. *Archives in Neurology, 47*, 529–533.

Jobling, A., & Cuskelly, M. (2002). *Life styles of adults with Down Syndrome Living at Home*. Whurr Publishers.

Kubo, M., & Ulrich, B. D. (2006). Early stage of walking: Development of control in and anteroposterior directions. *Journal of Motor Behavior, 38*, 229–237.

Lin, H. C., & Wuang, Y. P. (2012). Strength and agility training in adolescents with Down syndrome: A randomized controlled trial. *Research in Developmental Disabilities, 33*(6), 2236–2244.

Looper, J., & Ulrich, D. (2010). Effect of treadmill training and supramalleolar orthosis use on motor skill development in infants with Down syndrome: A randomized clinical trial. *Physical Therapy, 90*(3), 382–390.

Maraj, B. K. V., Bonertz, C. M., Kivi, J. J., Furler, B. L., Ringenbach, S. D., Mulvey, G. M. (2007). Cerebral specialization in individuals with Down syndrome: The ongoing development of a model. *Down Syndrome Quarterly, 9*, 7–16.

Maraj, B. K. V., Robertson, S. D., Welsh, T. N., Weeks, D. J., Chua, R., Heath, M., Roy, E. A., Simon, D. A., Weinberg, H., & Elliott, D. (2002). Verbal-motor behaviour in persons with Down syndrome. In M. Cuskelly, A. Jobling, & S. Buckley (Eds.), *Down syndrome across the life span* (pp. 175–193). Whurr Publishers Ltd.

Marchal, J. P., Maurice-Stam, H., Houtzager, B. A., van Rozenburg-Marres, S. L. R., Oostrom, K. J., Grootenhuis, M. A., & van Trotsenburg, A. P. (2016). Growing up with Down syndrome: Development from 6 months to 10.7 years. *Research in Developmental Disabilities, 59*, 437–450.

Nakano-Kobayashi, A., Awaya, T., Kii, I., Sumida, Y., Okuno, Y., Yoshida, S., Sumida, T., Inoue, H., Hosoya, T., Hagiwara, M., (2017*).* Prenatal neurogenesis induction therapy normalizes brain straucture and function in Down syndronme mice. *Proceedings of the National Academy of Sciences of the United States of America, 114*(38), 10268–10273.

O'Brien, J., Ottoboni, G., Tessari, A., & Setti, A. (2017). One bout of open skill exercise improves crossmodal perception and immediate memory in healthy older adults who habitually exercise, *PLoS ONE, 12*(6), 1–16.

Palisano, R. J., Walter, S. D., Russell, D. J., Rosenbaum, P. L., Gémus, M., Galuppi, B. E., & Cunningham, L. (2001). Gross motor function of children with down syndrome: Creation of motor growth curves. *Archives of Physical Medicine and Rehabilitation, 82*(4), 494–500.

Pastore, E., Marino, B., Calzolari, A., Digilio, C. M., Giannotti, A., & Turchetta, A. (2000). Clinical and cardiorespiratory assessment in children with Down syndrome without congenital heart disease. *Archives of Pediatric Adolescent Medicine, 154*(4), 408–410.

Penedo, F. J., & Dahn, J. R. (2005). Exercise and well-being: A review of mental and physical health benefits associated with physical activity. *Current Opinions in Psychiatry, 8*(2), 189–193.

Petzinger, G. M., Fisher, B. E., Van Leeuwen, J. E., Vukovic, M., Akopian, G., Meshul, C. K., Holschneider, D. P., Nacca, A., Walsh, J. P., Jakowec, M. W. (2010). Enhancing neuroplasticity in the basal ganglia: The role of exercise in parkinson's disease. Movement Disord*ers*, 25(1), S141–S145.

Piek, J., Dawson, L., Smith, L. M., & Gasson, N. (2008). The role of early fine and gross motor development on later motor and cognitive ability. *Human Movement Science, 27*(5), 668–681.

Pitetti, K. H., Climstein, M., Campbell, K. D., & Barrett, P. J. (1992). The cardiovascular capacities of adults with Down syndrome: A comparative study. *Medicine in Science and Sports Exercise, 24*(1), 13–19.

Pontifex, M. B., Saliba, B. J., Raine, L. B., Picchietti, D. L., Hillman, C. H. (2013). Exercise improves behavioral, neurocognitive, and scholastic performance in children with attention-deficit/hyperactivity disorder. *The Journal of Pediatrics, 162*(3), 543–551.

Ridgel, A. L., Vitek, J. L., & Alberts, J. L. (2009). Forced, not voluntary, exercise improves motor function in Parkinson's disease patients. *Neurorehabiltation and Neural Repair, 23*, 600–608.

Rigoldi, C., Galli, M., & Albertini, G. (2011). Gait development during lifespan in subjects with Down syndrome. *Research in Developmental Disabilities, 32*(1), 158–163.

Rimmer, J. H., Heller, T., Wang, E., & Valerio, I. (2004). Improvements in physical fitness in adults with Down syndrome. *American Journal of Mental Retardation, 109*(2), 165–174.

Ringenbach, S. D. R., Albert, A. R., Chen, C. C., & Alberts, J. L. (2014). Acute bouts of assisted cycling improves cognitive and upper extremity movement functions in adolescents with down syndrome. *Intellectual and Developmental Disabilities, 52*(2), 124–135.

Ringenbach, S., Arnold, N., Myer, B., Hayes, C., Nam, K., & Chen, C. C. (2021). Executive function improves following acute exercise in adults with Down syndrome. Brain Sciences, 11(5), 620. https://doi.org/10.3390/brainsci11050620.

Ringenbach, S. D. R., Beachy, C., & Mulvey, G. M. (2007). Persons with Down syndrome use similar strategies when using visual instructions for bimanual drumming. *Journal of Intellectual Disability Research, 51*, 953–961.

Ringenbach, S. D. R., Chen, C. C., Mulvey, G. M., & Jung, M. L. (2012). Unimanual and bimanual continuous movements benefit from visual instructions in persons with Down syndrome. *Journal of Motor Behavior, 44*(4), 233–239.

Ringenbach, S. D. R., Holzapfel, S. D., Arnold, N. E., Nam, K., Lopez, C., Chen, C.-C., Buman, M. P., Youngstedt, S. D., Teslevich, J., & Wallace, K. C. (2019). Assisted Cycling Therapy (ACT) improves adaptive behaviors in adolescents with Down syndrome. *Journal of Developmental and Physical Disabilities*, 32, 535–552. https://doi.org/10.1007/s10882-019-09706-z.

Ringenbach, S. D. R., Holzapfel, S. D., Mulvey, G. M., Richter, M., Jimenez, A., & Benson, A. (2016). The effects of Assisted Cycling Therapy (ACT) and voluntary cycling on reaction time and measures of executive function in adolescents with Down syndrome. *Journal of Intellectual Disability Research, 60*(11), 1073–1085.

Ringenbach, S. D. R., Mulvey, G. M., Van Gemmert, A. W. A., Stankus, A., & Maraj, B. K. V. (2009). Sensory feedback is beneficial for performance of continuous bimanual tasks for adults with Down syndrome. *Down Syndrome Quarterly, 11*, 3–9.

Ringenbach, S. D. R., Chen, C. C., Albert, A. R., Lichtsinn, K., & Alberts, J. L. (2013). Assisted Cycle Therapy (ACT): Implications for improvements in motor control. In M. Leitner & M. Fuchs (Eds.), *Motor behavior and control: New research* (pp. 103–114). Nova Science Publishers Inc.

Savelsbergh, G., van der Kamp, J., Ledebt, A., & Planinsek, T. (2000). Information-movement coupling in children with Down syndrome. In D. J. Weeks, R. Chua, & D. Elliott (Eds.), *Perceptual-motor behavior in Down syndrome* (pp. 251–271). Human Kinetics.

Schall, J. D. (2003). Neural correlates of decision processes: Neural and mental chronometry. *Current Opinion in Neurobiology, 13*(2), 182–186.

Schott, N., & Holfelder, B. (2015). Relationship between motor skill competency and executive function in children with Down's syndrome. *Journal of Intellectual Disability Research, 59*, 860–872.

Shields, N., Taylor, N. F., & Dodd, K. J. (2008). Effects of a community-based progressive resistance training program on muscle performance and physical function in adults with Down syndrome: A randomized controlled trial. *Archives Physical Medicine and Rehabilitation, 89*(7), 1215–1220.

Shields, N., Taylor, N., Wee, E., Wollersheim, D., O'Shea, S. D., Fernhall, B. (2013). A community-based strength straining programme increases muscle strength and physical activity in young people with Down syndrome: A randomized control trial. *Research in Developmental Disabilities, 34*(12), 4385–4394.

Silva, V., Campos, C., Sá, A., Cavadas, M., Pinto, J., Simões, P., Machado, S., Murillo-Rodriguez, E., & Barbosa-Rocha, N. (2017). Wii-based exercise program to improve physical fitness, motor proficiency and functional mobility in adults with Down syndrome. *Journal of Intellectual Disability Research, 61*(8), 755–765.

Smith, B. A., Kubo, M., Black, D. P., Holt, K. G., & Ulrich, B. D. (2007). Effect of practice on a novel task—walking on a treadmill: preadolescents with and without Down syndrome. *Physical Therapy, 87*, 766–777.

Smith, B. A., & Ulrich, B. D. (2008). Early onset of stabilizing strategies for gait and obstacles: Older adults with Down syndrome. *Gait & Posture, 28*(3), 448–455.

Spano, M., Mercuri, E., Rando, T., Panto, T., Gagliano, A., Henderson, S., & Guzzeta, F. (1999). Motor and perceptual-motor competence in children with Down syndrome: Variation in performance with age. *European Journal of Paediatric Neurology, 3*, 7–14.

Ulrich, D. A., Burghardt, A. R., Lloyd, M., Tiernan, C., & Hornyak, J. E. (2011). Physical activity benefits of learning to ride a two-wheel bicycle for children with Down syndrome: A randomized trial. *Physical Therapy, 91*(10), 1463–1473.

Ulrich, B. D., Haehl, V., Buzzi, U. H., Kubo, M., & Holt, K. G. (2004). Modeling dynamic resource utilization in populations with unique constraints: Preadolescents with and without Down syndrome. *Human Movement Science, 23*, 133–156.

Ulrich, D., Lloyd, M., Tiernan, C., Looper, J., & Angulo-Barroso, R. (2008). Effects of intensity of treadmill training on developmental outcomes and stepping in infants with Down syndrome: A randomized trial. *Physical Therapy, 88*(1), 114–22.

Ulrich, D. A., Ulrich, B. D., Angulo-Kinzler, R. M., & Yun, J. (2001). Treadmill training of infants with Down syndrome: Evidence-based developmental outcomes. *Pediatrics, 108*(5), 853–858.

Vimercati, S. L., Galli, M., Rigoldi, C., & Albertini, G. (2013). Obstacle avoidance in Down syndrome. *Journal of Electromyography and Kinesiology, 23*(2), 483–489.

Virji-Babul, N., & Brown, M. (2004). Stepping over obstacles: Anticipatory modifications in children with and without Down syndrome. *Experimental Brain Research, 159*(4), 487–490.

Weeks, D. J., Chua, R., & Elliott, D. (2000). *Perceptual-motor behavior in Down syndrome.* Human Kinetics.

Weiss, E. M., Siedentopf, C., Hofer, A., Deisenhammer, E. A., Hoptman, M. J., Kremser, C., Golaszewski, S., Felber, S., Fleischhacker, W. W., & Delazer, M. (2003). Brain activation pattern during a verbal fluency test in healthy male and female volunteers: a functional magnetic resonance imaging study. *Neuroscience Letters, 352*(3), 191–194.

Winders P. C. (1997). *Gross motor skills in children with Down syndrome.* Woodbine House.

Wuang, Y., Chiang, C., Su, C., & Wang, C. (2011). Effectiveness of virtual reality using Wii gaming technology in children with Down syndrome. *Research in Developmental Disabilities, 32*(1), 312–321.

Yanagisawa, H., Dan, I., Tsuzuki, D., Kato, M., Okamoto, M., Kyutoku, Y., & Soya, H. (2010). Acute moderate exercise elicits increased dorsolateral prefrontal activation and improves cognitive performance with Stroop test. *NeuroImage, 50*(4), 1702–1710.

SECTION 4

Comorbid Conditions

CHAPTER 16

Brain Aging and Alzheimer's Disease in Down Syndrome

Alex Helman, Kathryn Van Pelt, Frederick A. Schmitt, *and* Elizabeth Head

Abstract

People with Down syndrome (DS) are vulnerable to Alzheimer disease (AD), particularly over the age of 40 years due to the extra copy of chromosome 21 in the most common form of DS. Despite the prevalence of AD in people with DS, there are few clinical trials for people with DS. This gap highlights that persons with DS comprise an underserved, vulnerable population who develop AD neuropathology at an early age. This article reviews AD neuropathology in persons with DS and key genes associated with DS that are also thought to play a role in AD development. The potential roles of inflammation, cerebrovascular pathology, and white matter changes are also reviewed. Gaps in our understanding of AD in persons with DS and promising areas of investigation are identified. It will be critical to better understand the age-dependency of AD- associated events in persons with DS to identify novel targets for intervention and to determine the ages at which these pathways may be most modifiable.

Key Words: beta-amyloid, cerebrovascular pathology, chromosome 21 genes, neurofibrillary tangles, neuroinflammation, white matter integrity

Introduction

As improvements in medical technology continue, the life expectancy of people with Down Syndrome (DS) continues to increase. In 1929, a diagnosis of DS was associated with a life expectancy of around 9 years. However, people with DS are now living longer lives, with an average life span of about 60 years of age (Bittles & Glasson, 2004). As with the general population, the risk of developing health-related problems increases as people with DS get older (Bayen, Possin, Chen, Cleret de Langavant, & Yaffe, 2018). In particular, people with DS are at high risk of developing cognitive impairment and dementia associated with Alzheimer disease (AD) after the age of 50 years (Zigman, 2013; Zigman, Schupf, Sersen, & Silverman, 1996).

What Are Dementia and Alzheimer Disease?

Dementia is a term used to describe changes in cognition that affect daily function. There are many biological causes of dementia (i.e., the pathology that causes the dementia can vary), including vascular dementia, frontotemporal dementia, Lewy body disease, and, most commonly, Alzheimer disease (AD ; Plassman et al., 2007). The risk of AD rises with age, as 2% of people between 71 and 79 years are diagnosed with AD, 18% of those between 80 and 89 years, and 28% of people over 90 years (Plassman et al., 2007). There is a critical need to be able to diagnose people earlier in the disease process, prior to signs of significant cognitive change, as there are more opportunities (based on future clinical trials) to intervene with the most benefit. Consequently, the field has moved to the discussion of modifying the criteria for a clinical diagnosis of AD to primarily depend on biomarkers that can be obtained noninvasively. These biomarkers include the pathological accumulation of senile plaques and neurofibrillary tangles (NFT) in the brain as detected by cerebrospinal fluid (CSF) protein levels and/or neuroimaging using positron emission tomography (PET) that may show AD-associated changes prior to a person meeting criteria for a diagnosis of mild cognitive impairment or dementia (Jack et al., 2018). Ultimately, AD can only be confirmed at autopsy with neuropathological evidence of the presence of NFT, senile plaques (Aβ, which will be described), and neuron loss.

The first type of AD pathology that we see in the brain at autopsy are NFTs. NFTs are made up of a protein that has an important role in supporting the structure, forming a cytoskeleton, and assisting in the transport of proteins and organelles within the cell body and axons of neurons in the brain (Gao et al., 2018). In AD, this tau protein becomes abnormally hyperphosphorylated — in other words, lots of phosphate groups are added to the protein, and it leads to a twisting of the protein into paired helical filaments that disrupt normal neuronal function (Gendron & Petrucelli, 2009). These filaments fill the neuron and form NFT and neuropil threads (Fig. 16.1a).

The second type of AD pathology is senile plaques. Senile plaques are deposits of a toxic protein, beta-amyloid (Aβ), which aggregate outside and between neurons (Selkoe, 2001) (Fig. 16.1b). The Aβ protein can be of various lengths but typically is 40– 42 amino acids long and is cut from a longer beta-amyloid precursor protein (APP, which will be discussed in more detail shortly). The gene for APP is on chromosome 21, which leads to overexpression in people with full trisomy 21 because of the extra copy of the gene; this is thought to be the underlying mechanism for early onset AD in persons with DS (Doran et al., 2017; Prasher et al., 1998). Senile plaques can vary in size and appearance. Typically, plaques first form as diffuse fibrils that can be large and amorphous (Fig. 16.1c). Senile plaques can also take on a more compact form, with some having a dense core and associated NFT pathology. These smaller, denser plaques, which are called neuritic plaques or cored plaques (Fig. 16.1d), are typically observed in more severe stages of AD in persons with DS. When sufficient numbers of NFTs and senile plaques are observed affecting the hippocampus, underlying entorhinal cortex, and neocortex, a diagnosis of AD can be made.

Linking the breadth of AD pathology in the brain with the severity of dementia a person exhibits prior to death helps researchers test hypotheses about what types of brain

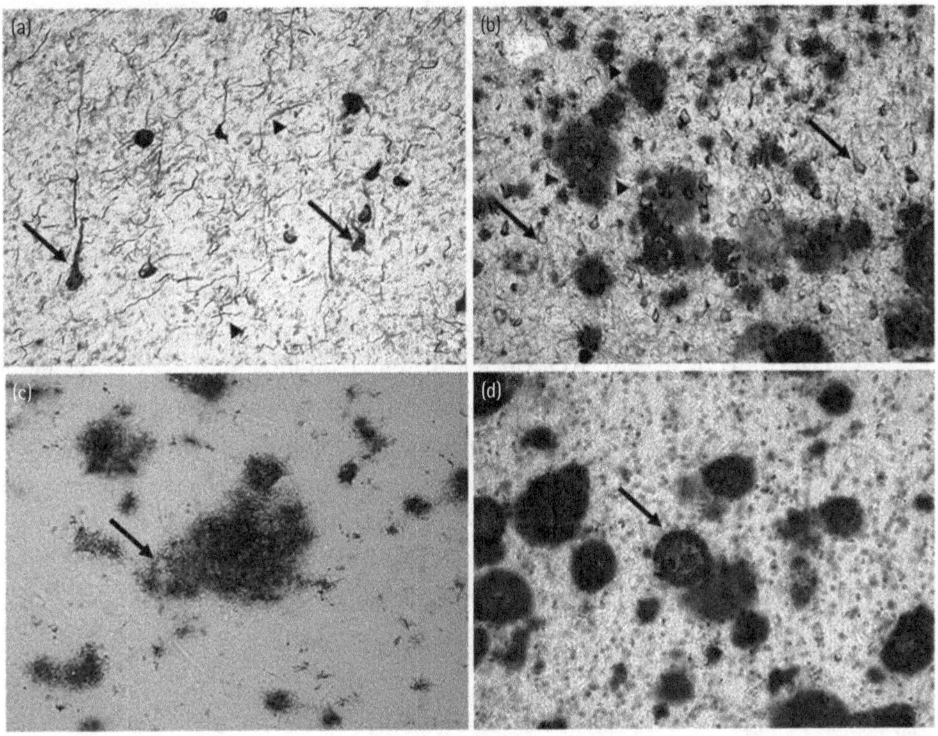

Figure 16.1. AD senile plaques and neurofibrillary tangles in persons with DS
(a) Neurofibrillary tangles (PHF-1 immunostaining; arrows) and neuropil threads (arrowheads) can be observed in the frontal cortex of a 46-year- old female with DS . (b) Aβ plaques (deposits—immunohistochemistry using an anti-Aβ42 antibody; arrowheads) are present in the space between neurons and neurofibrillary tangle bearing neurons (using anti-PHF-1 immunohistochemistry; arrows) in the frontal cortex of a 46-year- old female with DS. (c) Diffuse plaques are large amorphous deposits of Aβ that can show "holes" (immunohistochemistry with anti-Aβ42 antibody; arrow) where intact neurons can be found in a 48-year- old female with DS . (d) Compact or dense core (anti-Aβ42 antibody; arrow) Aβ plaques are observed in the frontal cortex of a 54-year old female with DS .

pathology might underlie specific cognitive deficits in people with AD. In the most commonly used scoring system, Braak staging, the severity and location of NFT and senile plaques are described, with higher "stages" being associated with more severe pathology (Braak & Braak, 1991). NFT pathology is scored on a scale of I–VI and senile plaques are scored as A, B, or C. Thal et al. (2002) have expanded the staging system for describing the extent and severity of senile plaques to 5 categories (phases 1– 5; Thal, Rub, Orantes, & Braak, 2002). Thus, a typical report from a neuropathologist will include information regarding the final diagnosis as well as the extent of senile plaques and NFTs.

AD Neuropathology in Persons With DS

AD pathology occurs in the brains of people with DS but at younger ages than typically observed in the non-DS population. Virtually all adults with DS develop the neuropathology for an AD diagnosis (Aβ and NFT) by the age of 40 years (Mann & Esiri, 1989;

Wisniewski, Howe, Williams, & Wisniewski, 1978; Wisniewski, Wisniewski, & Wen, 1985). However, most people with DS do not show signs of dementia until almost a decade later in their 50s. The mean age of diagnosis of dementia in people with DS (based upon a study of 839 people) was 55.8 years (Sinai et al., 2018). However, some adults with DS never develop clinical dementia although AD pathology is exhibited in their brains (Franceschi, Comola, Piattoni, Gualandri, & Canal, 1990; Head, Powell, Gold, & Schmitt, 2012; Head, Silverman, Patterson, & Lott, 2012; Schupf & Sergievsky, 2002), suggesting that certain factors (environmental or genetic) may modify age of onset, and may be protective, which could serve as targets for intervention.

As in late onset or sporadic AD(which is the most common form of dementia in the non-DS elderly population), Aβ and NFTs accumulate in the brain, but what is unique to people with DS is that it is strongly age-dependent (Fig. 16.2). In the general population, the age of onset of AD can vary widely—from 60 to 100 years. In contrast, in people with DS, a progressive accumulation of AD pathology begins in their 30s (Mann, 1988; Mann & Esiri, 1989; Wisniewski et al., 1985). Thus, based on the age of a person with DS we can make reasonable estimates of the extent of AD pathology in their brains.

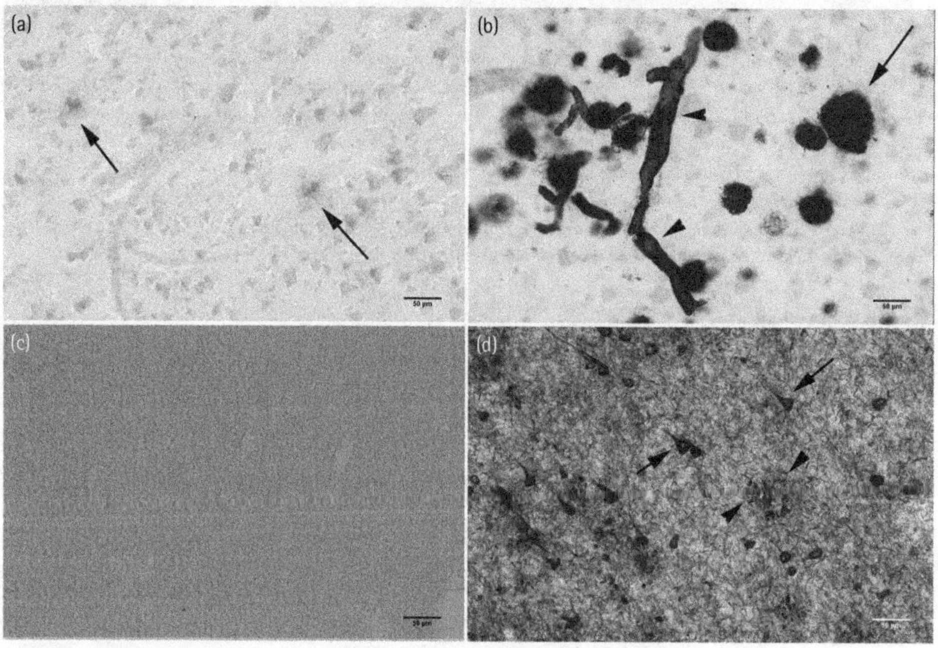

Figure 16.2. AD pathology increases with age in persons with DS
Immunoreactivity for Aβ (6E10) in the posterior cingulate cortex of **(a)** a young individual with DS (age = 39) with diffuse amyloid plaques (arrows) and **(b)** an individual with DSAD (age = 51) with amyloid plaques (arrows) and CAA (arrowheads). Tau pathology (AT8) also increases with age, as shown in the posterior cingulate cortex of **(c)** a young individual with DS (age = 25) and **(d)** an individual with DSAD (age = 51) with neuronal AT8 labeling (arrows) and neuropil AT8 labeling (arrowheads).

Although Braak and Thal staging of Aβ and NFTs are essential in evaluating AD severity and progression, this approach has not been systematically conducted in large numbers of brains from people with DS. Staging requires that multiple brain regions are available for assessment, but acquiring autopsy cases from people with DS is challenging, thereby limiting our numbers for systematic analyses. Although it is possible that AD neuropathology may develop and progress differently among individuals with DS as compared to those with sporadic AD, there is little evidence to support this. Indeed, in a recent study based on brains from 56 people with DS ranging in age from 0.1 to 76 years at death, Davidson and colleagues observed a similar pattern of NFT pathology as reported in sporadic AD (Davidson, Robinson, Prasher, & Mann, 2018). A systematic characterization of Aβ accumulation will also be helpful and represents a gap in our knowledge of how senile plaques spread in the brains of people with DS. Noninvasive *in vivo* imaging of Aβ and NFT by PET will significantly advance our understanding of AD progression and clinical correlations in people with DS.

Genetics of Senile Plaques in Persons With DS

Several genes associated with an increased risk of AD are located on chromosome 21. The most well studied of these is APP, which, when cleaved to Aβ, is implicated as a possible cause of AD in the general population (Hardy, 2006). APP is present in healthy neurons, but in persons with DS, its overexpression (the increased amounts of this protein that are being produced) leads to more production and, thus, accumulation of Aβ. Chromosome 21-related overexpression is thought to overwhelm the ability of neurons to clear excess APP (Mann & Esiri, 1989), and evidence from partial trisomy cases suggests that overexpression of APP is critical to the development of AD neuropathology among persons with DS (Doran et al., 2017; Prasher et al., 1998).

APP is processed and cleared within neurons in various ways, but the crucial processing step for the development of AD occurs at the cell surface. It is here that APP is either cleaved by enzymes, preventing the production of Aβ (Sisodia, 1992), or is cleaved to form Aβ (Fig. 16.3). The pathway that leads to the production of toxic Aβ from APP (amyloidogenic pathway) involves an initial cleavage by an enzyme, β-secretase (Nunan & Small, 2000; Selkoe, 1994), now identified as beta-amyloid cleaving enzyme 1 (BACE1 ; Vassar et al., 1999). This process is followed by an additional cleavage by another enzyme, γ-secretase (Nunan & Small, 2000; Selkoe, 1994), generating an APP intracellular domain (AICD) fragment along with Aβ (Multhaup, Huber, Buee, & Galas, 2015). In cases of familial AD (where affected people have a genetic mutation in one of several possible genes that leads to early- onset AD) and DS, Aβ accumulates throughout affected individuals' lifetimes, which causes AD pathology to develop earlier than in the sporadic AD population (Cohen et al., 2018). However, unlike familial AD, the accumulation of Aβ among persons with DS is caused by an overexpression of APP as a result of chromosome 21 triplication rather than a mutation in the gene itself (Wiseman et al., 2015).

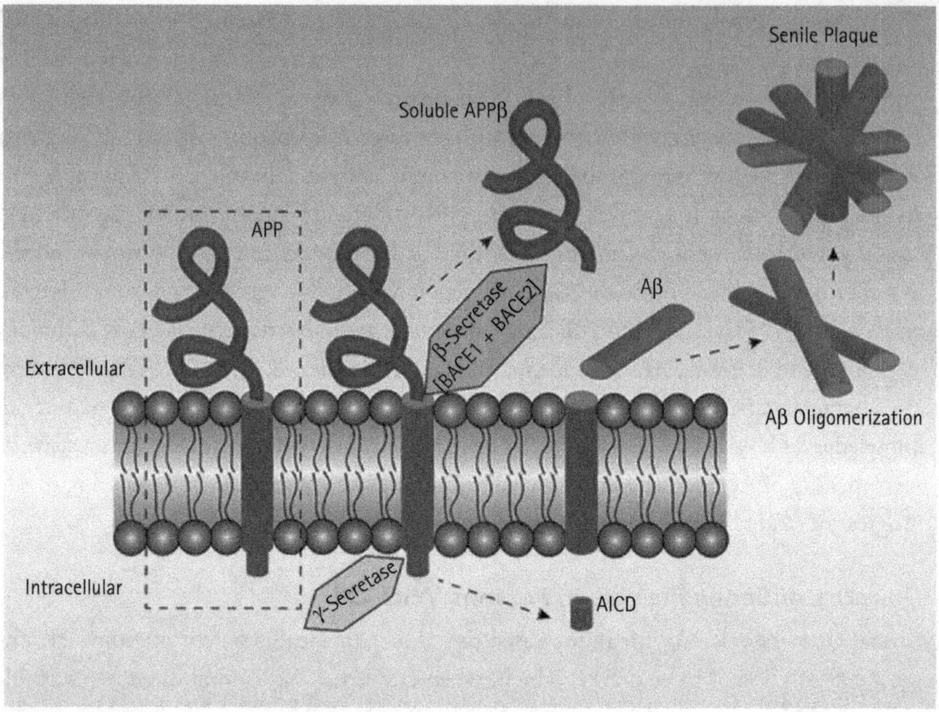

Figure 16.3. Senile Plaques, Aβ, and APP
APP is overexpressed due to triplication of chromosome 21 in persons with DS. The overexpression generates an abundance of APP that can be cleaved into Aβ. APP is cleaved by β-secretase and γ-secretase to create Aβ. Aβ will accumulate into oligomers and finally into senile plaques.

Overexpression of APP and subsequent production of the smaller Aβ protein is first caused by the actions of an enzyme called BACE1 (Vassar, 2004). Even in the presence of APP overexpression, BACE1 must be available to convert APP into Aβ (Vassar, 2004). Thus, the initial APP cleavage by BACE1 is thought to be the rate-limiting step in Aβ production. In sporadic AD, both BACE1 protein levels and enzymatic activity increase in regions where Aβ deposition occurs (Fukumoto, Cheung, Hyman, & Irizarry, 2002; Yang et al., 2003). The positive association between elevated BACE1, enzymatic activity, and Aβ deposition indicated BACE1 as a possible mechanism. Notably, for individuals with DS, BACE1 activity increases at a more rapid rate with age as compared to non-DS populations (Nistor et al., 2007). However, while BACE1 activity was higher among individuals with DS, no association was found between BACE1 activity and Aβ plaque burden (Nistor et al., 2007). Thus, the overexpression of APP, possibly in combination with higher BACE1 activity with age, is likely driving the early and rapid accumulation of Aβ in persons with DS.

In addition to BACE1, BACE2 may also play a role in the development of AD in persons with DS. BACE2 is a protein with a highly similar amino acid sequence (homology) to BACE1, and the gene for BACE2 is located on chromosome 21 (Acquati et al., 2000; Webb & Murphy, 2012). Initially, as BACE2 appears homologous to BACE1 it was thought to have a similar function in cleaving APP. Indeed, BACE2 can cleave APP (Farzan et al., 2000) and could play a role in Aβ production. However, despite an increase in BACE2 mRNA levels in persons with DS (Holler et al., 2012) due to the extra copy of chromosome 21, BACE2 does not appear to contribute significantly to the overproduction of Aβ in persons with DS (Barbiero et al., 2003; Cheon, Dierssen, Kim, & Lubec, 2008). Additionally, several groups of researchers have reported that BACE2 cleaves in the middle of the Aβ domain, causing a reduction in the amount of Aβ (Fluhrer et al., 2002; Sun, He, & Song, 2006). As BACE2's role in Aβ deposition in DS and AD is relatively unclear, further mechanistic studies on BACE2 and APP would be helpful. While both BACE1 and BACE2 have the potential to initiate Aβ production, BACE1 appears to be the primary driver of Aβ production in the AD (Ahmed et al., 2010) and DS brain. Therefore, while the potential for Aβ accumulation might be greater in DS patients due to the over expression of APP and increased BACE1 activity, plaque burden may be due not just to increased accumulation, but possibly also to changes in clearance and degradation mechanisms. Future research is needed to assess these possible mechanisms leading to Aβ accumulation in persons with DS.

Accumulation of Senile Plaques in the Brains of People With DS—When and Where

One of the earliest signs of accumulation of Aβ is in the form of diffuse senile plaques, which tend to systematically accumulate over the age of 30 years (Mann & Esiri, 1989; Figs. 16.1 and 16.2a, b), although some diffuse plaques are found in younger individuals. In an autopsy study of 29 people with DS ranging in age from 3 to 73 years old, plaques appeared earliest at age 12 years in the temporal cortex and were present in about half of the people under the age of 30 years (Lemere et al., 1996). Of note, the people with DS included in this study had been living in an institutionalized setting and are not typical of people with DS in today's society. In a second study, senile plaques were observed in a person with DS who was 8 years old (Leverenz & Raskind, 1998). The precise pattern of where and how Aβ accumulates is not fully understood among persons with DS, although Aβ first appears to accumulate in clusters, starting in the outer layers of the entorhinal and frontal cortices. For example, Azizeh et al. (2000) found that, as individuals with DS age, senile plaques spread into deeper cortical layers closer to the white matter (Azizeh et al., 2000). Similar to sporadic AD, the longer more toxic type of $Aβ_{42}$ (42 amino acids long) is the most prevalent form and appears in the cortex before the deposition of $Aβ_{40}$ (40 amino acids long—less toxic) is evident (Iwatsubo, Mann, Odaka, Suzuki, & Ihara, 1995). It is useful to determine where in the brain we see the first accumulation of Aβ, as it may provide us with clues as to which cognitive or behavioral signs we may see evolve first as a person may develop dementia. For example, Aβ appears to deposit in the cortex first, and in particular within the frontal cortex (Azizeh et al., 2000) with autopsy studies, which may suggest that executive dysfunction or behavioral changes such as apathy may be early signs of AD development in the brain.

In addition to measuring Aβ in the brain, we can also measure this protein in the blood. Peripheral changes in plasma Aβ may reflect the presence of plaques in sporadic AD (Mayeux et al., 2003). Individuals with sporadic AD have significantly higher $A\beta_{42}$, but not $A\beta_{40}$, levels in plasma during early stages of AD, but these levels decline thereafter as senile plaque pathology increases in the brain (Mayeux et al., 2003). In persons with DS, both $A\beta_{40}$ and $A\beta_{42}$ are elevated in the plasma (Mehta et al., 1998), but these levels are even higher in those individuals who develop dementia (Cavani et al., 2000; Schupf et al., 2001).

Visualizing Senile Plaques in the Brain in Living People

With the exciting development of positron emission tomography (PET) using ligands that bind to Aβ in vivo, more has been learned about the age of onset and clinical correlations of Aβ accumulation in the brain among persons with DS. The first of these ligands, Pittsburgh Compound B (PiB), was a breakthrough in the AD field (Cohen & Klunk, 2014). Autopsy studies of PiB binding reveal an affinity of PiB for senile plaques in DS (LeVine et al., 2017). PiB binding, representing Aβ accumulation in senile plaques, becomes evident around the age of 40 years in people with DS (notably much later than seen in autopsy studies), usually beginning in the striatum (Handen et al., 2012; Hartley et al., 2014; Lao et al., 2016, 2017). In DS, following PiB binding in the striatum, binding begins to appear in the rostral prefrontal-cingulo-parietal regions, then caudal frontal, rostral temporal, primary sensorimotor and occipital, and finally mediotemporal regions and the rest of the basal ganglia (Annus et al., 2016). This initial pattern of striatal PiB binding replicates what is seen in familial AD (Koivunen et al., 2008), but once Aβ pathology has appeared, Aβ pathology follows similar patterns of deposition to sporadic AD (Klunk et al., 2004). Notably, PiB binding is observed in people with DS who are not demented, suggesting a preclinical phase of the disease (Hartley et al., 2014; Lao et al., 2016). Striatal Aβ observed with PiB PET scans runs counter to observations in autopsy studies and it will be interesting to observe in future studies what clinical signs may correspond to pathology in this brain region. For example, we may predict that changes in motor function or gait may also be an early sign of AD pathology in people with DS (Anderson-Mooney, Schmitt, Head, Lott, & Heilman, 2016).

Aβ is critically involved with AD pathogenesis in persons with DS. The strongest evidence for this is from case studies of people with DS who were partially trisomic for chromosome 21, where only a piece of the chromosome was triplicated. Prasher et al. (1998) describe a 78-year old woman with DS who showed no signs of dementia and also no evidence for AD neuropathology who was later determined to be partial trisomy, and the APP gene was present in duplicate (Prasher et al., 1998). Similarly, Doran et al.

(2017) described a 72-year old man with partial trisomy who did not develop dementia for a 7-year period. He was negative for PiB binding and, at autopsy, showed typical aging and low levels of AD neuropathology (Doran et al., 2017). This person also had only two copies of the APP gene as opposed to that seen in full trisomy, suggesting that APP triplication is a critical step in early onset AD in persons with DS.

Genetics of Neurofibrillary Tangles in Persons With DS

Similar to sporadic AD, individuals with DS develop NFTs in addition to Aβ deposition (Burger & Vogel, 1973; Figs. 16.1 and 16.2c, d). NFTs accumulate in a similar pattern as in sporadic AD, in that they appear after plaques, with most NFT deposition occurring in the hippocampus, entorhinal cortex, and neocortex (Davidson et al., 2018; Hof et al., 1995; Hyman et al., 1995). The presence of hyperphosphorylated tau leads to NFTs, which eventually leads to neuronal death in vulnerable brain regions (Dickson, 2004; Wegiel et al., 2008). In sporadic AD, neuron loss in the superior temporal sulcus correlates with the number of NFTs (Gomez-Isla et al., 1997), indicating that NFT burden may contribute to neuron loss. Additionally, entorhinal cortical volume was 42% smaller in the brains of older people with DS as compared to the typically developing age-matched comparison group, and the older people with DS had 90% fewer neurons free of NFTs (Sadowski et al., 1999). Thus, NFTs may represent a significant cause of neuronal degeneration in aging and AD in people with DS. Any neuronal loss is concerning for those with DS, as a reduction in neurons would diminish an individual's neuronal and cognitive reserve, increasing susceptibility to AD.

Among persons with DS, NFTs clearly develop after the deposition of Aβ, which suggests that Aβ may drive the accumulation of NFTs (Davidson et al., 2018), as observed in mouse models of AD that deposit plaques and tangles (Oddo et al., 2008). As these events occur at an earlier age in people with DS, executive function and memory are compromised early during the development of AD in persons with DS. Further, the accumulation of NFTs may occur at an earlier age and faster rate in persons with DS because of overexpression of Dyrk1A and RCAN1, two genes on chromosome 21 (Guimera et al., 1996; Jung et al., 2011; Korenberg et al., 1990; Rahmani et al., 1989; Shindoh et al., 1996; Song et al., 1996).

Dyrk1A regulates a wide variety of neurodevelopmental processes (Tejedor & Hammerle, 2011). Dyrk1A is expressed in neurons across an individual's lifetime, including fetal development, suggesting that it plays an important role in neuron development, maturation, and aging (Wegiel et al., 2004). Among persons with DS, Dyrk1A is expressed at 1.5-fold higher protein (consistent with the extra copy of chromosome 21) and shows higher activity levels in the brain (Ferrer et al., 2005; Guimera, Casas, Estivill, & Pritchard, 1999; Kimura et al., 2007). Its overexpression and increased activity have significant implications for brain development, including dysregulation in the differentiation of neuronal progenitor cells (Tejedor & Hammerle, 2011). This, in turn, may lead to learning and cognitive deficits and motor skill impairments that are often seen in people with DS, as exemplified by both DYRK1A overexpressing mice and NFAT knockout mice (Ahn et al., 2006; Altafaj et al., 2001, 2008; Arron et al., 2006; Martinez de Lagran et al., 2004). Dyrk1A acts in synergy with another gene on chromosome 21, RCAN1, to impact some phenotypic characteristics of DS, including the development of AD pathology, specifically hyperphosphorylated tau (Jung et al., 2011).

The DYRK1A gene plays a major role in driving NFT pathogenesis in persons with DS (Ryoo et al., 2007; Wegiel et al., 2008, 2011). Dyrk1A directly and indirectly plays a key role in aging in people with DS through phosphorylation of tau. Directly, Dyrk1A phosphorylates tau at Thr212 and several other sites, which promotes tau to be further phosphorylated by another enzyme GSK-3β (which is not on chromosome 21; Liu et al., 2008). This leads to a hyperphosphorylated form of tau, which causes the loss of tau's biological function and stimulates the formation of NFTs. Indirectly, Dyrk1A inhibits calcineurin by phosphorylating RCAN1. Calcineurin typically dephosphorylates tau, but when inhibited by phosphorylated RCAN1, tau phosphorylation is enhanced (Song et al., 2013).

Another possible cause for the early presence of NFTs among persons with DS is the overexpression of RCAN1, which is also located on chromosome 21. RCAN1 levels are higher in people with DS and AD, and levels increase in the brain with aging. RCAN1 in turn hyperphosphorylates tau, creating NFTs and potentially leading to AD (Song et al., 2013). Both RCAN1 and DYRK1A are also upregulated by $A\beta_{42,}$ suggesting that all three of these proteins interact in some way to contribute to neurodegeneration (Kimura et al., 2007; Lloret et al., 2011). The conclusion from these studies is that not only is APP overexpression important for the development of senile plaques (Aβ) in people with DS, but also there are other genes that can make significant contributions to NFT accumulation (e.g., Dyrk1a and RCAN).

Region-Specific Neuron Loss

Aging- and disease-associated neuronal loss in people with DS occur in a similar pattern to that of AD. In AD, the loss of neurons is extensive, but not all areas of the brain are affected equally and a pattern of when and where neurons are lost has emerged. The causes of neuronal loss may be through multiple pathways including exposure to toxic Aβ, NFT, vascular dysfunction, or others (or a combination). Evidence from magnetic resonance imaging (MRI) studies among persons with DS have consistently indicated significant atrophy (loss of brain tissue volume) with age (Teipel & Hampel, 2006). As compared to sporadic AD brains, the brains of older people with DS had lower overall neuron loss but this was due to there being fewer neurons to lose in DS (Mann, 1988). This intriguing conclusion merits further study; is the smaller brain volume in people with DS leading to less neuronal reserve?

The frontal and temporal lobes are underdeveloped among persons with DS (Lee et al., 2016) and thus may pose an area of vulnerability to AD, as fewer neurons are available to lose before cortical circuitry is compromised. As individuals with DS age, neuronal loss preferentially occurs in the entorhinal cortex, hippocampus, temporal and frontal cortices, and basal forebrain nuclei (Ball & Nuttall, 1980; Hyman et al., 1995; Koran et al., 2014; Mann, Marcyniuk, Yates, Neary, & Snowden, 1988; Mullins et al., 2013; Sadowski et al., 1999; Schliebs & Arendt, 2011). The spread of neuronal loss is important to consider, as it may help us identify which cortical circuits are compromised first with age in DS, allowing us to select cognitive tasks to assess changes that are sensitive to the function of these circuits.

Neuron Loss in Subcortical Nuclei Associated With Neurotransmitters in Persons With DS

Neuron loss within specific areas of the brain shapes the neurochemistry. For example, the nucleus basalis of Meynert (nbM) in the basal forebrain is the major producer of acetylcholine (a neurochemical involved with memory), and is a common area of neuron loss in both AD and persons with DS. In AD, losses noted in autopsy cases in the nbM led to the "cholinergic hypothesis," which forms the foundation for AD-treatment drugs (i.e., anti-acetylcholinesterases) that increase the levels of acetylcholine by inhibiting the enzyme that breaks it down as treatments for AD (Terry & Buccafusco, 2003). Research in this area was active in the 1980s in autopsy cases from people with DS. In a small study comparing five brains from people with DS (16–56 years) to similarly-aged typically developing persons without DS, Casanova et al. (1985) observed 29% fewer neurons in the nbM across the life span, and the oldest individual with DS also had the lowest number of neurons in the nbM. Conversely, Mann et al. (1985) found that neuron numbers in the nbM were similar between autopsy cases of younger persons with DS and those without DS, but were significantly lower in people with DS over 50 years of age (Mann, Yates, Marcyniuk, & Ravindra, 1985). Therefore, a reduction in the number of nbM neurons is likely among middle- aged and older individuals with DS, and consequent acetylcholine losses may contribute to the development of cognitive decline and dementia.

Another specific brain region with significant neuron loss both in AD and DS is the locus coeruleus (LC; Mann, Yates, & Marcyniuk, 1984). The LC is a small nucleus in the brainstem, containing neurons that are primarily responsible for the synthesis of noradrenaline with extensive projections throughout the brain. Neuron loss in this region in persons with DS (Marcyniuk, Mann, Yates, & Ravindra, 1988) follows an identical pattern to that of sporadic AD (Mann et al., 1985; Marcyniuk, Mann, & Yates, 1986). In cases of young persons with DS (<50 years), neuron number in the LC is similar to age-matched non-DS comparison cases but begins to decline with middle age in persons with DS (Mann et al., 1985). The loss of LC neurons in persons with DS with age and

AD suggests that disease progression involves a loss of norepinephrine to support synaptic transmission, leading to impaired attention and memory.

Signs of Neuron Loss or Dysfunction—White Matter Degeneration

In addition to AD neuropathology and neuron losses in specific brain regions, aging people with DS display increased white matter degeneration. White matter degeneration reflects pathology or losses of the axons from neurons connecting various parts of the brain and can lead to impaired connectivity in cortical circuits required for intact learning and memory. Losing neurons can also lead to losses in axons and thus white matter integrity. Evidence from neuroanatomical MRI studies indicates that adults with DS have lower white matter volumes (thus, fewer axon bundles or unhealthy smaller bundles) than typically developing people without DS (Raz et al., 1995; Teipel et al., 2004; White, Alkire, & Haier, 2003).

A noninvasive means to detect white matter degeneration in the brain, prior to autopsy, is through neuroimaging. One neuroimaging protocol, diffusion tensor imaging (DTI), measures the diffusion of water molecules along axons to give information about how intact the neuronal axons of the white matter are, alternatively known as white matter integrity. When axons are intact, water molecules move in a straight line (or show little scatter) but when white matter is pathological, water molecules will move in multiple directions as measured by fractional anisotropy. In people with DS, the white matter appears to be less intact, even at 35 years of age and continues to break down as compared to age-matched people without DS (Basser, Pajevic, Pierpaoli, Duda, & Aldroubi, 2000; Fenoll et al., 2017; Powell et al., 2014). White matter integrity losses were more exaggerated in those people with DS with dementia as compared to non demented persons with DS (Powell et al., 2014). However, white matter integrity did not change with age among a study of non demented individuals with DS (Fenoll et al., 2017), suggesting that early changes in white matter integrity in individuals with DS may be due in part to developmental differences and that these changes are more severe with the development of AD neuropathology.

Cerebrovascular Pathology With Age in DS

In addition to senile plaques, NFTs, neuron loss, changes in neurochemistry, and losses of white matter integrity, vascular pathology may contribute to cognitive decline and dementia in persons with DS. Vascular contributions to cognitive impairment and dementia (VCID) are widely considered the second most common form of dementia after AD, and VCID is estimated to co-occur in as many as 40%– 50% of AD cases (Bowler, Munoz, Merskey, & Hachinski, 1998; Kammoun et al., 2000; Langa, Foster, & Larson, 2004). The most obvious consequence of VCID is stroke, but most people with VCID have much more subtle brain changes, including multiple small strokes, chronic cerebral hypoperfusion (reduced blood flow to the brain), cerebrovascular occlusions, cerebral microhemorrhages, and cerebral amyloid angiopathy (CAA; Levine & Langa, 2011; Wilcock, Schmitt, & Head, 2016). Vascular factors likely lower the age of onset of dementia and accelerate the progression of neurodegenerative diseases, but the ways that AD and VCID pathologies interact are not yet known.

Although VCID is a major contributing factor to dementia in the general population, particularly in sporadic AD, it is relatively unexplored among persons with DS. Key risk factors that contribute to VCID include atherosclerosis (fatty deposits in arteries that lead to narrowing and reduced blood flow) and hypertension (high blood pressure), both of which can lead to heart attacks and strokes. People with DS represent a unique group in which to study the cerebrovascular features of aging and AD because these risk factors are rare in this cohort. For example, in a study of people with DS ranging from 40 to 66 years old, atherosclerosis was absent or rare when compared with similarly aged people without DS but with intellectual disability (Murdoch, Rodger, Rao, Fletcher, & Dunnigan, 1977; Yla-Herttuala, Luoma, Nikkari, & Kivimaki, 1989). The second major risk factor for cerebrovascular disease is high blood pressure. In children and younger adults with DS, lower blood pressure is consistently found (Draheim, Geijer, & Dengel, 2010; Draheim, McCubbin, & Williams, 2002; Rodrigues et al., 2011) relative to typically developing cohorts without DS. In contrast to the general population, blood pressure does not increase (hypertension) with age among people with DS. When directly compared with a cohort with other causes of intellectual disability, people with DS showed significantly lower blood pressure (Murdoch et al., 1977). Thus, the lack of development of hypertension in DS is not related to intellectual disability per se, nor most likely lifestyle, but has a biological basis.

Despite these apparent protective factors for the blood vessels in the brain, cerebrovascular pathology is found among persons with DS. In addition to significant AD pathology, including NFTs and Aβ plaques, people with DS often have a buildup of Aβ in medium to smaller size arteries, known as cerebral amyloid angiopathy (CAA; Reijmer, van Veluw, & Greenberg, 2016). CAA causes changes to the blood vessels and is a major risk factor for both micro and macrohemorrhages (Vinters, 1987). Cerebral amyloid angiopathy in DS is consistently reported in the literature (Belza & Urich, 1986; Donahue & Steinfeld, 1998; Mendel, Bertrand, Szpak, Stepien, & Wierzba-Bobrowicz, 2010; Naito, Sekijima, & Ikeda, 2008; Fig. 16.4), and Carmona-Iragui et al. (2017) found that people with DS have more severe CAA observed by MRI than those with both sporadic and autosomal dominant AD. Carriers of the APOE *E4* allele are at a higher risk for CAA in the general population and in individuals with AD without DS (Greenberg et al., 1996; Rannikmae, Samarasekera, Martinez-Gonzalez, Al-Shahi Salman, & Sudlow, 2013), but not among individuals with DS with AD (Carmona-Iragui et al., 2017). Further, in people with DS who were demented, 38.5% showed evidence of lobar microbleeds and 15.4% had intracerebral hemorrhage, both of which were higher in extent and severity compared to persons with sporadic AD, indicating a possible genetic vulnerability (Carmona-Iragui et al., 2017).

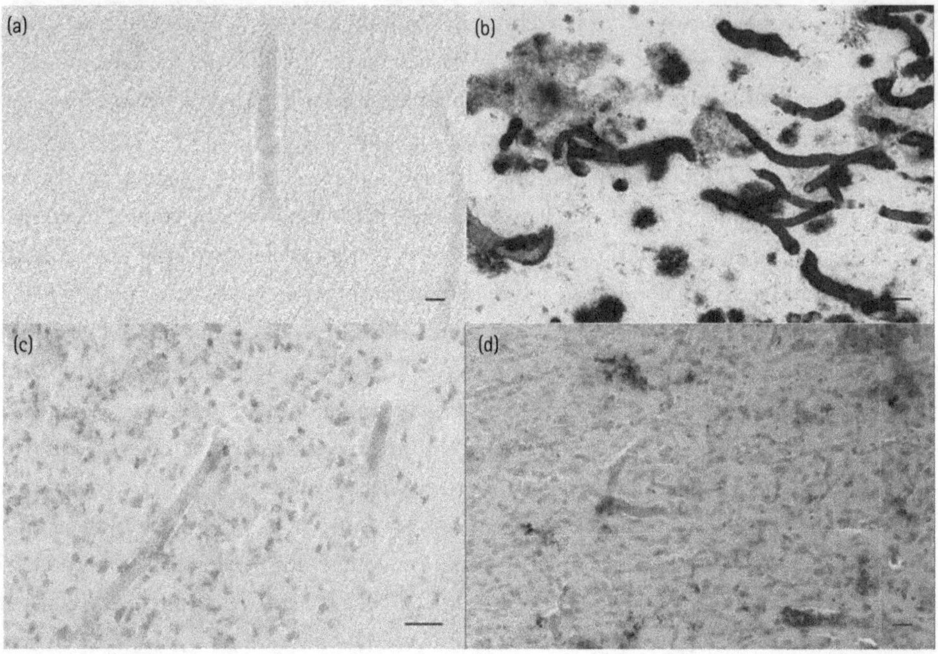

Figure 16.4. Vascular neuropathology in persons with DS
$A\beta_{1-40}$ stain shows that CAA pathology increases in the occipital cortex from a **(a)** young individual with DS (age = 25) to **(b)** a person with DSAD (age = 51). This increase in CAA correlates with an increase in microhemorrhages, shown with Prussian blue staining, from **(c)** a young subject with DS (age = 39) to **(d)** an older subject with DSAD (age = 57).

To systematically characterize how cerebrovascular pathology increases with age in people with DS and how it may be linked to cognitive decline, our laboratory has focused on characterizing cerebrovascular pathology in persons with DS. In a collaborative project, autopsy samples from 32 people with DS with an average age of 55.2 years were compared with sporadic AD cases (n = 80, average age of 76 years) and non demented, non-DS typically developing comparison cases (n = 37, average age of 80.3 years; Head et al., 2017). The extent of atherosclerosis (obstruction of arteries in the Circle of Willis), arteriolosclerosis (thickening of the small arteries), and the extent of CAA were determined as being mild, moderate, or severe. The brains of people with DS had little atherosclerosis (75% showed none) or arteriolosclerosis (97% showed none) but extensive CAA (8% showed none). In contrast, the brains of people with AD showed significant atherosclerosis (42% showed none) and arteriolosclerosis (54% showed none) but less CAA (28% showed none) than people with DS. Relative to comparison cases of typically developing brains, the brains of people with DS had less atherosclerosis, but more CAA. Although the brains of AD patients and typically developing comparison brains were significantly older than the DS cases, which could account for more frequent observations of atherosclerosis and arteriolosclerosis, CAA was far more frequent even in the younger

DS cohort. This study suggests that CAA is a prominent form of blood vessel pathology in the aging brain among persons with DS.

The consequences of CAA in persons with DS may be impaired blood vessel function such the compromise of blood vessel dilation and contribution and thus, reduced blood flow to the brain. Reduced blood flow to the brain can lead to a loss of required levels of glucose critical for brain function. CAA and the impaired function of blood vessels may lead to abnormalities in the white matter of the brain because of less blood perfusing these brain regions (Back et al., 2011; Chao et al., 2013; Erten-Lyons et al., 2013). Further, CAA can also lead to small bleeds or microhemorrhages in the brain. To address this latter hypothesis, we have characterized the extent of microhemorrhages in DS as a function of age and when AD neuropathology is present. In these ongoing autopsy studies, we have observed microhemorrhages in aged DS brains that may correspond to CAA (Fig. 16.4c, d; unpublished data). Yet, despite the presence of CAA and microhemorrhages, the frequency of overt strokes was remarkably low in people with DS, leading to the hypothesis that perhaps some protective factor could be identified (Buss et al., 2016).

Thus, as we uncover more of the different neuropathologies that may contribute to cognitive decline for people with DS, the consideration of cerebrovascular pathology as a risk factor that potentially affects the age of onset or rate of decline should be considered.

Neuroinflammation

Cerebrovascular pathology may have implications for the development of inflammation in the brain. If microhemorrhages occur with age in the brains of persons with DS, the proteins in the blood may leak into the brain (Vinters, 1987). These proteins from the periphery may drive inflammation in the brain, which may be exacerbated due to genetic contributions to neuroinflammation in persons with DS (Wilcock, 2012). Neuroinflammation is associated with increased numbers and sizes of microglia and astrocytes in the brain, which in turn, secrete more inflammatory molecules that lead to a cycle of increasing inflammation. Several genes on chromosome 21 are associated with immune system function (Wilcock, 2012; Wilcock & Griffin, 2013). In autopsy studies of the brains of persons with DS, neuroinflammation is associated with AD neuropathology. For example, C1q, the first protein in the classical complement pathway, a cascade pathway leading to inflammation, is increased in DS brains with AD neuropathology (Head et al., 2001; Stoltzner et al., 2000). In addition, IL-1β, a key pro-inflammatory cytokine, is increased in the brains of persons with DS along with S100β (Griffin et al., 1989). Microglial cells, key mediators of inflammation in the brain, show morphological changes in persons with DS that suggest the degeneration of these cells in association with increased NFT accumulation (Xue & Streit, 2011). Thus, increasing numbers of NFTs may also drive microglial activation, and the release of toxic chemicals, which also may stimulate degeneration in these same microglial cells (Cagnin et al., 2001).

In a study by Wilcock et al. (2015) of autopsy cases of persons with DS with a range of ages, RNA levels of several key neuroinflammatory proteins were quantified and revealed a distinct profile in the DS brain with AD neuropathology (Wilcock et al., 2015). CD86 and FCGR1β were uniquely increased only in individuals with DS with AD, indicating immune complexes may form that can activate microglial cells and toll-like receptors (Wilcock et al., 2015). Increased CD86 and FCGR1β RNA expression has been observed only rarely in sporadic AD. The implications of this study indicate that reducing CD86 or FCGR1β, possibly through anti-inflammatory pharmacological interventions, might be a novel treatment to test in clinical trials for AD, specifically among persons with DS. However, the unique neuroinflammatory profile in aging adults with DS might also serve as a cautionary note when considering immunotherapeutics because this treatment can lead to elevated CD86 and FCGR1β that exacerbate inflammation in persons with DS, which could lead to adverse events (Head & Schmitt, 2014).

Another inflammation-associated molecule that may be important for people with DS is S100β, a small astrocyte-derived protein implicated in the growth of neurons and proliferation and differentiation of glia (Selinfreund, Barger, Welsh, & Van Eldik, 1990). The gene for S100β is located on chromosome 21 and is elevated throughout the lives of individuals with DS (Royston et al., 1999), with twice the number of astrocytes expressing S100β in people with DS at all ages as compared to a typically developing comparison group. While S100β is vital for growth and development of the central nervous system, elevated levels have significant negative consequences. Overexpression of S100β causes abnormal neuronal growth (Kligman & Marshak, 1985; Reeves et al., 1994) and is commonly found in astrocytes associated with Aβ plaques (Griffin et al., 1989; Mrak, Sheng, & Griffin, 1996). Transgenic mice that overexpress S100β have increased dendritic density in the hippocampus when young, but the density of the dendrites was drastically lower at one year of age (Whitaker-Azmitia et al., 1997). Similarly, human fetuses with DS initially have normal dendritic morphology, but dendritic development becomes stunted in infants with DS (Takashima, Becker, Armstrong, & Chan, 1981; Takashima, Iida, Mito, & Arima, 1994). This decrease in dendrites corresponds well with learning and memory deficits, suggesting that S100β may play a significant role in the progression of cognitive decline in aging individuals with DS.

In addition to S100β, several other genes on chromosome 21 are associated with inflammation including CXADR, ADAMTS1, ADAMTS5, TIAM1, IFNAR1, IFNAR2, IFNGR2, RIPK4, CBS and PRMT2 (Wilcock & Griffin, 2013). In a review of the potential role of these genes in the development of AD in people with DS, Wilcock and Griffin (2013) suggest that cytokines, neuroinflammatory molecules released by astrocytes, may drive some of the AD pathogenesis observed in persons with DS (Wilcock & Griffin, 2013). Furthermore, the triplication of inflammatory genes overexpressed due to trisomy 21 may lead to a complex immune profile among persons with DS that can lead to accelerated AD (Wilcock, 2012). Thus, inflammation in the brains of people with DS may contribute to developmental differences in the brain and may also accelerate AD pathogenesis.

Other Genes Associated With AD in Persons With DS

Although we have focused on only a few genes thought to be important for AD among people with DS, other genes may also play a role, such as those associated with oxidative stress and mitochondrial dysfunction (Lott, Head, Doran, & Busciglio, 2006; Pagano & Castello, 2012), compensatory genes (Head, Lott, Patterson, Doran, & Haier, 2007), and additional genes that may underlie cognitive deficits at younger ages (Sturgeon, Le, Ahmed, & Gardiner, 2012) that are all present on chromosome 21. There are clearly multiple possible mechanisms and pathways that either singly or in combination that may lead to early onset AD in people with DS. DS is complex, with genes that may be beneficial or detrimental being overexpressed and the manipulation of any of the gene products must be considered with care.

Future Directions

Our understanding of factors involved with AD progression among persons with DS is growing rapidly. There are fewer autopsy studies in this cohort primarily due to challenges in acquiring brain tissue and particularly tissue from clinically characterized people. In vivo imaging of Aβ and tau, which are noninvasive approaches, may improve our understanding of AD progression in persons with DS throughout the life span. New developments in the neuroimaging field will allow researchers and clinicians to see NFT and senile plaques in the brains of people while still alive.

There are now ligands that bind to tau in NFTs that can be seen by PET imaging and allow researchers to determine Braak stage in vivo (Schwarz et al., 2016). Using a PET ligand with high affinity for paired helical filaments (insoluble fibers composed of hyperphosphorylated tau), Schöll et al. (2016) showed that patterns of tau PET tracer retention corresponded well with Braak staging. The ability to visualize NFT pathology in vivo will help in the early diagnosis of AD both in the general population and in people with DS. Indeed, a recent pilot study observed NFT accumulation by PET neuroimaging in people with DS but NFTs were only observed after people had already accumulated senile plaques (also seen by PET imaging ; Rafii et al., 2017). Given that NFT pathology appears after senile plaques with age in persons with DS, it may be the case that NFTs occur closer in time to initial observations of clinical decline and could therefore be a more proximal biomarker of dementia.

Improved understanding of the pathological consequences of increased gene expression in DS and how this contributes to the development of dementia, particularly genes that are involved in neuroinflammation and cerebrovascular disease, will be important.

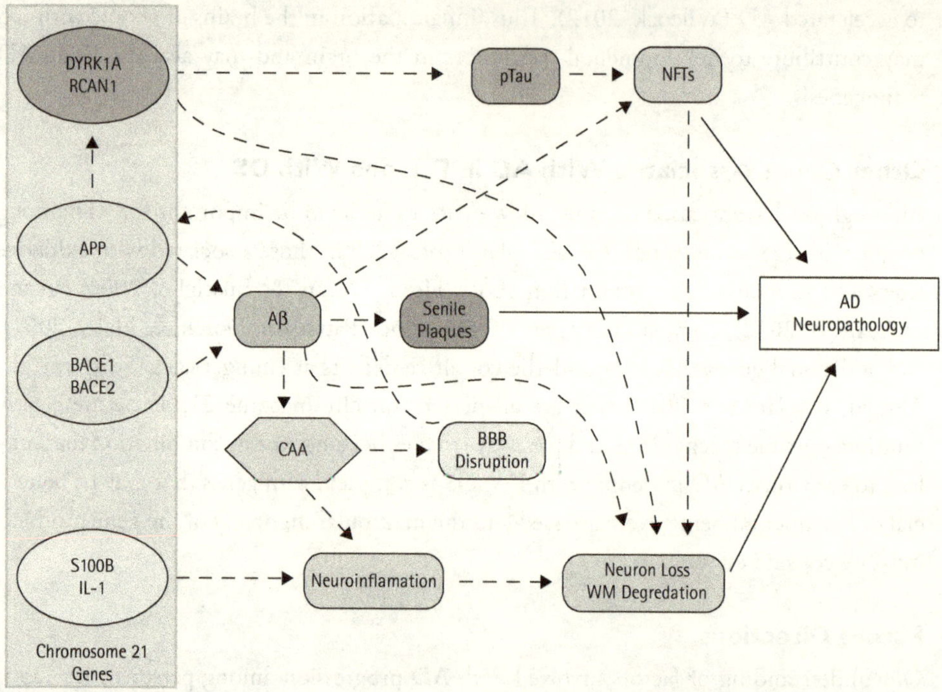

Figure 16.5. Hypothetical role for DS-associated verexpressed proteins and AD pathogenesis in persons with DS Triplication of chromosome 21 in individuals with DS leads to gene overexpression and increased protein expression (DYRK1A, RCAN1, APP, BACE2, S100β) that each engage different and overlapping AD pathologies. DYRK1A and RCAN 1 play a role in the accumulation of NFTs. APP and BACE2 (along with evidence for BACE1 activity increases in persons with DS) overexpression may lead to enhanced Aβ deposition both in senile plaques and in cerebral amyloid angiopathy (CAA). S100β (and associated increases in IL-1) may lead to increased neuroinflammation in persons with DS that may be exacerbated by CAA including CAA-induced compromise of the blood brain barrier (BBB). Aβ and NFTs along with neuroinflammation may combine to induce neuron loss and white matter degeneration.

As more molecular pathways are identified that are pathologically activated (or suppressed) in persons with DS, we can identify novel targets for interventions based on age. Figure 16.5 provides a summary of possible genetic processes leading to the development of AD in persons with DS.

The few clinical trials for AD in persons with DS (Ballard, Mobley, Hardy, Williams, & Corbett, 2016; Table 16.1) highlight the need to continue to enroll volunteers into longitudinal aging studies that involve clinical measures, neuroimaging, plasma or cerebrospinal fluid biomarkers, and autopsy. Given the unique and strong age dependency of AD neuropathology in persons with DS, we have an exciting opportunity to potentially prevent its occurrence once we identify the pathways that are critical at different age epochs. Prevention studies for AD in the general population are a challenge, as the age of onset can vary widely and no biomarkers definitively indicate if a person will develop the disease.

Table 16.1. Ongoing Clinical Trials for Aging Adults With Down Syndrome

Study Title	Purpose of Study	Cohort
A Phase Ib Multi-Center, Double-Blind, Randomized, Placebo-Controlled Dose Escalation Study of the Safety, Tolerability and Immunogenicity of ACI-24 in Adults with Down Syndrome	To examine the safety, tolerability, and immunogenicity of the ACI-24 vaccine	Adults with DS, ages 25–45
Nicotinic Treatment of Age-Related Cognitive Decline in Down Syndrome: An Open Label Pilot Trial	To ascertain the safety and tolerability of nicotine in DS patients and look for evidence of enhancements in cognitive function	Adults with DS with mild cognitive impairment
Phase II Multicenter 16-Week Randomized Double Blind Placebo-Controlled Evaluation of the Efficacy, Tolerability and Safety of Memantine Hydrochloride on Enhancing the Cognitive Abilities of Adolescents and Young Adults With Down Syndrome	To learn if memantine hydrochloride can help adolescents and young adults with Down syndrome	Children and adults with DS, ages 15–32

Note: Queried from ClinTrials.gov

Acknowledgments

EH and FAS are supported by Eunice Kennedy Shriver National Institute of Child Health and Development of the National Institutes of Health under award number R01HD064993. The content is solely the responsibility of the authors and does not necessarily represent the official views of the National Institutes of Health. The authors are grateful to Ms. Paula Thomason for careful editing of the manuscript.

References

Acquati, F., Accarino, M., Nucci, C., Fumagalli, P., Jovine, L., Ottolenghi, S., & Taramelli, R. (2000). The gene encoding DRAP (BACE2), a glycosylated transmembrane protein of the aspartic protease family, maps to the down critical region. *FEBS Letters*, *468*(1), 59–64. https://doi.org/10.1016/s0014-5793(00)01192-3

Ahmed, R. R., Holler, C. J., Webb, R. L., Li, F., Beckett, T. L., & Murphy, M. P. (2010). BACE1 and BACE2 enzymatic activities in Alzheimer's disease. *Journal of Neurochemistry*, *112*(4), 1045–1053. https://doi.org/10.1111/j.1471-4159.2009.06528.x

Ahn, K. J., Jeong, H. K., Choi, H. S., Ryoo, S. R., Kim, Y. J., Goo, J. S., Choi, S. Y., Han, J. S., Ha, I., & Song, W. J. (2006). DYRK1A BAC transgenic mice show altered synaptic plasticity with learning and memory defects. *Neurobiology of Disease*, *22*(3), 463–472. https://doi.org/10.1016/j.nbd.2005.12.006

Altafaj, X., Dierssen, M., Baamonde, C., Martí, E., Visa, J., Guimerà, J., Oset, M., González, J. R., Flórez, J., Fillat, C., & Estivill, X. (2001). Neurodevelopmental delay, motor abnormalities and cognitive deficits in transgenic mice overexpressing Dyrk1A (minibrain), a murine model of Down's syndrome. *Human Molecular Genetics*, *10*(18), 1915–1923. https://doi.org/10.1093/hmg/10.18.1915

Altafaj, X., Ortiz-Abalia, J., Fernández, M., Potier, M. C., Laffaire, J., Andreu, N., Dierssen, M., González-García, C., Ceña, V., Martí, E., & Fillat, C. (2008). Increased NR2A expression and prolonged decay of NMDA-induced calcium transient in cerebellum of TgDyrk1A mice, a mouse model of Down syndrome. *Neurobiology of Disease*, *32*(3), 377–384. https://doi.org/10.1016/j.nbd.2008.07.024

Anderson-Mooney, A. J., Schmitt, F. A., Head, E., Lott, I. T., & Heilman, K. M. (2016). Gait dyspraxia as a clinical marker of cognitive decline in Down syndrome: A review of theory and proposed mechanisms. *Brain and Cognition*, *104*, 48–57. https://doi.org/10.1016/j.bandc.2016.02.007

Annus, T., Wilson, L. R., Hong, Y. T., Acosta-Cabronero, J., Fryer, T. D., Cardenas-Blanco, A., Smith, R., Boros, I., Coles, J. P., Aigbirhio, F. I., Menon, D. K., Zaman, S. H., Nestor, P. J., & Holland, A. J. (2016). The pattern of amyloid accumulation in the brains of adults with Down syndrome. *Alzheimer's & Dementia: The Journal of the Alzheimer's Association*, *12*(5), 538–545. https://doi.org/10.1016/j.jalz.2015.07.490

Arron, J. R., Winslow, M. M., Polleri, A., Chang, C. P., Wu, H., Gao, X., Neilson, J. R., Chen, L., Heit, J. J., Kim, S. K., Yamasaki, N., Miyakawa, T., Francke, U., Graef, I. A., & Crabtree, G. R. (2006). NFAT dysregulation by increased dosage of DSCR1 and DYRK1A on chromosome 21. *Nature*, *441*(7093), 595–600. https://doi.org/10.1038/nature04678

Azizeh, B. Y., Head, E., Ibrahim, M. A., Torp, R., Tenner, A. J., Kim, R. C., Lott, I. T., & Cotman, C. W. (2000). Molecular dating of senile plaques in the brains of individuals with Down syndrome and in aged dogs. *Experimental Neurology*, *163*(1), 111–122. https://doi.org/10.1006/exnr.2000.7359

Back, S. A., Kroenke, C. D., Sherman, L. S., Lawrence, G., Gong, X., Taber, E. N., Sonnen, J. A., Larson, E. B., & Montine, T. J. (2011). White matter lesions defined by diffusion tensor imaging in older adults. *Annals of Neurology*, *70*(3), 465–476. https://doi.org/10.1002/ana.22484

Ball, M. J., & Nuttall, K. (1980). Neurofibrillary tangles, granulovacuolar degeneration, and neuron loss in Down Syndrome: Quantitative comparison with Alzheimer dementia. *Annals of Neurology*, *7*(5), 462–465. https://doi.org/10.1002/ana.410070512

Ballard, C., Mobley, W., Hardy, J., Williams, G., & Corbett, A. (2016). Dementia in Down's syndrome. *The Lancet. Neurology*, *15*(6), 622–636. https://doi.org/10.1016/S1474-4422(16)00063-6

Barbiero, L., Benussi, L., Ghidoni, R., Alberici, A., Russo, C., Schettini, G., Pagano, S. F., Parati, E. A., Mazzoli, F., Nicosia, F., Signorini, S., Feudatari, E., & Binetti, G. (2003). BACE-2 is overexpressed in Down's syndrome. *Experimental Neurology*, *182*(2), 335–345. https://doi.org/10.1016/s0014-4886(03)00049-9

Basser, P. J., Pajevic, S., Pierpaoli, C., Duda, J., & Aldroubi, A. (2000). In vivo fiber tractography using DT-MRI data. *Magnetic Resonance in Medicine*, *44*(4), 625–632. https://doi.org/10.1002/1522-2594(200010)44:4<625::aid-mrm17>3.0.co;2-o

Bayen, E., Possin, K. L., Chen, Y., Cleret de Langavant, L., & Yaffe, K. (2018). Prevalence of aging, dementia, and multimorbidity in older adults with down syndrome. *JAMA Neurology*, *75*(11), 1399–1406. https://doi.org/10.1001/jamaneurol.2018.2210

Belza, M. G., & Urich, H. (1986). Cerebral amyloid angiopathy in Down's syndrome. *Clinical Neuropathology*, *5*(6), 257–260.

Bittles, A. H., & Glasson, E. J. (2004). Clinical, social, and ethical implications of changing life expectancy in Down syndrome. *Developmental Medicine and Child Neurology*, *46*(4), 282–286. https://doi.org/10.1017/s0012162204000441

Bowler, J. V., Munoz, D. G., Merskey, H., & Hachinski, V. (1998). Fallacies in the pathological confirmation of the diagnosis of Alzheimer's disease. *Journal of Neurology, Neurosurgery, and Psychiatry*, *64*(1), 18–24. https://doi.org/10.1136/jnnp.64.1.18

Braak, H., & Braak, E. (1991). Neuropathological stageing of Alzheimer-related changes. *Acta Neuropathologica*, *82*(4), 239–259. https://doi.org/10.1007/BF00308809

Burger, P. C., & Vogel, F. S. (1973). The development of the pathologic changes of Alzheimer's disease and senile dementia in patients with Down's syndrome. *American Journal of Pathology*, *73*(2), 457–476.

Buss, L., Fisher, E., Hardy, J., Nizetic, D., Groet, J., Pulford, L., & Strydom, A. (2016). Intracerebral haemorrhage in Down syndrome: Protected or predisposed?. *F1000Research*, *5*, F1000 Faculty Rev-876. https://doi.org/10.12688/f1000research.7819.1

Cagnin, A., Brooks, D. J., Kennedy, A. M., Gunn, R. N., Myers, R., Turkheimer, F. E., Jones, T., & Banati, R. B. (2001). In-vivo measurement of activated microglia in dementia. *Lancet* (London, England), *358*(9280), 461–467. https://doi.org/10.1016/S0140-6736(01)05625-2

Carmona-Iragui, M., Balasa, M., Benejam, B., Alcolea, D., Fernández, S., Videla, L., Sala, I., Sánchez-Saudinós, M. B., Morenas-Rodriguez, E., Ribosa-Nogué, R., Illán-Gala, I., Gonzalez-Ortiz, S., Clarimón, J., Schmitt, F., Powell, D. K., Bosch, B., Lladó, A., Rafii, M. S., Head, E., Molinuevo, J. L., . . . Fortea, J. (2017). Cerebral amyloid angiopathy in Down syndrome and sporadic and autosomal-dominant Alzheimer's disease. *Alzheimer's & Dementia: The Journal of the Alzheimer's Association*, *13*(11), 1251–1260. https://doi.org/10.1016/j.jalz.2017.03.007

Casanova, M. F., Walker, L. C., Whitehouse, P. J., Price, D., (1985). Abnormalities of the nucleus basalis in Down's syndrome. *Annals of Neurology*, *18*(3), 310–313. doi: 10.1002/ana.410180306.

Cavani, S., Tamaoka, A., Moretti, A., Marinelli, L., Angelini, G., Di Stefano, S., Piombo, G., Cazzulo, V., Matsuno, S., Shoji, S., Furiya, Y., Zaccheo, D., Dagna-Bricarelli, F., Tabaton, M., & Mori, H. (2000). Plasma levels of amyloid beta 40 and 42 are independent from ApoE genotype and mental retardation in Down syndrome. *American Journal of Medical Genetics, 95*(3), 224–228.

Chao, L. L., Decarli, C., Kriger, S., Truran, D., Zhang, Y., Laxamana, J., Villeneuve, S., Jagust, W. J., Sanossian, N., Mack, W. J., Chui, H. C., & Weiner, M. W. (2013). Associations between white matter hyperintensities and β amyloid on integrity of projection, association, and limbic fiber tracts measured with diffusion tensor MRI. *PloS One, 8*(6), e65175. https://doi.org/10.1371/journal.pone.0065175

Cheon, M. S., Dierssen, M., Kim, S. H., & Lubec, G. (2008). Protein expression of BACE1, BACE2 and APP in Down syndrome brains. *Amino Acids, 35*(2), 339–343. https://doi.org/10.1007/s00726-007-0618-9

Cohen, A. D., & Klunk, W. E. (2014). Early detection of Alzheimer's disease using PiB and FDG PET. *Neurobiology of Disease, 72 Pt A*, 117–122. https://doi.org/10.1016/j.nbd.2014.05.001

Cohen, A. D., McDade, E., Christian, B., Price, J., Mathis, C., Klunk, W., & Handen, B. L. (2018). Early striatal amyloid deposition distinguishes Down syndrome and autosomal dominant Alzheimer's disease from late-onset amyloid deposition. *Alzheimer's & dementia: The Journal of the Alzheimer's Association, 14*(6), 743–750. https://doi.org/10.1016/j.jalz.2018.01.002

Davidson, Y. S., Robinson, A., Prasher, V. P., & Mann, D. (2018). The age of onset and evolution of Braak tangle stage and Thal amyloid pathology of Alzheimer's disease in individuals with Down syndrome. *Acta Neuropathologica Communications, 6*(1), 56. https://doi.org/10.1186/s40478-018-0559-4

Dickson D. W. (2004). Apoptotic mechanisms in Alzheimer neurofibrillary degeneration: Cause or effect?. *Journal of Clinical Investigation, 114*(1), 23–27. https://doi.org/10.1172/JCI22317

Donahue, B., & Steinfeld, A. (1998). Intracranial ependymoma in the adult patient: Successful treatment with surgery and radiotherapy. *Journal of Neuro-Oncology, 37*(2), 131–133. https://doi.org/10.1023/a:1005965328104

Doran, E., Keator, D., Head, E., Phelan, M. J., Kim, R., Totoiu, M., Barrio, J. R., Small, G. W., Potkin, S. G., & Lott, I. T. (2017). Down syndrome, partial trisomy 21, and absence of Alzheimer's disease: The role of APP. *Journal of Alzheimer's Disease: JAD, 56*(2), 459–470. https://doi.org/10.3233/JAD-160836

Draheim, C. C., Geijer, J. R., & Dengel, D. R. (2010). Comparison of intima-media thickness of the carotid artery and cardiovascular disease risk factors in adults with versus without the Down syndrome. *American Journal of Cardiology, 106*(10), 1512–1516. https://doi.org/10.1016/j.amjcard.2010.06.079

Draheim, C. C., McCubbin, J. A., & Williams, D. P. (2002). Differences in cardiovascular disease risk between nondiabetic adults with mental retardation with and without Down syndrome. *American Journal of Mental Retardation: AJMR, 107*(3), 201–211. https://doi.org/10.1352/0895-8017(2002)107<0201:DICDRB>2.0.CO;2

Erten-Lyons, D., Woltjer, R., Kaye, J., Mattek, N., Dodge, H. H., Green, S., Tran, H., Howieson, D. B., Wild, K., & Silbert, L. C. (2013). Neuropathologic basis of white matter hyperintensity accumulation with advanced age. *Neurology, 81*(11), 977–983. https://doi.org/10.1212/WNL.0b013e3182a43e45

Farzan, M., Schnitzler, C. E., Vasilieva, N., Leung, D., & Choe, H. (2000). BACE2, a beta -secretase homolog, cleaves at the beta site and within the amyloid-beta region of the amyloid-beta precursor protein. *Proceedings of the National Academy of Sciences of the United States of America, 97*(17), 9712–9717. https://doi.org/10.1073/pnas.160115697

Fenoll, R., Pujol, J., Esteba-Castillo, S., de Sola, S., Ribas-Vidal, N., García-Alba, J., Sánchez-Benavides, G., Martínez-Vilavella, G., Deus, J., Dierssen, M., Novell-Alsina, R., & de la Torre, R. (2017). Anomalous white matter structure and the effect of age in Down syndrome patients. *Journal of Alzheimer's Disease: JAD, 57*(1), 61–70. https://doi.org/10.3233/JAD-161112

Ferrer, I., Barrachina, M., Puig, B., Martínez de Lagrán, M., Martí, E., Avila, J., & Dierssen, M. (2005). Constitutive Dyrk1A is abnormally expressed in Alzheimer disease, Down syndrome, Pick disease, and related transgenic models. *Neurobiology of Disease, 20*(2), 392–400. https://doi.org/10.1016/j.nbd.2005.03.020

Fluhrer, R., Capell, A., Westmeyer, G., Willem, M., Hartung, B., Condron, M. M., Teplow, D. B., Haass, C., & Walter, J. (2002). A non-amyloidogenic function of BACE-2 in the secretory pathway. *Journal of Neurochemistry, 81*(5), 1011–1020. https://doi.org/10.1046/j.1471-4159.2002.00908.x

Franceschi, M., Comola, M., Piattoni, F., Gualandri, W., & Canal, N. (1990). Prevalence of dementia in adult patients with trisomy 21. *American Journal of Medical Genetics. Supplement, 7*, 306–308. https://doi.org/10.1002/ajmg.1320370760

Fukumoto, H., Cheung, B. S., Hyman, B. T., & Irizarry, M. C. (2002). Beta-secretase protein and activity are increased in the neocortex in Alzheimer disease. *Archives of Neurology, 59*(9), 1381–1389. https://doi.org/10.1001/archneur.59.9.1381

Gao, Y. L., Wang, N., Sun, F. R., Cao, X. P., Zhang, W., & Yu, J. T. (2018). Tau in neurodegenerative disease. *Annals of Translational Medicine, 6*(10), 175. https://doi.org/10.21037/atm.2018.04.23

Gendron, T. F., & Petrucelli, L. (2009). The role of tau in neurodegeneration. *Molecular Neurodegeneration, 4*, 13. https://doi.org/10.1186/1750-1326-4-13

Gómez-Isla, T., Hollister, R., West, H., Mui, S., Growdon, J. H., Petersen, R. C., Parisi, J. E., & Hyman, B. T. (1997). Neuronal loss correlates with but exceeds neurofibrillary tangles in Alzheimer's disease. *Annals of Neurology, 41*(1), 17–24. https://doi.org/10.1002/ana.410410106

Greenberg, S. M., Briggs, M. E., Hyman, B. T., Kokoris, G. J., Takis, C., Kanter, D. S., Kase, C. S., & Pessin, M. S. (1996). Apolipoprotein E epsilon 4 is associated with the presence and earlier onset of hemorrhage in cerebral amyloid angiopathy. *Stroke, 27*(8), 1333–1337. https://doi.org/10.1161/01.str.27.8.1333

Griffin, W. S., Stanley, L. C., Ling, C., White, L., MacLeod, V., Perrot, L. J., White, C. L., 3rd, & Araoz, C. (1989). Brain interleukin 1 and S-100 immunoreactivity are elevated in Down syndrome and Alzheimer disease. *Proceedings of the National Academy of Sciences of the United States of America, 86*(19), 7611–7615. https://doi.org/10.1073/pnas.86.19.7611

Guimera, J., Casas, C., Estivill, X., & Pritchard, M. (1999). Human minibrain homologue (MNBH/DYRK1): characterization, alternative splicing, differential tissue expression, and overexpression in Down syndrome. *Genomics, 57*(3), 407–418. https://doi.org/10.1006/geno.1999.5775

Guimerá, J., Casas, C., Pucharcòs, C., Solans, A., Domènech, A., Planas, A. M., Ashley, J., Lovett, M., Estivill, X., & Pritchard, M. A. (1996). A human homologue of Drosophila minibrain (MNB) is expressed in the neuronal regions affected in Down syndrome and maps to the critical region. *Human Molecular Genetics, 5*(9), 1305–1310. https://doi.org/10.1093/hmg/5.9.1305

Handen, B. L., Cohen, A. D., Channamalappa, U., Bulova, P., Cannon, S. A., Cohen, W. I., Mathis, C. A., Price, J. C., & Klunk, W. E. (2012). Imaging brain amyloid in nondemented young adults with Down syndrome using Pittsburgh compound B. *Alzheimer's & Dementia: The Journal of the Alzheimer's Association, 8*(6), 496–501. https://doi.org/10.1016/j.jalz.2011.09.229

Hardy J. (2006). Alzheimer's disease: The amyloid cascade hypothesis: An update and reappraisal. *Journal of Alzheimer's Disease: JAD, 9*(3 Suppl), 151–153. https://doi.org/10.3233/jad-2006-9s317

Hartley, S. L., Handen, B. L., Devenny, D. A., Hardison, R., Mihaila, I., Price, J. C., Cohen, A. D., Klunk, W. E., Mailick, M. R., Johnson, S. C., & Christian, B. T. (2014). Cognitive functioning in relation to brain amyloid-*β* in healthy adults with Down syndrome. *Brain: A Journal of Neurology, 137*(Pt 9), 2556–2563. https://doi.org/10.1093/brain/awu173

Head, E., Azizeh, B. Y., Lott, I. T., Tenner, A. J., Cotman, C. W., & Cribbs, D. H. (2001). Complement association with neurons and beta-amyloid deposition in the brains of aged individuals with Down Syndrome. *Neurobiology of Disease, 8*(2), 252–265. https://doi.org/10.1006/nbdi.2000.0380

Head, E., Lott, I. T., Patterson, D., Doran, E., & Haier, R. J. (2007). Possible compensatory events in adult Down syndrome brain prior to the development of Alzheimer disease neuropathology: Targets for nonpharmacological intervention. *Journal of Alzheimer's Disease: JAD, 11*(1), 61–76. https://doi.org/10.3233/jad-2007-11110

Head, E., Phelan, M. J., Doran, E., Kim, R. C., Poon, W. W., Schmitt, F. A., & Lott, I. T. (2017). Cerebrovascular pathology in Down syndrome and Alzheimer disease. *Acta Neuropathologica Communications, 5*(1), 93. https://doi.org/10.1186/s40478-017-0499-4

Head, E., Powell, D., Gold, B. T., & Schmitt, F. A. (2012). Alzheimer's Disease in Down Syndrome. *European Journal of Neurodegenerative Disease, 1*(3), 353–364.

Head, E., & Schmitt, F. A. (2014). Con: Are we ready to translate Alzheimer's disease-modifying therapies to people with down syndrome?. *Alzheimer's Research & Therapy, 6*(5-8), 61. https://doi.org/10.1186/s13195-014-0061-6

Head, E., Silverman, W., Patterson, D., & Lott, I. T. (2012). Aging and down syndrome. *Current Gerontology and Geriatrics Research, 2012*, 412536. https://doi.org/10.1155/2012/412536

Hof, P. R., Bouras, C., Perl, D. P., Sparks, D. L., Mehta, N., & Morrison, J. H. (1995). Age-related distribution of neuropathologic changes in the cerebral cortex of patients with Down's syndrome. Quantitative regional analysis and comparison with Alzheimer's disease. *Archives of Neurology, 52*(4), 379–391. https://doi.org/10.1001/archneur.1995.00540280065020

Holler, C. J., Webb, R. L., Laux, A. L., Beckett, T. L., Niedowicz, D. M., Ahmed, R. R., Liu, Y., Simmons, C. R., Dowling, A. L., Spinelli, A., Khurgel, M., Estus, S., Head, E., Hersh, L. B., & Murphy, M. P. (2012). BACE2 expression increases in human neurodegenerative disease. *American Journal of Pathology, 180*(1), 337–350. https://doi.org/10.1016/j.ajpath.2011.09.034

Hyman, B. T., West, H. L., Rebeck, G. W., Lai, F., & Mann, D. M. (1995). Neuropathological changes in Down's syndrome hippocampal formation. Effect of age and apolipoprotein E genotype. *Archives of Neurology, 52*(4), 373–378. https://doi.org/10.1001/archneur.1995.00540280059019

Iwatsubo, T., Mann, D. M., Odaka, A., Suzuki, N., & Ihara, Y. (1995). Amyloid beta protein (A beta) deposition: A beta 42(43) precedes A beta 40 in Down syndrome. *Annals of Neurology, 37*(3), 294–299. https://doi.org/10.1002/ana.410370305

Jack, C. R., Jr, Bennett, D. A., Blennow, K., Carrillo, M. C., Dunn, B., Haeberlein, S. B., Holtzman, D. M., Jagust, W., Jessen, F., Karlawish, J., Liu, E., Molinuevo, J. L., Montine, T., Phelps, C., Rankin, K. P., Rowe, C. C., Scheltens, P., Siemers, E., Snyder, H. M., Sperling, R., . . . Contributors (2018). NIA-AA Research Framework: Toward a biological definition of Alzheimer's disease. *Alzheimer's & Dementia: The Journal of the Alzheimer's Association, 14*(4), 535–562. https://doi.org/10.1016/j.jalz.2018.02.018

Jung, M. S., Park, J. H., Ryu, Y. S., Choi, S. H., Yoon, S. H., Kwen, M. Y., Oh, J. Y., Song, W. J., & Chung, S. H. (2011). Regulation of RCAN1 protein activity by Dyrk1A protein-mediated phosphorylation. *Journal of Biological Chemistry, 286*(46), 40401–40412. https://doi.org/10.1074/jbc.M111.253971

Kammoun, S., Gold, G., Bouras, C., Giannakopoulos, P., McGee, W., Herrmann, F., & Michel, J. P. (2000). Immediate causes of death of demented and non-demented elderly. *Acta Neurologica Scandinavica. Supplementum, 176*, 96–99. https://doi.org/10.1034/j.1600-0404.2000.00314.x

Kimura, R., Kamino, K., Yamamoto, M., Nuripa, A., Kida, T., Kazui, H., Hashimoto, R., Tanaka, T., Kudo, T., Yamagata, H., Tabara, Y., Miki, T., Akatsu, H., Kosaka, K., Funakoshi, E., Nishitomi, K., Sakaguchi, G., Kato, A., Hattori, H., Uema, T., . . . Takeda, M. (2007). The DYRK1A gene, encoded in chromosome 21 Down syndrome critical region, bridges between beta-amyloid production and tau phosphorylation in Alzheimer disease. *Human Molecular Genetics, 16*(1), 15–23. https://doi.org/10.1093/hmg/ddl437

Kligman, D., & Marshak, D. R. (1985). Purification and characterization of a neurite extension factor from bovine brain. *Proceedings of the National Academy of Sciences of the United States of America, 82*(20), 7136–7139. https://doi.org/10.1073/pnas.82.20.7136

Klunk, W. E., Engler, H., Nordberg, A., Wang, Y., Blomqvist, G., Holt, D. P., Bergström, M., Savitcheva, I., Huang, G. F., Estrada, S., Ausén, B., Debnath, M. L., Barletta, J., Price, J. C., Sandell, J., Lopresti, B. J., Wall, A., Koivisto, P., Antoni, G., Mathis, C. A., . . . Långström, B. (2004). Imaging brain amyloid in Alzheimer's disease with Pittsburgh Compound-B. *Annals of Neurology, 55*(3), 306–319. https://doi.org/10.1002/ana.20009

Koivunen, J., Verkkoniemi, A., Aalto, S., Paetau, A., Ahonen, J. P., Viitanen, M., Någren, K., Rokka, J., Haaparanta, M., Kalimo, H., & Rinne, J. O. (2008). PET amyloid ligand [11C]PIB uptake shows predominantly striatal increase in variant Alzheimer's disease. *Brain: Journal of Neurology, 131*(*Pt 7*), 1845–1853. https://doi.org/10.1093/brain/awn107

Koran, M. E., Hohman, T. J., Edwards, C. M., Vega, J. N., Pryweller, J. R., Slosky, L. E., Crockett, G., Villa de Rey, L., Meda, S. A., Dankner, N., Avery, S. N., Blackford, J. U., Dykens, E. M., & Thornton-Wells, T. A. (2014). Differences in age-related effects on brain volume in Down syndrome as compared to Williams syndrome and typical development. *Journal of Neurodevelopmental Disorders, 6*(1), 8. https://doi.org/10.1186/1866-1955-6-8

Korenberg, J. R., Kawashima, H., Pulst, S. M., Ikeuchi, T., Ogasawara, N., Yamamoto, K., Schonberg, S. A., West, R., Allen, L., & Magenis, E. (1990). Molecular definition of a region of chromosome 21 that causes features of the Down syndrome phenotype *American Journal of Human Genetics, 47*(2), 236–246.

Langa, K. M., Foster, N. L., & Larson, E. B. (2004). Mixed dementia: Emerging concepts and therapeutic implications. *JAMA, 292*(23), 2901–2908. https://doi.org/10.1001/jama.292.23.2901

Lao, P. J., Betthauser, T. J., Hillmer, A. T., Price, J. C., Klunk, W. E., Mihaila, I., Higgins, A. T., Bulova, P. D., Hartley, S. L., Hardison, R., Tumuluru, R. V., Murali, D., Mathis, C. A., Cohen, A. D., Barnhart, T. E., Devenny, D. A., Mailick, M. R., Johnson, S. C., Handen, B. L., & Christian, B. T. (2016). The effects of normal aging on amyloid-β deposition in nondemented adults with Down syndrome as imaged by carbon 11-labeled Pittsburgh compound B. *Alzheimer's & Dementia: The Journal of the Alzheimer's Association, 12*(4), 380–390. https://doi.org/10.1016/j.jalz.2015.05.013

Lao, P. J., Handen, B. L., Betthauser, T. J., Mihaila, I., Hartley, S. L., Cohen, A. D., Tudorascu, D. L., Bulova, P. D., Lopresti, B. J., Tumuluru, R. V., Murali, D., Mathis, C. A., Barnhart, T. E., Stone, C. K., Price, J. C., Devenny, D. A., Mailick, M. R., Klunk, W. E., Johnson, S. C., & Christian, B. T. (2017). Longitudinal changes in amyloid positron emission tomography and volumetric magnetic resonance imaging in the nondemented Down syndrome population. *Alzheimer's & Dementia* (Amsterdam, Netherlands), *9*, 1–9. https://doi.org/10.1016/j.dadm.2017.05.001

Lee, N. R., Adeyemi, E. I., Lin, A., Clasen, L. S., Lalonde, F. M., Condon, E., Driver, D. I., Shaw, P., Gogtay, N., Raznahan, A., & Giedd, J. N. (2016). Dissociations in cortical morphometry in youth with Down syndrome: Evidence for reduced surface area but increased thickness. *Cerebral Cortex* (New York, N.Y.: 1991), *26*(7), 2982–2990. https://doi.org/10.1093/cercor/bhv107

Lemere, C. A., Blusztajn, J. K., Yamaguchi, H., Wisniewski, T., Saido, T. C., & Selkoe, D. J. (1996). Sequence of deposition of heterogeneous amyloid beta-peptides and APO E in Down syndrome: Implications for initial events in amyloid plaque formation. *Neurobiology of Disease*, *3*(1), 16–32. https://doi.org/10.1006/nbdi.1996.0003

Leverenz, J. B., & Raskind, M. A. (1998). Early amyloid deposition in the medial temporal lobe of young Down syndrome patients: A regional quantitative analysis. *Experimental Neurology*, *150*(2), 296–304. https://doi.org/10.1006/exnr.1997.6777

Levine, D. A., & Langa, K. M. (2011). Vascular cognitive impairment: Disease mechanisms and therapeutic implications. *Neurotherapeutics: The Journal of the American Society for Experimental Neurotherapeutics*, *8*(3), 361–373. https://doi.org/10.1007/s13311-011-0047-z

LeVine, H., 3rd, Spielmann, H. P., Matveev, S., Cauvi, F. M., Murphy, M. P., Beckett, T. L., McCarty, K., Lott, I. T., Doran, E., Schmitt, F., & Head, E. (2017). Down syndrome: Age-dependence of PiB binding in postmortem frontal cortex across the lifespan. *Neurobiology of Aging*, *54*, 163–169. https://doi.org/10.1016/j.neurobiolaging.2017.03.005

Liu, F., Liang, Z., Wegiel, J., Hwang, Y. W., Iqbal, K., Grundke-Iqbal, I., Ramakrishna, N., & Gong, C. X. (2008). Overexpression of Dyrk1A contributes to neurofibrillary degeneration in Down syndrome. *FASEB Journal: Official Publication of the Federation of American Societies for Experimental Biology*, *22*(9), 3224–3233. https://doi.org/10.1096/fj.07-104539

Lloret, A., Badia, M. C., Giraldo, E., Ermak, G., Alonso, M. D., Pallardó, F. V., Davies, K. J., & Viña, J. (2011). Amyloid-β toxicity and tau hyperphosphorylation are linked via RCAN1 in Alzheimer's disease. *Journal of Alzheimer's Disease: JAD*, *27*(4), 701–709. https://doi.org/10.3233/JAD-2011-110890

Lott, I. T., Head, E., Doran, E., & Busciglio, J. (2006). Beta-amyloid, oxidative stress and down syndrome. *Current Alzheimer Research*, *3*(5), 521–528. https://doi.org/10.2174/156720506779025305

Mann D. M. (1988). The pathological association between Down syndrome and Alzheimer disease. *Mechanisms of Ageing and Development*, *43*(2), 99–136. https://doi.org/10.1016/0047-6374(88)90041-3

Mann, D. M., & Esiri, M. M. (1989). The pattern of acquisition of plaques and tangles in the brains of patients under 50 years of age with Down's syndrome. *Journal of the Neurological Sciences*, *89*(2–3), 169–179. https://doi.org/10.1016/0022-510x(89)90019-1

Mann, D. M., Marcyniuk, B., Yates, P. O., Neary, D., & Snowden, J. S. (1988). The progression of the pathological changes of Alzheimer's disease in frontal and temporal neocortex examined both at biopsy and at autopsy. *Neuropathology and Applied Neurobiology*, *14*(3), 177–195. https://doi.org/10.1111/j.1365-2990.1988.tb00880.x

Mann, D. M., Yates, P. O., & Marcyniuk, B. (1984). Alzheimer's presenile dementia, senile dementia of Alzheimer type and Down's syndrome in middle age form an age related continuum of pathological changes. *Neuropathology and Applied Neurobiology*, *10*(3), 185–207. https://doi.org/10.1111/j.1365-2990.1984.tb00351.x

Mann, D. M., Yates, P. O., Marcyniuk, B., & Ravindra, C. R. (1985). Pathological evidence for neurotransmitter deficits in Down's syndrome of middle age. *Journal of Mental Deficiency Research*, *29*(Pt 2), 125–135. https://doi.org/10.1111/j.1365-2788.1985.tb00320.x

Marcyniuk, B., Mann, D. M., & Yates, P. O. (1986). The topography of cell loss from locus caeruleus in Alzheimer's disease. *Journal of the Neurological Sciences*, *76*(2–3), 335 345. https://doi.org/10.1016/0022-510x(86)90179-6

Marcyniuk, B., Mann, D. M., Yates, P. O., & Ravindra, C. R. (1988). Topography of nerve cell loss from the locus caeruleus in middle aged persons with Down's syndrome. *Journal of the Neurological Sciences*, *83*(1), 15–24. https://doi.org/10.1016/0022-510x(88)90016-0

Martínez de Lagrán, M., Altafaj, X., Gallego, X., Martí, E., Estivill, X., Sahún, I., Fillat, C., & Dierssen, M. (2004). Motor phenotypic alterations in TgDyrk1a transgenic mice implicate DYRK1A in Down syndrome motor dysfunction. *Neurobiology of Disease, 15*(1), 132–142. https://doi.org/10.1016/j.nbd.2003.10.002

Mayeux, R., Honig, L. S., Tang, M. X., Manly, J., Stern, Y., Schupf, N., & Mehta, P. D. (2003). Plasma A[beta]40 and A[beta]42 and Alzheimer's disease: Relation to age, mortality, and risk. *Neurology, 61*(9), 1185–1190. https://doi.org/10.1212/01.wnl.0000091890.32140.8f

Mehta, P. D., Dalton, A. J., Mehta, S. P., Kim, K. S., Sersen, E. A., & Wisniewski, H. M. (1998). Increased plasma amyloid beta protein 1-42 levels in Down syndrome. *Neuroscience Letters, 241*(1), 13–16. https://doi.org/10.1016/s0304-3940(97)00966-x

Mendel, T., Bertrand, E., Szpak, G. M., Stępień, T., & Wierzba-Bobrowicz, T. (2010). Cerebral amyloid angiopathy as a cause of an extensive brain hemorrhage in adult patient with Down's syndrome: A case report. *Folia neuropathologica, 48*(3), 206–211.

Mrak, R. E., Sheng, J. G., & Griffin, W. S. (1996). Correlation of astrocytic S100 beta expression with dystrophic neurites in amyloid plaques of Alzheimer's disease. *Journal of Neuropathology and Experimental Neurology, 55*(3), 273–279. https://doi.org/10.1097/00005072-199603000-00002

Mullins, D., Daly, E., Simmons, A., Beacher, F., Foy, C. M., Lovestone, S., Hallahan, B., Murphy, K. C., & Murphy, D. G. (2013). Dementia in Down's syndrome: An MRI comparison with Alzheimer's disease in the general population. *Journal of Neurodevelopmental Disorders, 5*(1), 19. https://doi.org/10.1186/1866-1955-5-19

Multhaup, G., Huber, O., Buée, L., & Galas, M. C. (2015). Amyloid Precursor Protein (APP) Metabolites APP Intracellular Fragment (AICD), Aβ42, and Tau in Nuclear Roles. *Journal of Biological Chemistry, 290*(39), 23515–23522. https://doi.org/10.1074/jbc.R115.677211

Murdoch, J. C., Rodger, J. C., Rao, S. S., Fletcher, C. D., & Dunnigan, M. G. (1977). Down's syndrome: An atheroma-free model?. *British Medical Journal, 2*(6081), 226–228. https://doi.org/10.1136/bmj.2.6081.226

Naito, K. S., Sekijima, Y., & Ikeda, S. (2008). Cerebral amyloid angiopathy-related hemorrhage in a middle-aged patient with Down's syndrome. *Amyloid: The International Journal of Experimental and Clinical Investigation: The Official Journal of the International Society of Amyloidosis, 15*(4), 275–277. https://doi.org/10.1080/13506120802524981

Nistor, M., Don, M., Parekh, M., Sarsoza, F., Goodus, M., Lopez, G. E., Kawas, C., Leverenz, J., Doran, E., Lott, I. T., Hill, M., & Head, E. (2007). Alpha- and beta-secretase activity as a function of age and beta-amyloid in Down syndrome and normal brain. *Neurobiology of Aging, 28*(10), 1493–1506. https://doi.org/10.1016/j.neurobiolaging.2006.06.023

Nunan, J., & Small, D. H. (2000). Regulation of APP cleavage by alpha-, beta- and gamma-secretases. *FEBS Letters, 483*(1), 6–10. https://doi.org/10.1016/s0014-5793(00)02076-7

Oddo, S., Caccamo, A., Tseng, B., Cheng, D., Vasilevko, V., Cribbs, D. H., & LaFerla, F. M. (2008). Blocking Abeta42 accumulation delays the onset and progression of tau pathology via the C terminus of heat shock protein70-interacting protein: A mechanistic link between Abeta and tau pathology. *The Journal of Neuroscience: The Official Journal of the Society for Neuroscience, 28*(47), 12163–12175. https://doi.org/10.1523/JNEUROSCI.2464-08.2008

Pagano, G., & Castello, G. (2012). Oxidative stress and mitochondrial dysfunction in Down syndrome. *Advances in Experimental Medicine and Biology, 724*, 291–299. https://doi.org/10.1007/978-1-4614-0653-2_22

Plassman, B. L., Langa, K. M., Fisher, G. G., Heeringa, S. G., Weir, D. R., Ofstedal, M. B., Burke, J. R., Hurd, M. D., Potter, G. G., Rodgers, W. L., Steffens, D. C., Willis, R. J., & Wallace, R. B. (2007). Prevalence of dementia in the United States: The aging, demographics, and memory study. *Neuroepidemiology, 29*(1–2), 125–132. https://doi.org/10.1159/000109998

Powell, D., Caban-Holt, A., Jicha, G., Robertson, W., Davis, R., Gold, B. T., Schmitt, F. A., & Head, E. (2014). Frontal white matter integrity in adults with Down syndrome with and without dementia. *Neurobiology of Aging, 35*(7), 1562–1569. https://doi.org/10.1016/j.neurobiolaging.2014.01.137

Prasher, V. P., Farrer, M. J., Kessling, A. M., Fisher, E. M., West, R. J., Barber, P. C., & Butler, A. C. (1998). Molecular mapping of Alzheimer-type dementia in Down's syndrome. *Annals of Neurology, 43*(3), 380–383. https://doi.org/10.1002/ana.410430316

Rafii, M. S., Lukic, A. S., Andrews, R. D., Brewer, J., Rissman, R. A., Strother, S. C., Wernick, M. N., Pennington, C., Mobley, W. C., Ness, S., Matthews, D. C., & Down Syndrome Biomarker Initiative and the Alzheimer's Disease Neuroimaging Initiative (2017). PET imaging of Tau pathology and relationship to

Amyloid, longitudinal MRI, and cognitive change in Down syndrome: Results from the Down Syndrome Biomarker Initiative (DSBI). *Journal of Alzheimer's Disease: JAD*, *60*(2), 439–450. https://doi.org/10.3233/JAD-170390

Rahmani, Z., Blouin, J. L., Creau-Goldberg, N., Watkins, P. C., Mattei, J. F., Poissonnier, M., Prieur, M., Chettouh, Z., Nicole, A., & Aurias, A. (1989). Critical role of the D21S55 region on chromosome 21 in the pathogenesis of Down syndrome. *Proceedings of the National Academy of Sciences of the United States of America*, *86*(15), 5958–5962. https://doi.org/10.1073/pnas.86.15.5958

Rannikmäe, K., Samarasekera, N., Martînez-Gonzâlez, N. A., Al-Shahi Salman, R., & Sudlow, C. L. (2013). Genetics of cerebral amyloid angiopathy: systematic review and meta-analysis. *Journal of Neurology, Neurosurgery, and Psychiatry*, *84*(8), 901–908. https://doi.org/10.1136/jnnp-2012-303898

Raz, N., Torres, I. J., Briggs, S. D., Spencer, W. D., Thornton, A. E., Loken, W. J., Gunning, F. M., McQuain, J. D., Driesen, N. R., & Acker, J. D. (1995). Selective neuroanatomic abnormalities in Down's syndrome and their cognitive correlates: Evidence from MRI morphometry. *Neurology*, *45*(2), 356–366. https://doi.org/10.1212/wnl.45.2.356

Reeves, R. H., Yao, J., Crowley, M. R., Buck, S., Zhang, X., Yarowsky, P., Gearhart, J. D., & Hilt, D. C. (1994). Astrocytosis and axonal proliferation in the hippocampus of S100b transgenic mice. *Proceedings of the National Academy of Sciences of the United States of America*, *91*(12), 5359–5363. https://doi.org/10.1073/pnas.91.12.5359

Reijmer, Y. D., van Veluw, S. J., & Greenberg, S. M. (2016). Ischemic brain injury in cerebral amyloid angiopathy. *Journal of Cerebral Blood Flow and Metabolism: Official Journal of the International Society of Cerebral Blood Flow and Metabolism*, *36*(1), 40–54. https://doi.org/10.1038/jcbfm.2015.88

Rodrigues, A. N., Coelho, L. C., Goncalves, W. L., Gouvea, S. A., Vasconcellos, M. J., Cunha, R. S., & Abreu, G. R. (2011). Stiffness of the large arteries in individuals with and without Down syndrome. *Vascular Health and Risk Management*, *7*, 375–381. https://doi.org/10.2147/VHRM.S21273

Royston, M. C., McKenzie, J. E., Gentleman, S. M., Sheng, J. G., Mann, D. M., Griffin, W. S., & Mrak, R. E. (1999). Overexpression of s100beta in Down's syndrome: Correlation with patient age and with beta-amyloid deposition. *Neuropathology and Applied Neurobiology*, *25*(5), 387–393. https://doi.org/10.1046/j.1365-2990.1999.00196.x

Ryoo, S. R., Jeong, H. K., Radnaabazar, C., Yoo, J. J., Cho, H. J., Lee, H. W., Kim, I. S., Cheon, Y. H., Ahn, Y. S., Chung, S. H., & Song, W. J. (2007). DYRK1A-mediated hyperphosphorylation of Tau. A functional link between Down syndrome and Alzheimer disease. *Journal of Biological Chemistry*, *282*(48), 34850–34857. https://doi.org/10.1074/jbc.M707358200

Sadowski, M., Wisniewski, H. M., Tarnawski, M., Kozlowski, P. B., Lach, B., & Wegiel, J. (1999). Entorhinal cortex of aged subjects with Down's syndrome shows severe neuronal loss caused by neurofibrillary pathology. *Acta Neuropathologica*, *97*(2), 156–164. https://doi.org/10.1007/s004010050968

Schliebs, R., & Arendt, T. (2011). The cholinergic system in aging and neuronal degeneration. *Behavioural Brain Research*, *221*(2), 555–563. https://doi.org/10.1016/j.bbr.2010.11.058

Schöll, M., Lockhart, S. N., Schonhaut, D. R., O'Neil, J. P., Janabi, M., Ossenkoppele, R., Baker, S. L., Vogel, J. W., Faria, J., Schwimmer, H. D., Rabinovici, G. D., & Jagust W. J. (2016). PET Imaging of Tau deposition in the aging human brain. *Neuron*, *89*(5), 971–982.

Schupf, N., Patel, B., Silverman, W., Zigman, W. B., Zhong, N., Tycko, B., Mehta, P. D., & Mayeux, R. (2001). Elevated plasma amyloid beta-peptide 1-42 and onset of dementia in adults with Down syndrome. *Neuroscience Letters*, *301*(3), 199–203. https://doi.org/10.1016/s0304-3940(01)01657-3

Schupf, N., & Sergievsky, G. H. (2002). Genetic and host factors for dementia in Down's syndrome. *The British Journal of Psychiatry: The Journal of Mental Science*, *180*, 405–410. https://doi.org/10.1192/bjp.180.5.405

Schwarz, A. J., Yu, P., Miller, B. B., Shcherbinin, S., Dickson, J., Navitsky, M., Joshi, A. D., Devous, M. D., Sr, & Mintun, M. S. (2016). Regional profiles of the candidate tau PET ligand 18F-AV-1451 recapitulate key features of Braak histopathological stages. *Brain: A Journal of Neurology*, *139*(Pt 5), 1539–1550. https://doi.org/10.1093/brain/aww023

Selinfreund, R. H., Barger, S. W., Welsh, M. J., & Van Eldik, L. J. (1990). Antisense inhibition of glial S100 beta production results in alterations in cell morphology, cytoskeletal organization, and cell proliferation. *Journal of Cell Biology*, *111*(5 Pt 1), 2021–2028. https://doi.org/10.1083/jcb.111.5.2021

Selkoe D. J. (1994). Normal and abnormal biology of the beta-amyloid precursor protein. *Annual Review of Neuroscience*, *17*, 489–517. https://doi.org/10.1146/annurev.ne.17.030194.002421

Selkoe D. J. (2001). Alzheimer's disease: Genes, proteins, and therapy. *Physiological Reviews, 81*(2), 741–766. https://doi.org/10.1152/physrev.2001.81.2.741

Shindoh, N., Kudoh, J., Maeda, H., Yamaki, A., Minoshima, S., Shimizu, Y., & Shimizu, N. (1996). Cloning of a human homolog of the Drosophila minibrain/rat Dyrk gene from "the Down syndrome critical region" of chromosome 21. *Biochemical and Biophysical Research Communications, 225*(1), 92–99. https://doi.org/10.1006/bbrc.1996.1135

Sinai, A., Mokrysz, C., Bernal, J., Bohnen, I., Bonell, S., Courtenay, K., Dodd, K., Gazizova, D., Hassiotis, A., Hillier, R., McBrien, J., McCarthy, J., Mukherji, K., Naeem, A., Perez-Achiaga, N., Rantell, K., Sharma, V., Thomas, D., Walker, Z., Whitham, S., . . . Strydom, A. (2018). Predictors of age of diagnosis and survival of Alzheimer's disease in Down syndrome. *Journal of Alzheimer's Disease: JAD, 61*(2), 717–728. https://doi.org/10.3233/JAD-170624

Sisodia S. S. (1992). Beta-amyloid precursor protein cleavage by a membrane-bound protease. *Proceedings of the National Academy of Sciences of the United States of America, 89*(13), 6075–6079. https://doi.org/10.1073/pnas.89.13.6075

Song, W. J., Song, E. A., Choi, S. H., Baik, H. H., Jin, B. K., Kim, J. H., & Chung, S. H. (2013). Dyrk1A-mediated phosphorylation of RCAN1 promotes the formation of insoluble RCAN1 aggregates. *Neuroscience Letters, 554*, 135–140. https://doi.org/10.1016/j.neulet.2013.08.066

Song, W. J., Sternberg, L. R., Kasten-Sportès, C., Keuren, M. L., Chung, S. H., Slack, A. C., Miller, D. E., Glover, T. W., Chiang, P. W., Lou, L., & Kurnit, D. M. (1996). Isolation of human and murine homologues of the Drosophila minibrain gene: human homologue maps to 21q22.2 in the Down syndrome "critical region." *Genomics, 38*(3), 331–339. https://doi.org/10.1006/geno.1996.0636

Stoltzner, S. E., Grenfell, T. J., Mori, C., Wisniewski, K. E., Wisniewski, T. M., Selkoe, D. J., & Lemere, C. A. (2000). Temporal accrual of complement proteins in amyloid plaques in Down's syndrome with Alzheimer's disease. *American Journal of Pathology, 156*(2), 489–499. https://doi.org/10.1016/S0002-9440(10)64753-0

Sturgeon, X., Le, T., Ahmed, M. M., & Gardiner, K. J. (2012). Pathways to cognitive deficits in Down syndrome. *Progress in Brain Research, 197*, 73–100. https://doi.org/10.1016/B978-0-444-54299-1.00005-4

Sun, X., He, G., & Song, W. (2006). BACE2, as a novel APP theta-secretase, is not responsible for the pathogenesis of Alzheimer's disease in Down syndrome. *FASEB journal: Official publication of the Federation of American Societies for Experimental Biology, 20*(9), 1369–1376. https://doi.org/10.1096/fj.05-5632com

Takashima, S., Becker, L. E., Armstrong, D. L., & Chan, F. (1981). Abnormal neuronal development in the visual cortex of the human fetus and infant with down's syndrome. A quantitative and qualitative Golgi study. *Brain Research, 225*(1), 1–21. https://doi.org/10.1016/0006-8993(81)90314-0

Takashima, S., Iida, K., Mito, T., & Arima, M. (1994). Dendritic and histochemical development and ageing in patients with Down's syndrome. *Journal of Intellectual Disability Research: JIDR, 38*(Pt 3), 265–273. https://doi.org/10.1111/j.1365-2788.1994.tb00394.x

Teipel, S. J., Alexander, G. E., Schapiro, M. B., Möller, H. J., Rapoport, S. I., & Hampel, H. (2004). Age-related cortical grey matter reductions in non-demented Down's syndrome adults determined by MRI with voxel-based morphometry. *Brain: A Journal of Neurology, 127*(Pt 4), 811–824. https://doi.org/10.1093/brain/awh101

Teipel, S. J., & Hampel, H. (2006). Neuroanatomy of Down syndrome in vivo: A model of preclinical Alzheimer's disease. *Behavior Genetics, 36*(3), 405–415. https://doi.org/10.1007/s10519-006-9047-x

Tejedor, F. J., & Hämmerle, B. (2011). MNB/DYRK1A as a multiple regulator of neuronal development. *The FEBS Journal, 278*(2), 223–235. https://doi.org/10.1111/j.1742-4658.2010.07954.x

Terry, A. V., Jr, & Buccafusco, J. J. (2003). The cholinergic hypothesis of age and Alzheimer's disease-related cognitive deficits: Recent challenges and their implications for novel drug development. *Journal of Pharmacology and Experimental Therapeutics, 306*(3), 821–827. https://doi.org/10.1124/jpet.102.041616

Thal, D. R., Rüb, U., Orantes, M., & Braak, H. (2002). Phases of A beta-deposition in the human brain and its relevance for the development of AD. *Neurology, 58*(12), 1791–1800. https://doi.org/10.1212/wnl.58.12.1791

Vassar R. (2004). BACE1: The beta-secretase enzyme in Alzheimer's disease. *Journal of Molecular Neuroscience: MN, 23*(1–2), 105–114. https://doi.org/10.1385/JMN:23:1-2:105

Vassar, R., Bennett, B. D., Babu-Khan, S., Kahn, S., Mendiaz, E. A., Denis, P., Teplow, D. B., Ross, S., Amarante, P., Loeloff, R., Luo, Y., Fisher, S., Fuller, J., Edenson, S., Lile, J., Jarosinski, M. A., Biere, A. L., Curran, E., Burgess, T., Louis, J. C., . . . Citron, M. (1999). Beta-secretase cleavage of Alzheimer's amyloid precursor protein by the transmembrane aspartic protease BACE. *Science* (New York, N.Y.), *286*(5440), 735–741. https://doi.org/10.1126/science.286.5440.735

Vinters H. V. (1987). Cerebral amyloid angiopathy. A critical review. *Stroke, 18*(2), 311–324. https://doi.org/10.1161/01.str.18.2.311

Webb, R. L., & Murphy, M. P. (2012). β-Secretases, Alzheimer's disease, and Down syndrome. *Current Gerontology and Geriatrics Research, 2012*, 362839. https://doi.org/10.1155/2012/362839

Wegiel, J., Dowjat, K., Kaczmarski, W., Kuchna, I., Nowicki, K., Frackowiak, J., Mazur Kolecka, B., Wegiel, J., Silverman, W. P., Reisberg, B., Deleon, M., Wisniewski, T., Gong, C. X., Liu, F., Adayev, T., Chen-Hwang, M. C., & Hwang, Y. W. (2008). The role of overexpressed DYRK1A protein in the early onset of neurofibrillary degeneration in Down syndrome. *Acta Neuropathologica, 116*(4), 391–407. https://doi.org/10.1007/s00401-008-0419-6

Wegiel, J., Kaczmarski, W., Barua, M., Kuchna, I., Nowicki, K., Wang, K. C., Wegiel, J., Yang, S. M., Frackowiak, J., Mazur-Kolecka, B., Silverman, W. P., Reisberg, B., Monteiro, I., de Leon, M., Wisniewski, T., Dalton, A., Lai, F., Hwang, Y. W., Adayev, T., Liu, F., . . . Gong, C. X. (2011). Link between DYRK1A overexpression and several-fold enhancement of neurofibrillary degeneration with 3-repeat tau protein in Down syndrome. *Journal of Neuropathology and Experimental Neurology, 70*(1), 36–50. https://doi.org/10.1097/NEN.0b013e318202bfa1

Wegiel, J., Kuchna, I., Nowicki, K., Frackowiak, J., Dowjat, K., Silverman, W. P., Reisberg, B., DeLeon, M., Wisniewski, T., Adayev, T., Chen-Hwang, M. C., & Hwang, Y. W. (2004). Cell type- and brain structure-specific patterns of distribution of minibrain kinase in human brain. *Brain Research, 1010*(1–2), 69–80. https://doi.org/10.1016/j.brainres.2004.03.008

Whitaker-Azmitia, P. M., Wingate, M., Borella, A., Gerlai, R., Roder, J., & Azmitia, E. C. (1997). Transgenic mice overexpressing the neurotrophic factor S-100 beta show neuronal cytoskeletal and behavioral signs of altered aging processes: Implications for Alzheimer's disease and Down's syndrome. *Brain Research, 776*(1–2), 51–60. https://doi.org/10.1016/s0006-8993(97)01002-0

White, N. S., Alkire, M. T., & Haier, R. J. (2003). A voxel-based morphometric study of nondemented adults with Down Syndrome. *NeuroImage, 20*(1), 393–403. https://doi.org/10.1016/s1053-8119(03)00273-8

Wilcock D. M. (2012). Neuroinflammation in the aging down syndrome brain; lessons from Alzheimer's disease. *Current Gerontology and Geriatrics Research, 2012*, 170276. https://doi.org/10.1155/2012/170276

Wilcock, D. M., & Griffin, W. S. (2013). Down's syndrome, neuroinflammation, and Alzheimer neuropathogenesis. *Journal of Neuroinflammation, 10*, 84. https://doi.org/10.1186/1742-2094-10-84

Wilcock, D. M., Hurban, J., Helman, A. M., Sudduth, T. L., McCarty, K. L., Beckett, T. L., Ferrell, J. C., Murphy, M. P., Abner, E. L., Schmitt, F. A., & Head, E. (2015). Down syndrome individuals with Alzheimer's disease have a distinct neuroinflammatory phenotype compared to sporadic Alzheimer's disease. *Neurobiology of Aging, 36*(9), 2468–2474. https://doi.org/10.1016/j.neurobiolaging.2015.05.016

Wilcock, D. M., Schmitt, F. A., & Head, E. (2016). Cerebrovascular contributions to aging and Alzheimer's disease in Down syndrome. *Biochimica et Biophysica Acta, 1862*(5), 909–914. https://doi.org/10.1016/j.bbadis.2015.11.007

Wiseman, F. K., Al-Janabi, T., Hardy, J., Karmiloff-Smith, A., Nizetic, D., Tybulewicz, V. L., Fisher, E. M., & Strydom, A. (2015). A genetic cause of Alzheimer disease: Mechanistic insights from Down syndrome. Nature reviews. *Neuroscience, 16*(9), 564–574. https://doi.org/10.1038/nrn3983

Wisniewski, K., Howe, J., Williams, D. G., & Wisniewski, H. M. (1978). Precocious aging and dementia in patients with Down's syndrome. *Biological Psychiatry, 13*(5), 619–627.

Wisniewski, K. E., Wisniewski, H. M., & Wen, G. Y. (1985). Occurrence of neuropathological changes and dementia of Alzheimer's disease in Down's syndrome. *Annals of Neurology, 17*(3), 278–282. https://doi.org/10.1002/ana.410170310

Xue, Q. S., & Streit, W. J. (2011). Microglial pathology in Down syndrome. *Acta Neuropathologica, 122*(4), 455–466. https://doi.org/10.1007/s00401-011-0864-5

Yang, L. B., Lindholm, K., Yan, R., Citron, M., Xia, W., Yang, X. L., Beach, T., Sue, L., Wong, P., Price, D., Li, R., & Shen, Y. (2003). Elevated beta-secretase expression and enzymatic activity detected in sporadic Alzheimer disease. *Nature Medicine, 9*(1), 3–4. https://doi.org/10.1038/nm0103-3

Ylä-Herttuala, S., Luoma, J., Nikkari, T., & Kivimäki, T. (1989). Down's syndrome and atherosclerosis. *Atherosclerosis, 76*(2–3), 269–272. https://doi.org/10.1016/0021-9150(89)90110-x

Zigman W. B. (2013). Atypical aging in Down syndrome. *Developmental Disabilities Research Reviews, 18*(1), 51–67. https://doi.org/10.1002/ddrr.1128

Zigman, W. B., Schupf, N., Sersen, E., & Silverman, W. (1996). Prevalence of dementia in adults with and without Down syndrome. *American Journal of Mental Retardation: AJMR, 100*(4), 403–412.

CHAPTER

17 Co-occurrence of Autism Spectrum Disorder and Down Syndrome

Cory Shulman

Abstract

Autism spectrum disorder (ASD) refers to a heterogeneous condition characterized by deficits in social communication and the presence of restricted, repetitive, and stereotypic behaviors, interests, or activities. While some neurodevelopmental disorders have a well-established correlation with ASD, people continue to believe that because individuals with Down syndrome are characteristically perceived as affectionate and engaging, a diagnosis of ASD is contradictory. However, some people with Down syndrome indeed do meet diagnostic criteria for ASD and this chapter examines the research literature regarding Down syndrome and ASD, presenting information regarding the establishment of a diagnosis of ASD in individuals with Down syndrome and research techniques to understand the dual diagnosis of ASD and Down syndrome. Behavioral manifestations of ASD in Down syndrome are presented and research methodologies which address possible underlying mechanisms in Down syndrome and ASD are surveyed. Finally, the need for specification of behavioral profiles for individuals with a dual diagnosis of Down syndrome and ASD, in order to design and implement appropriate therapeutic interventions, is highlighted. Once a person with Down syndrome is diagnosed with ASD, he or she should automatically receive a combined treatment approach incorporating direct instruction, natural environment teaching, and incidental teaching. The manifestation of ASD in individuals with Down syndrome can shed light on our understanding of how ASD and intellectual disability are associated and what impact these diagnoses have on individuals and their families. This knowledge can help shape public policy and our research agenda in the areas of ASD, intellectual impairment, and Down syndrome.

Key Words: Down syndrome, autism spectrum disorder, ASD, dual diagnosis, assessment, research methodologies, co-occurring conditions, dual diagnosis

Introduction

Autism spectrum disorder (ASD) refers to a heterogeneous condition characterized by deficits in social communication and the presence of restricted, repetitive, and stereotypic behaviors, interests, or activities (American Psychological Association [APA], 2013). The heterogeneity of ASD expresses itself in the severity of the ASD symptoms as well as the co-occurrence of ASD and other disorders. While some neurodevelopmental disorders have a well-established correlation with ASD, ASD is underdiagnosed among persons with Down syndrome. This may be partially due to the fact that individuals with Down syndrome are characteristically perceived as being affectionate and outgoing, which would appear to be incompatible with an ASD diagnosis (Fidler, 2005; Roizen, 2001), which manifests itself in difficulties interacting with others (Constantino & Charman, 2016; Mundy, Sigman, Ungerer, & Sherman, 1986). Thus, the behavioral phenotypes of individuals with Down syndrome and those with ASD seem contradictory (Ghaziuddin, Tsai, & Ghaziuddin, 1992; Hepburn, Philofsky, Fidler, & Rogers, 2008; Howlin, Wing, & Gould, 1995; Rasmussen, Borjesson, Wentz, & Gillberg, 2001). However, some people with Down syndrome are not friendly, affectionate, or extroverted (Fidler, 2005; Kent, Evans, Paul, & Sharp, 1999), and among the 10–20% of persons with Down syndrome who display significant behavioral problems (Chapman & Hesketh, 2000; Flynt & Yule, 1994), some may have undiagnosed co-occurring ASD. Therefore, the purpose of this chapter is to examine the literature regarding Down syndrome and ASD, presenting what we know about how individuals with Down syndrome and ASD compare to those with Down syndrome only and to those individuals with ASD without Down syndrome (Hamner et al., 2019; Wester Oxelgren et al., 2019).

The observation that many individuals with Down syndrome tend to be engaging and affectionate has been postulated as a protective factor against developing psychiatric disorders as compared to others with intellectual disabilities of a different etiology (Dykens, 2007; Mantry et al., 2008). In a large study comparing adults with intellectual disability who were matched on chronological age and developmental quotient, 360 adults with Down syndrome displayed lower rates of aggression, antisocial behavior, property destruction, disturbing others at night, attention seeking, untruthfulness, and excessive activity than 1829 adults with intellectual disability with various other etiologies, including fragile X, tuberous sclerosis, Prader-Willi, and others (Collacott, Cooper, Branford, & McGrother, 1998). Although individuals with Down syndrome have recognized language impairments, their social communication and ability to establish relationships have been found to be comparable to typically developing individuals matched for mental age by some researchers (e.g., Laws & Bishop, 2004). Others have specified some social processing deficits in recognizing facial expressions, particularly surprise and fear (Hippolyte, Barisnikov, & Van der Linden, 2008; Williams, Wishart, Pitcairn, & Willis, 2005; Wishart & Pitcairn, 2000). As compared to typically developing children matched for overall mental age, children with Down syndrome appear to spend more of their time involved in functional and symbolic play and request objects and help more frequently (Kasari & Freeman, 2001). These findings help to explain the fact that children with Down syndrome and ASD had better interactional skills with their peers than children with ASD only (Hamner et al., 2019).

Autism Spectrum Disorder

Over the last 40 years, the definition of autism has undergone major transformations that have shaped our current understanding of the autism spectrum. With the changes in the conceptualization of ASD, the diagnostic process no longer simply relates to the question "is this ASD or not?" but rather must involve consideration of the fact that ASD is associated with genetic syndromes, including fragile X, Angelman, Cornelai de Lange, 22q11 deletion, Phelan-McDermid, and others (Coleman & Gillberg, 2012). During the past more than 70 years since autism was first coined as a diagnostic term by Dr. Leo Kanner (1943), many attempts have been made to operationalize its clinical manifestations. The developments in diagnosis of autism are reflected in changing terminology used over the years. From the monolithic perception of "autism," the field has dealt with "pervasive developmental disorders" and "autistic disorders," culminating in 2013 with the inclusive term of ASD. Since much of the research presented here deals with the terminology in use when the research was performed, the term "autism" appears as well as "ASD" throughout the paper. Findings reported from earlier research will be discussed with the term autism if the findings reflect something essential to that time in the history of our understanding of ASD, whereas the term ASD will be used if the findings are still relevant today, even if it was not used in the original studies.

ASD is used to describe a constellation of behaviorally identified criteria that cluster together in various patterns and severities. Kanner (1943) and Asperger (1944) first identified autism as a diagnostic category over 75 years ago. Although Kanner's original description of autism was more widely known and influential in American psychiatry, Kanner's and Asperger's work appeared almost simultaneously, possibly emerging from their common Austrian professional milieu and through shared colleagues (for a review, see Silberman, 2015). Since Kanner's original description based on the profiles of 11 children with unusual social interaction, difficulties in communication, and focused and repetitive behaviors, much effort has gone into characterizing the diagnostic criteria of autism. The history of diagnosing autism reflects the need for specification of the phenomenological characteristics of autism, or in other words, the presence or absence of those behaviors that define it.

Although ASD is one of the most common neurodevelopmental disorders, with one in every 59 individuals in the US identified as having ASD (Baio et al., 2018; Fombonne, 2018), it is also quite heterogeneous, making the identification and diagnosis of ASD a complex process. Autism was first conceptualized as a neurodevelopmental disorder, which appears in early childhood and continues throughout the lifespan, in the third edition of the *Diagnostic and Statistical Manual of Mental Disorders* (*DSM*; APA, 1980). In 1980, around the time that research about comorbidity of Down syndrome and autism began, the American Psychiatric Association defined autism as a pervasive developmental disorder for the first time and attempted to classify different types of autism based on the age of onset. The subtypes of autism consisted of early infantile autism, early childhood onset autism, residual autism, and atypical autism, a sub-threshold category (APA, 1980). In the *DSM-IIIR* (APA, 1987) the category Pervasive Developmental Disorders was retained, but the subcategories based on age of onset were eliminated. Instead, a diagnosis of autism was established when the individual met eight of the 16 characteristics in three areas of impairments (i.e., social impairment, communication and symbolic dysfunction and repetitive and restrictive behaviors). With these revisions (APA, 1987), the diagnostic concept of autism became substantially broader and the prevalence of autism increased (Fombonne, 2009). With the publication of the fourth edition of the *DSM* (APA, 1994), five syndromes appeared under the umbrella of pervasive developmental disorders (i.e., autism, childhood disintegrative disorder, Rett syndrome, Asperger syndrome, and pervasive developmental disorder—not otherwise specified), all characterized by marked social impairments and repetitive, restrictive behaviors. These editions of the *DSM* made it difficult to establish dual diagnoses of autism in children with other neurodevelopmental disorders (e.g., attention deficit disorder) and other intellectual impairments (e.g., Down syndrome), as the diagnosis of autism was based on establishing a differential diagnosis among the Pervasive Developmental Disorder syndromes. The fifth edition of the *DSM* (2013) combines the syndromes under one overarching spectrum of autism disorders and is both more specific, making it easier to determine if an individual meets ASD diagnostic criteria, and broader, allowing for individuals with other diagnoses to receive an additional diagnosis of ASD.

Currently, the diagnostic criteria for ASD are based on the fifth edition of the *DSM* (*DSM-5*; APA, 2013) and address some of the challenges of diagnosing ASD that have arisen over the years. The changes in the newest edition are based on research findings and emphasize that diagnoses should rely on information collected through the use of standardized diagnostic instruments, resulting in a reliable and valid diagnostic category (Volkmar, Reichow, Westphal, & Mandell, 2014). The most outstanding change is expressed in the inclusion of five distinct pervasive developmental disorders which appeared in the *DSM-IV* (APA, 1994, 2000) within one overarching category of ASD. Thus, autistic disorder, Asperger's disorder, Rett's disorder, childhood disintegrative disorder, and pervasive developmental disorder—not otherwise specified are no longer separate diagnostic classifications under the heading of pervasive developmental disorders, thereby eliminating the need for differential diagnosis within the autism spectrum. In addition, the *DSM-5* diagnostic criteria for ASD moved from a triad of impairments (impairments in social interactions, in communication, and repetitive restrictive patterns of behavior) to a dyad of impairments by combining the social and communication domains into a domain of impairments in social communication. Another significant change is the necessity of meeting all three of the social communication criteria, so that all individuals with a diagnosis of ASD share a core of similar impairments in social communication.

While the *DSM* is accepted primarily in the United States, the World Health Organization (WHO), which sees its primary responsibility as achieving an international approach to public health, issued the *International Classification of Diseases* (*ICD*; WHO, 1992, 2004). Health professionals from over 180 countries shared knowledge and experience to establish the diagnostic criteria as they appear in the *ICD-10*. With regard to ASD, a purposeful endeavor was undertaken to unify the *DSM-IV* (1994) and the *ICD-10* (1992) criteria as much as possible with the aim of clarifying autism symptomatology worldwide. Despite the similarities in ASD diagnostic criteria, *ICD-10* criteria are accepted in European countries and are typically the basis on which countries make their own local adaptations (e.g., Chinese Classification of Mental Disorders (CCMD); Chen, 2002).

While the definition of ASD has evolved over time, the core symptoms have remained largely the same. In the *DSM-5* (APA, 2013), social communication criteria are defined as (1) deficits in social-emotional reciprocity or the exchange of social behaviors, which include difficulties sharing enjoyment and interests with others, difficulties sustaining a back-and-forth in conversation, and reduced initiating and responding to social interaction; (2) deficits in using and understanding nonverbal communication; and (3) deficits in understanding and maintaining social relationships, which includes having interest in peers, understanding the nature of friendships and other common relationships, understanding social cues and norms, and sharing imaginative play with peers. Restricted, repetitive behaviors and fixated interests include (1) repetitive or stereotyped motor movements or use of objects (e.g., lining up objects, repetitive interest in parts of objects) and/or speech (e.g., echolalia, idiosyncratic speech); (2) difficulties with changes in routines or rigid patterns of verbal or nonverbal behavior; (3) fixated, narrow interests that are unusual in intensity (e.g., perseverative interest in dinosaurs or anime) or focus (e.g., strong attachment to or preoccupation with unusual objects); and (4) unusual responses to sensory aspects of the environment, including both unusual interest in and seeking of sensory input (e.g., visual fascination with moving objects, excessive smelling or touching of objects) and being highly sensitive or aversive to sensory input (e.g., unable to tolerate ordinary noises or textures).

Diagnostic criteria in *DSM-5* are accompanied by specifiers and modifiers, which are expected to provide information that is relevant to service decisions for the individual and to identify subgroupings of ASD. The system of specifiers for ASD includes a functional severity score across a three-level scale (requiring support, requiring substantial support, requiring very substantial support), based on the impact of ASD symptoms on everyday functioning. The specifiers, modifiers and severity scores help characterize the presentation of ASD in a particular individual. In addition, the specifiers and modifiers include information about accompanying intellectual disability; other neurodevelopmental, mental, behavioral, genetic and/or medical conditions; language impairment; and environmental factors. As the *ICD-10* (WHO, 1992, 2004) has not yet published its latest revision, its diagnostic criteria remain the triad of impairments which characterized the diagnostic criteria of ASD in the *DSM-IV* (APA, 1994, 2000).

Diagnostic Assessment in ASD

The heterogeneity of ASD complicates the diagnostic assessment process, necessitating a multidisciplinary assessment. Because ASD is a behavioral disorder with no medical test, the team should include an experienced clinician with specific and extensive expertise in diagnosing and treating ASD, as the diagnosis of ASD is impacted by the clinician's experience and skill in identifying characteristics of ASD and other typical and atypical presentations and by the instruments used to measure these behaviors. The consensus best-practice guidelines for diagnostic evaluation of ASD recommend a multidisciplinary evaluation that gathers information across multiple sources, including at a minimum direct observation of the child, a detailed parent interview for historical and current status, and direct assessment of developmental/cognitive skills (Esler & Ruble, 2015; Hammond, Campbell, & Ruble, 2013; Huerta & Lord, 2012; Ozonoff, Goodlin-Jones, & Solomon, 2005). The diagnosis of ASD is more challenging when the individual being evaluated has some form of intellectual disability (Bölte & Poustka, 2002; Osterling, Dawson, & Munson, 2002). Care must be taken to ensure that the observed behaviors are not just the result of profound intellectual impairment; conversely, caution should be exercised not to assume that observed behaviors are the result of severe intellectual disability only.

Recommendations include conducting a standardized assessment of the individual's development in cognitive, adaptive, and language skills regardless of the age at which the evaluation is conducted. When assessing cognitive abilities, one essential consideration is that individuals with ASD have the greatest difficulty on tests involving the use of social language skills (Dawson et al., 2010), imitation (Rogers, Hepburn, Stackhouse, & Wehner, 2003), and joint attention (Mundy, Sigman, & Kasari, 1994). Their scores on these types of tasks are likely to be lower than scores on tasks requiring skills that are often strengths in individuals with ASD (e.g., perception, rote memory). Information obtained about the individual's behavior and functioning in natural settings, such as from educational or employment frameworks, complements the information gathered during the diagnostic assessment and can be very helpful in making the diagnosis. Assessment should be an ongoing, carefully designed multidisciplinary process that captures the individual's functional, cognitive, intellectual, and language abilities and behavioral profile.

Diagnostic Instruments in ASD

The instruments used to establish the diagnosis are the central component of the diagnostic evaluation, as they are the conduit of pertinent information regarding the individual being assessed and the method of measurement. The correct instruments need to be chosen in order to avoid mismeasurement and/or misinformation. Better instruments yield more accurate, reliable, and valid information that can ultimately inform both researchers and clinicians. A short survey of the most widely used measures follows, focusing on some of the strengths and weaknesses of each.

The Autism Diagnostic Observation Schedule, second edition (ADOS-2: Lord et al., 2000) is considered the gold-standard instrument in diagnosing ASD as it is based on clinical observation and direct testing of the individual's behavior during semistructured activities which allow for the assessment of communication, social interaction, restrictive and repetitive behaviors and play in younger children, and imagination in adolescents and adults. It is comprised of five modules and the clinician chooses the appropriate module according to the individual's age and expressive language ability. Each module takes between 45–60 minutes to administer, and since the individual's levels of development and speech are taken into account in choosing the correct module, the issues that arise during the assessment are not considered to be the sequelae of developmental delay or language and speech limitations. Each module consists of a variety of structured and unstructured activities that are designed to elicit the social communication and repetitive behavior symptoms of ASD relevant to the language level and age appropriate to that module. Examiners take notes during the ADOS-2 administration and the codes are rated immediately following administration. Guidelines are provided for deciding on the rating for each code and algorithms are provided for formulating ADOS-2 classifications. The ADOS ratings provide summary scores but they are one part of the multidisciplinary evaluation of individuals for whom there is a suspicion of ASD, and although they provide a classification, the professionals involved in the evaluation must decide on the final diagnosis using their best clinical judgment. The ADOS-2 scores can be mapped onto the *DSM-5* diagnostic criteria for ASD.

The Autism Diagnostic Interview-Revised (ADI-R: Rutter, LeCouteur, & Lord, 2003), another gold-standard instrument for diagnosing ASD, is an extended, semistructured interview of a parent or caregiver who is knowledgeable about the individual's behavior, development, and functioning currently and in the past, focusing on the period from 4 to 5 years of age. The individual being assessed must have a mental age of at least 2 years. The ADI-R is administered by an experienced clinician and produces information needed to diagnose ASD, as well as characterizing current behavior patterns. It consists of 93 questions focusing primarily on developmental and medical history, language and communication, reciprocal social interactions, and restricted and repetitive behaviors, including preoccupations and interests. The interview takes approximately 1 1/2 to 3 hours to complete. The interviewer records and codes detailed responses of the informant using the interview protocol. After the protocol is coded, the codes are transferred to the appropriate algorithm depending upon the purpose of the interview. The two algorithms are used for different purposes: (1) a diagnostic algorithm for establishing an ASD diagnosis and (2) a current behavior algorithm for characterizing present behavior patterns. The diagnostic algorithm generates a classification of either ASD or nonspectrum. However, even the ADOS-2 and the ADI-R are limited in their ability to accurately diagnose ASD in individuals with profound intellectual impairment (Charman & Gotham, 2013; Gotham, Risi, Pickles, & Lord, 2007; Risi et al., 2006), so that they are not reliable when assessing very severely intellectually impaired children with Down syndrome.

The Childhood Autism Rating Scale, second edition (CARS-2; Schopler, van Bourgondien, Wellman & Love, 2010) comprises three forms. The CARS-2 standard form is for ages 6 and younger with an estimated IQ of 79 or lower. The second form, the

CARS-2 high functioning version, is designed for those 6 and older with an estimated IQ of 80 or higher. The third version of the CARS-2 questionnaire is for parents or caregivers, and is designed to assist in gathering information regarding behaviors related to ASD. Each version of the CARS-2 consists of 15 items associated with the diagnosis of ASD.

When assessing for possible co-occurring ASD in children with Down syndrome, one essential consideration is that many very young children who undergo an ASD assessment also have some general developmental delay. The complexity of understanding the overlap between ASD and intellectual disability is more pronounced in younger children, for whom distinguishing social-communication limitations above and beyond global developmental delays is difficult even for the most experienced clinicians (Bishop, Thurm, Farmer, & Lord, 2016). The common features of individuals with intellectual disability only and those with intellectual disability and ASD include cognitive and language delays, difficulties in behavioral regulation, aggressive outbursts, and/or self-injurious behavior. Despite the many similarities, there are also some key distinctions that may be helpful in establishing a differential or dual diagnosis. Often the cognitive profile of individuals with intellectual disability only will be more evenly distributed than the more scattered cognitive profile of individuals with intellectual disability and ASD. Likewise, although language and communication skills are delayed in intellectual disability without ASD, these individuals experience fewer atypical behaviors and manifest more compensatory strategies. Social skills and adaptive functioning in individuals with intellectual disability tend to be similar to their mental age, whereas in individuals with intellectual disability and ASD they tend to be lower than expected based on mental age (Perry, Flanagan, Geier, & Freeman, 2009). Early history can also be quite informative for differential diagnosis. Parents of both groups often become concerned because of delayed language development and/or delayed crawling/walking (Bishop et al., 2016), but parents of children with ASD often describe social concerns such as poor eye contact, limited social smiling, and difficulty engaging, whereas parents of children with intellectual disability typically describe appropriate eye contact and report that their children can play simple reciprocal games with adults.

Adapting the ASD Assessment for Individuals With Down Syndrome

In an attempt to clarify some of these overlapping diagnostic issues in children with ASD and Down syndrome, Hamner et al. (2019) assessed co-occurring ASD in children (mean chronological age 6 years old) with Down syndrome using the ADOS for groups of children with ASD and Down syndrome, ASD only, and Down syndrome only. They found specific cognitive profiles for each group, with those with ASD and Down syndrome exhibiting greater cognitive impairment on both verbal and nonverbal measures. In addition, those with ASD and Down syndrome had less social impairment with peers than those with ASD only. A similar pattern was reported by Starr, Berument, Tomlins, Papanikolaou, and Rutter (2005), who noted that individuals with both Down syndrome and ASD tended to show sociability and emotional responsiveness with more reciprocity and a wider range of facial expressions than is typically displayed in individuals with ASD without Down syndrome, which may point to a possible reason for missing ASD in those with Down syndrome. Many of these phenomena are also seen in individuals with fragile X and ASD (Abbeduto, McDuffie, & Thurm, 2014), which may lead to appropriate research in individuals with Down syndrome and ASD.

Screening for Autism Spectrum Disorder Among Persons With Down Syndrome

The Autism Spectrum Screening Questionnaire (ASSQ; Ehlers, Gillberg, & Wing, 1999), which was originally developed to study the prevalence of Asperger syndrome, has been used with individuals with Down syndrome (Kent et al., 1999). The subjectivity of such instruments must be recognized, as recommended cutoffs vary somewhat from country to country and are dependent on whether parents or teachers are used as informants. Taking into consideration that the ASSQ is not a diagnostic instrument but rather a screener, several items were identified as characterizing those individuals with Down syndrome who went on to get an autism diagnosis according to *ICD-10* diagnostic criteria for autism. They included "clumsy with ill-coordinated movements and gestures," "compulsory repetitive behaviors," "lives in a world of own," and "has restricted idiosyncratic interests." These items may help develop a screener or adapt one already in use for use with young children with Down syndrome who may be at risk for ASD.

Ortiz et al. (2017) also tried to address the need for understanding early signs of ASD in children with Down syndrome in order to be able to screen for possible ASD in young children with Down syndrome. They used the Modified Checklist for Autism in Toddlers (M-CHAT; Robins, Fein, Barton, & Green, 2001), a screener for ASD, with the ADI-R (Rutter et al., 2003), a diagnostic instrument, to gather information about 10 children with Down syndrome with suspected ASD. The researchers watched and coded a 1- or 2-hour videotape of the child in natural interactions and identified six items as possible warning signs of ASD in Down syndrome children between the ages of birth and 5 years of age (Ortiz et al., 2017). They included (1) lack of shared attention, (2) lack of interest in others, (3) absence of gaze integration, (4) absence of imitation, (5) rituals such as repetitive actions or repetitive sentences, and (6) stereotypies. The findings from this study suggest the possibility of establishing a diagnosis of ASD in children with Down syndrome under the age of 5 years.

Diagnosing an Autism Spectrum Disorder in Down Syndrome

ASD in young children with Down syndrome may be overlooked, with the behavioral characteristics of ASD attributed to intellectual impairment. Differentiating young children with Down syndrome and ASD from those with Down syndrome alone may be especially challenging, as many professionals may believe that the social communication issues and behaviors seen in children with Down syndrome are attributable to the cognitive delays related to Down syndrome and not the result of autistic symptomatology. This is particularly salient in the domain of repetitive and restrictive patterns of behavior. For example, motor stereotypies and/or specific areas of interest have been documented in children with Down syndrome without a suspicion of co-occurring ASD (Harris, Mahone, & Singer, 2008). In order to address this difficulty, more developmentally sensitive criteria need to be established. This can be achieved by characterizing developmental and behavioral profiles associated with the dual diagnosis of Down syndrome and ASD. Researchers need to specify behaviors that appear in individuals with Down syndrome only, those with a diagnosis of ASD only, and those with both Down syndrome and ASD. Unfortunately, much of the published research on ASD in individuals with Down syndrome has not been based on comprehensive assessments as recommended for the diagnosis of ASD (Nachshen et al., 2008; Zwaigenbaum et al., 2009). In one example, Capone (2001, 2003) and Capone, Goyal, Ares, and Lannigan (2006) used the Aberrant Behavior Checklist (ABC; Aman & Singh, 1994) to describe differences in behavioral profiles among individuals with Down syndrome, those with ASD and those with Down syndrome and ASD, thus characterizing similarities and differences in these groups. Although the assessments reported in these studies did not follow best practices for ASD evaluations, they are informative, capturing correlated phenotypic differences among those with ASD and those with Down syndrome.

When parents of children with Down syndrome report that their child is not developing similarly to other children with Down syndrome (Capone, 2003), ASD should be considered as a possible co-occurring condition if the concerns are in the social communication domain and/or reflect repetitive and restricted behavior patterns. Parental reports of children with Down syndrome who are subsequently diagnosed with comorbid ASD depicted their children as seeming to prefer to play alone, often in an odd manner, not using language communicatively, and exhibiting repetitive behaviors, sometimes accompanied by obsessions (Reilly, 2009). This behavior is similar to the behavior reported by parents of children with ASD when they arrive for a diagnostic assessment (Lord, Rutter, & LeCouteur, 1994). Awareness of the possibility of an ASD–Down syndrome comorbid assessment facilitates the opportunity to provide intervention as early as possible. As early intervention among children with ASD is associated with better outcomes, children with Down syndrome who also have ASD must also be diagnosed as early as possible in order to begin interventions (Dawson et al., 2010).

ASD can be diagnosed as early as 2 years of age but that diagnosis usually occurs much later in children with severe developmental delay, typically around 5 or 6 years of age (Johnson & Myers, 2007; Mandell, Novak, & Zubritsky, 2005). The implications of not identifying ASD in children with Down syndrome are significant for both the individuals with Down syndrome and their families (Hodapp, Ricci, Ly, & Fidler, 2003; Kent et al., 1999). A failure to diagnose ASD in children with Down syndrome may result in inappropriate educational placement for these children and unnecessary emotional hardship for their parents (Ghaziuddin, 2000; Warner, Howlin, Salomone, Moss, & Charman, 2017). Without the ASD diagnosis, parents are prevented from accessing supports and interventions available to families with children with ASD (Bromley, Hare, Davison, & Emerson, 2004; Johnson & Myers, 2007; Moes & Frea, 2002; Siklos, & Kerns, 2006). Although the current trend is to diagnose ASD as early as possible, the early identification of ASD is not without its difficulties and dilemmas. These challenges may be even more complex in relation to identifying ASD in the population of individuals with Down syndrome. The difficulties inherent in the early diagnosis of ASD include the fact that some of the behaviors specified as criteria for a diagnosis of ASD may not be present in very young children or even in older children with significant developmental delay, such as those with Down syndrome, because they have not yet developed the prerequisite skills necessary for the behaviors associated with a diagnosis of ASD (Chawarshka & Volkmar, 2005; Stone et al., 1999). Despite this developmental gap, early recognition of possible ASD in young children with Down syndrome should remain a priority (Kent et al., 1999; Remington et al., 2007; Russa, Matthews, & Owen-DeSchryver, 2015).

Behavioral Profiles of Individuals With Co-occurring Down Syndrome and ASD

Once the comorbid diagnoses of ASD and Down syndrome have been established, the characterization of the profile of abilities and disabilities, and strengths and weaknesses, of the individual is necessary in order to inform intervention. In one example, Capone et al. (2006) used the ABC (Aman & Singh, 1994), to assess the behavioral profiles of 471 individuals with Down syndrome. Using *DSM-IV* criteria for pervasive developmental disorders, they identified 61 individuals who met diagnostic criteria for autism. The profiles that emerged from the ABC revealed that the persons with autism and Down syndrome had elevated scores on all the subscales of the ABC as compared to the persons with Down syndrome only, indicating more behavior problems. The hyperactivity and inappropriate speech subscales were not helpful in differentiating among the groups. The social items were most sensitive in identifying those with autism and Down syndrome. In a continuation of this study with 127 individuals with Down syndrome, Carter, Capone, Gray, Cox, and Kaufmann (2007) found that the dual diagnosis group of persons with autism and Down syndrome experienced more behavior problems and more difficulties as indicated by the Autism Behavior Checklist (Krug, Arick, & Almond, 1980). This measure differentiated between the persons with Down syndrome only and the persons with Down syndrome and autism. The persons with dual diagnosis were characterized as more anxious and more withdrawn than any of the other groups. These findings reinforce the claim that autism in individuals with Down syndrome is identifiable, with different manifestations than the behavioral profiles of individuals with Down syndrome or autism only.

Cognitive and Adaptive Functioning in Individuals With Down Syndrome and ASD

Although most individuals with Down syndrome tend to function in the moderate range of intellectual impairment (Hodapp, Evans & Gray, 1997; Myers & Pueschal, 1991; Roizen, 2001), many of the individuals with a dual diagnosis of Down syndrome and ASD appear to be more cognitively impaired, but still with considerable variability. For example, in the studies of intellectual disability, those with Down syndrome and ASD were in the moderate, severe, or profound level of impairment (Capone et al., 2006; Carter et al., 2007; Hepburn et al., 2008; Ghaziuddin, 2000; Kent et al., 1999; Rasmussen et al., 2001), while none of the individuals with Down syndrome only functioned in the profound range, with approximately a third functioning in the severe range, a little over a third in the moderate range, and a little under a third in the mild range. In some of these studies, the type of Down syndrome (e.g., trisomy, mosaicism) was not mentioned, whereas in others all types were included. For example, in the Rasmussen study, three of the 25 individuals diagnosed with both autism and Down syndrome had mosaicism, which is associated with higher cognitive functioning among individuals with Down syndrome only (Fishler & Koch, 1991).

In addition to comparing intellectual functioning profiles, Dressler, Perelli, Bozza, and Bargagna (2011) studied adaptive behavior in people with Down syndrome only, autism only, and both Down syndrome and autism. Using the Vineland Adaptive Behavior Scales (VABS; Sparrow & Cicchetti, 1985) and the Childhood Autism Rating Scale (CARS; Schopler, Reichler, & Renner, 2002) and *DSM-IV-TR* (APA, 2000) criteria for autism, they examined adaptive functioning in eight individuals with autism without Down syndrome, eight with Down syndrome without autism, and eight with co-occurring autism and Down syndrome, in order to investigate characteristics that might be important in distinguishing the autism phenotype in Down syndrome. The groups were matched on age (around 22 years), sociocultural background, gender and ethnic group, although not on intellectual impairment, as the participants with both autism and Down syndrome functioned at a significantly lower cognitive level, with 75% of the group manifesting severe intellectual disability. Dressler et al. reported that the profile of adaptive functioning of participants with autism and Down syndrome was more like the profile of the persons with Down syndrome than of those with autism. Similarly, the persons with autism and Down syndrome showed similar strengths on items on the CARS in the areas of imitating and relating to the participants with Down syndrome only, revealing better social skills than those with ASD only. Both groups differed significantly from the persons with ASD only. Conversely, the persons with dual diagnosis autism and Down syndrome were more impaired in adaptive functioning than the persons with Down syndrome only, suggesting that the comorbidity of ASD in Down syndrome may be related to lower intellectual and adaptive functioning. The specific pattern of adaptive functioning for individuals with Down syndrome and ASD was more similar to that of the individuals with

Down syndrome only than to that of the individuals with ASD only, which may make the diagnosis of ASD in individuals with Down syndrome more challenging.

Etiologies

There are many theories about the pathogenesis of ASD in individuals with Down syndrome. In a number of case reports, an increased prevalence of medical difficulties in individuals with Down syndrome is suggested as being associated with the presence of ASD. For example, 11 of the 25 participants in Rasmussen et al.'s (2001) study of autism and Down syndrome reported medical complications during pregnancy as well as other complex medical issues, such as infantile spasms, early hypothyroidism, and evidence of brain injury after complicated heart surgery. These findings suggest that either Down syndrome is a potent risk factor for ASD when other risk genes for ASD are present or that something about the chromosomal abnormality in Down syndrome may predispose individuals with Down syndrome toward autistic traits. For example, Capone (2003) found that individuals with comorbid Down syndrome and autism were significantly more likely than gender and chronological and mental age matched groups of persons with Down syndrome only or with autism only to have additional medical problems including congenital heart failure, anatomical gastrointestinal tract abnormalities, seizures, severe hypotonia, motor delay and other neurological findings, ophthalmological issues, and respiratory problems including sleep apnea. However, the number of matched pairs was small and, as a result, these findings need to be replicated.

One of the documented risk factors for ASD among individuals with Down syndrome is a family history of the broader ASD phenotype and/or of psychiatric difficulties. In an attempt to specify these correlated profiles, Ghaziuddin (2000) examined 11 subjects with Down syndrome who were diagnosed with autism based on *DSM-III-R* criteria (APA, 1987) and obtained a detailed family history from the biological parents using an adapted version of the Family History Schedule (Bolton et al., 1994), an investigator-based interview designed to identify the presence of developmental disorders, abnormalities of emotional development, and psychiatric disorders in first- and second-degree relatives. Among the 22 parents of the persons in the comorbid Down syndrome and autism group, six fathers and one mother met the broader autism phenotype based on the Family History Schedule as compared with one in the comparison group of parents who had a child with Down syndrome without autism. Among the 11 biological siblings in the comorbid Down syndrome and autism group, two had a history of speech problems severe enough to require treatment, two had a diagnosis of intellectual disability, and one had Down syndrome. There were also 11 biological siblings in the Down syndrome without autism group, and none of these siblings had a history of communication or social difficulties requiring intervention. Rasmussen et al. (2001) reported that five out of 25 individuals with Down syndrome and autism had one or more first- or second-degree relatives who had a diagnosis of autism, severe attention deficits, or learning disorders.

Similar problems among relatives, but to a less severe degree, were reported for another eight of the participants.

History of Research in Comorbidity of Down Syndrome and Autism Spectrum Disorder

The research on ASD among persons with Down syndrome can be divided into four categories, the first three of which involve research from the perspective of Down syndrome. The first category focuses on the characteristics of ASD that are found in individuals with Down syndrome; the second category consists of studies based on the identification of individuals with Down syndrome with a dual diagnosis of Down syndrome and ASD; the third category includes research on psychiatric issues in individuals with Down syndrome, including ASD as one of the many psychiatric issues which can occur concomitantly with Down syndrome; and the fourth category is focused on ASD and Down syndrome from the perspective of ASD.

The primary goal of the research in the first category is to identify and specify characteristics of ASD that are found in individuals with Down syndrome. The purpose is to assess behavioral manifestations of ASD, such as social impairments and abnormal behaviors associated with autism, as they appear in individuals with Down syndrome. For example, Bregman and Volkmar (1988) examined autistic social dysfunction in individuals with Down syndrome, with a focus on the social manifestations related to a diagnosis of autism only, and Coleman (1986) described children with Down syndrome with autistic features, following Wing and Gould's (1978, 1979) methodology of characterizing autistic behaviors in individuals with intellectual disability using a systematic recording of behaviors associated with autism. This line of research led to the second category, comprising studies focused on individuals with Down syndrome with a dual diagnosis of Down syndrome and ASD. These studies reflected the changing and broadening diagnostic criteria for autism. For example, Ghaziuddin (1997) found a higher rate of autistic-like characteristics among family members of those with Down syndrome and autism as compared to family members of those with Down syndrome only. Still from the perspective of Down syndrome, the third category of research is not focused specifically on autism at all but rather includes the investigation of psychiatric issues in individuals with Down syndrome, including autism as one of the many possible comorbidities. For example, Dykens et al. (2015) reviewed the differential rates of psychiatric disorders in children and adults with Down syndrome as compared to other disabilities and reported on the many gaps in the research and treatment of mental health concerns in people with Down syndrome. They reported relatively low rates of severe problems in children, and well-documented risks of depression and Alzheimer's disease in older adults with Down syndrome. They emphasized the need to assess possible co-occurring conditions such as ASD in individuals with Down syndrome at all ages. Similarly, Lund (1988) and Myers and Pueschel (1991) both investigated psychiatric aspects in Down syndrome and found a 22% overall frequency of psychiatric disorders. Disruptive behaviors, anxiety disorders, and repetitive behaviors characterized the individuals with Down syndrome under the age of 20 years, while major depressive disorders and increased prevalence of dementia were found among the individuals with Down syndrome older than 20 years. Neither Lund nor Myers and Pueschel included a diagnosis of ASD in their profiles, as their primary focus was persons with Down syndrome rather than those with ASD. In contrast, ASD researchers Gillberg, Persson, Grufman, and Themnér (1986) broadened their examination of psychiatric disorders in mildly and severely impaired urban children and adolescents with intellectual disability, including those with Down syndrome, and found that autism-like behaviour was common among those with the most severe intellectual disability. More research is needed in order to understand the relationship between severe intellectual impairment and ASD, specifically with regard to the overlap between intellectual disability and the social communication and behavioral impairments that are at the core of ASD.

The final category of research is focused on those with a dual diagnosis of Down syndrome and ASD through an ASD lens. This research stream emerged from Howlin et al.'s (1995) follow-up study of the original Wing and Gould (1979) study of autism characteristics in children with intellectual disability. Howlin et al. addressed the difficulties of actually diagnosing autism in children with Down syndrome and not simply looking for "autistic characteristics," in an attempt to identify possible etiological mechanisms. This led to the investigation of nonspecific etiology of intellectual disability and ASD (Hamdan et al., 2011), as well as establishing associations between ASD and genetic syndromes such as fragile X syndrome (August & Lockhart, 1984; Hagerman, Hoem, & Hagerman, 2010), tuberous sclerosis (Smalley, 1998; Wiznitzer, 2004), Lesch-Nyhan syndrome (Nyhan, 1973), and Angelman syndrome (Baker et al., 2018). This line of research conceptualizes the relationship between intellectual disability and ASD as one of intellectual disability being a possible etiology of ASD (Rutter & Schopler, 1987).

In research searching for other possible explanations for the co-occurrence of ASD and Down syndrome, Bolton and Rutter (1990) examined autism and Down syndrome within a population of children with autism and conceptualized autism and Down syndrome as one example of the possibility that the chromosomal disorders involved in Down syndrome may be involved in the etiology of autism. Similarly, Gillberg (1992) presented subgroups in autism by describing behavioral phenotypes based on medical conditions, including Down syndrome (Gillberg & Coleman, 1996). These research approaches can also be considered from a dimensional rather than a categorical perspective, considering autism characteristics and behaviors in genetic and neurodevelopmental disorders without categorically diagnosing autism as a co-occurring condition, but rather considering the quality of social impairment and restrictive repetitive behavioral profiles. This would enable researchers and clinicians alike to relate to the dimensionality of the distributions of autistic characteristics as they manifest themselves in genetic syndromes (Abbeduto et al., 2014; Bölte, Westerwald, Holtmann, Freitag, & Poustka, 2011; Constantino & Todd, 2003; Loesch et al., 2007; Ronald, Happé, & Plomin, 2005; Skuse, 2007).

Methodologies Used in the Study of Comorbid Down Syndrome and ASD

The study of co-occurring ASD and Down syndrome has been characterized by a variety of methodologies, which may compromise the generalizability of the findings. The investigation of comorbid Down syndrome and ASD began with the publication of case studies, continued with epidemiological studies of the prevalence of comorbid ASD and Down syndrome, and today is characterized by comparison studies of the differences among individuals with Down syndrome and ASD, those with Down syndrome without ASD, and those with ASD without Down syndrome. The advantages and limitations of each of these methodologies are discussed below.

Case Studies

The earliest studies of autism in individuals with Down syndrome were based on case reports. In some of the first case studies, Wakabayashi (1979) and Bregman and Volkmar (1988) reported co-occurring autism diagnosed in intellectually impaired children. Similarly, Ghaziuddin et al. (1992) described children with Down syndrome who met criteria for an autism diagnosis according to *DSM-III-R* (APA, 1987), noting that their stereotypic and repetitive behaviors were similar to the more complex rituals and routines seen in individuals with autism and not simply those typically associated with moderate or severe intellectual disability. Howlin et al. (1995) described the social profiles of boys with a dual diagnosis of Down syndrome and autism whose social relationships were underdeveloped, showing diminished shared attention, empathy, and shared enjoyment. Their relationships with peers were especially problematic as they were characterized by aggression, resistance, and/or withdrawal. Ghaziuddin (1997) presented case studies of adults with Down syndrome and autism, all of whom had severe intellectual impairment and met autism diagnostic criteria based on *DSM-III-R* criteria (APA, 1987). Kent et al. (1999) were the first to also include early developmental information about participants in their case studies. For example, they presented a nonverbal 19-year old male with Down syndrome who fulfilled *ICD-10* criteria for Childhood Autism (WHO, 1992, 2004) and expressed his needs by leading someone by the hand to what he wanted. This young man's parents reported that from infancy he had avoided eye contact with others, seemingly preferred his own company to being with others, and did not even show interest in what others were doing. They noted he had always demonstrated a lack of empathy, did not display imitative or symbolic play, and exhibited stereotyped movements and a marked resistance to change from a very early age. These case studies provided the basis for continuing investigation of the co-occurrence of Down syndrome and autism by describing the individuals and specifying the variables to be addressed in further research.

Prevalence Studies

There have been many attempts to ascertain the co-occurrence of Down syndrome and ASD, with reported prevalence of ASD among individuals with Down syndrome from the past 30 years ranging between 1 and 5%, (Capone, 2003; Ghaziuddin et al., 1992; Lowenthal, Paula, Schwartzman, Brunoni, & Mercadante, 2007; Moss, Richards, Nelson, & Oliver, 2013), with the higher prevalence rates in more recent research. Rubenstein et al. (2018) reported ASD and co-occurring conditions between the years 2002–2010 and found rising prevalence rates of Down syndrome in children aged 8 years old with ASD, indicating that ASD does manifest itself in children with Down syndrome and practitioners must be made especially aware of the need to look for signs of ASD in children with Down syndrome.

The findings from prevalence studies on the incidence of Down syndrome and ASD have been influenced by differences in sample size, age range of the participants, diagnostic instruments, informants, and the diagnostic criteria employed (Kent et al., 1999; Lowenthal et al., 2007; Richards, Jones, Groves, Moss, & Oliver, 2015), which is especially problematic as the diagnostic criteria for ASD have changed simultaneously with the research conducted on the prevalence of Down syndrome and ASD. The changes in ASD criteria have made for inconsistencies in the research findings. In addition to the methodological difficulties inherent in the study of the prevalence of ASD in individuals with Down syndrome, the diagnosis of ASD alongside a diagnosis of Down syndrome is difficult to ascertain because accepted standardized ASD diagnostic instruments were not used consistently. Thus, many of the findings presented here reflect research based on a range of often outdated diagnostic criteria. For example, Wing and Gould (1979) carried out an epidemiological study of 35,000 children under the age of 15 years utilizing the Medical Research Council's Handicaps, Behavior, and Skills interview schedule (HBS; Wing & Gould, 1982), which is not an accepted diagnostic instrument. Similarly, they categorized the children who participated in the study as meeting diagnostic criteria for Kanner's autism or autism spectrum disorder, at a time when the differentiation between these diagnoses for autism was not standardized. For example, using the revised HBS (Wing, 1982), which is a profile of adaptive functioning rather than a *DSM-III* validated diagnostic instrument, 5–11% of children with Down syndrome were found to have autism symptoms (Ghaziuddin et al., 1992; Lund, 1988; Turk, 1992). In an attempt to address some of these methodological issues, Kent et al. (1999) had parents of the children complete the ASSQ (Ehlers & Gillberg, 1993), a 27-item questionnaire. Unfortunately this instrument was designed to screen for social deficits associated with autism in individuals without intellectual impairment, which makes it less than ideal for screening children with Down syndrome who have intellectual impairment. After screening, a diagnosis was established based on an interview with the parents, after which the CARS (Schopler et al., 2002) was completed by the examiner. Using this technique, 12% of the participants met criteria for autism spectrum according to the *ICD-10* criteria (WHO, 1992).

Continuing to study the prevalence of autism in individuals with Down syndrome, Lowenthal et al. (2007) screened 180 individuals with Down syndrome using the Autism Screening Questionnaire (ASQ; Berument, Rutter, Lord, Pickles, & Bayley, 1999), which is based on the autism diagnostic criteria of both the *DSM-IV* (APA, 1994) and the *ICD-10* (WHO, 1992, 2004), while Hepburn et al. (2008) used the gold-standard assessment instruments, the ADOS (Lord et al., 2000) and the ADI-R (Rutter et al., 2003), in order to characterize ASD behavioral profiles of 20 two-year old children with Down syndrome. In the Hepburn et al. study, five toddlers with Down syndrome met diagnostic criteria on the ADOS-G, and none of the toddlers with Down syndrome met ASD diagnostic criteria according to the ADI-R, although many of the children exhibited behaviors associated with autism.

Research regarding prevalence rates of psychiatric disorders in individuals with intellectual impairments, including Down syndrome, typically included information about co-occurring ASD as it was considered a psychiatric condition. However, the gold-standard diagnostic instruments were not used, perhaps biasing the prevalence rates. The prevalence reported in these studies may not reflect the true prevalence of ASD in individuals with Down syndrome, as the goal of such studies was to determine susceptibility of persons with Down syndrome to psychiatric disorders and not to identify the prevalence of ASD. A summary of the numbers of participants in prevalence studies is presented in Table 17.1.

Group Comparison Studies

Comparisons of groups of individuals with Down syndrome only, ASD only, and those with a dual diagnosis of ASD and Down syndrome allows for the assessment of relationships among the variables identified in previous case studies. For example, developmental regression was described in case studies and has been reported in individuals with Down syndrome alone as well as in individuals with autism alone and those with Down syndrome and ASD (Davidovitch, Glick, Holtzman, Tirosh, & Safir, 2000; Parr et al., 2011; Rogers, 2004). Regression is strictly defined as a documented deterioration or loss of a previously acquired skill in the developmental domains of language, communication, and social skills (Pickles et al., 2009). It has been documented among children with autism and Down syndrome at up to 40%, higher than in either autism or Down syndrome alone. For example, Hickey and Patterson (2006) found that 54% (8) of a cohort of 15 children with autism and Down syndrome had a history of regression, as compared to an estimated 21–33% of individuals with autism who have a developmental history of regression (Lainhart et al., 2002; Lord, Shulman, & DiLavore, 2004; Werner & Dawson, 2005). The criterion for these studies was regression occurring sometime between 18 and 21 months of age. Typically, regression was reported retrospectively by parents when interviewed, using instruments such as the ADI-R (Rutter et al., 2003).

Table 17.1. The Percentages of ASD and Down Syndrome			
Study	Number of participants	Number of individuals with Down syndrome and ASD	Percentage
Gath & Gumley (1986)	193 with Down syndrome	2	1%
McMahon & Ritvo (1989)	241 with autism	3	1%
Myers & Pueschel (1991)	497 with Down syndrome	5	1%
Collacott, Cooper, Branford, & McGrother (1998)	371 with Down syndrome	8	2%
Li, Chen, Lai, Hsu, & Wang (1993)	104 with autism, 12 with chromosomal abnormalities	2 of 12 with chromosomal abnormalities	17%
Kielinen, Rantala, Timonen, Linna, & Moilanen (2004)	187 children with autism	7	3.7%
Lowenthal, Paula, Schwartzman, Brunoni, & Mercadante (2007)	180 children with Down syndrome	10	5.5%
Hepburn, Philofsky, Fidler, & Rogers (2008)	20 toddlers with Down syndrome	1	5%
Warner, Moss, Smith, & Howlin (2014)	499 children with Down syndrome	183	36%

Castillo et al. (2008) also used the ADI-R parent interview in order to characterize regression patterns in children with ASD with and without Down syndrome, in an attempt to determine whether regression in ASD had a different clinical presentation when it occurred in children with Down syndrome. Twelve children with documented regression and a diagnosis of autism were matched on gender and chronological and mental ages to 12 children with documented regression and a dual diagnosis of autism and Down syndrome. The groups, with average ages from 4–18 years (M = 9.8; SD = 5.8), were also matched on the type of loss (e.g., language loss, skill loss). Castillo et al. concluded that regression occurs at a significantly later age in children with a dual diagnosis of ASD and Down syndrome than in children with a diagnosis of ASD only. The profile of regression in the autism only group and the autism and Down syndrome group was similar, with the timing of the regression the only differentiating characteristic.

Summary and Conclusions

A diagnosis of ASD in individuals with Down syndrome contrasts with the widespread perception that individuals with Down syndrome are personable, social, and outgoing. However, a subgroup of individuals with Down syndrome meet the diagnostic criteria for ASD and consequently are likely to need different interventions, services, and supports to realize their potential and maximize their quality of life. This raises the question whether individuals with Down syndrome and ASD constitute a qualitatively different group of individuals within those who have Down syndrome, or whether there is a continuum of autistic behaviors among those with Down syndrome. Evidence from recent studies of individuals with fragile X syndrome suggests that a spectrum or continuum of autistic behaviors best describes the traits seen in fragile X, as opposed to a dichotomous, definite classification of "autism" or "not autism" (Abbeduto et al., 2014; Clifford et al., 2007). One methodology which can be used to inform this perspective is to examine autism characteristics and behaviors in genetic and neurodevelopmental disorders without categorically diagnosing ASD as a co-occurring condition, but rather considering the quality of social impairment and presence of restrictive repetitive behavioral profiles, thereby focusing on the severity of the symptoms and their effect on adaptive functioning of autistic characteristics in genetic syndromes (Constantino & Todd, 2003; Ronald et al., 2005; Skuse, 2007). This approach is likely to be useful in contributing to an increased understanding of the manifestation and extent of autism behaviors in individuals with Down syndrome and in members of other populations.

The delineation of specific behavioral profiles is important for the proper design and implementation of therapeutic interventions for children with Down syndrome (Capone, 2003; Ji, Capone, & Kaufmann, 2011). Some preliminary findings characterize the dual diagnosis group as more anxious and more withdrawn than either the Down syndrome only or ASD only group. In addition, individuals with Down syndrome and ASD appear to be clumsier, use fewer gestures, evidence more repetitive behaviors, and have restricted areas of interest. These issues require intervention. Therefore, once a person with Down syndrome is diagnosed with ASD, he or she should receive treatment and educational interventions appropriate for individuals with ASD. The benefits of this policy were documented by Kroeger and Nelson (2006), who describe how a combined treatment approach incorporating direct instruction, natural environment teaching, and incidental teaching can be effective in increasing and maintaining responsive and spontaneous speech in a child with Down syndrome diagnosed with ASD.

There is also a need for continued work to examine whether ASD expression in a comorbid diagnosis of Down syndrome and ASD expression without Down syndrome are similar. Investigating whether alternative explanations may account for the social and communication difficulties associated with an ASD diagnosis in people with Down syndrome (Hepburn et al., 2008) can add to the recognition of overlapping conditions and of different pathways and mechanisms in the pathogenesis of ASD. Understanding both Down syndrome and ASD through a developmental lens would enrich our understanding, as developmental level and its impact on autism symptomatology is an essential starting point (Brunsdon & Happé, 2014; Howlin et al., 1995; Joseph, Tager-Flusberg, & Lord, 2002). The fact that ASD is diagnosed more frequently in lower-functioning individuals may point to some of the autism symptoms being related to developmental level, as increased autistic features are adversely related to cognitive functioning (Wing & Gould, 1978). In addition, developmental level is likely to have an impact on response to treatment. There is still much to be learned about the manifestation of ASD in individuals with Down syndrome, and a total population epidemiological sample of individuals with Down syndrome, employing reliable and valid diagnostic instruments, is essential in order to further clarify prevalence rates of ASD among those with Down syndrome and to specify the clinical manifestation of ASD in individuals with Down syndrome.

References

Abbeduto, L., McDuffie, A., & Thurman, A. J. (2014). The fragile X syndrome–autism comorbidity: What do we really know? *Frontiers in Genetics, 5*, 355.

Aman, M. G., & Singh, N. (1994). *Aberrant Behavior Checklist. Community (ABC)*. East Aurora, NY: Slosson Educational Publications.

American Psychiatric Association. (1980). *Diagnostic and statistical manual of mental disorders* (3rd ed.). Washington, DC: Author.

American Psychiatric Association. (1987). *Diagnostic and statistical manual of mental disorders* (3rd ed.–revised.). Washington, DC: Author.

American Psychiatric Association. (1994). *Diagnostic and statistical manual of mental disorders* (4th ed.). Washington, DC: Author.

American Psychiatric Association. (2000). *Diagnostic and statistical manual of mental disorders* (4th ed.–TR). Washington, DC: Author.

American Psychiatric Association. (2013). *Diagnostic and statistical manual of mental disorders* (5th ed.). Washington, DC: Author.

Asperger, H. (1944). Die "Autistischen Psychopathen" im kindesalter. *European Archives of Psychiatry and Clinical Neuroscience, 117*(1), 76–136.

August, G. J., & Lockhart, L. H. (1984). Familial autism and the fragile-X chromosome. *Journal of Autism and Developmental Disorders, 14*(2), 197–204.

Baio, J., Wiggins, L., Christensen, D. L., Maenner, M. J., Daniels, J., Warren, Z., . . . Durkin, M. S. (2018). Prevalence of autism spectrum disorder among children aged 8 years—autism and developmental disabilities monitoring network, 11 sites, United States, 2014. *MMWR Surveillance Summaries, 67*(6), 1.

Baker, E. K., Godler, D. E., Bui, M., Hickerton, C., Rogers, C., Field, M., . . . Bretherton, L. (2018). Exploring autism symptoms in an Australian cohort of patients with Prader-Willi and Angelman syndromes. *Journal of Neurodevelopmental Disorders, 10*(1), 24.

Berument, S. K., Rutter, M., Lord, C., Pickles, A., & Bailey, A. (1999). Autism screening questionnaire: Diagnostic validity. *The British Journal of Psychiatry, 175*(5), 444–451.

Bishop, S. L., Thurm, A., Farmer, C., & Lord, C. (2016). Autism spectrum disorder, intellectual disability, and delayed walking. *Pediatrics, 137*(3), e20152959.

Bölte, S., & Poustka, F. (2002). The relation between general cognitive level and adaptive behavior domains in individuals with autism with and without co-morbid mental retardation. *Child Psychiatry & Human Development, 33*(2), 165–172.

Bölte, S., Westerwald, E., Holtmann, M., Freitag, C., & Poustka, F. (2011). Autistic traits and autism spectrum disorders: The clinical validity of two measures presuming a continuum of social communication skills. *Journal of Autism and Developmental Disorders, 41*(1), 66–72.

Bolton, P., Macdonald, H., Pickles, A., Rios, P., Goode, S., Crowson, M., . . . Rutter, M. (1994). A case-control family history study of autism. *Journal of child Psychology and Psychiatry, 35*(5), 877–900.

Bolton, P., & Rutter, M. (1990). Genetic influences in autism. *International Review of Psychiatry, 2*(1), 67–80.

Bregman, J. & Volkmar, F. (1988). Autistic social dysfunction and Down syndrome. *Journal of the American Academy of Child and Adolescent Psychiatry, 27*(4), 440–441.

Bromley, J., Hare, D. J., Davison, K., & Emerson, E. (2004). Mothers supporting children with autistic spectrum disorders: Social support, mental health status and satisfaction with services. *Autism, 8*(4), 409–423.

Brunsdon, V. E., & Happé, F. (2014). Exploring the "fractionation" of autism at the cognitive level. *Autism, 18*(1), 17–30.

Capone, G. T. (2001). Down syndrome and autistic spectrum disorder: A look at what we know. *Down's Syndrome Association newsletter*.

Capone, G. T. (2003). Down syndrome and autistic spectrum disorders. In W. I. Cohen, L. Nadel, & M. E. Madnick (Eds.). *Down syndrome: Visions for the 21st century* (pp. 327–336). New York, NY: Wiley.

Capone, G., Goyal, P., Ares, W., & Lannigan, E. (2006). Neurobehavioral disorders in children, adolescents, and young adults with Down syndrome. *American Journal of Medical Genetics Part C: Seminars in Medical Genetics, 142*(3), 158–172.

Carter, J. C., Capone, G. T., Gray, R. M., Cox, C. S., & Kaufmann, W. E. (2007). Autistic-spectrum disorders in Down syndrome: Further delineation and distinction from other behavioral abnormalities. *American Journal of Medical Genetics Part B: Neuropsychiatric Genetics, 144*(1), 87–94.

Castillo, H., Patterson, B., Hickey, F., Kinsman, A., Howard, J. M., Mitchell, T., & Molloy, C. A. (2008). Difference in age at regression in children with autism with and without Down syndrome. *Journal of Developmental & Behavioral Pediatrics, 29*(2), 89–93.

Chapman, R. S., & Hesketh, L. J. (2000). Behavioral phenotype of individuals with Down syndrome. *Developmental Disabilities Research Reviews, 6*(2), 84–95.

Charman, T., & Gotham, K. (2013). Measurement issues: Screening and diagnostic instruments for autism spectrum disorders—lessons from research and practise. *Child and Adolescent Mental Health, 18*(1), 52–63.

Chawarska, K., & Volkmar, F. R. (2005). Autism in infancy and early childhood. *Handbook of autism and pervasive developmental disorders, 1*, 223–246.

Chen, Y. F. (2002). Chinese classification of mental disorders (CCMD-3): Towards integration in international classification. *Psychopathology, 35*(2–3), 171–175.

Clifford, S., Dissanayake, C., Bui, Q. M., Huggins, R., Taylor, A. K., & Loesch, D. Z. (2007). Autism spectrum phenotype in males and females with fragile X full mutation and premutation. *Journal of Autism and Developmental Disorders, 37*(4), 738–747.

Coleman M. (1986). Down's syndrome children with autistic features. *Down Syndrome Papers and Abstracts for Professionals 9*(3), 1–2.

Coleman, M., & Gillberg, C. (2012). *The autisms*. New York, NY: Oxford University Press.

Collacott, R. A., Cooper, S. A., Branford, D., & McGrother, C. (1998). Behaviour phenotype for Down's syndrome. *The British Journal of Psychiatry, 172*(1), 85–89.

Constantino, J. N., & Charman, T. (2016). Diagnosis of autism spectrum disorder: Reconciling the syndrome, its diverse origins, and variation in expression. *The Lancet Neurology, 15*(3), 279–291.

Constantino, J. N., & Todd, R. D. (2003). Autistic traits in the general population: A twin study. *Archives of General Psychiatry, 60*(5), 524–530.

Davidovitch, M., Glick, L., Holtzman, G., Tirosh, E., & Safir, M. P. (2000). Developmental regression in autism: Maternal perception. *Journal of Autism and Developmental Disorders, 30*(2), 113–119.

Dawson, G., Rogers, S., Munson, J., Smith, M., Winter, J., Greenson, J., . . . Varley, J. (2010). Randomized, controlled trial of an intervention for toddlers with autism: The Early Start Denver Model. *Pediatrics, 125*(1), e17–e23.

Dressler, A., Perelli, V., Bozza, M., & Bargagna, S. (2011). The autistic phenotype in Down syndrome: Differences in adaptive behaviour versus Down syndrome alone and autistic disorder alone. *Functional Neurology, 26*(3), 151–159.

Dykens, E. M. (2007). Psychiatric and behavioral disorders in persons with Down syndrome. *Developmental Disabilities Research Reviews, 13*(3), 272–278.

Dykens, E. M., Shah, B., Davis, B., Baker, C., Fife, T., & Fitzpatrick, J. (2015). Psychiatric disorders in adolescents and young adults with Down syndrome and other intellectual disabilities. *Journal of Neurodevelopmental Disorders, 7*(1), 9.

Ehlers, S., & Gillberg, C. (1993). The epidemiology of Asperger syndrome: A total population study. *Journal of Child Psychology and Psychiatry, 34*(8), 1327–1350.

Ehlers, S., Gillberg, C., & Wing, L. (1999). A screening questionnaire for Asperger syndrome and other high-functioning autism spectrum disorders in school age children. *Journal of Autism and Developmental Disorders, 29*(2), 129–141.

Esler, A. N., & Ruble, L. A. (2015). DSM-5 diagnostic criteria for autism spectrum disorder with implications for school psychologists. *International Journal of School & Educational Psychology, 3*(1), 1–15.

Fidler, D. J. (2005). The emerging Down syndrome behavioral phenotype in early childhood: Implications for practice. *Infants & Young Children, 18*(2), 86–103.

Fishler, K., & Koch, R. (1991). Mental development in Down syndrome mosaicism. *American Journal on Mental Retardation, 96*(3), 345–351.

Flynt, J., & Yule, W. (1994). Behavioural phenotypes. In M. Rutter, E. Taylor, & L. Hersov (Eds.), *Child and adolescent psychiatry: Modern approaches* (3rd ed., pp. 666–687). London, UK: Blackwell.

Fombonne, E. (2009). Epidemiology of pervasive developmental disorders. *Pediatric Research, 65*(6), 591–598.

Fombonne, E. (2018). The rising prevalence of autism. *Journal of Child Psychology and Psychiatry, 59*(7), 717–720.

Gath, A., & Gumley, D. (1986). Behaviour problems in retarded children with special reference to Down's syndrome. *The British Journal of Psychiatry, 149*(2), 156–161.

Ghaziuddin, M. (1997). Autism in Down syndrome: Family history correlates. *Journal of Intellectual Disability Research, 41*, 86–91.

Ghaziuddin, M. (2000). Autism in Down's syndrome: A family history study. *Journal of Intellectual Disability Research, 44*(5), 562–566.

Ghaziuddin, M., Tsai, L. Y., & Ghaziuddin, N. (1992). Autism in Down's syndrome: Presentation and diagnosis. *Journal of Intellectual Disability Research, 36*(5), 449–456.

Gillberg, C. (1992). Subgroups in autism: Are their behavioral phenotypes typical of underlying medical conditions? *Journal of Intellectual Disabilities Research, 36*, 201–214.

Gillberg, C., Persson, E., Grufman, M., & Themnér, U. (1986). Psychiatric disorders in mildly and severely mentally retarded urban children and adolescents: Epidemiological aspects. *The British Journal of Psychiatry, 149*(1), 68–74.

Gillberg, C., & Coleman, M. (1996). Autism and medical disorders: A review of the literature. *Developmental Medicine & Child Neurology, 38*(3), 191–202.

Gillberg, J. C., Gillberg, C., & Ahlsén, G. (1994). Autistic behaviour and attention deficits in tuberous sclerosis: A population-based study. *Developmental Medicine & Child Neurology, 36*(1), 50–56.

Gotham, K., Risi, S., Pickles, A., & Lord, C. (2007). The Autism Diagnostic Observation Schedule: Revised algorithms for improved diagnostic validity. *Journal of Autism and Developmental Disorders, 37*(4), 613.

Hagerman, R., Hoem, G., & Hagerman, P. (2010). Fragile X and autism: Intertwined at the molecular level leading to targeted treatments. *Molecular Autism, 1*(1), 12.

Hamdan, F. F., Daoud, H., Piton, A., Gauthier, J., Dobrzeniecka, S., Krebs, M. O., . . . Wang, Z. (2011). De novo SYNGAP1 mutations in nonsyndromic intellectual disability and autism. *Biological Psychiatry, 69*(9), 898–901.

Hammond, R. K., Campbell, J. M., & Ruble, L. A. (2013). Considering identification and service provision for students with autism spectrum disorders within the context of response to intervention. *Exceptionality, 21*(1), 34–50.

Hamner, T., Hepburn, S., Zhang, F., Fidler, D., Robinson, C. R., Robins, D. L., & Lee, N. R. (2019). Cognitive profiles and autism symptoms in comorbid Down syndrome and autism spectrum disorder. *Journal of Developmental and Behavioral Pediatrics, 41*(3), 172–179.

Harris, K. M., Mahone, E. M., & Singer, H. S. (2008). Nonautistic motor stereotypies: Clinical features and longitudinal follow-up. *Pediatric neurology, 38*(4), 267–272.

Hepburn, S., Philofsky, A., Fidler, D. & Rogers, S. (2008). Autism symptoms in toddlers with Down syndrome. *Journal of Applied research in Intellectual Disabilities, 21*, 48–57.

Hickey, F. J., & Patterson, B. (2006). Dual diagnosis of Down syndrome and autism. *International Journal on Disability and Human Development, 5(*4), 365–368.

Hippolyte, L., Barisnikov, K., & Van der Linden, M. (2008). Face processing and facial emotion recognition in adults with Down syndrome. *American Journal on Mental Retardation, 113*(4), 292–306.

Hodapp, R. M., Evans, D., & Gray, F. L. (1997). Cognitive functioning in adolescents with Down syndrome: Theoretical and practical issues. *Adolescents with Down syndrome: toward a more fulfilling life* (pp. 91–98). Baltimore, MD: Paul H. Brookes.

Hodapp, R. M., Ricci, L. A., Ly, T. M., & Fidler, D. J. (2003). The effects of the child with Down syndrome on maternal stress. *British Journal of Developmental Psychology, 21*(1), 137–151.

Howlin, P., Wing, L. & Gould, J. (1995). The recognition of autism in children with Down syndrome: Implications for intervention. *Developmental Medicine and Child Neurology, 37*, 406–414.

Huerta, M., & Lord, C. (2012). Diagnostic evaluation of autism spectrum disorders. *Pediatric Clinics of North America, 59*(1), 103–111.

Ji, N. Y., Capone, G. T., & Kaufmann, W. E. (2011). Autism spectrum disorder in Down syndrome: Cluster analysis of Aberrant Behaviour Checklist data supports diagnosis. *Journal of Intellectual Disability Research, 55(*11), 1064–1077.

Johnson, C. P., & Myers, S. M. (2007). Identification and evaluation of children with autism spectrum disorders. *Pediatrics, 120*(5), 1183–1215.

Joseph, R. M., Tager-Flusberg, H., & Lord, C. (2002). Cognitive profiles and social-communicative functioning in children with autism spectrum disorder. *Journal of Child Psychology and Psychiatry, 43*(6), 807–821.

Kanner, L. (1943). Autistic disturbances of affective contact. *Nervous Child, 2*(3), 217–250.

Kasari, C., & Freeman, S. F. (2001). Task-related social behavior in children with Down syndrome. *American Journal on Mental Retardation, 106*(3), 253–264.

Kent, L., Evans, J., Paul, M., & Sharp, M. (1999). Comorbidity of autism spectrum disorders in children with Down syndrome. *Developmental Medicine and Child Neurology, 41*, 152–158.

Kielinen, M., Rantala, H., Timonen, E., Linna, S. L., & Moilanen, I. (2004). Associated medical disorders and disabilities in children with autistic disorder: A population-based study. *Autism, 8*(1), 49–60.

Kroeger, K. A., & Nelson, W. M., III. (2006). A language programme to increase the verbal production of a child dually diagnosed with Down syndrome and autism. *Journal of Intellectual Disability Research, 50*(2), 101–108.

Krug, D. A., Arick, J., & Almond, P. (1980). Behavior checklist for identifying severely handicapped individuals with high levels of autistic behavior. *Journal of Child Psychology and Psychiatry, 21*(3), 221–229.

Lainhart, J. E., Ozonoff, S., Coon, H., Krasny, L., Dinh, E., Nice, J., & McMahon, W. (2002). Autism, regression, and the broader autism phenotype. *American Journal of Medical Genetics, 113*(3), 231–237.

Laws, G., & Bishop, D. V. M. (2004). Verbal deficits in specific language impairment and Down syndrome: A comparative review. *International Journal of Language and Communication Disorders, 39*, 423–451.

Li, S. Y., Chen, Y. C. J., Lai, T. J., Hsu, C. Y., & Wang, Y. C. (1993). Molecular and cytogenetic analyses of autism in Taiwan. *Human Genetics, 92*(5), 441–445.

Loesch, D. Z., Bui, Q. M., Dissanayake, C., Clifford, S., Gould, E., Bulhak-Paterson, D., . . . Huggins, R. M. (2007). Molecular and cognitive predictors of the continuum of autistic behaviours in fragile X. *Neuroscience & Biobehavioral Reviews, 31*(3), 315–326.

Lord, C., Risi, S., Lambrecht, L., Cook, E. H., Leventhal, B. L., DiLavore, P. C., . . . Rutter, M. (2000). The autism diagnostic observation schedule—Generic: A standard measure of social and communication deficits associated with the spectrum of autism. *Journal of Autism and Developmental Disorders, 30*(3), 205–223.

Lord, C., Rutter, M., DiLavore, P. C., Risi, S., Gotham, K., & Bishop, S. (2012). *Autism diagnostic observation schedule: ADOS-2*. Los Angeles, CA: Western Psychological Services.

Lord, C., Rutter, M., & Le Couteur, A. (1994). Autism Diagnostic Interview–Revised: A revised version of a diagnostic interview for caregivers of individuals with possible pervasive developmental disorders. *Journal of Autism and Developmental Disorders, 24*(5), 659–685.

Lord, C., Shulman, C., & DiLavore, P. (2004). Regression and word loss in autistic spectrum disorders. *Journal of Child Psychology and Psychiatry, 45*(5), 936–955.

Lowenthal, R., Paula, C. S., Schwartzman, J. S., Brunoni, D., & Mercadante, M. T. (2007). Prevalence of pervasive developmental disorder in Down's syndrome. *Journal of Autism and Developmental Disorders, 37*(7), 1394–1395.

Lund, J. (1988). Psychiatric aspects of Down's syndrome. *Acta Psychiatrica Scandinavica, 78*(3), 369–374.

Mandell, D. S., Novak, M. M., & Zubritsky, C. D. (2005). Factors associated with age of diagnosis among children with autism spectrum disorders. *Pediatrics, 116*(6), 1480–1486.

Mantry, D., Cooper, S. A., Smiley, E., Morrison, J., Allan, L., Williamson, A., . . . Jackson, A. (2008). The prevalence and incidence of mental ill-health in adults with Down syndrome. *Journal of Intellectual Disability Research, 52*(2), 141–155.

McMahon, W., & Ritvo, A. (1989). The UCLA-University of Utah epidemiologic survey of autism: Prevalence. *American Journal of Psychiatry, 146*(2), 194–199.

Moes, D. R., & Frea, W. D. (2002). Contextualized behavioral support in early intervention for children with autism and their families. *Journal of Autism and Developmental Disorders, 32*(6), 519–533.

Moss, J., Richards, C., Nelson, L., & Oliver, C. (2013). Prevalence of autism spectrum disorder symptomatology and related behavioural characteristics in individuals with Down syndrome. *Autism, 17*(4), 390–404.

Mundy, P., Sigman, M., & Kasari, C. (1994). Joint attention, developmental level, and symptom presentation in autism. *Development and Psychopathology, 6*(3), 389–401.

Mundy, P., Sigman, M., Ungerer, J., & Sherman, T. (1986). Defining the social deficits of autism: The contribution of non-verbal communication measures. *Journal of Child Psychology and Psychiatry, 27*(5), 657–669.
Myers, B. A., & Pueschel, S. M. (1991). Psychiatric disorders in persons with Down syndrome. *The Journal of Nervous and Mental Disease, 179*(10), 609–613.
Nachshen, J., Garcin, N., Moxness, K., Tremblay, Y., Hutchinson, P., Lachance, A., . . . Caron, C. (2008). *Screening, assessment, and diagnosis of autism spectrum disorders in young children: Canadian best practice guidelines*. Montreal, Quebec: Miriam Foundation.
Nyhan, W. L. (1973). The Lesch-Nyhan syndrome. *Annual Review of Medicine, 24*(1), 41–60.
Ortiz, B., Videla, L., Gich, I., Alcacer, B., Torres, D., Jover, I., . . . Videla, S. (2017). Early warning signs of autism spectrum disorder in people with Down syndrome. *International Medical Review on Down Syndrome, 21*(1), 3–11.
Osterling, J. A., Dawson, G., & Munson, J. A. (2002). Early recognition of 1-year-old infants with autism spectrum disorder versus mental retardation. *Development and Psychopathology, 14*(2), 239–251.
Ozonoff, S., Goodlin-Jones, B. L., & Solomon, M. (2005). Evidence-based assessment of autism spectrum disorders in children and adolescents. *Journal of Clinical Child and Adolescent Psychology, 34*(3), 523–540.
Parr, J. R., Le Couteur, A., Baird, G., Rutter, M., Pickles, A., Fombonne, E., . . . International Molecular Genetic Study of Autism Consortium. (2011). Early developmental regression in autism spectrum disorder: Evidence from an international multiplex sample. *Journal of Autism and Developmental Disorders, 41*(3), 332–340.
Perry, A., Flanagan, H. E., Geier, J. D., & Freeman, N. L. (2009). Brief report: The Vineland Adaptive Behavior Scales in young children with autism spectrum disorders at different cognitive levels. *Journal of Autism and Developmental Disorders, 39*(7), 1066–1078.
Pickles, A., Simonoff, E., Conti-Ramsden, G., Falcaro, M., Simkin, Z., Charman, T., . . . Baird, G. (2009). Loss of language in early development of autism and specific language impairment. *Journal of Child Psychology and Psychiatry, 50*(7), 843–852.
Rasmussen, P., Borjesson, O., Wentz, E., & Gillberg, C. (2001). Autistic disorders in Down syndrome: Background factors and clinical correlates. *Developmental Medicine and Child Neurology, 43*, 750–754.
Reilly, C. (2009). Autism spectrum disorders in Down syndrome: A review. *Research in Autism Spectrum Disorders, 3*(4), 829–839.
Remington, B., Hastings, R. P., Kovshoff, H., Degli Espinosa, F., Jahr, E., Brown, T., . . . Ward, N. (2007). Early intensive behavioral intervention: Outcomes for children with autism and their parents after two years. *American Journal on Mental Retardation, 112*(6), 418–438.
Richards, C., Jones, C., Groves, L., Moss, J., & Oliver, C. (2015). Prevalence of autism spectrum disorder phenomenology in genetic disorders: A systematic review and meta-analysis. *The Lancet Psychiatry, 2*(10), 909–916.
Risi, S., Lord, C., Gotham, K., Corsello, C., Chrysler, C., Szatmari, P., . . . Pickles, A. (2006). Combining information from multiple sources in the diagnosis of autism spectrum disorders. *Journal of the American Academy of Child & Adolescent Psychiatry, 45*(9), 1094–1103.
Robins, D. L., Fein, D., Barton, M. L., & Green, J. A. (2001). The Modified Checklist for Autism in Toddlers: An initial study investigating the early detection of autism and pervasive developmental disorders. *Journal of Autism and Developmental Disorders, 31*(2), 131–144.
Rogers, S. J. (2004). Developmental regression in autism spectrum disorders. *Developmental Disabilities Research Reviews, 10*(2), 139–143.
Rogers, S. J., Hepburn, S. L., Stackhouse, T., & Wehner, E. (2003). Imitation performance in toddlers with autism and those with other developmental disorders. *Journal of Child Psychology and Psychiatry, 44*(5), 763–781.
Roizen, N. J. (2001). Down syndrome: Progress in research. *Mental Retardation and Developmental Disabilities Research Reviews, 7*(1), 38–44.
Ronald, A., Happé, F., & Plomin, R. (2005). The genetic relationship between individual differences in social and nonsocial behaviours characteristic of autism. *Developmental Science, 8*(5), 444–458.
Rubenstein, E., Schieve, L., Wiggins, L., Rice, C., Braun, K. V. N., Christensen, D., . . . Lee, L. C. (2018). Trends in documented co-occurring conditions in children with autism spectrum disorder, 2002–2010. *Research in Developmental Disabilities, 83*, 168–178.
Russa, M. B., Matthews, A. L., & Owen-DeSchryver, J. S. (2015). Expanding supports to improve the lives of families of children with autism spectrum disorder. *Journal of Positive Behavior Interventions, 17*(2), 95–104.
Rutter, M., Le Couteur, A., & Lord, C. (2003). *Autism diagnostic interview–revised*. Los Angeles, CA: Western Psychological Services.

Rutter, M., & Schopler, E. (1987). Autism and pervasive developmental disorders: Concepts and diagnostic issues. *Journal of Autism and Developmental Disorders, 17*(2), 159–186.
Schopler, E., Reichler, R. J., & Renner, B. R. (2002). *The childhood autism rating scale (CARS).* Los Angeles, CA: Western Psychological Services.
Schopler, E., Van Bourgondien, M. E., Wellman, G. J., & Love, S. R. (2010). *CARS-2: Childhood autism rating scale* (2nd ed.). Los Angeles: Western Psychological Services.
Silberman, S. (2015). *Neurotribes: The legacy of autism and the future of neurodiversity.* New York: Penguin.
Siklos, S., & Kerns, K. A. (2006). Assessing need for social support in parents of children with autism and Down syndrome. *Journal of Autism and Developmental Disorders, 36*(7), 921–933.
Skuse, D. H. (2007). Rethinking the nature of genetic vulnerability to autistic spectrum disorders. *Trends in Genetics, 23*(8), 387–395.
Smalley, S. L. (1998). Autism and tuberous sclerosis. *Journal of Autism and Developmental Disorders, 28*(5), 407–414.
Sparrow, S. S., & Cicchetti, D. V. (1985). Diagnostic uses of the Vineland adaptive behavior scales. *Journal of Pediatric Psychology, 10*(2), 215–225.
Starr, E. M., Berument, S. K., Tomlins, M., Papanikolaou, K., & Rutter, M. (2005). Brief report: Autism in individuals with Down syndrome. *Journal of Autism and Developmental Disorders, 35*(5), 665–673.
Stone, W. L., Lee, E. B., Ashford, L., Brissie, J., Hepburn, S. L., Coonrod, E. E., & Weiss, B. H. (1999). Can autism be diagnosed accurately in children under 3 years? *The Journal of Child Psychology and Psychiatry and Allied Disciplines, 40*(2), 219–226.
Turk, J. (1992). Children with Down's syndrome and fragile X syndrome: A comparison study. In *Society for the Study of Behavioural Phenotypes: 2nd Symposium Abstracts.* Oxford, UK: SSBP.
Volkmar, F. R., Reichow, B., Westphal, A., & Mandell, D. S. (2014). Autism and the autism spectrum: Diagnostic concepts. In F. R. Volkmar, S. Rogers, R. Paul, & K. A. Pelphrey, (Eds.). *Handbook of autism and pervasive developmental disorders* (4th ed., pp. 3–27). Hoboken, NJ: Wiley.
Wakabayashi, S. (1979). A case of infantile autism associated with Down's syndrome. *Journal of Autism and Developmental Disorders, 9*(1), 31–36.
Warner, G., Howlin, P., Salomone, E., Moss, J., & Charman, T. (2017). Profiles of children with Down syndrome who meet screening criteria for autism spectrum disorder (ASD): A comparison with children diagnosed with ASD attending specialist schools. *Journal of Intellectual Disability Research, 61*(1), 75–82.
Warner, G., Moss, J., Smith, P., & Howlin, P. (2014). Autism characteristics and behavioural disturbances in ~500 children with Down's syndrome in England and Wales. *Autism Research, 7*(4), 433–441.
Werner, E., & Dawson, G. (2005). Validation of the phenomenon of autistic regression using home videotapes. *Archives of General Psychiatry, 62*(8), 889–895.
Wester Oxelgren, U., Åberg, M., Myrelid, Å., Annerén, G., Westerlund, J., Gustafsson, J., & Fernell, E. (2019). Autism needs to be considered in children with Down syndrome. *Acta Paediatrica, 108*(11), 2019–2026.
Williams, K. R., Wishart, J. G., Pitcairn, T. K., & Willis, D. S. (2005). Emotion recognition by children with Down syndrome: Investigation of specific impairments and error patterns. *American Journal on Mental Retardation, 110*(5), 378–392.
Wing, L. (1982). *Schedule of handicaps, behavior and skills.* London, UK: Medical Research Council.
Wing, L., & Gould, J. (1978). Systematic recording of behaviors and skills of retarded and psychotic children. *Journal of Autism and Childhood Schizophrenia, 8*(1), 79–97.
Wing, L., & Gould, J. (1979). Severe impairments of social interaction and associated abnormalities in children: Epidemiology and classification. *Journal of Autism and Developmental Disorders, 9*(1), 11–29.
Wishart, J. G., & Pitcairn, T. K. (2000). Recognition of identity and expression in faces by children with Down syndrome. *American Journal on Mental Retardation, 105*(6), 466–479.
Wiznitzer, M. (2004). Autism and tuberous sclerosis. *Journal of Child Neurology, 19*(9), 675–679.
World Health Organization. (1992). *International classification of diseases* (10th revision). Geneva: World Health Organization.
World Health Organization. (2004). *ICD-10: International statistical classification of diseases and related health problems* (10th revision, 2nd ed.). Geneva: World Health Organization.
Zwaigenbaum, L., Bryson, S., Lord, C., Rogers, S., Carter, A., Carver, L., . . . Fein, D. (2009). Clinical assessment and management of toddlers with suspected autism spectrum disorder: Insights from studies of high-risk infants. *Pediatrics, 123*(5), 1383–1391.

CHAPTER

18 Sleeping to Dream, Develop, and Resist Decline: Down Syndrome and Sleep Across the Lifespan

Katharine Hughes*, Payal Khosla*, Lauren Pisani, Goffredina Spanò, *and* Jamie Edgin

Abstract

Sleep quality is increasingly recognized as a potential factor influencing healthy cognitive and neural development across the lifespan. It is becoming more recognized as an important factor for persons with Down syndrome, and this chapter describes the most recent literature regarding sleep disturbance, its correlates, and findings from animal models in this population. The authors discuss the relation of poor sleep to behavioral, brain, and cognitive dysfunction and highlight the family consequences for altered sleep in children with Down syndrome. These pervasive sleep deficits have the potential to derail cognitive development during critical periods for language learning and could also exacerbate age-related cognitive decline. The authors hope that this compilation of evidence regarding sleep deficits in persons with Down syndrome will help facilitate more treatment studies for sleep disorders in this population, including treatments aimed at poor sleep in infants, as well as mid-adulthood, which may lessen or delay the impact of the pathological progression of Alzheimer's disease. Methodological challenges to sleep research are discussed, and future directions for this field are highlighted.

Key Words: Down syndrome, sleep, neurocognitive outcomes, behavioral outcomes, Alzheimer's disease, mouse models

Sleep's function has long been a mystery, with philosophers and researchers alike debating its potential utility as a period of physical repair, exploration of dreams and memories, or perhaps as having no important function at all. In part, this debate persists because sleep is a physiological state that fools our expectations. Why would a physically quiet and peaceful organism's brain be experiencing a neural firestorm or the clearing of neuropathology? Because of this outward lack of utility, sleep quality has been somewhat under-recognized as an important factor that could influence development in developmental disorders such as Down syndrome (DS). Here we argue that sleep might be as important a brain state as attentional awareness or executive control and that for developmental disorders that present with life-long sleep disturbance, sleep may result in a bottleneck on healthy developmental outcomes. Beyond influencing cognitive development, sleep has the potential to exacerbate the neuropathological progression of atypical aging and dementia, with sleep disturbances observed decades prior to dementia onset (Esbensen, 2016; Fernandez & Edgin, 2013).

The presence of sleep disturbance is a key component of the cognitive and physical phenotype of people with Down syndrome (Breslin, Edgin, Bootzin, Goodwin, & Nadel, 2011; Shott et al., 2006), and its function and correlated skills are important to study across the lifespan of individuals with this syndrome. People with Down syndrome have substantially higher rates of sleep disorders across their lifespan, and these sleep disturbances are present during developmental stages that may be particularly vulnerable to insult, including the early years of neurodevelopment and during the aging years, during which people with Down syndrome have increased rates of Alzheimer's disease (AD). Specifically, 50–80% of individuals with Down syndrome show clinically significant levels of obstructive sleep apnea (OSA) even as infants (Breslin et al., 2014; Dyken, Lin-Dyken, Poulton, Zimmerman, & Sedars, 2003; Shott et al., 2006), leading them to be vulnerable during the earliest years of rapid cognitive and language development. People with Down syndrome show substantially higher rates of AD than the typical population (see Startin, Zaman, & Strydom, this volume; Zigman & Lott, 2007), and show high rates of sleep disturbance during the years at which they are at risk for decline. In typical individuals, sleep disturbances have been shown to relate to the neuropathological processes of AD, as reflected in Holth et al.'s (2019) finding of significant increases in the accumulation of tau and Beta-amyloid proteins in the cerebrospinal fluid of typical adults aged 30–60 years following a night of sleep deprivation. Given these findings, more research is required to examine sleep's role in development and decline. These data are important to better understand the sources of atypical cognition in this population and for the development of comprehensive treatment options.

Several theories regarding the functions of sleep have been proposed during the last 50 years and, as we learn more, sleep deficits seem to be a fundamental characteristic of a number of developmental disorders, including Down syndrome. For instance, rapid eye movement (REM) sleep, which predominates in early development, has long been considered to play a role in brain development and learning (Blumberg, 2003; Crick & Mitchison, 1983; Roffwarg, Muzio, & Dement, 1966). In this context, Hobson and Stickgold (1995) referred to sleep as the "beloved teacher" in their discussion of Wilson and McNaughton's (1994) provocative suggestion that a rodent's place cell firing patterns acquired during navigation were reactivated—with some modification—during sleep. Wilson and McNaughton's findings, in conjunction with those of others (Louie & Wilson, 2001; Peigneux et al., 2004), led to the active systems consolidation theory, in which sleep is thought to provide a period of active replay to strengthen and integrate memories encoded during the day through a series of hippocampal-cortical interactions (Diekelmann & Born, 2010). Further, recent work suggests that sleep may help support both new learning as well as abstraction through the forgetting of irrelevant detail (Poe, 2017).

In total, these theoretical perspectives and associated empirical studies suggest sleep is an ideal state for the resetting of synaptic connectivity as well as the repair of daily physiological wear and tear of the body and brain. Specifically, data from animal models and humans suggest that the neuropathology associated with AD may be cleared during slow wave (or deep) sleep (SWS; reviewed in Winer & Mander, 2018). In this context, states of persistent sleep disturbance leave the brain vulnerable, as neither this neural "housekeeping" nor new learning are conducted in an efficient manner. Therefore, in conditions with life-long sleep impairments—and we argue this impairment *is* life long in persons with Down syndrome—there is potential for poor sleep, which in turn may have a major impact on the developing nervous system and learning.

The causal role of sleep in driving change in cognition and behavior—while originally controversial—is becoming clearer through ongoing research. That is, a key question for this field has been whether chronically poor sleep patterns are causally related to cognitive and developmental outcomes, or are they merely correlated? Sleep manipulations and treatments are now more frequently conducted in typically developing (TD) groups, so data suggesting a causal role for sleep in learning and healthy development is accumulating. In terms of cognitive outcomes, evidence from studies in which sleep is manipulated (i.e., the presence of naps) suggests that young children need to sleep shortly after learning to retain initially fragile memories (Gómez, Bootzin, & Nadel, 2006). Other work has shown that memory reactivation or stimulation of the electroencephalogram (EEG) power of sleep states may enhance long-term retention (Rudoy, Voss, Westerberg, & Paller, 2009). Finally, treatment of sleep disorders, such as OSA, which is highly prevalent among persons with Down syndrome, has shown only preliminary evidence of cognitive and behavioral benefits, such as improved verbal knowledge in one published abstract (Hill, Fairley, Williams, Cooper, & Riha, 2015). While data show that sleep may causally relate to some memory and cognitive functions across some populations, this evidence is currently scarce among people with Down syndrome. Therefore, more experimental studies are needed to determine the causal relationship between sleep deficits and developmental outcomes in this population.

A careful examination of the importance of sleep among persons with Down syndrome also requires a transactional approach (Bronfenbrenner, 1977), in which the individual's developmental trajectory is examined in reference to sleep's complex relationships with brain development, cognition, behavior, and the social environment. In this chapter, we present evidence that sleep disturbance is present across the lifespan in persons with Down syndrome, may affect critical periods for cognitive development and decline, and could potentially be a source of variability in healthy family dynamics.

Fundamentals of Sleep

Sleep is a dynamic physiological state, with a long history of data showing sleep's influence on typical children's learning, behavior, emotions, and family functioning (Gómez,

Newman-Smith, Breslin, & Bootzin, 2011). Sleep can be organized into states of non-rapid eye movement (NREM) and REM sleep (Mindell & Owens, 2015); these states occur in repetitive, ordered cycles across the course of the night, also referred to as the architecture of sleep. NREM sleep is a time during which the brain is active and body movements are minimal (Mindell & Owens, 2015). It is subdivided into Stage 1, Stage 2, and Stage 3 sleep. Stage 1 sleep occurs as we transition from the sleep-wake state and lasts between 30 seconds to 5 minutes per cycle. It is characterized by involuntary muscle contractions, recollection of fragmented images, and the lowest arousal threshold of sleep states (Mindell & Owens, 2015). Stage 2 sleep is considered "true" sleep, and duration ranges from 5 to 25 minutes per cycle. It is differentiated from the other sleep stages by slower brain wave activity and includes characteristic EEG features of sleep spindles and K-complexes, as well as a halt in eye movements (Mindell & Owens, 2015; National Institute of Neurological Disorders & Stroke, 2014). Stage 3 sleep is referred to as "deep" sleep, delta sleep, or slow wave sleep (SWS), and lasts about 30 to 45 minutes per cycle (Mindell & Owens, 2015). Its key elements include decreased respiration, increased parasympathetic activity, and highest arousal threshold (Mindell & Owens, 2015). EEG activity during this stage consists of delta waves, hence the name "delta sleep." NREM sleep is followed by REM sleep, which is characterized by multiple changes in physiological and neural functioning. For example, while there is an absence of movement in most muscles and of normal thermoregulation, the brain is metabolically active (Mindell & Owens, 2015). Humans dream during REM sleep and the periodic eye movements observed are characteristic of this stage.

The quality and quantity of sleep changes with age. Infants spend approximately 14–15 hours per day sleeping at 6 months of age, at which point they already exhibit sleep characteristics such as NREM and REM sleep (Ednick et al., 2009; Gómez & Edgin, 2015; Ohayon, Carskadon, Guilleminault, & Vitiello, 2004). REM sleep characterizes 50% of sleep in newborns but is significantly reduced to 25–30% in adolescents and adults; children also produce more SWS (Stage 3), which is reduced in later childhood and adulthood (Mindell & Owens, 2015). In contrast, over a single night of sleep, adults experience sleep cycles approximately 4–6 times, with each cycle lasting 90 to 110 minutes, sleeping substantially less and with less deep sleep than children.

While the longitudinal developmental profile of sleep disturbance has not yet been tracked in persons with Down syndrome, we know that they are at risk for generalized as well as specific sleep issues (Breslin et al., 2011; Carter, McCaughey, Annaz, & Hill, 2009). These difficulties cause Down syndrome to be one of the few conditions with a lifespan prevalence of sleep disorders, allowing us to better understand how sleep may influence outcomes during key developmental periods. Further, we assert that a lifespan treatment regimen is required for the sleep difficulties faced by these individuals, as they are diverted from a typical developmental pathway so early in life, with potentially cascading influences on cognitive and behavioral milestones.

Measurement of Sleep in Persons With Down Syndrome

Sleep is a multidimensional construct and comprehensive assessments of the integrity of sleep states should include measurements of peripheral (i.e., heart rate and oxygen level) and neural physiology (i.e., EEG). Polysomnography (PSG) is considered a gold standard assessment for sleep, which includes pulse oximetry, EEG, and respiratory measurements. In order to best understand sleep patterns in pediatric populations, multiple converging assessments are required, such as assessments of sleep physiology as well as circadian rhythms. In a sleep study of 23 children with Down syndrome aged 8–19 years, Konstantinopoulou et al. (2016) found that 87% of participants had OSA when measured with PSG. A number of researchers have examined subjective reports of sleep gathered from caregiver reports that provide an important view of the sleep profile from the caregiver's perspective. Of all the parent-reported measures, the Children's Sleep Habits Questionnaire (CSHQ) appears to be the most reliable and accurate representation of child sleep behaviors (Esbensen & Hoffman, 2017). However, the extent to which caregiver reports can identify some key aspects of the sleep profile (i.e., particularly OSA) is debated (Esbensen, Hoffman, Stansberry, & Shaffer, 2018). For example, in a study of parent reported sleep issues and PSG, of the 69% of parents who reported no sleep issues, 54% of their children had abnormal sleep; whereas of the parents who did report sleep problems, only 36% of their children had abnormal sleep profiles (Shott et al., 2006). Thus, while parent reports may underestimate OSA prevalence, they may be important indicators of problems in other sleep domains, such as bedtime routines, sleep anxiety, or the presence of parasomnias (i.e., night terrors).

PSG is the most accurate measure of sleep because it captures the necessary physiology; however, it is a taxing assessment for both the participant and the administrator. Another assessment of sleep that is far less demanding is actigraphy, a wrist monitor that measures light levels and movement. Actigraphy, as a proxy for sleep, measures movement via an accelerometer. Although some concerns have been raised over how effective this measure is, including its sensitivity to detect waking intervals, relatively strong correlations have been found between actigraphy and PSG-based measures in people with Down syndrome (Esbensen et al., 2018).

In summary, multimethod assessments are required to capture the complete picture regarding sleep difficulties in persons with Down syndrome. PSG is the gold standard assessment, but researchers wishing to gather data from fully representative cohorts may find measurement with actigraphy and parent report measures sufficient to yield instructive data, with consideration of their limitations. Future work should include the development of a set of required outcome measures for sleep studies, so that researchers can consistently report similar outcome variables.

Sleep Profile in Persons With Down Syndrome

Sleep deficits are apparent across the lifespan among persons with Down syndrome and represent a complex constellation of symptoms, including increased rates of OSA and sleep fragmentation (Nisbet, Phillips, Hoban, & O'Brien, 2015). OSA is the most commonly reported sleep disturbance in persons with Down syndrome. It is a sleep disorder involving respiratory dysfunction in which typical breathing is disturbed by intermittent airway collapses due to low muscle tone, obesity, and altered craniofacial structure. In the typical population, 2% of children are diagnosed with OSA (Beck & Marcus, 2009). The rates among children with Down syndrome are substantially higher, with reported prevalence rates of 30–80% (Dyken et al., 2003; Shott et al., 2006) that continue to be observed across the lifespan among groups recruited both from medical clinics and from the community (Breslin et al., 2014).

The evidence from initial cross-sectional studies has confirmed that children and adults with Down syndrome display sleep disturbances during critical periods in development (Churchill, Kieckhefer, Landis, & Ward, 2012; Nisbet et al., 2015). For example, the role of sleep in language learning and abstraction has been extensively examined in typical children, indicating that quality sleep is a predictor of vocabulary and grammar acquisition (Gómez et al., 2006). Sleep is disturbed by conditions such as OSA and elevated arousal indices in at least 50% of individuals with Down syndrome during this period of language learning (Shott et al., 2006), with our work demonstrating a relationship between OSA, sleep disturbance, and verbal knowledge acquisition (Breslin et al., 2014; Spanò et al., 2018).

We have previously suggested that sleep disturbance is an important factor to consider in the progression to AD in persons with Down syndrome (Fernandez & Edgin, 2013). Specifically, in older adults with Down syndrome, rates of OSA may be higher given increases in obesity and muscle tone reductions across age, with Trois et al. (2009) reporting that a clinic-based sample of 87.5% of adults with Down syndrome had moderate-severe OSA. A comorbid diagnosis of dementia was more common among a group of older adults with Down syndrome with behavioral sleep disturbances in a previous study (Esbensen, 2016). The finding of links between SWS and the clearance of AD neuropathology (Winer & Mander, 2018) and of reduced SWS in children with OSA and Down syndrome are concerning (Breslin et al., 2014). Reduced SWS could possibly decrease the clearance of AD neuropathology and increase the likelihood of AD in persons with Down syndrome as they continue to age. Accordingly, research is needed to examine if the established links between sleep quality and the AD neuropathology are also present in people with Down syndrome.

In Esbensen, Beebe, Byars, and Hoffman's (2016) review of sleep in a clinic-based group of persons with Down syndrome aged 5–21 years, only 48% had undergone PSG, with 61% showing no sleep problem, 27% showing OSA, 3.5% showing a behavioral sleep disturbance (BSD), and 8.6% showing both. Of the individuals with sleep disorders of any origin, 60% had some form of treatment. Those with OSA, or combined OSA and BSD, were more likely to be treated with continuous positive airway pressure (CPAP) or have a history of tonsillectomy and adenoidectomy surgery, whereas those with BSD alone were more likely to be treated with medication (Esbensen et al., 2016). These findings are indicative of the common occurrence of disordered sleep profiles of children, adolescents, and young adults with Down syndrome.

The sleep deficits among persons with Down syndrome are not confined to apnea. While likely a product of OSA as well as other factors, sleep is fragmented in persons with Down syndrome, resulting in more shifts in sleep stages and poor maintenance of sleep states. Levanon, Tarasiuk, and Tal (1999) reported a 30% increase in the number of stage shifts per hour from "deeper" to "lighter" sleep stages of NREM and increased arousals in children with Down syndrome as compared to TD participants with primary snoring (i.e., a disordered sleep profile). In a community prevalence study among children with Down syndrome from birth to 18 years, Carter, McCaughey, Annaz, and Hill (2009) found that at least 40% of participants with Down syndrome, aged 4–18 years, woke once in the night, 28% woke up at least twice, and 48% transitioned to another bed. Of school-aged children with Down syndrome, 70% exhibited daytime tiredness on two or more days per week and 50% fell asleep in the car during the preceding week. Using actigraphy, Ashworth, Hill, Karmiloff-Smith, and Dimitriou (2013) found that children with Down syndrome exhibited greater sleep fragmentation with more frequent and longer night wakings as well as restlessness compared to TD children and children with Williams syndrome (WS) of the same age.

In terms of sleep architecture, persons with Down syndrome exhibit a unique sleep phenotype characterized by alterations of the sleep macro-architecture, including abnormalities in NREM sleep compared to chronological age-matched individuals with other genetic disorders (i.e., fragile X Syndrome [FXS], WS), as well as reduced REM sleep and lower sleep efficiency compared to TD children (Ferri et al., 1997; Miano et al., 2008). Miano et al. (2008) also found those with Down syndrome showed a greater percentage of Stage 1 sleep (6.1%), whereas both Stage 2 (39.9%) and REM sleep (5.73%) were reduced in comparison to TD participants matched on chronological age. The REM deficit is one of the most studied aspects of the sleep profile in both humans (Diomedi et al., 1999; Miano et al., 2008) and mouse models of Down syndrome (Colas, London, Gharib, Cespuglio, & Sarda, 2004) and extends beyond deficits primarily associated with sleep apnea (Nisbet et al., 2015). Across a number of studies, REM sleep has been shown to be consistently reduced in people with Down syndrome when compared to TD individuals, and more recent data have suggested important memory functions may be linked to REM sleep (Boyce, Glasgow, Williams, & Adamantidis, 2016; Spanò et al., 2018). Breslin et al. (2014) also suggested that SWS was specifically reduced in persons with Down syndrome and OSA, in relation to those with Down syndrome without OSA, which could be reflective of the frontal cortex involvement when OSA is present (D'Rozario et al., 2017).

Sleep deficits appear to begin in infancy and persist throughout the lifespan in persons with Down syndrome. Data recently collected in our own work shows sleep deficits measured with movement monitoring via actigraphy at 6, 12, 18, and 24-month age points in 59 infants with Down syndrome and controls (Khosla et al., 2019). The children were enrolled via hospital settings, community events, and word-of-mouth across the United States. At each time point, the parents completed detailed phone interviews regarding medical history, family background, child sleep quality, and developmental milestones. The graph of sleep efficiency is presented in Figure 19.1, showing a clear divergence in the sleep patterns in infants with Down syndrome at all four ages. As PSG studies of sleep in persons with Down syndrome are rare, the relation between these deficits and OSA in infancy is unclear. However, Goffinski et al. (2015) suggested that at least 30% of infants with Down syndrome may have moderate-severe OSA. Therefore, from our preliminary data and other published studies we have evidence that sleep is impaired in Down syndrome early in infancy and during ages of important developmental milestones.

In another study from our group utilizing data from our cohort, Fernandez et al. (2017) suggested that while sleep states may be fragmented in young children, the circadian or daily rhythms of these individuals are relatively unimpaired. Although infants and toddlers with Down syndrome slept less and had reduced sleep efficiency as compared to their age-matched TD peers, daily rhythms, as well as the development of these rhythms, were not significantly different between the groups.

Comparisons with other groups with intellectual disability (ID) have also highlighted an increased severity of sleep deficits specifically in persons with Down syndrome. Using PSG, Miano et al. (2008) examined the sleep profile in adolescents with Down syndrome in comparison to a group with FXS and chronologically age-matched TD participants. The participants with Down syndrome showed lower sleep efficiency, greater wake after sleep onset, and a reduced percentage of Stage 2 NREM sleep when compared to the

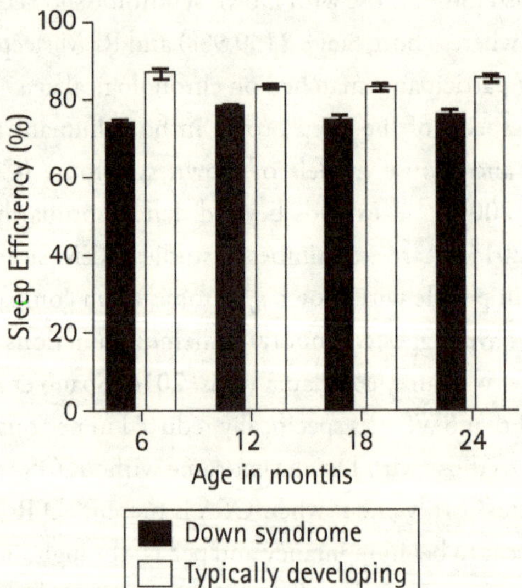

Figure 19.1. Patterns of total overnight sleep efficiency in children with and without Down syndrome.

participants with FXS. Similarly, Ashworth et al. (2013) used parent reports and actigraphy to compare school-aged children with Down syndrome to peers with WS. School-aged children wore an Actiwatch mini for one week, supported by parent completion of a sleep diary and the CSHQ. From the actigraphy data, the TD children had a later bedtime as compared to both the other groups. The children with WS had longer sleep latency, whereas the children with Down syndrome spent more time in bed, had a longer assumed sleep time, more night waking, longer wake after sleep onset, lower sleep efficiency, spent more time moving around, and had more fragmentation/restlessness. However, actual sleep time was not significantly different between any of the three groups. On the CSHQ, the children with Down syndrome had higher scores for bedtime resistance, parasomnias, and sleep duration as compared to the TD children, as well as elevated scores for sleep anxiety, night waking, sleep disordered breathing (SDB), and a higher total score as compared to both the TD and WS groups. In contrast, the children with WS had a higher score for sleep onset, night waking, and sleep duration as compared to the TD children. These findings suggest specific and severe impairment in sleep quality in persons with Down syndrome in comparison to other groups with ID.

In total, data regarding the sleep profile among persons with Down syndrome suggest elevated rates of OSA and other deficits across the lifespan. Further, these deficits are observed in developmental windows that could severely impact children's learning or an individual's ability to withstand cognitive decline. People with Down syndrome seem to show greater sleep deficits as compared to some other syndromes associated with ID. However, more work is required to track the links between sleep and developmental outcomes, including longitudinal investigations across key points of vulnerability. We have noted two such points in this chapter already, and others may be possible. For instance, as adolescence is a time of heightened sleep difficulty in the typical population, as well as a period of extreme neural plasticity and synaptic pruning, sleep during this period may also be altered among people with Down syndrome, with lasting effects on brain development.

Sleep Effects in Animal Models

Sleep has also been extensively studied in animal models of Down syndrome. Animal models have proven essential in furthering our understanding of the cause and progression of many human conditions, and they have been particularly important in driving the development of treatment protocols in Down syndrome (see Moyer & Reeves, this volume; Aziz & Haydar, this volume). They can be manipulated both genetically and behaviorally in ways that are not possible in the human population. There are both strengths and weaknesses to this methodology. The manipulations permitted are a strength, whereas the natural differences in both genetics and sleep between humans and model animals are a weakness, such as the structure of multiple sleeps in a 24-hour period commonly observed in many animals. Within the context of these benefits and shortcomings, we review the ways that mouse models of Down syndrome have been used to inform our understanding of sleep architecture and the neurologic consequences of these changes, with the following outcomes.

The Ts65Dn mouse model is trisomic for the majority of mouse chromosome 16, containing about 140 genes that are represented on human chromosome 21 (Hsa21) and implicated in the phenotype of Down syndrome, as well as some additional genes that are not on the Hsa21 (Davisson, Schmidt, & Akeson, 1990; Korenburg et al., 1994). As in the human data reported by Fernandez et al. (2017), circadian rhythms are mostly normal in Ts65Dn mice, as compared to control litter mates, and do not affect sleep-driven behaviors such as nest building (Heller et al., 2014; Ruby et al., 2010). However, Ts65Dn mice do appear to have reduced overall sleep time, specifically impacting their NREM sleep time, which mimics the findings among humans (Colas et al., 2008). Ts65Dn mice show increased activity as compared to control mice in the first hours of darkness, which could be equated to the early waking and hyperactivity observed in children with Down syndrome (Escorihuela et al., 1995). The Ts65Dn model is historically the most commonly used model and recapitulates many of the gross features of sleep architecture seen in children with Down syndrome. It may, therefore, be a useful model for examining how sleep can affect behavior and cognition across the lifespan.

The sleep patterns of two animal models with partial, but not full trisomy (i.e., Ts65Dn and Ts1Cje mice) have also been compared (Sago et al., 1998). Ts65Dn and Ts1Cje mice were implanted with EEG and electromyogram (EMG) electrodes at 3 months of age and recorded for 72 hours, including baseline and sleep deprivation conditions. The Ts65Dn mice had longer waking bouts and decreased NREM durations as compared to the control mice. REM and NREM sleep had increased theta power frequencies, with NREM also displaying reduced delta power. Following sleep deprivation, the Ts65Dn mice displayed increased latency time compared to first sleep and increased NREM amounts compared to the control mice. In contrast, the Ts1Cje mice showed no differences in natural sleep rhythms or spectral profiles. Following sleep deprivation, these mice also displayed increased sleep latency, although no altered sleep profiles were observed. These different sleep profiles appear to be due to the different genotypes, and the subsequent neuroanatomical changes, in these two models (Colas et al., 2008).

Other researchers have investigated the impact of aging on sleep in Down syndrome models and have identified patterns of sleep in aged mice that compare to patterns observed in older persons with Down syndrome. For example, Levenga, Peterson, Cain, and Hoeffer (2018) implanted Dp(16)1Yey/+ mice, aged 12–14 months, with EEG and EMG electrodes and recorded for 24 hours. During the light phase, when animals should sleep, the transgenic mice were significantly more active than the control mice and overall had significantly lower levels of NREM sleep, which could be compared to increased night waking and sleep fragmentation observed in humans. During NREM sleep, the transgenic mice had increased alpha and beta power and reduced delta power (the frequency band most prevalent in SWS) when compared to the control mice in both the light and dark phases. Therefore, these animal models showed similar sleep deficits to people with Down syndrome during the vulnerable period of aging that is associated with AD onset.

The recently developed Tc1 mouse model has the majority of Hsa21 (the human chromosome, although a mosaic distribution) present in the genome. When Tc1 mice were exposed to light-dark, dark-dark, and light-light conditions, they were significantly more active in the dark phase compared to wild type mice, replicating wake time hyperactivity from previous studies, whereas the number of immobile episodes were significantly greater in the light phase, suggesting fragmented sleep patterns (Heise et al., 2015).

Overall, the findings from mouse models with different genetic components of trisomy 21 generally recapitulate some sleep features seen in humans with Down syndrome. Reduced sleep duration with specific impact on NREM sleep appears to be a consistent finding across models, both of which are also observed in humans, suggesting some validity of these models in representing human sleep deficits. The models reflect consistently delayed sleep onset and increased activity in periods of waking. Furthermore, EEG findings of altered power frequencies in mouse models of Down syndrome suggest potential streams of human research to investigate whether these power shifts are observed among humans. Manipulations of EEG power in sleep in mice, and studies of this effect on behavior and cognition, would enable us to associate these changes to long-term alterations observed among persons with Down syndrome. Circadian rhythms were not significantly different between DS and wild type mice, as was also found for the daily rhythms of young children and infants with Down syndrome (Fernandez et al., 2017).

In total, the availability of representative animal models is important for future work on the mechanisms of sleep disturbance among persons with Down syndrome. Given the difficulty in measuring sleep with EEG among humans, findings from animal models could be useful for developing hypotheses regarding the brain states that may contribute to sleep-dependent learning deficits in persons with Down syndrome and correlations between sleep and cognition in this group. One very recent study is an elegant start toward this aim. Alemany-González et al. (2020) recently explored the link between functional connectivity disturbances during sleep and wake and memory retention in Ts65Dn mice. Abnormal synchrony was observed across wake and sleep, including decreased sharp wave ripples and REM sleep abnormalities. This study was the first to suggest disturbances in the neural physiology of sleep may relate to memory impairment in animal models of DS.

Sleep and Daytime Behavior in Persons With Down Syndrome

The correlation between sleep and daytime behavioral outcomes among persons with Down syndrome has been assessed in several studies. The majority of past research has included correlational data; only preliminary data from Hill, Fairley, Williams, Cooper, and Riha (2015) have suggested change in behavior associated with sleep treatment. Using parent-report measures of sleep and development, Churchill, Kieckhefer, Bjornson, and

Herting (2015) investigated correlations between sleep disturbances and daily life habits among 110 children with Down syndrome and 29 TD children, aged 5–18 years. Across all these ages, the children with Down syndrome exhibited significantly earlier bedtimes, early weekend wake time, and more weekday hours of sleep. Statistically significant differences also emerged on the CSHQ, although the profile was affected by age. The children with Down syndrome aged 5–12 years experienced more night wakings, parasomnias, and a higher total CSHQ score compared to TD children of the same age, while the children with Down syndrome aged 13–18 years experienced shorter sleep durations and more parasomnias, sleep-disordered breathing (SDB), and daytime sleepiness compared to the age-matched TD group. Regardless of age, the children with Down syndrome scored significantly lower on all daily life habit scores, and these deficits were correlated with sleep disturbances. In particular, SDB was found to be significantly correlated with all 12 life skill domains except for communication. These results suggest that parent-reported estimates of sleep disturbance are related to daily function in children with Down syndrome, including functional activities such as personal care and quality of relationships.

Other evidence suggests that sleep may relate to aspects of temperament and behavioral regulation in ways that could lead to day-to-day functional impairments in young children with Down syndrome. Lukowski and Milojevich (2017) compared parent-reported sleep problems and temperament between children with Down syndrome, aged 18–53 months, and TD children, aged 15–28 months. The children with Down syndrome adhered to a consistent bedtime less frequently, often did not fall asleep within 20 minutes after going to bed, were more likely to snore loudly during sleep, had reduced total sleep time during the night, and were more likely to appear tired and fall asleep during daytime activities. They also received lower scores for effortful control, attentional focusing, attentional shifting, cuddliness, and inhibitory control. According to regression models, sleep mediated the association between group and temperament outcomes, specifically levels of effortful and inhibitory control, indicating an association between sleep and behavior (Lukowski & Milojevich, 2017).

The effects of sleep disorders on behavior have also been studied in older adults. For example, Esbensen (2016) examined comorbidities associated with sleep apnea and behavioral sleep disturbances (BSD) based on age and level of intellectual and developmental disabilities, including a group of 75 adults with Down syndrome, aged 37–65 years. The older adults with Down syndrome and BSD were more likely to have clinical diagnoses of anxiety and depression, while the younger adults with Down syndrome and BSD were more likely to be diagnosed with dementia as compared to the adults without BSD. In addition, the adults with BSD exhibited more generalized behavior issues and asocial behavior problems, such as socially offensive and uncooperative behavior, thereby highlighting how sleep continues to affect behavioral and health problems into adulthood and can be considered a lifespan concern.

Despite these findings, the relationships between sleep disturbance and daytime attention, effortful control, or behavioral problems in persons with Down syndrome have been equivocal. In particular, statistically significant associations between poor sleep and daytime behavior problems or inattention have not been found with objective sleep measures such as actigraphy or PSG. Joyce and Dimitriou (2017) assessed SDB among younger children with Down syndrome and TD children aged 24–59 months with cardiorespiratory polygraphy. The children's parents completed the Strengths and Difficulties questionnaire (SDQ; five subscales reporting on emotional symptoms, conduct problems, hyperactivity, peer problems, and prosocial behavior). The children with Down syndrome had higher apnea-hypopnea index (AHI), desaturation index, baseline and minimum oxygen level, and slept 1 hour longer on average, resulting from increased daytime sleep. According to regression models, sleep did not predict performance on the SDQ among the children with Down syndrome, but the TD children with high and low AHI had significantly different scores on subscales of the strengths and difficulties questionnaire. These findings suggest that the children with Down syndrome were generally impaired across parent-reported sleep data and in behavior, but these observed impairments were not associated with PSG sleep measures. Similar negative findings have been reported in other studies with objective measures of sleep in relation to attention and behavior in Down syndrome (Breslin et al., 2014; Edgin et al., 2015).

In total, these studies indicate mixed findings concerning the relation between sleep, daytime behavior, attention, and problem behaviors in persons with Down syndrome. From the studies conducted in children with Down syndrome to date, parent-reported sleep may show more consistent relationships with daytime behavioral outcomes than do studies with objective measures. Therefore, more research is needed with multimethod sleep assessment to best understand the nature of these associations. Examinations of causal pathways via experimental or longitudinal study designs are also required. To this effect, longitudinal studies which include sleep and behavior may help us understand the stability of each of these functions and whether sleep patterns may affect outcomes over time within individuals. To date, we know of no published longitudinal work of this nature in persons with Down syndrome.

Sleep and Neurocognition Across Development and Aging in Down Syndrome

In this section, we review literature relating to correlations between sleep and cognition across the lifespan in persons with Down syndrome. Studies have been conducted in the toddler through adult years, but as of the publication of this chapter none have been focused on the relation between sleep and cognition in individuals with Down syndrome at risk for AD (i.e., aged >40 years). Studying how poor sleep may relate to cognition at points during development is essential to understanding which cognitive and neural systems may be particularly vulnerable to sleep disturbance, and these may include periods of rapid developmental progression or decline.

In one of the first studies to examine links between sleep and cognition in Down syndrome, Andreou, Galanopoulou, Gourgoulianis, Karapetsas, and Molyvdas (2002) tested the relationship between SDB and cognition in twelve individuals with Down syndrome aged 17–30 years who presented with oxygen saturation (SaO_2) less than 95% (M = 86%) and apneas greater than 10 per hour (M = 28.75). Increased incidence of apneas was associated with decreased achievement on Set A of the Ravens Progressive Matrices, which was related to performance in the orientation subtest of the Mini-Mental State test. Andreou et al. concluded that the increased apneas were related to impairments in visuoperceptual skills, as Set A is specifically used to test visuoperception linked to right hemispheric functioning. Although one of the first studies to examine sleep's relation to cognition in Down syndrome, Andreou et al. examined a limited set of cognitive outcomes, and more studies were required to continue to understand correlations between sleep and frequently studied cognitive domains (i.e., language) in this group.

In order to examine the relationship between sleep and cognition in early development, Edgin et al. (2015) characterized sleep, language development, and behavior in toddlers with Down syndrome and TD toddlers, aged 26–64 months. Objective measures of sleep were collected through actigraphy, while subjective measures included a sleep diary and the CSHQ. Actigraphy revealed significant sleep disturbances in the toddlers with Down syndrome, including reduced sleep efficiency. Consequently, the group was divided into toddlers with Down syndrome who were poor sleepers (PS; SE < 80%), and good sleepers (GS; SE ≥ 80%), with 66% of the toddlers with Down syndrome classified as poor sleepers. The children in the PS group displayed significantly shorter sleep time, greater minutes of wake after sleep onset, and a higher fragmentation index. The parents also reported significantly more sleep-disordered breathing among toddlers with Down syndrome versus TD children. Language measures indicated that the toddlers in the PS group, as compared to the GS group, had 190 fewer words on average as well as impairments in word combination, sentence length, vocalizations, and length of longest utterance blindly recorded coded from objective measures gathered in the home environment. This evidence suggests that cognition is correlated with sleep disturbances even among very young children with Down syndrome. The relation between sleep and communication deficits in young children with Down syndrome have now been replicated in D' Souza, D'Souza, Horváth, Plunkett, and Karmiloff-Smith (2020) and Arias-Trejo, Angulo-Chavira, Demara, Figueroa, and Edgin (2021).

In Breslin et al. (2014), we described the correlation between OSA and performance on the Arizona Cognitive Test Battery (Edgin et al., 2010) in children with Down syndrome aged 7–12 years. Using PSG, we found that the children with Down syndrome with OSA (defined as an AHI > 1.5) had impaired executive function and a verbal IQ nine points lower than those without apnea. These results are unique because the comparison was between children of the same age and background factors (i.e., a matched sample of children < 12 years) who differed only on OSAS status, defined by PSG. The evidence from this study suggests links between OSA in children with Down syndrome and cognitive functions that also appear to be impaired in the typical population of children with OSA.

Lukowski, Slonecker, and Milojevich (2020) recently tested the relationship between parent reported sleep problems and recall memory in toddlers with and without Down syndrome using a deferred imitation paradigm. The children were presented with four three-step event sequences during an initial session that included a baseline phase and a modeling phase, in which the researcher modeled each sequence of actions twice in succession, immediately followed by asking the child to imitate the presented sequence to demonstrate encoding. A second session occurred one month after. Frequent sleep problems were found to be positively associated with increased forgetting of individual target actions and temporal order information by the children with Down syndrome, while sleep problems were not predictive of forgetting in the TD children.

Lee and colleagues have recently examined the neural correlates of sleep disturbance in Down syndrome, finding cross-brain volumetric reductions (i.e., total, frontal, parietal, temporal, and left hippocampus brain volumes) in children with Down syndrome with higher caregiver reports of sleep disturbance (Lee, Perez, Hamner, Adeyemi, & Clasen, 2020). These findings are consistent with other neural studies of sleep disorders in TD children, which have found correlations between OSA and white matter development in the hippocampus (Cha et al., 2017). Studies of the neural correlates of sleep in humans with Down syndrome are rare, and Lee's study is the only study we found in which sleep was examined alongside neuroimaging data in children with Down syndrome. Therefore, more work should examine the relationship between sleep and brain development among persons with Down syndrome across the lifespan to better understand how sleep problems may influence development at the neural level.

Two recent studies have suggested links between sleep disturbance and brain development and neurocognition in adults with Down syndrome. Chen, Spanò, and Edgin (2013) explored the association between sleep, measured via questionnaire (Simonds & Parraga, 1982), and executive function among adolescents and adults with Down syndrome aged 14–31 years. The participants who exhibited poor sleep and had higher SDB, as measured via caregiver ratings, also produced significantly fewer words in verbal fluency and completed fewer trials on the knock-tap test, a measure of rule-shifting. These results suggest that executive function abilities in adolescence and early adulthood are associated with sleep profiles.

In another recent study Cody et al. (2020) examined sleep, Beta-amyloid levels, and AD-related cognitive decline in 47 nondemented adults with Down syndrome (aged 26–56 years). Global and striatal Beta-amyloid accumulation was measured using Pittsburgh Compound-B (PiB) positron emission tomography (PET) imaging and sleep was measured with actigraphy. The mean length of night-time awakenings across all participants was found to be associated with higher levels of striatal Beta-amyloid and decreased cognitive performance on executive functioning and motor planning and coordination tasks. However, when adjusting for chronological age, only the association between length of awakenings and executive function performance remained significant. Overall, these findings support the association between disrupted sleep, Beta-amyloid accumulation, and cognitive features of preclinical AD in persons with Down syndrome. Given these associations and potential impact of sleep in the vulnerable period of cognitive decline, future work should test the relation of the full spectrum of sleep disturbance, including OSA-related symptoms, on the rate of cognitive decline in adults in middle adulthood, a period in which poor sleep may be of greater impact because of the increasing neuropathology of AD among persons with Down syndrome.

The findings from our lab and others generally support the hypothesis that sleep correlates with cognition and brain development across the lifespan in persons with Down syndrome. These results highlight the importance of examining early life divergence from the typical trajectory sleep's potential influence on the progression of cognitive decline. However, these findings contradict those of Churchill et al. (2012) and Joyce and Dimitriou (2017), who did not find the typical relationship between sleep measures and the emergence of communication abilities among children with Down syndrome. Reasons for the disparities might be the use of a questionnaire-based assessment rather than an empirical measure by Churchill et al. (2015) and the focus on outcomes of pulse oximetry rather than PSG or actigraphy by Joyce and Dimitriou (2017). The inconsistencies across studies serve as an impetus to conduct more research in this area that may speak to the specific associations between sleep and cognitive domains (i.e., is language most affected?) and to identify the developmental age periods for which sleep disturbance may be of most impact. Furthermore, until recently, the literature on sleep in people with Down syndrome lacked experimental manipulations of sleep and learning, which can help determine the specific impact of sleep intervals on the retention of new knowledge. This methodology allows for an estimate of sleep's role better than correlational data, so we can see learning in "real time" in relation to sleep stages and quality. We review the existing literature employing these designs in the next section.

Studies of Sleep-Dependent Learning and Memory in Down Syndrome

While the findings of studies of sleep treatments have suggested some causal links between sleep treatment and improved cognitive outcomes in persons with Down syndrome (Hill et al., 2015), another study design that is useful for highlighting sleep's role is the direct comparison of memory retention across intervals with and without sleep (i.e., studies of sleep-dependent learning). In these studies, learning opportunities are manipulated in relation to sleep intervals to examine the effect on cognition.

In the first sleep-dependent learning study published in persons with Down syndrome, Ashworth, Hill, Karmiloff-Smith, and Dimitriou (2017) examined retention patterns in school-aged children who were TD or had Down syndrome or WS. The children were tested on a novel animal names task to examine the effects of sleep-dependent learning. After a learning phase, the participants were tested on the animal names and then retested after wake and sleep intervals (after 12 and 24 hours). Half of the participants were trained in the morning and retested after a wake interval then again after a sleep interval (wake/sleep condition). The other half were trained in the evening then retested after a sleep interval and then again after a wake interval (sleep/wake condition). In both conditions, the TD group showed significant improvement (remembered more words) following the sleep period, but no significant change in the score was found after the wake interval. In contrast, the children with Down syndrome did not show significant improvement after sleep or wake periods, although the group with Down syndrome trained in the morning had overall stronger performance than the group trained before sleep. These findings suggest that children with Down syndrome do not have the same sleep-dependent learning benefits as typical children, and that they may actually show better levels of retention across wake intervals. Of interest was that this pattern of sleep-dependent learning deficits was not observed in the children with WS. This study represents an advance, as it involved a direct comparison of retention across sleep and wake intervals. However, the manipulation was between subjects and different children were studied in the sleep and wake conditions. This design may have resulted in differences in background factors, a possibly learning, across training groups. Further, neither sleep quality nor physiology was measured, thereby precluding the gathering of the information regarding the neurophysiological mechanisms underlying these sleep-related learning deficits in people with Down syndrome.

In a study with findings that mirror those of Ashworth et al. (2017) and expand on them with the measurement of nap PSG after learning, Spanò et al. (2018) found that young children with Down syndrome (average age 4.5 years) also showed reduced sleep-dependent learning in comparison to typical controls. Specifically, in a within-participants design, children with Down syndrome showed equivalent retention to the TD children matched on nonverbal IQ raw score, across 5-minute and 4-hour wake delays, but were impaired only when they napped. This pattern of impairment was evident at 4 hours as well as 24 hours later. These findings suggest that some processes of sleep in naps may interfere with memory consolidation in toddlers with Down syndrome such that they do not experience the benefit from sleeping directly after learning that is observed among TD children. The primary difference in the sleep neurophysiology in the persons with Down syndrome was reductions in REM sleep; more research is needed to understand links between disordered sleep and outcomes in Down syndrome using designs of this nature that incorporate objective measures of sleep as well as designs directly comparing various long-term retention intervals.

In another recent study from our laboratory, we suggested that sleep-dependent learning deficits are not present under all conditions in persons with Down syndrome, and understanding the factors relating to these impairments may help reveal the best strategies for supporting learning in persons with Down syndrome. Sakhon, Edwards, Luongo, Murphy, and Edgin (2018) found evidence for unimpaired memory retention for a small set of novel words in adolescents and young adults with Down syndrome, aged 11–28 years. In this study, the participants with Down syndrome retained these labels for 1 week and their levels of retention did not relate to sleep quantity or quality. Unlike previous sleep-dependent memory manipulations, the set size of this study was very small and the children were retested on materials at both delay periods, which could have led to early consolidation and resistance to loss over time. We are now undertaking research to determine if children with Down syndrome may benefit from repeated testing, as the findings from this study suggest they could retain information under those conditions. Such work may support educational strategies that maximize retention even when sleep is poor.

In total, correlational and experimental data suggest that poor sleep impacts knowledge acquisition in Down syndrome, particularly learning and producing new words. Treatment (i.e., experimental) studies are required to determine how sleep intervention may impact word acquisition in order to further probe the causal nature of these deficits. Overall, these studies illustrate mixed evidence associated with altered sleep profiles in persons with Down syndrome, but most of the published work suggests that sleep correlates with profiles of learning, communication, and behavior. Some contradictory evidence emphasizes a need for studies with larger samples and consistent, well-validated sleep measures and cognitive outcomes. Consistent with this goal, the field must continue to develop valid and reliable measures that tap into neurocognitive performance among children with Down syndrome at different ages.

Further, research has suggested a developmental trajectory for sleep's effects on learning that parallels the development of the hippocampus, and therefore sleep's effects may be reliant on different neural systems (i.e., cortex vs. hippocampus; Gómez & Edgin, 2015) at some developmental stages. Thus, depending on the developmental state, we might expect that people with Down syndrome may show different patterns of impairment in sleep-dependent learning. Most extant data in this population have been collected at single "snapshots" in time, and in order to best understand these relationships and how sleep may support learning across development, more work is needed that spans larger age ranges and includes longitudinal investigations.

Effect on the Family

Sleep's effects may extend beyond the direct influences on the child with Down syndrome to also affect the family including parent and sibling sleep and mental health. Cotton and Richdale (2006) examined parental perceptions of child sleep and family stress in children with autism, familial intellectual disability (FID), Prader-Willi syndrome, Down syndrome, and in TD children. The parents completed questionnaires on demographics, medical history, severity of intellectual disability, and sleep. A variety of sleep behaviors including daytime napping, excessive daytime sleepiness, settling habits, night waking, bedtime routines, and presence and severity of sleep issues were measured using questions in yes/no format, 100-mm visual analogue scales, and sleep behavior descriptions. Overall, parent-reported sleep problems were four times more likely in the children with developmental disorders than TD children, and children with autism were the most likely to exhibit a sleep problem. Although the severity of sleep problems did not differ across groups, the types of sleep problems varied. The children with Down syndrome or FID presented with sleep maintenance problems while the children with autism displayed settling difficulties or cosleeping behaviors, and the children with Prader-Willi syndrome were more likely to exhibit daytime sleepiness and/or excessive tiredness. However, sleep maintenance difficulties and night waking (particularly prevalent in the children with Down syndrome) were associated with a family's well-being, indicating there are consequences of impaired sleep on the family.

From the literature on typical children, we know poor sleep may also affect other aspects of family functioning, specifically the quality of dyadic relationships within the family (i.e., marital, sibling, etc.), home environment, and employment (Dahl & El-Sheikh, 2007). For instance, night-time crying during the infancy period is found to significantly influence both marital relationships and many parents' own sleep (Meijer & van den Witenboer, 2007). Among typical children aged 2–12 years with more than one sleep issue, correlations were found between child sleep problems and daytime sleepiness in parents, and some of these associations could relate to parental stress or functioning (Boergers, Hart, Owens, Streisand, & Spirito, 2007).

Considering research from the TD population, we can speculate about the role of sleep in families with children with DS in the home (Boergers et al., 2007; El-Sheikh, Buckhalt, Mize, & Acebo, 2006; Meijer & van den Witenboer, 2007). Parents of children with Down syndrome with sleep problems are also likely to experience daytime tiredness, which could further impact functioning around the home, childcare, and employment. Given the persistent nature of sleep difficulties in persons with Down syndrome, more research should be focused on the broader influence of poor sleep on family dynamics in persons with Down syndrome. Research addressing this question is currently lacking in persons with Down syndrome specifically and could provide important information for therapeutic intervention.

Treatments and Impacts for Intervention

Fortunately, sleep problems are treatable through several means, and exciting new methodologies for treating sleep apnea in persons with Down syndrome have been reported and many are still under investigation (Diercks et al., 2016). However, we would be remiss not to highlight, given the potential impact of sleep on cognition and behavioral outcome measures, the importance of considering this domain in future research investigations in this population. We therefore recommend the careful consideration of sleep deficits when designing behavioral and pharmacological interventions across the lifespan for persons with Down syndrome. We have illustrated the importance of this recommendation for both people with and without Down syndrome and highlight the ongoing and planned pharmacological interventions for memory impairment in people with Down syndrome (reviewed in Fernandez & Edgin, 2016). The studies presented in this review strongly suggest that sleep should be more seriously considered as an important source of variability influencing development among persons with Down syndrome across the lifespan. Given efforts to characterize the extent to which persons with Down syndrome may respond to clinical intervention, including approaches to understanding the progression of AD which are currently underway, we assert that future studies will be better informed if they also consider, and adequately measure, sleep. In addition, for better understanding of the causal nature of disordered sleep on features of Down syndrome, future interventions should include measurements of sleep to determine how treatment effects may be moderated by sleep deficits. Given the data suggesting that sleep is an important brain state for knowledge acquisition, we also argue that sleep itself should be considered a "neurocognitive" endpoint in future clinical trials of this syndrome.

Conclusion and Future Directions

In conclusion, the impact of sleep on behavioral, neurocognitive, and developmental outcomes is imperative to address, due to its potential to impact quality of life for persons with Down syndrome. While sleep is impaired at greater levels across the lifespan in persons with Down syndrome in relation to persons with other developmental disorders, sleep issues are not restricted to this community. Commonly, these issues are often overlooked in all groups due to cultural and societal misconceptions regarding the functions and importance of sleep. However, among people with Down syndrome, this oversight may leave individuals vulnerable to further cognitive delays during critical developmental periods. We have provided an in-depth illustration of how sleep may impact those with Down syndrome and their families across the lifespan. The evidence highlights differences in sleep behaviors and associated developmental outcomes, although the causal nature of these links requires further investigation with treatment studies (Breslin et al., 2014; Churchill et al., 2015; Edgin et al., 2015; Esbensen, 2016). Representative animal models are available and could be used to gain detail regarding the precise mechanisms linking sleep deficits to cognitive and neural difficulties. What is also evident is that most previous research on sleep and development in persons with Down syndrome has been focused on associations solely in pediatric groups. Given links between sleep and AD in the typical population, more research is needed to assess sleep's role in the progression of cognitive decline in older adults with Down syndrome (see Startin, Zaman, & Strydom, this volume for general information on AD in persons with Down syndrome). The implications for future research are many, but for brevity we would prioritize the following future directions:

1. *Measuring sleep across age and intellectual disability.* Objective sleep assessment (i.e., PSG) is required to obtain an understanding of the extent of sleep impairment in individuals with Down syndrome across the lifespan, and these assessments are not currently routinely used in clinical or research practice in this population. Anecdotally, some families may take months to years to gain access to a clinical sleep study. Variability in sleep patterns have been reported in studies relying on subjective measures such as parent-report, objective measures such as actigraphy and polysomnographic studies, or both (Andreou et al., 2002; Cotton & Richdale, 2006; Edgin et al., 2015). The academic and clinical sleep communities are familiar with the limitations of these measures, particularly inaccurate reporting, inconsistent or absent validation across age groups, inconsistent participant compliance, and the time and financial resources required to complete these measures (Andreou et al., 2002; Breslin et al., 2011; Cotton & Richdale, 2006; Goodlin-Jones, Tang, Liu, & Anders, 2008; Levanon et al., 1999). Researchers are now more frequently incorporating actigraphy monitors and sleep diaries, and there is a need to closely evaluate data collected from such studies (Acebo et al., 1999; Ashworth et al., 2013, 2015; Edgin et al., 2015). For example, to allow for cross-study comparison and actigraphy validation, number of days worn and types of algorithms used to calculate different sleep parameters should be specified. Similarly, administering PSG is key to furthering validation of in-home sleep assessments and determining whether clinical referral may be the next step to diagnosis of sleep problems, including OSA. As a full picture of the validity of these measures emerges, we will be able to characterize sleep profiles across the lifespan, as well as across different forms of ID. These profiles will allow us to determine how different sleep problems relate to different phenotypes, and thus how to intervene to best ameliorate developmental impairments and possible cognitive decline in aging.

2. *Timing and effectiveness of sleep interventions.* In some persons with Down syndrome sleep is disordered across the lifespan. As such, the efficacy of different surgical and non-surgical interventions must be considered, as well as which intervention is appropriate at different developmental time points while considering the physical and neurological features of the individual. As persons with Down syndrome are at risk for moderate to severe sleep problems across the lifespan, follow-up evaluations and treatment plans may be required even if an individual received treatment at an earlier point in development. Novel treatment strategies are currently being tested, and while some of them are promising, they may not be effective at all stages of development. In our view, future work should aim to provide findings which identify (a) the key age periods in which sleep most critically impacts the development of individuals with Down syndrome, and (b) treatments that can be best delivered at these ages.

Although more research is required before we fully understand the complete role of sleep disturbances across the lifespan in Down syndrome, we have illustrated the relevance and potential contribution of this field of investigation. What is clear from the work presented here is that sleep measurement in persons with Down syndrome is not an impossible endeavor and, given the extent of sleep difficulties in this population, future research should aim to include sleep measures. The studies described throughout this chapter suggest the ways in which neural "housekeeping", development, and learning might be derailed across development and in adulthood for people with Down syndrome because of poor sleep. The consequences of disturbing this "beloved teacher" of sleep could affect many domains, and, as such, sleep's role deserves additional research in people with Down syndrome across the lifespan.

Acknowledgement

*Hughes and Khosla contributed equally to this manuscript, this contribution was funded through grants from the Bill and Melinda Gates Foundation, the Foundation Jerome Lejeune, and National Institute of Child Health & Human Development (NICHD). We would like to thank members of the Down syndrome Research Group for comments on a final draft of the paper.

References

Acebo, C., Sadeh, A., Seifer, R., Tzischinsky, O., Wolfson, A. R., Hafer, A., & Carskadon, M. A. (1999). Estimating sleep patterns with activity monitoring in children and adolescents: How many nights are necessary for reliable measures? *Sleep*, *22*(1), 95–103.

Alemany-González, M., Gener, T., Nebot, P., Vilademunt, M., Dierssen, M., & Puig, M. V. (2020). Prefrontal–hippocampal functional connectivity encodes recognition memory and is impaired in intellectual disability. *Proceedings of the National Academy of Sciences*, *117*(21), 11788–11798.

Andreou, G., Galanopoulou, C., Gourgoulianis, K., Karapetsas, A., & Molyvdas, P. (2002). Cognitive status in Down syndrome individuals with sleep disordered breathing deficits (SDB). *Brain & Cognition*, *50*(1), 145–149.

Arias-Trejo, N., Angulo-Chavira, A. Q., Demara, B., Figueroa, C., & Edgin, J. (2021). The influence of sleep on language production modalities in preschool children with Down syndrome. *Journal of Sleep Research*, *30*(3), e13120.

Ashworth, A., Hill, C. M., Karmiloff-Smith, A., & Dimitriou, D. (2013). Cross syndrome comparison of sleep problems in children with Down syndrome and Williams syndrome. *Research in Developmental Disabilities*, *34*(5), 1572–1580.

Ashworth, A., Hill, C. M., Karmiloff-Smith, A., & Dimitriou, D. (2015). The importance of sleep: Attentional problems in school-aged children with Down syndrome and Williams syndrome. *Behavioral Sleep Medicine*, *13*(6), 455–471.

Ashworth, A., Hill, C. M., Karmiloff-Smith, A., & Dimitriou, D. (2017). A cross-syndrome study of the differential effects of sleep on declarative memory consolidation in children with neurodevelopmental disorders. *Developmental Science*, *20*(2), e12383.

Beck, S. E., & Marcus, C. L. (2009). Pediatric polysomnography. *Sleep Medicine Clinics*, *4*(3), 393–406.

Blumberg, M. S. (2003). Hippocampal theta in the newborn rat is revealed under conditions that promote REM sleep. *Journal of Neuroscience*, *23*(4), 1114–1118.

Boergers, J., Hart, C., Owens, J. A., Streisand, R., & Spirito, A. (2007). Child sleep disorders: Associations with parental sleep duration and daytime sleepiness. *Journal of Family Psychology*, *21*(1), 88.

Boyce, R., Glasgow, S. D., Williams, S., & Adamantidis, A. (2016). Causal evidence for the role of REM sleep theta rhythm in contextual memory consolidation. *Science, 352*(6287), 812–816.

Breslin, J. H., Edgin, J. O., Bootzin, R. R., Goodwin, J. L., & Nadel, L. (2011). Parental report of sleep problems in Down syndrome. *Journal of Intellectual Disability Research, 55*(11), 1086–1091.

Breslin, J., Spanò, G., Bootzin, R., Anand, P., Nadel, L., & Edgin, J. (2014). Obstructive sleep apnea syndrome and cognition in Down syndrome. *Developmental Medicine & Child Neurology, 56*(7), 657–664.

Bronfenbrenner, U. (1977). Toward an experimental ecology of human development. *American Psychologist, 32*(7), 513–531.

Carter, M., McCaughey, E., Annaz, D., & Hill, C. M. (2009). Sleep problems in a Down syndrome population. *Archives of Disease in Childhood, 94* (4), 308–310.

Cha, J., Zea-Hernandez, J. A., Sin, S., Graw-Panzer, K., Shifteh, K., Isasi, C. R., . . . Arens, R. (2017). The effects of obstructive sleep apnea syndrome on the dentate gyrus and learning and memory in children. *Journal of Neuroscience, 37*(16), 4280–4288.

Chen, C. C. J., Spanò, G., & Edgin, J. O. (2013). The impact of sleep disruption on executive function in Down syndrome. *Research in Developmental Disabilities, 34*(6), 2033–2039.

Churchill, S. S., Kieckhefer, G. M., Bjornson, K. F., & Herting, J. R. (2015). Relationship between sleep disturbance and functional outcomes in daily life habits of children with Down syndrome. *Sleep, 38*(1), 61–71.

Churchill, S. S., Kieckhefer, G. M., Landis, C. A., & Ward, T. M. (2012). Sleep measurement and monitoring in children with Down syndrome: A review of the literature, 1960–2010. *Sleep Medicine Reviews, 16*(5), 477–488.

Cody, K. A., Piro-Gambetti, B., Zammit, M. D., Christian, B. T., Handen, B. L., Klunk, W. E., . . . Hartley, S. L. (2020). Association of seep with cognition and β-amyloid accumulation in adults with Down syndrome. *Neurobiology of Aging, 93*, 44–51.

Colas, D., London, J., Gharib, A., Cespuglio, R., & Sarda, N. (2004). Sleepwake architecture in mouse models for Down syndrome. *Neurobiology of Disease, 16*(2), 291–299.

Colas, D., Valletta, J. S., Takimoto-Kimura, R., Nishino, S., Fujiki, N., Mobley, W. C., & Mignot, E. (2008). Sleep and EEG features in genetic models of Down syndrome. *Neurobiology of Disease, 30*(1), 1–7.

Cotton, S., & Richdale, A. (2006). Brief report: Parental descriptions of sleep problems in children with autism, Down syndrome, and Prader-Willi syndrome. *Research in Developmental Disabilities, 27*(2), 151–161.

Crick, F., & Mitchison, G. (1983). The function of dream sleep. *Nature, 304*(5922), 111–114.

Dahl, R. E., & El-Sheikh, M. (2007). Considering sleep in a family context: Introduction to the special issue. *Journal of Family Psychology, 21*(1), 1–3.

Davisson, M. T., Schmidt, C., & Akeson, E. C. (1990). Segmental trisomy of murine chromosome 16: A new model system for studying Down syndrome. *Progress in Clinical & Biological Research, 360*, 263.

Diekelmann, S., & Born, J. (2010). The memory function of sleep. *Nature Reviews Neuroscience* , *11*(2), 114.

Diercks, G. R., Keamy, D., Kinane, T. B., Skotko, B., Schwartz, A., Grealish, E., . . . Hartnick, C. J. (2016). Hypoglossal nerve stimulator implantation in an adolescent with Down syndrome and sleep apnea. *Pediatrics, 137*(5).

Diomedi, M., Curatolo, P., Scalise, A., Placidi, F., Caretto, F., & Gigli, G. L. (1999). Sleep abnormalities in mentally retarded autistic subjects: Down's syndrome with mental retardation and normal subjects. *Brain & Development, 21*(8), 548–553.

D'Rozario, A. L., Cross, N. E., Vakulin, A., Bartlett, D. J., Wong, K. K., Wang, D., & Grunstein, R. R. (2017). Quantitative electroencephalogram measures in adult obstructive sleep apnea—Potential biomarkers of neurobehavioural functioning. *Sleep Medicine Reviews, 36*, 29–42.

D'Souza, D., D'Souza, H., Horváth, K., Plunkett, K., & Karmiloff-Smith, A. (2020). Sleep is atypical across neurodevelopmental disorders in infants and toddlers: A cross-syndrome study. *Research in Developmental Disabilities, 97*, 103549.

Dyken, M. E., Lin-Dyken, D. C., Poulton, S., Zimmerman, M. B., & Sedars, E. (2003). Prospective polysomnographic analysis of obstructive sleep apnea in Down syndrome. *Archives of Pediatrics & Adolescent Medicine, 157*(7), 655–660.

Edgin, J. O., Mason, G. M., Allman, M. J., Capone, G. T., DeLeon, I., Maslen, C., . . . Nadel, L. (2010). Development and validation of the Arizona Cognitive Test Battery for Down syndrome. *Journal of Neurodevelopmental Disorders, 2*(3), 149–164.

Edgin, J. O., Tooley, U., Demara, B., Nyhuis, C., Anand, P., & Spanò, G. (2015). Sleep disturbance and expressive language development in preschool-age children with Down syndrome. *Child Development, 86*(6), 1984–1998.

Ednick, M., Cohen, A. P., McPhail, G. L., Beebe, D., Simakajornboon, N., & Amin, R. S. (2009). A review of the effects of sleep during the first year of life on cognitive, psychomotor, and temperament development. *Sleep, 32*(11), 1449–1458.

El-Sheikh, M., Buckhalt, J. A., Mize, J., & Acebo, C. (2006). Marital conflict and disruption of children's sleep. *Child Development, 77*(1), 31–43.

Esbensen, A. J. (2016). Sleep problems and associated comorbidities among adults with Down syndrome. *Journal of Intellectual Disability Research, 60*(1), 68–79.

Esbensen, A. J., Beebe, D. W., Byars, K. C., & Hoffman, E. K. (2016). Use of sleep evaluations and treatments in children with Down syndrome. *Journal of Developmental & Behavioral Pediatrics, 37*(8), 629–636.

Esbensen, A. J., & Hoffman, E. K. (2017). Reliability of parent report measures of sleep in children with Down syndrome. *Journal of Intellectual Disability Research, 61*(3), 210–220.

Esbensen, A. J., Hoffman, E. K., Stansberry, E., & Shaffer, R. (2018). Convergent validity of actigraphy with polysomnography and parent reports when measuring sleep in children with Down syndrome. *Journal of Intellectual Disability Research, 62*(4), 281–291.

Escorihuela, R. M., Fernández-Teruel, A., Vallina, I. F., Baamonde, C., Lumbreras, M. A., Dierssen, M., . . . Flórez, J. (1995). A behavioral assessment of Ts65Dn mice: A putative Down syndrome model. *Neuroscience Letters, 199*(2), 143–146.

Fernandez, F., & Edgin, J. O. (2013). Poor sleep as a precursor to cognitive decline in Down syndrome: A hypothesis. *Journal of Alzheimer's Disease & Parkinsonism, 3*(2), 124.

Fernandez, F., & Edgin, J. O. (2016). Pharmacotherapy in Down's syndrome: Which way forward? *The Lancet Neurology, 15*(8), 776–777.

Fernandez, F., Nyhuis, C. C., Anand, P., Demara, B. I., Ruby, N. F., Spanò, G., . . . Edgin, J. O. (2017). Young children with Down syndrome show normal development of circadian rhythms, but poor sleep efficiency: A cross-sectional study across the first 60 months of life. *Sleep Medicine, 33*, 134–144.

Ferri, R., Curzi-Dascalova, L. I. L. I. A., Del Gracco, S., Elia, M., Musumeci, S., & Stefanini, M. (1997). Respiratory patterns during sleep in Down's syndrome: Importance of central apnoeas. *Journal of Sleep Research, 6*(2), 134–141.

Goffinski, A., Stanley, M. A., Shepherd, N., Duvall, N., Jenkinson, S. B., Davis, C., . . . Roper, R. J. (2015). Obstructive sleep apnea in young infants with Down syndrome evaluated in a Down syndrome specialty clinic. *American Journal of Medical Genetics Part A, 167*(2), 324–330.

Gómez, R. L., Bootzin, R. R., & Nadel, L. (2006). Naps promote abstraction in language-learning infants. *Psychological Science, 17*(8), 670–674.

Gómez, R. L., & Edgin, J. O. (2015). Sleep as a window into early neural development: Shifts in sleep-dependent learning effects across early childhood. *Child Development Perspectives, 9*(3), 183–189.

Gómez, R. L., Newman-Smith, K. C., Breslin, J. H., & Bootzin, R. R. (2011). Learning, memory, and sleep in children. *Sleep Medicine Clinics, 6*(1), 45–57.

Goodlin-Jones, B. L., Tang, K., Liu, J., & Anders, T. F. (2008). Sleep patterns in preschool-age children with Autism, developmental delay, and typical development. *Journal of the American Academy of Child & Adolescent Psychiatry, 47*(8), 930–938.

Heise, I., Fisher, S. P., Banks, G. T., Wells, S., Peirson, S. N., Foster, R. G., & Nolan, P. M. (2015). Sleep-like behavior and 24-h rhythm disruption in the Tc1 mouse model of Down syndrome. *Genes, Brain & Behavior, 14*(2), 209–216.

Heller, H. C., Salehi, A., Chuluun, B., Das, D., Lin, B., Moghadam, S., . . . Colas, D. (2014). Nest building is impaired in the Ts65Dn mouse model of Down syndrome and rescued by blocking 5HT2a receptors. *Neurobiology of Learning & Memory, 116*, 162–171.

Hill, E. A., Fairley, D. M., Williams, L. J., Cooper, S. A., & Riha, R. L. (2015). A prospective, randomised, controlled trial of CPAP in adults with Down syndrome. *European Respiratory Journal, 46*(59).

Hobson, J. A., & Stickgold, R. (1995). Sleep: Sleep the beloved teacher? *Current Biology, 5*(1), 35–36.

Holth, J. K., Fritschi, S. K., Wang, C., Pedersen, N. P., Cirrito, J. R., Mahan, T. E., . . . Lucey, B. P. (2019). The sleep-wake cycle regulates brain interstitial fluid tau in mice and CSF tau in humans. *Science, 363*(6429), 880–884.

Joyce, A., & Dimitriou, D. (2017). Sleep-disordered breathing and cognitive functioning in preschool children with and without Down syndrome. *Journal of Intellectual Disability Research, 61*(8), 778–791.

Khosla, P. (2019). *A family systems approach to sleep patterns in Down syndrome* (Unpublished doctoral dissertation, University of Arizona).

Konstantinopoulou, S., Tapia, I. E., Kim, J. Y., Xanthopoulos, M. S., Radcliffe, J., Cohen, M. S., . . . Zemel, B. (2016). Relationship between obstructive sleep apnea cardiac complications and sleepiness in children with Down syndrome. *Sleep Medicine, 17*, 18–24.

Korenberg, J. R., Chen, X. N., Schipper, R., Sun, Z., Gonsky, R., Gerwehr, S., . . . Disteche, C. (1994). Down syndrome phenotypes: The consequences of chromosomal imbalance. *Proceedings of the National Academy of Sciences, 91*(11), 4997–5001.

Lee, N. R., Perez, M., Hamner, T., Adeyemi, E., & Clasen, L. S. (2020). A preliminary examination of brain morphometry in youth with Down syndrome with and without parent-reported sleep difficulties. *Research in Developmental Disabilities, 99*, 103575.

Levanon, A., Tarasiuk, A., & Tal, A. (1999). Sleep characteristics in children with Down syndrome. *The Journal of Pediatrics, 134*(6), 755–760.

Levenga, J., Peterson, D. J., Cain, P., & Hoeffer, C. A. (2018). Sleep behavior and EEG oscillations in Aged Dp (16) 1Yey/+ Mice: A Down syndrome model. *Neuroscience, 376*, 117–126.

Louie, K., & Wilson, M. A. (2001). Temporally structured replay of awake hippocampal ensemble activity during rapid eye movement sleep. *Neuron, 29*(1), 145–156.

Lukowski, A. F., & Milojevich, H. M. (2017). Sleep problems and temperament in young children with Down syndrome and typically developing controls. *Journal of Intellectual Disability Research, 61*(3), 221–232.

Lukowski, A. F., Slonecker, E. M., & Milojevich, H. M. (2020). Sleep problems and recall memory in children with Down syndrome and typically developing controls. *Research in Developmental Disabilities, 96*, 103512.

Meijer, A. M., & van den Wittenboer, G. L. (2007). Contribution of infants' sleep and crying to marital relationship of first-time parent couples in the 1st year after childbirth. *Journal of Family Psychology, 21*(1), 49.

Miano, S., Bruni, O., Elia, M., Scifo, L., Smerieri, A., Trovato, A., . . . Ferri, R. (2008). Sleep phenotypes of intellectual disability: A polysomnographic evaluation in subjects with Down syndrome and Fragile-X syndrome. *Clinical Neurophysiology, 119*(6), 1242–1247.

Mindell, J. A., & Owens, J. A. (2015). *A clinical guide to pediatric sleep: Diagnosis and management of sleep problems*. Philadelphia, PA: Wolters Kluwer.

National Institute of Neurological Disorders & Stroke. (2014). *Brain basics: Understanding sleep*. Retrieved from http://www.ninds.nih.gov/disorders/brain_basics/understanding_sleep.html

Nisbet, L. C., Phillips, N. N., Hoban, T. F., & O'Brien, L. M. (2015). Characterization of a sleep architectural phenotype in children with Down syndrome. *Sleep & Breathing, 19*(3), 1065–1071.

Ohayon, M. M., Carskadon, M. A., Guilleminault, C., & Vitiello, M. V. (2004). Meta-analysis of quantitative sleep parameters from childhood to old age in healthy individuals: Developing normative sleep values across the human lifespan. *Sleep, 27*(7), 1255–1274.

Peigneux, P., Laureys, S., Fuchs, S., Collette, F., Perrin, F., Reggers, J., . . . Luxen, A. (2004). Are spatial memories strengthened in the human hippocampus during slow wave sleep? *Neuron, 44*(3), 535–545.

Poe, G. R. (2017). Sleep is for forgetting. *Journal of Neuroscience, 37*(3), 464–473.

Roffwarg, H. P., Muzio, J. N., & Dement, W. C. (1966). Ontogenetic development of the human sleep-dream cycle. *Science, 152*(3722), 604–619.

Ruby, N. F., Fernandez, F., Zhang, P., Klima, J., Heller, H. C., & Garner, C. C. (2010). Circadian locomotor rhythms are normal in Ts65Dn "Down syndrome" mice and unaffected by pentylenetetrazole. *Journal of Biological Rhythms, 25*(1), 63–66.

Rudoy, J. D., Voss, J. L., Westerberg, C. E., & Paller, K. A. (2009). Strengthening individual memories by reactivating them during sleep. *Science, 326*(5956), 1079.

Sago, H., Carlson, E. J., Smith, D. J., Kilbridge, J., Rubin, E. M., Mobley, W. C., . . . Huang, T. T. (1998). Ts1Cje, a partial trisomy 16 mouse model for Down syndrome, exhibits learning and behavioral abnormalities. *Proceedings of the National Academy of Sciences, 95*(11), 6256–6261.

Sakhon, S., Edwards, K., Luongo, A., Murphy, M., & Edgin, J. (2018). Small sets of novel words are fully retained after 1-week in typically developing children and Down syndrome: A fast mapping study. *Journal of the International Neuropsychological Society, 24*(9), 955–965.

Shott, S. R., Amin, R., Chini, B., Heubi, C., Hotze, S., & Akers, R. (2006). Obstructive sleep apnea: Should all children with Down syndrome be tested? *Archives of Otolaryngology—Head & Neck Surgery, 132*(4), 432–436.

Simonds, J. F., & Parraga, H. (1982). Prevalence of sleep disorders and sleep behaviors in children and adolescents. *Journal of the American Academy of Child Psychiatry, 21*(4), 383–388.

Spanò, G., Gómez, R. L., Demara, B. I., Alt, M., Cowen, S. L., & Edgin, J. O. (2018). REM sleep in naps differentially relates to memory consolidation in typical preschoolers and children with Down syndrome. *Proceedings of the National Academy of Sciences, 115*(46), 11844–11849.

Trois, M. S., Capone, G. T., Lutz, J. A., Melendres, M. C., Schwartz, A. R., Collop, N. A., & Marcus, C. L. (2009). Obstructive sleep apnea in adults with Down syndrome. *Journal of Clinical Sleep Medicine, 5*(4), 317–323.

Wilson, M. A., & McNaughton, B. L. (1994). Reactivation of hippocampal ensemble memories during sleep. *Science, 265*(5172), 676–679.

Winer, J. R., & Mander, B. A. (2018). Waking up to the importance of sleep in the pathogenesis of Alzheimer disease. *JAMA Neurology, 75*(6), 654–656.

Zigman W. B., & Lott I. T. (2007). Alzheimer's disease in Down syndrome: Neurobiology and risk. *Mental Retardation & Developmental Disabilities Reviews, 13*(3), 237–246.

SECTION 5

Interventions and Future Directions

CHAPTER

19 Communication and Language Interventions for Children With Down Syndrome

Steven F. Warren, Shelley L. Bredin-Oja, Laura J. Hahn, *and* Nancy Brady

Abstract

Delayed and disordered speech and language development are among the primary challenges for young children with Down syndrome. Common sources of these delays include frequent ear infections and fluctuating hearing loss early in life, significant oral motor impairments, and delayed onset of joint attention and related cognitive skills. This chapter is focused on the early childhood period up to 8 years of age because most of the intervention research has been conducted during this period. The review is limited to two types of intervention: milieu teaching (MT) and augmentative and alternative communication (AAC) because much of the published research has focused on these two approaches. The review reveals the strengths and weaknesses of the research to date. Four directions for future research are proposed, most importantly combining MT and AAC approaches in a single flexible model of early communication and language intervention for young children with DS.

Key Words: Down syndrome, early communication, language development, augmentative communication, milieu teaching, parenting, single-subject designs, randomized controlled trials

In this chapter, we review the published research literature on communication and language intervention for children with Down syndrome (DS). Delayed and disordered speech and language development are among the primary features of DS. Common sources of these delays include frequent ear infections and fluctuating hearing loss in the first few months of life, oral motor impairments that affect speech development (i.e., low muscle tone in the tongue, lips, and cheeks; enlarged tongue), and delayed onset of joint attention and related cognitive skills (Sterling & Warren, 2008; also, see Abbeduto et al., this volume). As DS is diagnosed prior to, or, at birth, there is an opportunity to start communication intervention soon thereafter.

This chapter is focused primarily on the early childhood period of development up to 8 years because the bulk of communication and language intervention research has been conducted during this age period. We have not attempted a comprehensive review of all communication and language intervention studies, but rather a review of two types of interventions: milieu teaching (MT) and augmentative and alternative communication (AAC) studies. The reason for limiting our review to these two approaches is straightforward—much of the research on communication and language interventions with individuals with DS is connected to these interventions. The research on MT and related intervention approaches has progressed sufficiently so that we will focus primarily on intervention studies with a randomized clinical trial (RCT) design. These designs are based on random assignment of subjects such that each subject has an equal chance of being assigned to any one of the treatment conditions. This generally ensures that both known and unknown variables are evenly distributed across conditions, thus allowing an objective analysis of treatment effects. Our other focus is on AAC approaches because of their steadily increasing use with children with DS. However, to date most of the relevant research for AAC interventions is based on small-*N* single-subject design studies and non-randomized group designs with a wide range of children. Consequently, this limitation will be addressed in our review. In the final part of the chapter, we address several pressing issues that need to be considered for research on communication and language intervention to lead to better outcomes for children with DS.

As noted by Abbeduto et al. (this volume) in the chapter on language development, children with DS generally demonstrate both areas of relative strength (i.e., receptive language, social skills, visual-spatial processing) and areas of relative weakness (i.e., expressive language, verbal working memory, executive functioning, aspects of motor functioning, and speech intelligibility) within the language domain. This behavioral profile of strengths and weaknesses is probabilistic and has not necessarily translated into a *unique* intervention approach with individuals with DS but has influenced the choice of specific intervention targets and priorities (e.g., expressive vocabulary, early signs). For example, visual-spatial abilities are often described as a strength in children with DS relative to their verbal language skills (Yang, Conners, & Merrill, 2014) and may help a child learn vocabulary effectively from signs or graphic symbols, two forms of AAC. Thus, awareness of these relative strengths and weaknesses obviously should be a consideration in developing and adapting intervention approaches for children with DS. This perspective led the National Down Syndrome Society to recommend the use of AAC approaches, such as total communication (signing while speaking), picture or graphic symbol systems, or speech-generating devices (SGDs), as a transitional communication system with young children with DS (Kumin, 1999).

Because of our focus on RCTs, much of the research discussed here was published after the 1990s. Research published earlier than this was often focused on characterizing the development of children with DS (e.g., Cicchetti & Beeghly, 1990; Dodd, 1976) and on small-*N* single-subject design studies (e.g., Guess, Sailor, Rutherford, & Baer, 1968; Guess, 1969). Many of the earliest studies involved applied behavioral analytic techniques primarily with older children who resided in residential institutions (e.g., Halle, Baer, & Spradlin, 1981; Spradlin, Karlan, & Wetherby, 1976). However, beginning in the 1980s a clear trend toward more "community-based approaches" such as early intervention programs, and a focus on intervention with younger children emerged (e.g., Warren & Rogers-Warren, 1985). Many of these studies included children with intellectual disabilities other than DS. Small mixed-etiology studies have made it difficult to generalize the results of these interventions to any specific etiology associated with intellectual disability. Fortunately, the publication of several RCTs in the past two decades have included relatively large numbers of children with DS and have allowed the analysis of intervention effects specifically for these children.

To support our focus on MT and AAC intervention approaches for children with DS, we include three tables with key summary information for the studies discussed. This includes the level of evidence for each study based on a hierarchy for group designs (Darrah, Hickman, O'Donnell, Vogtle, & Wiart, 2008) and another for single-subject designs (Logan, Hickman, Harris, & Heriza, 2008). The hierarchies are described in detail in Table 19.1, while a summary of the RCTs is presented in Table 19.2, and a summary of studies with single-subject designs in Table 19.3. Finally, we present a summary of group design AAC studies that did not meet the definition of a randomized clinical trial in Table 19.4. The discussion of each general area of research begins with an overview followed by brief reviews of the specific studies. We conclude by characterizing of the strengths and weaknesses of research and recommendations for future directions.

Table 19.1. Levels of Evidence for Group and Single-Subject Design Studies

Level	Intervention (group) studies	Single-subject research design studies
I	Systematic review of randomized controlled trials (RCTs) Large RCT (with narrow confidence intervals—n > 100)	Randomized controlled N-of-1 (RCT), alternating treatment design (ATD), and concurrent or nonconcurrent multiple baseline design (MBDs) generalizability if ATD is replicated across three or more subjects and the MBD consists of a minimum of three subjects, behaviors, or settings
II	Smaller RCTs (with wider confidence intervals—n < 100) Systematic reviews of cohort studies	Nonrandomized, controlled, concurrent MBD; generalizability if design consists of a minimum of three subjects, behaviors, or settings
III	Cohort study with concurrent control group Systematic reviews of case control studies	Nonrandomized, noncontrolled, concurrent MBD; generalizability if design consists of a minimum of three subjects, behaviors, or settings
IV	Cohort study without concurrent control groupCase series	Nonrandomized, controlled, with at least three phases (ABA, ABAB, BAB, etc.); generalizability if replicated across three or more different subjects
V	Case-control study Expert opinion Case study or report	Nonrandomized, controlled AB design; generalizability if replicated across three or more different subjects

Table 19.2. Summary of Randomized Clinical Trials

Study	Level of Evidence	Intervention	Participants	Age Range	Duration	Intensity	Outcome of Interest	Effect Size
Fey et al., 2006	II	I = PMT/RE C = No Tx	I = 13 DS/ 12 DD C = 13 DS/13 DD	24–33 months	6 months	4 weekly 20 min PMT sessions + 8 1-hour RE sessions	Mother—linguistic mapping/recasting Child—rate of communication acts	Mother DD only group (r_G) = 0.49 DS only—*ns* Child Total group d = 0.68 DS only d = 0.65
Fey et al., 2013	II	I = High intensity PMT or MT/ RE C = Low intensity PMT or MT/ RE	I = 19 DS/14 DD C = 16 DS/15 DD	18–27 months	9 months	High intensity = 5 hours per week Low intensity = 1 hour per week RE = 9 1-hour sessions within 1st 3 months of study	Mother—follow-in comments, linguistic mapping/recasting, facilitating play and social interaction Child—rate of communication acts, number of different words (understood, spoken, signed + spoken)	Mother (total group)f ollow-in comments d = 0.40 linguistic maps/recasts d = 0.65 play/social interaction d = 0.40 Child (high object interest) rate of communication acts—*ns* different words g = 0.71 to 0.82
Girolametto et al., 1998	II	I = HPC = No Tx	I = 6 DS C = 6 DS	29–46 months	13 weeks	9 2.5-hour evening sessions + 4 home visits	Mother—talkativeness, complexity, labeling, focused target word use Child—target word use	Unable to calculate
Karaaslan & Mahoney, 2013	II	I = RTC = BAU	I = 7 DS C = 8 DS	24–72 months	6 months	1.5—2 hour weekly sessions	Mother—interactive behavior (responsiveness, affect, directiveness) Child—interactive behavior (attention, initiation) Screening measures of language	Mother responsiveness g = 0.62 affect g = 0.68 directiveness g = 0.42 Child attention g = 0.63 initiation g = 0.68 language screeners g = 0.42 & 1.14

Romski et al., 2010	II	I = AC-I or AC-O C= SC	N = 62, 18 DS/33 DD AC-I = 21 AC-O = 20 C = 21	21–40 months	12 weeks	2 30-minute weekly sessions	Mother—MLU, mean length of turn in utterances, total turns Child—number of augmented and/or spoken words, MLU, TTR, mean length of turn in utterances, total turns, proportion of intelligible utterances	Mother MLU η^2 =0.26 ML turns η^2 = 0.17 Total turns η^2 = 0.27 Child Augmented words η^2 = 0.11 Spoken words η^2 = 0.04 MLU η^2s = 0.15 TTR η^2s = 0.26 ML turn η^2 = 0.14 Total turns η^2 = 0.26 Intelligibility η^2 = 0.59
Warren et al., 2008	II	I = ?MT/RE followed by MT/REC = MT/RE	See Fey et al., 2006	See Fey et al., 2006	6 months	I = 4 weekly 20 min PMT sessions + 8 1-hour RE sessions followed by weekly 45-min MT sessions + 6 1-hour RE sessions C = weekly 45-min MT sessions + 6 1-hour RE sessions	Mother—linguistic mapping/recasting, and contingent responses Child—rate of communication acts, rate of different words	Mother linguistic map/recast - *ns* contingent responses - *ns* Child rate of communication acts—*ns* rate of different words—*ns*

(*continued*)

Table 19.2. *Continued*

Study	Level of Evidence	Intervention	Participants	Age Range	Duration	Intensity	Outcome of Interest	Effect Size
Yoder & Warren, 1998	II	I = PMT C = RSG	N = 58 4 DS/54 DD I = 28 C = 30	17–32 months	6 months	4 weekly 20 min sessions	Mother—responsivity to child acts Child—number of intentional communication acts	Child number of intentional communication acts—*ns*Interaction between maternal responsivity and group on child acts $R^2 = 0.08$
Yoder & Warren, 2002	II	I = PMT/RE C = BAU	I = 8 DS/10 DDC = 9 DS/9 DD	Mean of 22 months	6 months	3 or 4 weekly 20 min PMT sessions + 12 parent sessions	Mother—optimal response to child acts Child—rate of communication acts, rate of different words	Motherresponsiveness $d = 0.61$ Child rate of communication acts—*ns* rate of different words—*ns*
Yoder et al., 2014	II	See Fey et al., 2013					Child (DS etiology)—number of spoken words	$g = 0.55$

Note. I = intervention; C = comparison; PMT = prelinguistic milieu teaching; MT = milieu teaching; RE = responsivity education; HP = Hanen program; EMT = enhance milieu teaching; RT = responsive teaching; BAU = business as usual; AC-I = augmented communication input; AC-O = augmented communication output; SC = spoken communication; RSG = responsive small group; DS = Down syndrome; DD = developmental delay; ASD = autism spectrum disorder; MLU = mean length of utterance; NDW = number of different words; TTR = type token ratio; (r_G) = Glass rank-biserial correlation coefficient; d = Cohen's d; g = Hedge's g; η^2 = eta squared; R^2 = R^2 change; ns = not significant.

Table 19.3. Summary of Single-Subject Designs

Study	Level of Evidence	Design	Intervention	Sample	Age Range	Duration	Intensity	Outcome of Interest
Biggs et al., 2017	II	Multiple probe across-participants with phase for generalization	Peer support arrangement	2 DS/1 DD/1 AS	10–16 years			Communicative acts with peers
Dada & Alant, 2009	II	Multiple probe across 3 activities replicated across participants	Aided language stimulation	1 DS/3 CP	8–12 years	3 weeks	5 sessions	Target vocabulary acquisition
Harris & Reichle, 2004	II	Multiple probe across activities/sets with maintenance	Aided language stimulation	2 DS/1 DD	3;10–5;4 years			Symbol comprehension and production
Lanter et al., 2016	V Case study	AB design with follow-up phase forgeneralization	Modeling to establish requesting behaviors	1 DS	7;8 years	10 weeks	20min biweekly sessions	Functional requesting behavior
Warren et al., 1993 Experiment 1	Feasibility study	Multiple baseline across training targets	Prelinguistic milieu teaching	1 DS	20 months	60 sessions	25min session 4 days a week	Requesting, commenting, vocal imitation
Warren et al., 1993 Experiment 2	II	Multiple baseline across participants	Prelinguistic milieu teaching	1 DS/3 DD	23–30 months		25min session 4 days a week	Requesting, commenting, intentional communication Changes in teachers (requests for communication, turn taking)

(*continued*)

Table 19.3 *Continued*

Study	Level of Evidence	Design	Intervention	Sample	Age Range	Duration	Intensity	Outcome of Interest
Wright et al., 2013	II	Multiple-baseline across participants	EMT+JASPER	4 DS	23–29 months	10 weeks	20–30min biweekly sessions	Child language: spontaneous, imitated and prompted sign or spoken word Parents use of total and unique modeled signs Joint Engagement
Yoder et al., 1994	II	Multiple baseline across participants	Prelinguistic milieu teaching	2 DS/2 DD	21–27 months		25min session 4 days a week	Adult: linguistic mapping, requests for communication Child: intentional prompted requests, intentional self-initiated requests, other intentional communication (comments, protests, greetings), preintentional signals

Note. DS = Down syndrome; DD = developmental disability; AS = Angelman syndrome; CP = cerebral palsy; EMT = enhance milieu teaching; JASPER = joint attention, symbolic play, and emotional regulation.

Table 19.4. Summary of AAC Non-Randomized Group Designs

Study	Level of Evidence	Design	Intervention	Sample	Age Range	Duration	Intensity	Outcome of Interest
Bruno & Trembath, 2006	IV	One-group pretest-posttest design	Aided language stimulation	1 DS/8 DD	4;8–14;5 years	5 days	2 45-min sessions daily	Syntactic complexity
Foreman & Crews, 1998	IV	Simple repeated measures Latin square design	Multimodal AAC use	19 DS	2–4 years	4 days	3 teaching sessions: (1) initial teaching session, (2) 15min later post-teaching session; (3) 24hrs later follow-up	Object naming
Launonen (1996)	IV	Nonrandomized, noncontrolled longitudinal design	Early signing project	29 DS	6 months-3 years; follow-up at age 4, 5, & 8	2.5 years	25 sessions + daily training sessions by parents	Expressive vocabulary (spoken and signed) Early communication milestone The Portage Assessment Scale (social, language, self-help, cognitive, and motor)

Note. DS = Down syndrome; DD = developmental disability.

The Milieu Teaching Model

The term "milieu teaching" was first defined by Hart and Rogers-Warren (1978) as the integration of "training" into a child's natural "talking environment" (p. 198). They noted that the "milieu teaching model relies on communications that occur naturally in everyday environments" (Hart & Rogers-Warren, 1978, p. 199). This definition set up a distinct contrast between milieu teaching and the then-common practice of teaching communications skills in more directive one-to-one pull out sessions separated from the child's natural environment. In this chapter, we will use the term "milieu teaching" (MT) in a general way to represent a range of techniques and approaches that are more similar than different and, therefore, fit under the broad umbrella of "naturalistic" interventions.

The fundamental premises of the conceptual model underlying MT language intervention are that rate and quality of language input matters in terms of child development, and that how input is provided also matters (Brady, Bredin-Oja, & Warren, 2008; Kaiser, Yoder, & Keetz, 1992). According to this model, optimal language acquisition emerges during interactive exchanges between a child who initiates frequently and other people (e.g., parents) in their environment who respond in a way that serves as a learning scaffold for the child. Common techniques include embedding instruction into developmentally appropriate activities and contexts, following the child's attentional lead; modeling, using time delay as a prompt to generate child initiations; and recasting and expanding child utterances. There is substantial research on the efficacy of each of these specific techniques with both typically and atypically developing children (Warren & Walker, 2004). In addition to MT, combinations of these procedures have been included in "focused stimulation" (Ellis Weismer & Robertson, 2006), "incidental teaching" (Hart & Risley, 1975), "enhanced milieu teaching" (Hancock & Kaiser, 2006), "prelinguistic milieu teaching" (Yoder & Warren, 2002), and "pivotal response training" (Koegel, Koegel, Harrower, & Carter, 1999). These approaches virtually always include at least some level of parent training as well as intervention provided directly to the child by a teacher/therapist and/or parents (e.g., Girolametto, Greenberg, & Manolson, 1986).

During the same general period as the development of the initial MT model, developmental psychologists began to challenge the then-dominant "innate model of linguistic development" that was supported by the linguist Noam Chomsky (e.g., Chomsky, 1957). This challenge came in part from studies of early parent-child interactions that revealed important effects of having a highly responsive mother (e.g., Schiefelbusch & Lloyd, 1974; Snow, 1977). Parental responsivity has been broadly defined as a healthy, growth-producing relationship characterized by warmth, nurturance, and stability, as well as specific behaviors, such as consistent positive comments and expansions of child initiations (Shonkoff & Phillips, 2000; Spiker, Boyce, & Boyce, 2002). Substantial evidence indicates that a parent who is highly responsive to his young child will use some of the same techniques as MT without training. These "techniques" included following the child's attentional lead, providing a lot of conversational turn-taking, modeling, and expanding the child's utterances (Hart & Risley, 1992; Yoder & Warren, 1999a). Responsive parents provide a rich and dynamic language environment for their young children, and these children typically develop more complex and diverse language skills than their peers exposed to less responsive linguistic input (Dieterich, Assel, Swank, Smith, & Landry, 2006; Moody, Baker, & Blacher, 2018). This type of natural parental responsivity serves as a prototype for MT

Early in the 1980s, two psychologists at the University of Kansas, Betty Hart and Todd Risley, embarked on a now-famous longitudinal study of the cumulative effects of the early home language environment on a representative sample of 42 young children during their first 3 years of life (Hart & Risley 1992; 1995). This landmark study provided evidence of the enormous cumulative advantages of children who experienced lots of responsive conversation with their parents daily while on the way to acquiring relatively large vocabularies in the first 3 years of life as compared to children who experienced substantially lower levels of responsive parent-child interaction and acquired correspondingly smaller vocabularies. There has been no direct replications published of this study with children with DS or other developmental disabilities, but strong correlations between the language development of children with intellectual disabilities, including DS, and the "responsiveness" of their parents have been reported (e.g., Brady, Warren, Fleming, Keller, & Sterling, 2014; Mahoney, Finger, & Powell, 1985; Mahoney & Powell, 1988; Warren, Brady, Fleming & Hahn, 2017; Warren, Brady, Sterling, Fleming, & Marquis, 2010).

Taken together, the studies referenced above have revealed a range of effects associated with highly responsive parenting for children with various developmental challenges, including DS. This research supports an early intervention model that combines training to enhance parental responsiveness combined with some degree of direct intervention targeting child behaviors to create optimal communication and language learning environments early in the lives of children with neurodevelopmental disabilities, including children with DS (Brady et al., 2008). Thus, it should not be surprising that most of the intervention research reviewed in this chapter represents some version of MT combined with a responsive parent training component. Direct teacher/therapist intervention essentially "primes the pump" for learning by teaching new communication and language skills. These skills can then be expanded and reinforced by responsive parents and caregivers during their day-to-day interaction with the child (Warren & Brady, 2007).

Review of Milieu Teaching Studies and Parent Responsivity Randomized Clinical Trials

The MT approach is grounded in both developmental principles and specific techniques that have been shown to be effective with a wide variety of at-risk children (Warren & Walker, 2004). However, does the empirical data support the efficacy of this approach specifically for children with DS? This is obviously an important question. Therefore, in this section we summarize the results of the data so far. All the studies reviewed included children with DS. The first two studies reviewed involved only parent responsivity training.

We include them because teaching parents to employ responsivity techniques daily as a primary intervention approach can have substantial effects (i.e., Mahoney & Nam, 2011). We then review two small single-subject design MT studies followed by five true RCTs. In addition more specific, details about these studies are provided in Tables 19.2 and 19.3.

Girolametto, Weitzman, and Clements-Baartman (1998) conducted an RCT with 12 mothers and their children with DS (29 to 46 months) to examine the effects of a parent training program that incorporated focused stimulation (i.e., defined as frequent modeling of specifically targeted words during a parent-child interaction) as a technique. They found that the mothers in the intervention group labeled more different words and used focused stimulation more often than the mothers in the delayed-treatment control group. In addition, the children in the intervention group used twice as many targeted words as the children in the control group as measured by parent report and a free-play interaction. However, in contrast to findings from a similar study with late talkers (Girolametto, Pearce, & Weitzman, 1996), the two groups did not differ in terms of overall vocabulary size as measured by the MacArthur Communicative Development Index (Fenson et al., 1993), indicating that children with DS may have more difficulty learning words that are not specifically targeted by parents or teachers. These findings suggest that "parent responsivity" as a specific intervention by itself may be insufficient to spur meaningful language development.

In a second study of teaching responsive interactions to parents of children with DS, Karaaslan and Mahoney (2013) conducted an RCT with 15 Turkish mothers and their 2- to 6-year-old children as compared to a business-as-usual control group, all of whom had DS. The intervention, termed responsive teaching (RT), differs from other parent interventions (e.g., Kaiser & Roberts, 2013) as the parents are discouraged from directly prompting their child to produce a communicative act. Instead, the parents are encouraged to model behaviors that are at the child's current level of functioning to increase initiations, exploration, and joint attention behavior by the child. Karaaslan and Mahoney (2013) found that the parents in the treatment group increased their use of responsive strategies after 6 months of training. Additionally, the children in the treatment group increased their level of interactive engagement and these changes were highly correlated with their mothers' responsiveness. The children in the treatment group also made significant gains on two screening measures of development—the Turkish version of the Denver Developmental Screening Test-II (Denver-II; Anlar & Yalaz, 1996) and the Ankara Developmental Screening Inventory (ADSI; Savasir, Sezgin, & Erol, 1995). Significant gains were reported for both the language specific domain and the personal-social (or social-emotional) domain. The findings of this study stand out as a strong endorsement of the potential of a parent responsivity approach.

Additional single-subject design studies provided evidence of effects of combining responsivity training with MT for children with DS (Warren, Yoder, Gazdag, Kim, & Jones, 1993; Yoder, Warren, Kim, & Gazdag, 1994). In one, Warren et al. (1993) reported on two experiments with a combined total of five children, two of whom had DS, while in another Yoder et al. (1994) studied four children, two with DS. In these studies, the intervention was directly administered by a trained staff member and the generalization of effects were measured with both teachers and parents. In both cases, the intervention targeting prelinguistic forms of requesting (i.e., vocalizations and/or gestures paired with eye gaze) led to greater use of these forms separate from the intervention context, and the teachers and parents of these children increased their reciprocal interactions by contingently responding to the child's intentional communication acts. See Table 19.3 for a summary.

Randomized Controlled Trials of Milieu Teaching

The promising findings from the Warren and Yoder single-subject studies led to an RCT of 58 children between 17 and 32 months with developmental delays, four of whom had DS (Yoder & Warren, 1998, 1999a, 1999b, 2001). The children were randomly assigned to one of two treatment conditions: prelinguistic milieu teaching/milieu teaching (PMT/MT) or responsive small group (RSG). In PMT/MT, the adults followed the child's attentional lead and used specific prompts to communicate. In the RSG condition, which did not include any prompts to communicate, the adult played with the child in a highly responsive manner. No main effects were found for the treatment group, although a significant interaction between the type of intervention the child received and his or her mother's pretreatment style of interacting was found. Specifically, the children with mothers who were already highly responsive made greater gains if they received specific prompts to communicate during PMT. Conversely, the children whose mothers were not highly responsive made greater gains if they participated in the RSG treatment with a highly responsive teacher. These findings highlighted the importance of having a highly responsive adult with whom the child can interact. All the subsequent studies of PMT/MT by the Warren and Yoder team included a component to teach parents to be responsive.

Yoder and Warren (2002) conducted another RCT of PMT/MT with 39 toddlers (mean age of 22 months), 17 of whom had DS, that combined clinician led MT intervention with a parent education component focused on increasing responsivity to their child's prelinguistic communication bids. They found that the parent training enhanced the level of responsivity of parents in the intervention group as compared to the control group. The implications for lexical growth and number of requests by children were less clear. No main effects were found for the treatment group, but certain child characteristics predicted growth. In particular, the children with DS appeared to have slower growth trajectories for requests if they were enrolled in PMT. Additionally, the children who began the study with infrequent canonical vocalizations had steeper growth curves for comments and lexical density (i.e., rate of different words) if they participated in the treatment group, whereas the children with relatively high pre-experimental levels of canonical vocalizations had steeper growth curves if they were in the control group. Yoder and

Warren hypothesized that children who already produce a high number of prelinguistic communication acts and canonical vocalizations are better suited for an intervention that is focused on linguistic targets. Regarding the unexpected finding for slower growth in the children with DS, Yoder and Warren noted that the participating children with DS appeared more likely to resist teaching prompts by interventionists, and this resistance may have contributed to the slow growth. They suggested that interventionists accept a less complex communication act, such as a coordinated gaze shift, when children with DS react negatively to an adult "holding out" for a more complex act.

With these two caveats in mind, Fey et al. (2006) sought to replicate the treatment findings of Yoder and Warren (2002) in an RCT with a relatively large sample size. Fifty-one toddlers (24 to 33 months of age) with developmental delay and their parents participated in either a 6-month treatment group consisting of PMT implemented by a clinician combined with responsivity education for parents or a no-treatment control group. Twenty-six of these children had DS and they were evenly split between the two randomly assigned groups. Fey et al. made several key changes to the procedures prior to the start of the trial. One, they only included children with low rates of canonical vocalizations and prelinguistic comments to ensure that the intervention did not target behaviors already in the child's repertoire. Two, they modified the initial targets for some children by first accepting less complex communication acts for requesting before requiring more complex communication acts, such as a gaze shift plus a vocalization or gesture, that were targeted by Yoder and Warren (2002). Three, they responded to a child's vocalization that clearly referenced an object with a linguistic map (e.g., a child says "da" while looking at a ball and the adult responds by saying "ball" or "the ball"). Four, they employed speech-language pathologists as the interventionists on the basis that they may have been more adept than para-professionals at making subtle changes in response to children's reactions to the intervention. The speech language pathologists, who were certified in the Hanen parent training program called *It Takes Two to Talk* (Manolson, 1992), also provided the parent responsivity instruction. The parents were taught to follow their child's attentional lead, wait for their child to produce a communicative act, then respond to their child's communication acts by adding words, and to use focused stimulation. After 6 months of intervention, Fey et al. found a main effect for children in the treatment group in the form of a significant increase in their rate of intentional prelinguistic acts, such as gestures and vocalizations. Furthermore, the children with DS in the treatment group showed just as much gain in prelinguistic communication as children with other etiologies, indicating that the adjustments to the intervention made by Fey et al. (e.g., initially accepting a less complex communication act) benefitted the children with DS.

Warren et al. (2008) studied this same cohort of 51 children (Fey et al., 2006) and their parents at two additional time points; after a 6-month wait period following the initial 6 months of treatment or no treatment (Time 3), then followed by a 6-month additional course of intervention for all children (Time 4). This design allowed Warren et al.

to determine if the initial boost in prelinguistic communication experienced by the treatment group maintained or strengthened after a period of time. In addition, they hypothesized that the initial focus on prelinguistic targets would result in an increase in linguistic targets (i.e., spoken words) during the final 6 months of intervention, a full year after the children entered the study. However, they found no significant effect of intervention on spoken word targets measured at 6- and 12-months post intervention. Thus, no evidence was found for the anticipated boost from targeting early communication behaviors.

The null findings reported by Warren et al (2008) led Fey, Yoder, Warren, and Bredin-Oja (2013) to consider whether intervention that was more intense and longer in duration might make a meaningful difference. Thus, they conducted an RCT on the impact of differential treatment intensity with 64 children aged 18–27 months with mixed etiologies associated with intellectual disability, 35 of whom had DS, and their parents. The children were randomly assigned to either a high intensity group (i.e., 5 hours per week of direct instruction) or a low intensity group (i.e., 1 hour per week of direct instruction) of MT teaching provided by a skilled clinician. The mothers of the children in both groups (high and low intensity) received an equal amount of responsivity education. Once again, no main effect was found for the intervention. That is, more intense and longer duration intervention failed to produce significant gains in spoken words, although a moderating treatment effect for children who had a greater interest in objects was found (Fey et al., 2013). Specifically, the children who played with more toys learned more spoken words if they received the higher intensity level of intervention. The children with low interest in toys did not differ in their number of spoken words acquired, regardless of treatment group. Thus, providing more intervention for children who showed little interest in toys, regardless of their diagnosis, did not help them make gains in spoken language.

The limited findings of the Fey et al. (2013) RTC led Yoder, Woynaroski, Fey, and Warren (2014) to conduct a reanalysis of this same RCT that was specifically focused on the role that the children with DS played in the outcome reported by Fey et al. (2013). Thus Yoder et al. re-analyzed the data using a more complex growth model that included a quadratic parameter to identify nonlinear trends in development. This type of analysis allowed for the detection of acceleration or deceleration in spoken word growth both between and within groups of children with or without DS by treatment condition. The findings indicated that the children with DS showed accelerated growth if they were enrolled in the high intensity group. The same effect for intensity was not found for the other children who had a variety of other etiologies associated with intellectual disability. The re-analysis also confirmed that the child's level of interest in toys continued to be a moderating factor. Yoder et al. (2014) also replicated Girolametto et al.'s (1998) finding that children with DS generally had a slower growth trajectory for development of spoken words as compared to a group of children with different etiologies associated with intellectual disability.

What Have We Learned From These Milieu Teaching Studies?

Based on this review, we have identified five general themes regarding spoken word development in children with DS. One, high levels of parent responsivity positively impacts communication growth in children with DS (e.g., Yoder & Warren, 1998, 1999a, 1999b, 2001). Two, parents can be taught to be highly responsive (Fey et al., 2006; Girolametto et al., 1998; Karaaslan & Mahoney, 2013; Yoder & Warren, 2002). Three, children with DS may learn intentional communication behaviors similarly to other children with intellectual disabilities (Fey et al., 2006; Warren et al., 1993; Yoder et al., 1994), although their development of spoken words is generally at a slower rate (Girolametto et al., 1998; Warren et al., 2008; Yoder et al., 2014). Four, children with DS may need to be taught specific words more directly and may struggle to generalize word learning skills to other words that are not targeted (Girolametto et al., 1998). Five, young children with DS need even more intensive levels of intervention to make significant gains in speech and language development (Yoder et al., 2014), and/or perhaps different interventions than those reviewed here.

A disappointing but clear outcome from this series of studies on MT interventions is that they seldom resulted in significant gains in spoken language in children with DS, at least as measured by standardized tests or spoken language samples collected in nontrained contexts. However, this measure may be difficult to impact and the gains in spoken words directly targeted in intervention should not be discounted. Perhaps more important in considering these outcomes is the relatively small amount of intervention provided to these children and the small sample sizes in most of the studies. We will revisit these important issues later in the chapter.

Alternative and Augmentative Communication

AAC refers to communication that includes nonspeech modes such as gestures, signs, visual symbols or speech-generating devices to augment or replace speech). It is not a general intervention approach like MT. Rather, it represents various means of communication that can be embedded with MT techniques or other intervention approaches. Thus, AAC is a set of strategies that individuals with limited or no spoken language can use to either replace or supplement their spoken language so they can communicate with others. It can be used by individuals as their primary mode of communication for a limited period or throughout life. Further, AAC can be used during any stage of language development. For example, it can be used to accelerate early language development by providing children with a functional way to communicate their needs and wants and to help bridge the transition to spoken language (Charlop-Christy, Carpenter, Le, LeBlanc, & Kellet, 2013; Kumin, 2003; Millar, Light, & Schlosser, 2006). For individuals who have acquired some speech, AAC can continue to augment expressive communication, which increases their ability to have successful communication interactions with others.

Historically, AAC was sometimes viewed as the last resort for speech-language intervention (Vanderheiden & Harris-Vanderheiden, 1976). Fortunately, that myth faded away as research revealed that AAC does not hinder speech and language development, that there are no required skills necessary to use some form of AAC, and that children of any age can benefit from AAC (Romski & Sevcik, 2005). Children with DS are likely candidates for AAC early in childhood due to several characteristics that affect speech development. These characteristics include frequent ear infections associated with otitis media with effusion that may cause fluctuating chronic hearing loss; low muscle tone that affects eating and speech skills; and delays in imitation, turn-taking, auditory, tactile, oral motor, and cognitive skills (see Abbeduto et al., this volume). There is increasing evidence that the effects of these challenges can be ameliorated by making functional communication easier to acquire early in development through the provision of "aided AAC interventions" (O'Neill, Light, & Pope, 2018). These "aided techniques" mostly overlap with MT techniques and include the use of modeling, time delay, open-ended questions, contingent responding, prompting (spoken, gestural), and expansions and recasting (O'Neill et al., 2018). Due to the range of communication challenges that these children face early in development, the National Down Syndrome Society has long advocated for the use of AAC early in development for individuals with DS (Kumin, 1999). However, while AAC may be frequently used in clinical and educational applications, evidence concerning its empirical effectiveness is still primarily based on case studies and small-*N* experimental studies (Romski, Sevcik, Barton-Hulsey, & Whitmore, 2015).

Review of AAC Research

Although most children with DS eventually learn to communicate with speech, AAC can improve communication for many individuals especially early in development. AAC can be an effective mode of communication for children with DS because the onset of their spoken language is typically delayed, and poor intelligibility is common (Barnes et al., 2009; Stoel-Gammon, 2001). In addition, children with DS often have stronger receptive language abilities as compared to their expressive language skills, starting early in development (Price, Roberts, Vandergrift, & Martin, 2007; Roberts, Price, & Malkin, 2007). Language comprehension may support the use of AAC because children can harness their comprehension skills for learning visual representations.

AAC is often embedded in early language interventions for children with DS, such as MT discussed above. In the following sections, we provide examples of AAC approaches that have been used to promote language and communication development in children with intellectual and developmental disabilities, including children with DS.

Picture Exchange Communication Systems

Picture exchange communication systems (PECS) involve teaching children to select pictures and exchange them with a partner in order to communicate (Bondy, & Frost,

1994). As children advance in their language skills, they are taught to combine pictures to create basic sentences that then can be exchanged to make requests and to comment. When using PECS, children may have a binder containing their symbol set (i.e., a set of vocabulary words represented in pictures) that allows them to search for the symbols needed to communicate that can be placed on the sentence strip (i.e., a Velcro strip). PECS has been used with children with intellectual and developmental disabilities, including those with DS (Branson & Demchak, 2009; Hart & Banda, 2010). However, PECS is not always easily used because it requires that the child have the binder containing their symbol set with them, and the binder may not always contain the symbol a child needs to communicate, especially when they are in a new setting. Conversely, a benefit of PECS for early language learning is that the initial exchange can be taught directly with physical prompting, leading to immediate success with initiations of requests.

Most of the research on PECS has been focused on children with ASD. For example, in an RCT of a teacher-implemented PECS intervention, Howlin, Gordon, Pasco, Wade, and Charman (2007) found increased rates of initiated communication for students with ASD assigned to a PECS intervention. A meta-analysis of single-case research studies conducted with individuals with ASD showed that PECS resulted in small to moderate gains in communication rates, but negligible gains in speech (Flippin, Reszka, & Watson, 2010). While the research on the use of PECS with individuals with DS is limited, evidence from single-subject studies suggests that children with DS may benefit from language interventions that use pictures to promote functional communication (Kern, Gallagher, Starosta, Hickman, & George, 2006; Lanter et al., 2016; Schwartz, Garfinkle, & Bauer, 1998). For example, in a single-subject study, a 7-year-old boy with DS was taught to use a picture-based strategy to increase his functional requesting behaviors (Lanter et al., 2016). See Table 19.3 for a summary of these studies.

Graphic systems. Graphic symbols were used with children with intellectual and developmental disabilities, including DS, before the development of PECS and continue to be a useful form of AAC (i.e., Dada & Alant, 2009). Like PECS, graphic systems also are picture-symbol based, but instead of physically exchanging the picture, the child selects a symbol by touching it or by selecting with an alternative mode, such as eye gaze, for those with limited motor abilities. Like PECS, graphic systems help to promote word learning by linking a word to its referent that is represented in the picture (e.g. Hunt, Alwell, & Goetz, 1991). The graphic symbols may be available through low-tech options, such as a communication board or visual classroom schedule, or high-tech options, such as computers, or dedicated electronic devices. Recent advances in technology have made graphic systems widely available due to the increase in affordable tablet computers.

Graphic systems may be particularly effective for children with DS because they capitalize on the relative visual strengths associated with DS (Clibbens, Powell, & Atkinson, 2002; Kumin, 2003, Miller, 1999). Often, graphic symbol use is taught via the use of aided language stimulation/MT techniques (Dada & Alant, 2009; Harris & Reichle,

2004) with children with DS. Aided language stimulation is an AAC technique where the communication partner uses the child's AAC system to communicate with the child. Using a single-subject multiple probe design, Harris and Reichle (2004) examined symbol comprehension and symbol production (object labeling) using aided language stimulation in three preschool-age children (3;10–5;4 years) with moderate intellectual disability, including one child with DS, who all had less than 30 spoken words. All three of the children showed increases in both comprehension and productions skills during the intervention phase and these skills were maintained following the intervention (Harris & Reichle, 2004). See Table 19.3 for a summary.

Aided language stimulation has been used to investigate vocabulary acquisition with four 8- to 12-year-olds with little to no functional speech (less than 15 intelligible words), including one child with DS, in a single-subject multiple probe design (Dada & Alant, 2009). Dada and Alant measured vocabulary acquisition as the number of target vocabulary words that the children acquired during the intervention phase. All the children acquired the target vocabulary words and maintained their performance once the aided language stimulation was removed from the intervention, suggesting that the augmented input facilitated vocabulary acquisition. See Table 19.3 for a summary.

Speech-generating devices. Speech-generating devices (SGDs) are electronic devices that allow the user to select a symbol—like graphic systems—or type out a message that the device will then speak aloud. SGDs are increasingly more accessible due to the affordability of tablet computers and the development of applications ("apps") by AAC device companies that can be downloaded to these devices. In an RCT of young children with developmental delay (age 21 to 40 months), which included 18 children with DS, Romski et al. (2010) found significantly greater spoken vocabulary gains for children taught with SGDs as compared to a speech-only condition (See Table 19.2 for a summary).

SGDs may be effective for several reasons, particularly in the early phases of intervention. One, SGDs provide auditory information to communication partners; therefore, they may be a more successful form of AAC because potential communication partners have an easier time knowing when the child is communicating. Two, teaching communication partners strategies for facilitating communication for children who use SGDs, including children with DS, can increase turn-taking between parents and children, possibly improving parent-child interactions (Kent-Walsh, Binger, & Hasham, 2010). Three, the use of SGDs for children with DS may support peer relationships because other children can hear their response instead of having to interpret the symbols without speech output, making the interaction more natural (Batorowicz, Stadskleiv, von Tetzchner, & Missiuna, 2016; Biggs, Carter, & Gustafson, 2017; Thiemann-Bourque, 2012; Thiemann-Bourque, McGuff, & Goldstein, 2017). For example, Biggs et al. (2017) examined a peer support arrangement—an evidence-based intervention designed to increase peer interactions (Carter et al., 2016; Carter, Moss, Hoffman, Chung, & Sisco, 2011)—with a multiple probe-across-participants design that included four 12- to 15-year old children with intellectual disability, including two youth with DS, who used SGDs. Increases in peer interactions, including increases in initiated communication acts, were found for all four of the youth (see Table 19.3 for a summary). Four, communication with SGDs may be effective because of the clarity of the speech. Speech produced with SGDs may be more intelligible and hence more effective for some children who speak but are highly unintelligible.

Manual sign systems. Manual sign systems (e.g., sign language) were originally developed for individuals who are deaf, but they have also been successfully taught to infants and very young children with DS (e.g., Clibbens et al., 2002; Miller, 1992; Thompson, Cotnoir-Bichelman, McKerchar, Tate, & Dancho, 2007). Manual sign systems can be used alone or with speech (i.e., total communication). One concern associated with sign language is that it requires that communication partners also know sign language (Mirenda & Bopp, 2003). Thus, the lack of general knowledge of sign language may limit opportunities for successful communication interactions. For children with DS, sign language may be difficult to acquire initially due to delays in fine motor skills. This lack of dexterity in the fingers and hands may make some of their signs look very similar, leading to problems with accurately interpreting their meaning (Reichle, Cooley Hidecker, Brady, & Terry, 2003). Nevertheless, sign language remains one of the most popular forms of AAC for young children with DS, particularly when used as a transitional communication system during early childhood (Clibbens, 2001; Kay-Raining Bird & Chapman, 1994; Kay-Raining Bird, Gaskell, Babineau, & Macdonald, 2000; Kumin, 2003).

Perhaps one reason why parents and professionals may teach children with DS to sign is that they often show strengths in use of gestures (Caselli et al., 1998; Franco & Wishart, 1995). Sign language is a form of symbolic communication that builds upon gesture use and could therefore take advantage of this gestural strength. There is some evidence that when vocabulary counts include both signed and spoken words, young children with DS may have vocabularies similar to mental-age matched typically developing peers (Deckers, Van Zaalen, Van Balkom, & Verhoeven., 2017; Te Kaat, 2013; Zampini & D'Odorico, 2011). For example, Miller (1992) examined vocabulary growth in children with DS in comparison to typically developing children. When both signed and spoken vocabularies were considered together, the total vocabulary size was similar between children with and without DS between the ages of 11 and 17 months. However, after 17 months the rapidly growing spoken vocabularies of typically developing children outpaced the total vocabularies (signed + spoken) of children with DS (see Table 19.3 for a summary).

Launonen (1996) conducted a signing intervention for children with DS from 1 to 3 years of age that provided 2.5 years of intervention with follow-up at 4 and 5 years (Launonen, 1996) and at 8 years. The study involved a control group design, but assignment to treatment or control group was not randomized. The children in the control group (n = 12) received standard early intervention services, whereas the children in the intervention group (n = 12) received sign language instruction in addition to the early intervention. Launonen found significant differences in gains in language scores as measured by a nonstandardized comprehensive test developed for use in Finland, where the study took place. Follow-up scores at age 8 years indicated significant differences in social interaction, language comprehension, reading, and writing skills (see Table 19.4 for a summary). Thus, as an early communication intervention, sign language may have long-term benefits for language and other developmental outcomes (i.e., social skills, cognition, and learning).

Combining sign language and speech may also be an effective mode of communication during early language development. In one example, Wright, Kaiser, Reikowsky, and Roberts (2013) examined the use of a blended naturalistic communication intervention (enhanced milieu teaching; Hancock & Kaiser, 2006) combined with another intervention termed "joint attention symbolic play and emotion regulation" (Kasari, Freeman, & Paparella, 2006) in a multiple baseline design across participants aimed at increasing speech and language use by four young children with DS (23–29 months). Following stable baselines, 20 sessions of the combined intervention were implemented with each child. Clear and systematic effects were seen for sign production—increases followed the introduction of intervention for each child following stable baselines. In addition, intervention effects for sign use generalized to children's homes. However, only minimal increases were noted in spoken words and these increases were not clearly related to the introduction of intervention. Thus, the intervention was successful for increasing communication through sign language but did not show similar effects for speech, suggesting once again that sign language may be initially easier to learn for children with DS than speech. See Table 19.3 for a summary.

Comparing forms of AAC. To select optimal forms of AAC, different forms (e.g., graphic systems to SGDs) have been compared in participants with DS. For example, Foreman and Crews (1998) examined word learning in 19 children with DS across three different forms of AAC: symbol (COMPIC–a computerized picture-system), sign language (Makaton + verbal), and multimodal (verbal + sign + symbol), as well as a verbal-only instruction condition. In this repeated measure study, each child was their own control and participated in all four treatments over the course of 4 successive days. The children were taught 12 words, three in each treatment. Foreman and Crews found that the children with DS learned significantly more words in the sign and multimodal treatments than in the symbol treatment. While slightly more words were learned via the multimodal condition than the sign condition, the difference between these two treatments was not significant. The children with DS did not produce any of the three words taught in the verbal instruction condition. These findings suggest that simultaneous instructions of speech instruction and AAC may help to facilitate word learning and early communication in persons with DS (see Table 19.4 for a summary).

In addition to examining what type of AAC supports early language learning in DS, AAC has also been investigated for its ability to support more complex language skills such as syntactic complexity. In one example, Bruno and Trembath (2006) examined whether syntactic performance improved when children with complex communication needs, including one child with DS, used either a manual communication board or a dynamic display SGD during an aidlanguage stimulation intervention. The overall findings indicated that the children improved their syntactic abilities when using either form of AAC during aided-language stimulation, and that this improvement was greatest for the children when they used the manual communication board. However, there was considerable variability in individual performance. Specifically, the child with DS showed a small increase in the number of morphemes when using both the manual communication board and the SGD, but no change in the subject + verb + object sentences or progressive verb tense sentences (i.e., subject + is + verb + ING + object) using either AAC type (see Table 19.4 for a summary). Obviously, more research on determining optimal types of AAC for promoting complex communication abilities for children with DS is needed. However, irrespective of type of AAC, a meta-analysis conducted by O'Neill et al. (2018) strongly supports the use of "aided" AAC, which brings together the strengths of MT-like procedures with the functionality of AAC for children with DS.

What Has Been Learned From AAC Research With Children With DS?

A variety of types of AAC have been used with children with DS and this literature is promising, especially when combined with MT techniques. The initial evidence indicates that AAC can support vocabulary development, comprehension, and expression (i.e., symbols, signs, or speech). However, research on AAC applications in DS has almost exclusively been carried out with small-*N* single-subject designs. Based on our literature search, the Romski et al. (2010) study is the only published AAC RCT that has included children with DS, as 18 of the 62 participants had DS. The average age for the entire group at the start was 29.6 months. In comparing SGD use for input and output versus a spoken language intervention, Romski et al. found that the participants learned more words when they were taught to use their SGD for expressive communication. However, information specifically about children with DS was not available at the time of this publication.

The relative lack of studies on AAC, especially RCTs, that provide information on outcomes specific to children with DS, preclude an estimation of the long-term effects of AAC use and an assessment of whether these effects are similar, or different, compared to children with other neurodevelopmental disorders. However, in consideration of some of the key aspects of DS behavioral phenotypes—relative weaknesses in aspects of motor functioning, speech intelligibility, expressive language, and executive functioning, and relative strengths in receptive language, social skills, and visual-spatial processing—at least some forms of AAC could be particularly effective for any child who is not meeting their communication needs exclusively with speech. Building on the Romski et al. (2010) study, RCTs with larger numbers of individuals with DS are needed to determine the generalized benefits of AAC.

General Discussion

The meaningful effects of the small number of RCT intervention studies aimed at enhancing vocal communication and language development of children with DS appear to be modest at best. In contrast, the bright spot in our present review is the relative effectiveness of AAC approaches on the language development of children with DS as indicated in O'Neill et al.'s (2018) meta-analysis. According to their analysis, the 19 children with DS included in their review generated promising results with very large effect sizes of 0.9 on average. While this research is promising, most of it is based on single-subject designs. In comparison, while early single-subject studies of MT approaches were positive as well (e.g., Warren et al. 1993; Yoder et al. 1994), the findings across the RCTs have been less so. Fortunately, scientific and clinical successes are often built on what is learned from failures and partial successes. In this final section, we propose four directions for future research. These are (a) refining further adaptations for the DS behavioral and cognitive phenotype, (b) recognizing the limitations of small, short, low dose RCTs, (c) studying the continued role of parental responsivity, and (d) moving from better quality small-*N* studies to larger RCTs.

Adapting to the Down Syndrome Behavior and Cognitive Phenotype

We noted at the outset of this chapter that the dynamic processes of change that lead to the DS behavioral phenotype during early childhood and beyond remains a work in progress (see Abbeduto, this volume; Fidler, Lunkenheimer, & Hahn, 2011; Jarrold, this volume). Based on the studies reviewed here, to make meaningful progress in the effectiveness of communication and language intervention, we recommend combining MT and SGD for young children with DS starting as early in development as feasible. The RCTs on MT specifically with children with DS suggest that these techniques can be effective while the research on SGDs support their use as a potentially effective communication modality in early childhood.

The Limitations of Small, Short, Low Dose Randomized Clinical Trials

The RCTs reviewed in this chapter were all preceded by small-*N* studies that demonstrated short-term impacts on targeted goals (e.g., vocabulary gains). However, the RCTs also had small participant numbers especially when considering the number of children with DS in each study (see Table 19.1). These small sample sizes largely preclude finding meaningful effects. For example, an ANCOVA design with two groups of 20 children with DS randomized to treatment and control groups, and a pretest as a covariate, would have 0.80 power to detect large effects of $d = 0.45$. Furthermore, the power would not be enough to detect even moderately sized effects (e.g., $d = 0.25$). If examining the power of detecting group differences in slopes in a multilevel model across four observations for two groups of 20 each, the power would only be enough for detecting large differences with effect sizes of Cohen's d close to 1.00 (Hedges & Okin, 1985. Clearly, relatively small sample sizes make the task of finding meaningful effects very difficult. In all other ways except sample size, the studies reviewed met appropriate standards for RCTs. They all appropriately implemented random assignment procedures. Other procedures used in these studies appear to be methodologically solid. Furthermore, several of the studies generated at least one potentially interesting outcome or secondary effect (e.g., children with DS made greater gains if they received 5 hours of intervention per week than if they received 1 hour per week; Yoder et al., 2014, Yoder, Woynaroski, Fey, Warren, & Gardner, 2015), suggesting some impact. Nevertheless, overall the reported results are disappointing across these studies.

There were other implicit limitations of these studies beyond the small sample sizes. The most obvious one was that in all cases, with the exception of Launonen (1996) which is not an RCT, the interventions were substantially less than a year in length and the weekly intervention dose and dose frequency were low compared to the amount of potential daily and weekly learning time available to the child (Warren et al., 2007). Perhaps a more reasonable comparison is the intervention dose and frequency reported by the most effective autism interventions. These intervention studies have frequently involved between 25 and 40 hours per week of direct intervention for up to 2 years (Reichow, 2012; Spreckley & Boyd, 2008). In comparison, the children in the high intensity conditions of the Fey et al. (2013) study (the most intensive intervention condition for children with DS that we reviewed) received just 5 hours of direct intervention per week for a total of 9 months and the low intensity comparison group received just 1 hour per week. The parents of children in both groups also received training in parent responsivity. If we assume that the children in the Fey et al. (2013) study also had 100 hours a week available (i.e., hours awake) to actively learn language, their high-intensity intervention represented just 5 percent of the total learning time available per week. Of course, these children were likely learning communication and language skills during the nontreatment time. But the cumulative difference between 5 hours per week of direct intervention for 9 months and 25 hours or more per week for 2 years that many children with ASD have received in numerous RCTs (Dawson & Bernier, 2013) is a massive difference. In addition, effective ASD interventions have often been focused on a range of other social and cognitive skills in addition to language (Dawson & Bernier, 2013) effectively combined in some cases with AAC (e.g., Kasari et al., 2006). That is, the interventions were more comprehensive. Finally, there is one weakness in retrospect that all but the Romski et al. studies shared—they did not attempt to combine AAC approaches with MT for the children with DS. Thus, the emphasis only on oral communication may have further limited their effectiveness.

In summary, the nine RCTs we reviewed were limited on several dimensions that may have reduced their chances of finding significant differences. Testing higher doses of intervention in sufficiently large samples of children with DS for longer periods of time would seem like a logical next step. However, there is an intermediary step that should be studied in greater depth first—the effects of combining MT (implemented by both clinicians a parents) with speech-focused AAC.

Responsive Parenting Is Necessary but Not Sufficient

There is substantial research indicating that responsive parenting is of great benefit for both typically and atypically developing children. This includes empirical evidence across a range of young children including those with DS (Karaaslan & Mahoney, 2013; Mahoney, Perales, Wiggers, & Herman, 2006) and other neurodevelopmental disorders, such as fragile X syndrome (e.g., Brady, Thiemann-Bourque, Fleming, & Matthews., 2013; Warren et al., 2010, 2017). In our work with children with fragile X syndrome, we have found that specific types of responsiveness that expand children's verbal initiations predict increased vocabulary and other communication skills over lengthy periods of time (i.e., early through middle childhood; Warren et al., 2017). Forms of parental responsivity are not mutually exclusive and have been shown across an array of studies with typically and atypically developing children to impact language and communication development as well as emotional, social, and cognitive development (Warren & Brady, 2007). In the case of children with DS, parental responsivity may be necessary, but not sufficient, to assure optimal language development given the complexities of Down syndrome. Thus, large doses of parent-generated MT from early in development onward should be viewed as part of any broader long-term education and treatment approach.

Moving From Small-N Studies to Larger RCTs

Small-*N* and single-subject studies, such as those we reviewed in the AAC section of this chapter, remain an essential part of our research toolbox. These studies have been critical for developing treatment procedures and determining their initial potential. However, they have various limitations and only single-subject research designs across a minimum of three subjects, behaviors, or settings can provide causal inferences; nonrandomized designs represent lower levels in terms of evidence and can only hint at causality (Logan et al., 2008). Table 19.2 provides a list of the single-subject design studies that we have reviewed in this chapter and the level of evidence they offer. As the table illustrates, many of the studies are at a moderately high level (i.e., level 2) of the hierarchy of evidence put forth by Logan et al. (2008), suggesting that these approaches may be ready for testing via larger scale group designs and RCTs. If researchers are going to continue to conduct single-subject design studies, there is a clear need for more rigorous designs such as randomized concurrent or nonconcurrent multiple baseline designs with no fewer than three replications (Logan et al., 2008).

The highest level of evidence for group designs (level 1) are meta-analyses that include substantial numbers of relatively large RCTs with 100 or more subjects (Darrah et al., 2008). A step below that are smaller RCTs with less than 100 participants (the level of each of the 8 RCTs we reviewed). It should be a near-term goal to conduct further level 2

RCTs with individuals with DS with much larger sample sizes and much longer intervention periods. We have identified an intervention that appears to be worthy of this effort—the combination of MT, AAC, and parent responsivity training.

A Modest Proposal

We suggest that one, or a consortium, of US federal agencies (e.g., National Institutes of Health, Institute of Education Sciences, CDC) join with one or more major foundations (e.g., NDSS, March of Dimes) to create and launch an initiative aimed at determining the true potential of enhanced communication interventions that combine MT, AAC (e.g., SGDs), and parent responsivity training aimed at accelerating the language and cognitive development of young children with DS. The RCTs that have been conducted to date were constrained because of funding caps that limited the size of the grants to support this research. Larger (e.g., 80 to 100 young children), longer (e.g., up to 2 years), broader (e.g., communication, language, cognitive, and social skills), more intense (e.g., 25 hours per week), comprehensive RCTs are quite feasible with appropriate funding. The primary limitation is getting adequate funding to conduct multisite randomized clinical trials with larger sample sizes, breadth, intensity, and length. The model used to propel autism treatment research forward provides a starting point for initiating this effort. A concentrated 10- to 15-year effort could lead to beneficial clinical and scientific knowledge for children with DS, and perhaps for other non-ASD neurodevelopmental disorders. This effort would require the type of leadership that eventually led to large amounts of funding being provided to test comprehensive early treatments for ASD. We know that young children with DS are at great risk for significantly impaired language and cognition. Perhaps the time is right to invest in larger scale, state-of-the art clinical trial research aimed at addressing this educational and health care disparity.

References

Anlar, B., & Yalaz, K. (1996). *Denver II gelişimsel tarama testi Türk çocuklarına uyarlanması ve standardizasyonu el kitabı [Turkish Manual for Denver II]*. Ankara, Turkey: Meteksan.

Barnes, E., Roberts, J., Long, S., Martin, G. E., Berni, M., Mandulak, K., & Sideris, J. (2009). Phonological accuracy and intelligibility in connected speech of boys with fragile X syndrome or Down syndrome. *Journal of Speech, Language, and Hearing Research, 52*, 1048–1061. doi:10.1044/1092-4388(2009/08-0001

Batorowicz, B., Stadskleiv, K., von Tetzchner, S., & Missiuna, C. (2016). Children who use communication aids instructing peer and adult partners during play-based activity. *Augmentative and Alternative Communication, 32*, 105–119. doi:10.3109/07434618.2016.1160150

Biggs, E. E., Carter, E. W., & Gustafson, J. (2017). Efficacy of peer support arrangements to increase peer interaction and AAC use. *American Journal on Intellectual and Developmental Disabilities, 122*, 25–48. doi:10.1352/1944-7558-122.1.25

Bondy, A. S., & Frost, L. A. (1994). The picture exchange communication system. *Focus on Autistic Behavior, 9*, 1–19.

Brady, N. C., Bredin-Oja, S. L., Warren, S. F. (2008). Prelinguistic and early language interventions for children with Down syndrome or fragile X syndrome. In J. Roberts, C. Chapman, & S. Warren (Eds.) *Speech and language development and intervention in Down syndrome and fragile X syndrome* (p. 173–193). Baltimore, MD: Brookes.

Brady, N. C., Thiemann-Bourque, K., Fleming, K., & Matthews, K. (2013). Predicting language outcomes for children learning augmentative and alternative communication: Child and environmental factors. *Journal of Speech, Language, and Hearing Research, 56*, 1595–1612. doi:10.1044/1092-4388(2013/12-0102)

Brady, N., Warren, S. F., Fleming, K., Keller, J., & Sterling, A. (2014). The effect of sustained maternal responsivity on later vocabulary development in children with fragile X syndrome. *Journal of Speech, Language, Hearing Research, 57*, 212–226. doi:101044.1092-4388(213/12-0341)

Branson, D., & Demchak, M. (2009). The use of augmentative and alternative communication methods with infants and toddlers with disabilities: A research review. *Augmentative and Alternative Communication, 25*, 274–286. doi:10.3109/07434610903384529

Bruno, J., & Trembath, D. (2006). Use of aided language stimulation to improve syntactic performance during a weeklong intervention program. *Augmentative and Alternative Communication, 22*, 300–313. doi:10.1080/07434610600768318

Carter, E. W., Asmus, J., Moss, C. K., Amirault, K. A., Biggs, E. E., Bolt, D., . . . Wier, K. (2016). Randomized evaluation of peer supports arrangements to support the inclusion of high school students with severe disabilities. *Exceptional Children, 82*, 209–233. doi:10.1177/0014402915598780

Carter, E. W., Moss, C. K., Hoffman, A., Chung, Y. C., & Sisco, L. (2011). Efficacy and social validity of peer support arrangements for adolescents with disabilities. *Exceptional Children, 78*, 107–125. doi:10.1177/001440291107800107

Caselli, M. C., Vicari, S., Longobardi, E., Lami, L., Pizzoli, C., & Stella, G. (1998). Gestures and words in early development of children with Down syndrome. *Journal of Speech, Language, and Hearing Research, 41*, 1125–1135. doi:10.1044/jslhr.4105.1125

Charlop-Christy, M. H., Carpenter, M., Le, L., LeBlanc, L. A., & Kellet, K. (2013). Using the picture exchange communication system (PECS) with children with autism: Assessment of PECS acquisition, speech, social-communicative behavior, and problem behavior. *Journal of Applied Behavior Analysis, 35*, 213–231. doi:10/1901/jaba.2002.35-213

Chomsky, N. (1957). *Syntactic structures*. The Hague: Mouton.

Cicchetti, D., & Beeghly, M. (Eds.). (1990). *Children with Down syndrome: A developmental perspective*. Cambridge, UK: Cambridge University Press.

Clibbens, J. (2001). Signing and lexical development in children with Down syndrome. *Down Syndrome Research and Practice, 7*, 101–105. doi:10.3104/reviews.119

Clibbens, J., Powell, G. G., & Atkinson, E. (2002). Strategies for achieving joint attention when signing to children with Down's syndrome. *International Journal of Language & Communication Disorders, 37*, 309–323. doi:10.1080/13682820210136287

Dada, S., & Alant, E. (2009). The effect of aided language stimulation on vocabulary acquisition in children with little or no functional speech. *American Journal of Speech-Language Pathology, 18*, 50–64. doi:10.1044/1058-0360(2008/07-0018)

Darrah, J., Hickman, R., O'donnell, M., Vogtle, L., & Wiart, L. (2008). AACPDM methodology to develop systematic reviews of treatment interventions (Revision 1.2). Milwaukee, WI: American Academy for Cerebral Palsy and Developmental Medicine.

Dawson, G., & Bernier, R. (2013). A quarter century of progress on the early detection and treatment of autism spectrum disorder. *Development and psychopathology, 25*(4 pt 2), 1455–1472. doi:10.1017/S0954579413000710

Deckers, S. R. J. M., Van Zaalen, Y., Van Balkom, H., & Verhoeven, L. (2017). Core vocabulary of young children with Down syndrome. *Augmentative and Alternative Communication, 33*, 77–86. doi:10.1080/07434618.2017.1293730

Dieterich, S. E., Assel, M. A., Swank, P., Smith, K. E., & Landry, S. H. (2006). The impact of early maternal verbal scaffolding and child language abilities on later decoding and reading comprehension skills. *Journal of School Psychology, 43*, 481–494. doi:10.1016/jsp.2005.10.003

Dodd, B. (1976). A comparison of the phonological systems of mental age matched, normal, severely subnormal and Down's syndrome children. *British Journal of Disorders of Communication, 11*, 27–42. doi:10.3109/13682827609011289

Ellis Weismer, S., & Robertson, S. (2006). Focused stimulation approach to language intervention. In R. McCauley & M. Fey (Eds.), *Treatment of language disorders in children* (pp. 175–201). Baltimore, MD: Brookes.

Fenson, L., Dale, P., Resnick, J., Thal, D., Bates, E., Hartung, J., & Reilly, J. (1993). The Macarthur communicative development inventory: Words and gestures. San Diego, CA: Center for Research in Language.

Fey, M. E., Warren, S. F., Brady, N., Finestack, L. H., Bredin-Oja, S. L., Fairchild, M., . . . Yoder, P. J. (2006). Early effects of responsivity education/prelinguistic milieu teaching for children with developmental delays and their parents. *Journal of Speech, Language, and Hearing Research, 49*, 526–547. doi:10.1044/1092-4388(2006/039)

Fey, M. E., Yoder, P. J., Warren, S. F., & Bredin-Oja, S. L. (2013). Is more better? Milieu communication teaching in toddlers with intellectual disabilities. *Journal of Speech, Language, and Hearing Research, 56*, 679–693. doi:10.1044/1092-4388(2012/12-0061)

Fidler, D. J., Lunkenheimer, E., & Hahn, L. (2011). Emerging behavioral phenotypes and dynamic systems theory. *International Review of Research in Developmental Disabilities, 40*, 17–42.

Flippin, M., Reszka, S., & Watson, L. (2010). Effectiveness of the picture exchange communication system (PECS) on communication & speech for children with autism spectrum disorders: A meta-analysis. *American Journal of Speech-Language Pathology, 19*, 178–195. doi:10.1044/1058-0360(2010/09-0022)

Foreman, P., & Crews, G. (1998). Using augmentative communication with infants and young children with Down syndrome. *Down Syndrome Research and Practice, 5*(1), 16–25. doi:10.3104/reports.71

Franco, F., & Wishart, J. G. (1995). Use of pointing and other gestures by young children with Down syndrome. *American Journal on Mental Retardation, 100*(2), 160–182.

Girolametto, L., Greenberg, J., & Manolson, H. (1986). Developing dialogue skills: The Hanen Early Language Parent Program. *Seminars in Speech and Language, 7*, 367–382. doi:10.1055/s-0028-1085235

Girolametto, L., Pearce, P. S., & Weitzman, E. (1996). Interactive focused stimulation for toddlers with expressive vocabulary delays. *Journal of Speech, Language, and Hearing Research, 39*, 1274–1283. doi:10.1044/jshr.3906.1274

Girolametto, L., Weitzman, E., & Clements-Baartman, J. (1998). Vocabulary intervention for children with Down syndrome: Parent training using focused stimulation. *Infant-Toddler Intervention: The Transdisciplinary Journal, 8*(2), 109–125

Guess, D. (1969). A functional analysis of individual differences in generalization between receptive and productive language in retarded children. *Journal of Applied Behavior Analysis, 2*, 55–64.

Guess, D., Sailor, W., Rutherford, G., & Baer, D. M. (1968). An experimental analysis of linguistic development: The productive use of the plural morpheme. *Journal of Applied Behavior Analysis, 1*(4), 297–306.

Halle, J. W., Baer, D. M., & Spradlin, J. E. (1981). Teachers' generalized use of delay as a stimulus control procedure to increase language use in handicapped children. *Journal of Applied Behavior Analysis, 14*(4), 389–409.

Hancock, T. B., & Kaiser, A. P. (2006). Enhanced milieu teaching. In R. McCauley & M. Fey (Eds.), *Treatment of language disorders in children* (pp. 203–233). Baltimore, MD: Brookes.

Harris, M. D., & Reichle, J. (2004). The impact of aided language stimulation on symbol comprehension and production in children with moderate cognitive disabilities. *American Journal of Speech-Language Pathology, 13*, 155–167. doi:10.1044/1058-0360(2004/016)

Hart, S. L., & Banda, D. R. (2010). Picture Exchange Communication System with individuals with developmental disabilities: A meta-analysis of single subject studies. *Remedial and Special Education, 31*, 476–488. doi:10.1177/0741932509338354

Hart, B., & Risley, T. R. (1975). Incidental teaching of language in the preschool. *Journal of Applied Behavior Analysis, 8*, 411–420. doi:10.1901/jaba.1975.8-411

Hart, B., & Risley, T. R. (1992). American parenting of language-learning children: Persisting differences in family-child interactions observed in natural home environments. *Developmental Psychology, 28*, 1096–1105. doi:10.1037/0012-1649.28.6.1096

Hart, B., & Risley, T. R. (1995). *Meaningful differences in the everyday experience of young American children.* Baltimore: Paul H. Brookes.

Hart, B., & Rogers-Warren, A. K. (1978). Milieu language training. In R. L. Schiefelbusch (Ed.), *Language intervention strategies* (Vol. 2, pp.193–235). Baltimore, MD: University Park Press.

Hedges, L.V., & Olkin, I. (1985). *Statistical Methods for Meta-Analysis*. Orlando, FL: Academic Press.

Howlin, P., Gordon, R. K., Pasco, G., Wade, A., & Charman, T. (2007). The effectiveness of Picture Exchange Communication System (PECS) training for teachers of children with autism: A pragmatic, group randomized controlled trial. *Journal of Child Psychology and Psychiatry, 48*, 473–481. doi:10.1111/j.1469-7610.2006.01707.x

Hunt, P., Alwell, M., & Goetz, L. (1991). Interacting with peers through conversation turn taking with a communication book adaptation. *Augmentative and Alternative Communication, 7*, 117–126. doi:10.1080/07434619112331275783

Kaiser, A. P., & Roberts, M. Y. (2013). Parent-implemented enhanced milieu teaching with preschool children who have intellectual disabilities. *Journal of Speech, Language, and Hearing Research, 56*, 295–309. doi:10.1044/1092-4388(2012/11-0231)

Kaiser, A. P., Yoder, P. J., & Keetz, A. (1992). Evaluating milieu teaching. In S. F. Warren & J. Reichle (Eds.), *Communication and language intervention series: Vol. 1. Causes and effects in communication and language intervention* (pp. 9–48). Baltimore, MD: Brookes.

Karaaslan, O., & Mahoney, G. (2013). Effectiveness of responsive teaching with children with Down syndrome. *Mental Retardation, 51*(6), 458–469.

Kasari, C., Freeman, S., & Paparella, T. (2006). Joint attention and symbolic play in young children with autism: A randomized controlled intervention study. *Journal of Child Psychology and Psychiatry, and Allied Disciplines, 47*, 611–620. doi:10.1111/j.1469-7610.2005.01567.x

Kay-Raining Bird, E., & Chapman, R. S. (1994). Sequential recall in individuals with Down syndrome. *Journal of Speech, Language, and Hearing Research, 37*, 1369–1380. doi:10.1044/jshr.3706.1369

Kay-Raining Bird, E., Gaskell, A., Babineau, M. D., & Macdonald, S. (2000). Novel word acquisition in children with Down syndrome: Does modality make a difference? *Journal of Communication Disorders, 33*, 241–266. doi:10.1016/S0021-9924(00)00022-8

Kent-Walsh, J., Binger, C., & Hasham, Z. (2010). Effects of parent instruction on the symbolic communication of children using augmentative and alternative communication during storybook reading. *Communication Disorders Quarterly, 30*, 49–61. doi:10.1177/1525740108320353

Kern, L., Gallagher, P., Starosta, K., Hickman, W., & George, M. (2006). Longitudinal outcomes of functional behavioral assessment-based intervention. *Journal of Positive Behavior Interventions, 8*, 67–78. doi:10.1177/10983007060080020501

Koegel, L., Koegel, R., Harrower, J., & Carter, C. (1999). Pivotal response intervention I: Overview of approach. *Journal of the Association for Persons with Severe Handicaps, 24*, 174–185. doi:10.2511/rpsd.24.3.174

Kumin, L. (1999). Comprehensive speech and language treatment for infants, toddlers, and children with Down syndrome. In T. J. Hassold & D. Patterson (Eds.), *Down syndrome: A promising future, together* (pp. 145–154). New York, NY: Wiley-Liss.

Kumin L. (2003). *Early communication skills for children with Down syndrome: A guide for parents and professionals*. Bethesda, MD: Woodbine House.

Lanter, E., Russell, S. D., Kuriakose, A., & Blevins, K. E. (2016). Incorporating AAC and general instructional strategies in requesting interventions: A case study in Down syndrome. *Communication Disorders Quarterly, 38*, 52–63. doi:10.1177/1525740115602093

Launonen, K. (1996). Enhancing communication skills of children with Down syndrome: Early use of manual signs. In S. von Tetzchner & M. Jensen (Eds.), *Augmentative and alternative communication: European perspectives* (pp. 213–231). Sussex, United Kingdom: Whurr Publishers.

Logan, L. R., Hickman, R. R., Harris, S. R., & Heriza, C. B. (2008). Single-subject research design: Recommendations for levels of evidence and quality rating. *Developmental medicine & child neurology, 50*, 99–103. doi:10.111/j.1469-8749.2007.02005.x

Mahoney, G., Finger, I., & Powell, A. (1985). Relationship of maternal behavioral style to the development of organically impaired mentally retarded infants. *American Journal of Mental Deficiency, 90*(3), 296–302.

Mahoney, G., & Nam, S. (2011). The parenting model of developmental intervention. In R. M. Hodapp (Ed.), *International review of research on mental retardation, 41* (pp. 73–125). New York, NY: Academic Press.

Mahoney, G., Perales, F., Wiggers, B., & Herman, B., (2006), Responsive teaching: Early intervention for children with Down syndrome and other disabilities. *Down Syndrome Research and Practice 11*, 18–28. doi:10.3104/perspectives.311

Mahoney, G., & Powell, A. (1988). Modifying parent-child interaction: Enhancing the development of handicapped children. *The Journal of Special Education, 22*, 82–96. doi:10.1177/002246698802200110

Manolson, A. (1992). *It takes two to talk: A parent's guide to helping children communicate*. Toronto, Canada: Hanen Centre.

Millar, D. C., Light, J. C., & Schlosser, R. W. (2006). The impact of augmentative and alternative communication intervention on the speech production disabilities: A research review. *Journal of Speech, Language, and Hearing Research, 49*, 248–264. doi:10.1044/1092-4388(2006/021)

Miller, J. F. (1992). Development of speech and language in children with Down syndrome. In I. T. Lott & E. McCoy (Eds.), *Down syndrome: Advances in medical care* (pp. 39–50). New York, NY: Wiley-Liss.

Miller, J. (1999). Profiles of language development in children with Down syndrome. In J. Miller, M. Leddy, & L. Leavitt (Eds.), *Improving the communication of people with Down syndrome* (pp. 11–40). Baltimore, MD: Brookes.

Mirenda, P., & Bopp, K. D. (2003). "Playing the game": Strategic competence in AAC. In J. C. Light, D. R. Beukelman, & J. Reichle (Eds.), *Communicative competence for individuals who use AAC: From research to effective practice* (pp. 401–437). Baltimore, MD: Brookes.

Moody, C., Baker, B., & Blacher, J. (2018). Contribution of parenting to complex syntax development in preschool children with developmental delays or typical development. *Journal of Intellectual Disability Research, 62*, 604–616. doi:10.1111/jir.12501Moody

O'Neill, T., Light, J., Pope, L. (2018). Effects of interventions that include aided augmentative and alternative communication input on the communication needs of individuals with complex communication needs: A meta-analysis. *Journal of Speech, Language, and Hearing Research, 61*, 1743–1765. doi:10.1044/2018_JSLHR-L-17-0132

Price, J., Roberts, J. E., Vandergrift, N., & Martin, G. (2007). Language comprehension in boys with fragile X syndrome and boys with Down syndrome. *Journal of Intellectual Disability Research, 51*(Pt 4), 318–326. doi:10.1111/j.1365-2788.2006.00881.x

Reichle, J., Cooley Hidecker, M., Brady, N., & Terry, N. (2003). Intervention strategies for communication: Using aided communication systems. In J. Light, D. R. Beukelman, & J. Reichle (Eds.), *Communicative competence for individuals who use AAC* (pp. 441–479). Baltimore, MD: Brookes.

Reichow, B. (2012). Overview of meta-analyses on early intensive behavioral intervention for young children with autism spectrum disorders. *Journal of Autism and Developmental Disorders, 42*, 512–520. doi:10.1007/s10803-011-1218-9

Roberts, J. E., Price, J., & Malkin, C. (2007). Language and communication development in Down syndrome. *Mental Retardation and Developmental Disabilities Research Reviews, 13*, 26–35. doi:10.1002/mrdd.20136

Romski, M., & Sevcik, R. A. (2005). Augmentative communication and early intervention: Myths and realities. *Infants & Young Children*, 18, 174–185. doi:10.1097/00001163-200507000-00002

Romski, M., Sevcik, R. A., Adamson, L. B., Cheslock, M., Smith, A., Barker, R. M., & Bakeman, R. (2010). Randomized comparison of augmented and nonaugmented language interventions for toddlers with developmental delays and their parents. *Journal of Speech Language and Hearing Research, 53*, 350–364. doi:10.1044/1092-4388 (2009/08-0156)

Romski, M., Sevcik, R. A., Barton-Hulsey, A., & Whitmore, A. S. (2015). Early intervention and AAC: What a difference 30 years makes. *Augmentative and Alternative Communication, 31*, 181–202. doi:10.3109/07434618.2015.1064163

Savasir, I., Sezgin, N., & Erol, N. (1995). *Ankara Developmental Screening Inventory (ADSI) Handbook*. Ankara: Ankara University, Faculty of Medicine.

Schiefelbusch, R. L., & Lloyd, L. L. (1974). *Language perspectives—Acquisition, retardation, and intervention.* Baltimore, MD: University Park Press.

Schwartz, I. S., Garfinkle, A. N., & Bauer, J. (1998). The Picture Exchange Communication System: Communicative outcomes for young children with disabilities. *Topics in Early Childhood Special Education, 18*, 144–159. doi:10.1177/027112149801800305

Shonkoff, J. P., & Phillips, D. A. (Eds.) (2000). *From Neurons to Neighborhoods: The Science of Early Childhood. Committee on Integrating the Science of Early Childhood Development, Board on Children, Youth, and Families. Commission on Behavioral and Social Sciences and Education*. Washington, DC: National Academy Press.

Snow, C. E. (1977). The development of conversation between mothers and babies. *Journal of child language, 4*(1), 1–22.

Spiker, D., Boyce, G. C., & Boyce, L. K. (2002). Parent-child interactions when young children have disabilities. *International Review of Research in Mental Retardation, 25*, 35–70.

Spradlin, J. E., Karlan, G. R., & Wetherby, B. (1976). Behavior analysis, behavior modification, and developmental disabilities. In L. Loyd (Ed.), *Communication assessment and intervention strategies* (pp. 227–263). Baltimore, MD: University Park Press.

Spreckley, M., & Boyd, R. (2008). Early childhood intervention for preschool children. What is the evidence for applied behavioural intervention (ABI) for preschool children with autism? A systematic review and meta-analysis. *Developmental Medicine & Child Neurology, 50*(113), 36–37.

Sterling, A., & Warren, S. F. (2008).). Communication and language development in infants and toddlers with Down syndrome and fragile X syndrome. In J. Roberts, C. Chapman, & S. Warren (Eds.), *Speech and language development and intervention in Down syndrome and fragile X syndrome* (pp. 53–76). Baltimore, MD: Brookes.

Stoel-Gammon, C. (2001). Down syndrome phonology: Developmental patterns and intervention strategies. *Down Syndrome Research and Practice, 7*, 93–100. doi:10.3104/reviews.118

Te Kaat, D. J. A., (2013). Expressieve woordenschat bij Downsyndroom [Expressive vocabulary in Down syndrome]. *Nederlands Tijdschrift Voor Logopedie, 8*, 6–10.

Thiemann-Bourque, K. (2012). Peer-mediated AAC instruction for young children with autism and other developmental disabilities. *Perspectives on augmentative and alternative communication, 21*(4), 159–166. doi:10.4/acc21.4.159

Thiemann-Bourque, K. S., McGuff, S., & Goldstein, H. (2017). Training peer partners to use a speech-generating device with classmates with autism spectrum disorder: Exploring communication outcomes across preschool contexts. *Journal of Speech, Language, and Hearing Research, 60*, 2648–2662. doi:10.1044/2017_JSLHR-L-17-0049

Thompson, R. H., Cotnoir-Bichelman, N. M., McKerchar, P. M., Tate, T. L., & Dancho, K. A. (2007). Enhancing early communication through infant sign training. *Journal of Applied Behavior Analysis, 40*, 15–23. doi:10.1901/jaba.2007.23-06

Vanderheiden, G. C., & Harris-Vanderheiden, D. (1976). Communication techniques and aids for the nonvocal severely handicapped (pp. 601–652). In L. L. Lloyd (Ed.), *Communication assessment and intervention strategies*. Baltimore, MD: University Park Press.

Warren, S. F., & Brady, N. C. (2007). The role of maternal responsivity in the development of children with intellectual disabilities. *Developmental Disabilities Research Reviews, 13*(4), 330–338.

Warren, S. F., Brady, N., Fleming, K., & Hahn, L. (2017). The effects of parenting on adaptive behavior in children with fragile X syndrome. *Journal of Autism and Developmental Disorders, 47*, 768–784. doi:10.1007/s10803-016-2999-7

Warren, S. F., Brady, N., Sterling, A., Fleming, K., & Marquis, J. (2010). Maternal responsivity predicts language development in young children with fragile X syndrome. *American Journal on Intellectual and Developmental Disabilities, 115*, 54–75. doi:10.1352/1944-7558-115.1.54

Warren, S. F., Fey, M. E., Finestack, L. H., Brady, N. C., Bredin-Oja, S. L., & Fleming, K. K. (2008). A randomized trial of longitudinal effects of low-intensity responsivity education/prelinguistic milieu teaching. *Journal of Speech, Language, and Hearing Research, 51*, 451–470. doi:10.1044/1092-4388(2008/033)

Warren, S., & Rogers-Warren, A. (1985). *Teaching functional language*. Austin, TX: Pro-Ed.

Warren, S. F., & Walker, D. (2004). Fostering early communication and language development. In D. M. Teti (Ed.), *Handbook of research methods in developmental science* (pp. 249–270). Oxford, UK: Blackwell Publishers.

Warren, S. F., Yoder, P. J., Gazdag, G. E., Kim, K., & Jones, H. A. (1993). Facilitating prelinguistic communication skills in young children with developmental delay. *Journal of Speech, Language, and Hearing Research, 36*, 83–97. doi:10.1044/jshr.3601.83

Wright, C. A., Kaiser, A. P., Reikowsky, D. I., & Roberts, M. Y. (2013). Effects of a naturalistic sign intervention on expressive language of toddlers with Down syndrome. *Journal of Speech Language and Hearing Research, 56*(3), 994. doi:10.1044/1092-4388 (2012/12-0060)

Yang, Y., Conners, F. A., & Merrill, E. C. (2014). Visuo-spatial ability in individuals with Down syndrome: Is it really a strength? *Research in developmental disabilities, 35*(7), 1473–1500. doi:10.1016/j.ridd.2014.04.002

Yoder, P. J., & Warren, S. F. (1998). Maternal responsivity predicts the prelinguistic communication intervention that facilitates generalized intentional communication. *Journal of Speech, Language, and Hearing Research, 41*, 1207–1219. doi:10.1044/jsljr.4105.1207

Yoder, P. J., & Warren, S. F. (1999a). Facilitating self-initiated proto-declaratives and proto-imperatives in prelinguistic children with developmental disabilities. *Journal of Early Intervention, 22*, 337–354. doi:10.1177/105381519902200408

Yoder, P. J., & Warren, S. F. (1999b). Maternal responsivity mediates the relationship between prelinguistic intentional communication and later language. *Journal of Early Intervention, 22*, 126–136. doi:10.1177/105381519902200205

Yoder, P. J., & Warren, S. F. (2001). Relative treatment effects of two prelinguistic communication interventions on language development in toddlers with developmental delays vary by maternal characteristics. *Journal of Speech, Language, and Hearing Research, 44*, 224–237. doi:10.1044/1092-4388(2001/019)

Yoder, P. J., & Warren, S. F. (2002). Effects of prelinguistic milieu teaching and parent responsivity education on dyads involving children with intellectual disabilities. *Journal of Speech, Language, and Hearing Research, 45*, 1158–1174. doi:10.1044/1092-4388(2002/094)

Yoder, P. J., Warren, S. F., Kim, K., & Gazdag, G. E. (1994). Facilitating prelinguistic communication skills in young children with developmental delay II: Systematic replication and extension. *Journal of Speech, Language, and Hearing Research, 37*, 841–851. doi:10.1044/jshr.3704.841

Yoder, P., Woynaroski, T., Fey, M., & Warren, S. (2014). Effects of dose frequency of early communication intervention in young children with and without Down syndrome. *American Journal on Intellectual and Developmental Disabilities, 119*, 17–32. doi:10.1352/1944-7558-119.1.17

Yoder, P. J., Woynaroski, T. G., Fey, M. E., Warren, S. F, & Gardner, E. (2015). Why dose frequency affects spoken vocabulary in preschoolers with Down syndrome. *American Journal on Intellectual and Developmental Disabilities, 120*, 302–314. doi:10.1352/1944-7558-120.4.302

Zampini, L., & D'Odorico, L. (2011). Gesture production and language development: A longitudinal study of children with Down syndrome. *Gesture, 11*(2), 174–193. doi:10.1075/gest.11.2.04zam

CHAPTER

20 Development of Dementia, Including Assessment and Interventions

Carla M. Startin, Shahid H. Zaman, *and* André Strydom

Abstract

Adults with Down syndrome show premature aging with a high risk of developing dementia, specifically Alzheimer's disease. Dementia in people with Down syndrome develops in addition to pre-existing intellectual disability, which poses difficulties in its diagnosis. Determining baseline function and conducting regular assessments are essential to detecting cognitive and functional decline. Comorbid conditions such as epilepsy and depression may also affect dementia presentation. As there is little evidence for effective pharmacological treatment of dementia in adults with Down syndrome, the identification of novel treatment targets is vital. In addition, a better understanding of the time course of the development of dementia will aid in better detection and monitoring of individuals showing early signs of cognitive decline. Early dementia-related changes may include prominent declines in behavior, personality disturbance, and early impairments in memory. Advances in neuroimaging and biomarker detection will further assist in understanding the time course of dementia development in people with Down syndrome.

Key Words: Down syndrome, Alzheimer's disease, dementia, cognitive decline, premature aging

Introduction

As medical and social care have improved over the last several decades, the life expectancy of people with Down syndrome has dramatically increased. With aging, it has become apparent that adults show an usually high risk of developing dementia, specifically Alzheimer's disease. Further, in many countries including both the United Kingdom and the United States, there is now a peak in the prevalence of Down syndrome in adults aged 40–55 years (Alexander et al., 2016; Presson et al., 2013). Health conditions associated with aging in adults with Down syndrome, including dementia, are therefore increasingly a major health issue. In addition to people with Down syndrome having an increased risk of dementia, this is one of several conditions that have an earlier age of onset in people with Down syndrome compared to the typically developing population. This supports the notion of premature aging in those with Down syndrome (Esbensen, 2010; McCarron,

Gill, McCallion, & Begley, 2005), and further contributes to the high prevalence of dementia in this population.

The increased risk of Alzheimer's disease in adults with Down syndrome is thought to be largely due to the overexpression of certain genes on chromosome 21, which are found in three copies in this population (Wiseman et al., 2015). In particular, the amyloid precursor protein (*APP*) gene is associated with the development of Alzheimer's disease. Evidence for this association comes from genetic and neuropathological studies. First, mutations in this gene are associated with early-onset autosomal dominant familial Alzheimer's disease in the typically developing population (Rovelet-Lecrux et al., 2006; Ryan et al., 2016; Zis & Strydom, 2018). Second, the protein product of the *APP* gene, amyloid-beta, forms characteristic deposits (amyloid-beta plaques) in the brains of individuals with Alzheimer's disease, and similar deposits are reported to be present in the brains of almost all adults with Down syndrome over the age of 30 years (Davidson, Robinson, Prasher, & Mann, 2018; Mann, 1988; Wisniewski, Wisniewski, & Wen, 1985; also see Helman et al., this volume). Despite this almost universal early development of neuropathology of Alzheimer's disease, there appears to be a delay of many years between the appearance of amyloid-beta deposits and tauopathy (the deposition of abnormal forms of tau protein in neurons) and the clinical presentation of dementia in individuals with Down syndrome. A similar delay occurs in the development of clinical symptoms in Alzheimer's disease in the typically developing population.

While adults with Down syndrome have an increased risk of developing dementia, with onset at a younger age as compared to the typically developing population, clinical presentation varies considerably in terms of the age of onset of the first signs and symptoms of dementia. A small percentage of people with Down syndrome are diagnosed with dementia as early as their mid-30s, while others reach their 70s without signs of cognitive decline (Sinai et al., 2018; Startin et al., 2016). Large variability also occurs between those with Down syndrome regarding the presence of conditions that are comorbid to or a differential diagnosis for dementia, such as epilepsy. Individuals with Down syndrome also have extensive premorbid variability in the severity of their intellectual functioning and disability level. The diagnosis of dementia therefore requires careful and considerate assessment. Nevertheless, the degree of variability in age of onset of dementia in people with Down syndrome suggests that some people show increased protection against dementia. The identification of resilience factors that modify the risk for and age of onset of dementia may therefore provide clues to how best to target treatments that can delay its onset in this population.

In this chapter, we will discuss the conceptualization of the issues that pose challenges to the diagnosis of dementia in people with Down syndrome. We first discuss the epidemiology of dementia in adults with Down syndrome. We will then consider the diagnosis of dementia, including diagnostic criteria and dementia assessments, as well as clinical aspects relating to potential comorbid conditions and potential treatments. We will next discuss the conceptual issues related to variability in the age of onset of dementia, including risk factors associated with this. We will discuss the neuropsychological changes that occur as dementia develops, as well as considering recent advances in neuroimaging and identifying potential biomarkers for dementia. We will conclude by considering how these advances will improve the detection and treatment of dementia.

Epidemiology of Dementia

Over the last 50 years, the average life expectancy of adults with Down syndrome has shown a dramatic increase. According to a Swedish population study of individuals with Down syndrome between 1969–1973, the median life expectancy was 3.6 years, and by 1999–2003 this had risen to 56.8 years (Englund, Jonsson, Zander, Gustafsson, & Anneren, 2013). Similarly, researchers of a U.K. population study of individuals with Down syndrome have estimated that the median life expectancy for babies born in 2011 is 58 years (Wu & Morris, 2013).

As the life expectancy of people with Down syndrome has increased it has become evident that these adults are at a greatly increased risk of the development of dementia, with this risk increasing with age. Similarly, the incidence (i.e., frequency of new cases in a given period of time) of dementia increases with age in people with Down syndrome, with Coppus et al. (2006) reporting an incidence per 100 person years of 2.53 for adults aged 45–49 years, 2.82 for those aged 50–54 years, 4.88 for those aged 55–59 years, and 13.31 for adults aged 60 and over in the Netherlands. McCarron, McCallion, Reilly, and Mulryan (2014) found the overall risk of developing dementia was 20% by age 50, 45% by age 55, and 80% by age 65 in a study cohort based in the Republic of Ireland. Similarly, the prevalence (i.e., cross-sectional rate) of dementia in adults with Down syndrome greatly increases with age, usually from fewer than 5% in adults aged under 40 up to around 40% in adults aged over 50 (Coppus et al., 2006; Holland, Hon, Huppert, Stevens, & Watson, 1998; Sekijima et al., 1998; Tyrrell et al., 2001; Van Buggenhout et al., 1999; Visser et al., 1997; see Table 20.1). Although the prevalence of dementia appears to decrease in some studies in adults over the age of 60 years, this is likely due to increased mortality associated with dementia (Coppus et al., 2006), with relative preservation of cognitive and functional ability being associated with better survival (Coppus, Evenhuis, Verberne, Visser, Oostra, et al., 2008). Furthermore, the mean age of dementia diagnosis has been reported to be around 55 years (McCarron et al., 2014; Sinai et al., 2018; Tyrrell et al., 2001; Visser et al., 1997), with a mean survival length after dementia diagnosis of approximately 6 years (McCarron et al., 2014).

Further underlying the development of dementia as a major health issue in adults with Down syndrome is a strong relationship between the presence of dementia and mortality (Coppus, Evenhuis, Verberne, Visser, Oostra, et al., 2008; Uppal, Chandran, & Potluri, 2015). In a Swedish population study of individuals with Down syndrome, Englund et al. (2013) found that dementia was a main or contributing cause of death in 30% of adults

Table 20.1. Results of Studies Investigating the Prevalence of Dementia in Adults With Down syndrome

	39 years and under	40–45 years	45–49 years	50–54 years	55–59 years	60 years and over
Coppus et al. (2006)	-	-	8.9%	17.7%	32.1%	25.6%
Holland et al. (1998)	20.7%	20.7%		40.0%		0.0%
Sekijima et al. (1998)	0.0%	16.3%		40.9%		0.0%
Tyrrell et al. (2001)	1.4%	5.7%		30.4%		41.7%
Van Buggenhout et al. (1999)	0.0%	11.1%		42.4%		0.0%
Visser et al. (1997)	0.0%	11.1%		65.9%		79.2%

aged over 40 years, and Hithersay et al. (2019) found in a U.K.-based longitudinal study that 70% of adults aged 36 and over who died had dementia, with crude mortality rates five times higher for those with dementia as compared to those without.

Diagnosis of Dementia

The diagnosis of dementia in people with Down syndrome is complex due to the presence of premorbid intellectual disability, which needs to be distinguished from any subsequent cognitive decline. In addition, the variability in this premorbid intellectual disability severity means that simply adjusting thresholds for assessments to measure cognitive decline from typically developing thresholds is insufficient to detect decline. Instead of a population-wide threshold to detect cognitive decline, as is used in the typically developing population, an individual threshold that takes into account premorbid cognitive abilities is needed for people with Down syndrome. As a result, clinicians are required to obtain detailed information on past and present functioning to detect the presence of presenting decline in cognitive and functional abilities. This typically involves collecting a reliable and detailed medical history (or longitudinal formal assessment of cognitive functioning, which may not be available or possible), determining whether any change in ability has occurred relative to an established baseline, and if so the extent of this, as well as excluding other potential causes of cognitive and functional decline such as hypothyroidism or depression.

Criteria for Dementia Diagnosis

The criteria for a dementia diagnosis include those from the *International Statistical Classification of Diseases and Related Health Problems* (currently *ICD–10*; World Health Organization [WHO], 1992) and the *Diagnostic and Statistical Manual of Mental Disorders* (currently *DSM–5*; American Psychiatric Association [APA], 2013). Such criteria have been developed for the general population, and so clinicians need to account for premorbid cognitive difficulties while assessing individuals with Down syndrome (Fletcher, Barnhill, McCarthy, & Strydom, 2016).

The *ICD–10* (10th ed.) criteria for dementia diagnosis consist of a decline in memory, along with a decline in other cognitive abilities (such as thinking and judgement, or in information processing leading to an impairment in everyday functioning), and decline in emotional control or social behavior (such as emotional instability and apathy), all of which must have been present for at least 6 months (WHO, 1992). The most recently released *DSM–5* (5th ed.; APA, 2013) criteria has split dementia into major and mild "neurocognitive disorder," to take account of less severe symptoms of decline that may nonetheless cause concern and could benefit from treatment. Major neurocognitive disorder requires significant cognitive decline while minor neurocognitive disorder requires modest cognitive decline in performance for at least one of six cognitive domains (complex attention, executive function, learning and memory, language, perceptual-motor function, and social cognition). In addition, in order to be considered a major neurocognitive disorder, this decline must interfere with everyday activities, such as the regular work or activities the individual takes part in, or their ability to live independently. Prior to the development of the *DSM–5*, the *DSM–IV* (4th ed.; APA, 1994) criteria for dementia included memory decline, along with either aphasia, apraxia, agnosia, or executive function disturbance, with these impairments resulting in an impairment in social or everyday functioning and having occurred gradually. The newer *DSM–5* criteria may improve reliability in individuals with premorbid cognitive impairment as compared to the older *DSM–IV* criteria, as the older criteria require memory decline in addition to other cognitive changes while the newer criteria acknowledge that some types of dementia may not present with memory decline initially. However, caution is advised when applying criteria for mild neurocognitive disorder as it may be difficult to distinguish a moderate change in abilities from pre-existing impairments in those with an intellectual disability (Fletcher et al., 2016).

Sheehan et al. (2015) reported that for adults with Down syndrome who had undergone a clinical assessment, clinical impression of dementia status by a clinician blind to the individual's original diagnosis correlated better with a diagnosis of dementia given by the individual's usual clinical team than strict application of either *ICD–10* or *DSM–IV* classification. Over time, the number of adults meeting *ICD–10* or *DSM–IV* criteria for dementia increased. Sheehan et al. concluded that these findings indicate that when clinicians use their knowledge of dementia presentation in people with Down syndrome they are able to diagnose dementia earlier than if they were relying on the classical descriptions of dementia found in the diagnostic systems, and clinicians showed high levels of inter-rater reliability in their judgments. Accordingly, an experienced clinician's diagnosis of dementia in individuals with Down syndrome should be considered to be reliable and valid.

Dementia Assessment

Although dementia among people with Down syndrome is characterized by a decline in cognitive and everyday functioning, similar to the criteria for dementia in the typically developing population, mainstream norm-based tests such as the Mini-Mental State Examination (MMSE) are not suitable for use because they are based on the assumption that the premorbid level of functioning is within a typical range (Strydom et al., 2013). In some adults with Down syndrome, the presence of a more severe intellectual disability, or vision or hearing problems, also causes difficulties with using such tests. To account for these difficulties, comprehensive recommendations for the assessment, diagnosis, treatment, and follow-up of dementia in adults with an intellectual disability should be consulted where relevant (Moran et al., 2013).

Due to the premorbid presence of intellectual disability in those with Down syndrome, longitudinal changes should be measured to reliably detect cognitive decline. As poor performance on a single assessment of cognitive abilities could be due to a low premorbid cognitive ability, to poor engagement as a result of low motivation or fatigue, or to a decline in cognitive function, longitudinal assessments are essential to determine if cognitive decline has occurred. A baseline assessment should be taken prior to the start of any changes (typically by the age of 30), and performance at either subsequent regular assessments, such as every 2 years after the age of 40, or if there is a change in clinical presentation compared to this baseline (British Psychological Society [BPS], 2015). This allows changes to be detected over time. If decline is observed other aging-related conditions should be considered and ruled out where possible, through taking a detailed medical, psychiatric, and social history, considering prescribed medications, and performing a medical workup (including blood tests to detect hypothyroidism, a mental health assessment to exclude depression, hearing and vision tests to detect sensory impairments, and potentially a screen for obstructive sleep apnea).

Where possible, cognitive functioning should be evaluated through direct assessment. Although there is no universal agreement regarding the ideal battery to use, several cognitive batteries with a particular focus on memory measures have been developed to assess those abilities relevant to the development of dementia in people with intellectual disability (Crayton, Oliver, Holland, Bradbury, & Hall, 1998; Hon, Huppert, Holland, & Watson, 1999; Walsh et al., 2015). Repeated assessment using such batteries allows for the detection of changes over time.

For both those who can and cannot engage in a cognitive assessment, then information collected from informants using standardized questionnaires to assess changes related to the development of dementia allows for changes in everyday functioning to be assessed. Informant measures have been suggested to be more sensitive to the diagnosis of dementia as compared to some simple short cognitive assessments (Deb & Braganza, 1999; Jamieson-Craig, Scior, Chan, Fenton, & Strydom, 2010; McCarron et al., 2014), though these may be less sensitive to more subtle changes in the period before diagnosis.

Informant assessments are invaluable for assessing individuals who are unable to engage in direct cognitive assessment.

One questionnaire that may be used for informant assessment to obtain information about new symptoms and changes in abilities typically associated with dementia is the Cambridge Examination of Mental Disorders of Older People with Down's syndrome and others with Intellectual Disabilities (CAMDEX–DS; Ball et al., 2004). Screening tools that may be used include the Dementia Screening Questionnaire for Individuals with Intellectual Disabilities (DSQIID; Deb, Hare, Prior, & Bhaumik, 2007) and the Dementia Scale for Down Syndrome (DSDS; Gedye, 1995; Huxley, Prasher, & Haque, 2000). Other screening tools such as the Dementia Questionnaire for People with Learning Disabilities (DLD), previously known as the Dementia Questionnaire for Persons with Mental Retardation (DMR; Evenhuis, 1996) are used to assess abilities at one time point and so ideally require repeated use over time to detect changes.

Comorbid Conditions

The presence of comorbid medical conditions can complicate and pose a challenge for the diagnosis of dementia in people with Down syndrome. The presence of comorbidities during dementia diagnosis and treatment must be considered, as health comorbidities have been reported to be more prevalent among adults with Down syndrome and dementia as compared to those without dementia, and the number of such comorbidities increases with dementia progression (McCarron et al., 2005).

Epilepsy and Seizures

One potential comorbid condition that clinicians must consider during the assessment and diagnosis of dementia in people with Down syndrome is epilepsy. In addition to considering a pre-existing diagnosis of epilepsy, the development of seizures during adulthood is commonly associated with dementia in adults with Down syndrome (Coppus et al., 2006; McCarron et al., 2014; Tyrrell et al., 2001; Van Buggenhout et al., 1999). Almost half of adults with Down syndrome and dementia may develop seizures after the age of 35 years, with seizure onset a median time of 2 years following dementia diagnosis (Gholipour, Mitchell, Sarkis, & Chemali, 2017). Diffuse electroencephalogram (EEG) atypicalities may be demonstrated after the onset of dementia, followed by the development of myoclonic seizures, which are typically associated with myoclonic jerks and a diffuse epileptiform EEG pattern upon awakening (De Simone, Puig, Gelisse, Crespel, & Genton, 2010; d'Orsi, Specchio, & Apulian Study Group on Senile Myoclonic, 2014). Eventually, tonic-clonic seizures may develop as the dementia progresses (De Simone et al., 2010). The presence of seizures may also exacerbate the rate of cognitive decline in individuals with Down syndrome and dementia (Lott et al., 2012), in addition to causing potential distress to the individual and their care team. Due to the strong association between developing both seizures and dementia in Down syndrome, the onset of seizures in older adults should trigger an assessment for dementia, and the consideration of seizure development will aid in the diagnosis of dementia for those with Down syndrome.

Depression

Another common comorbidity in adults with Down syndrome and dementia is depression (Coppus et al., 2006). Antidepressant use is thought to be associated with a delayed dementia onset and increased longevity (Tsiouris, Patti, & Flory, 2014). Emphasizing the need to consider depression as a possible confounder of cognitive decline, Wark, Hussain, and Parmenter (2014) reported that some individuals with Down syndrome and dementia show an increase in functioning following a decline, and this may represent undiagnosed depression exaggerating the cognitive decline rather than a reversal of the decline. This finding indicates the importance of diagnosing depression in individuals with Down syndrome who may show signs of dementia, with undiagnosed depression potentially contributing to the previously discussed difficulties in diagnosing dementia in this population.

Other Comorbidities

A number of other comorbidities should also be considered during the assessment and diagnosis of dementia in people with Down syndrome. Such comorbidities may be premorbid and can pose a difficulty for detecting true irreversible cognitive decline or they may exacerbate the development of cognitive decline.

Treatable comorbidities that may result in apparent cognitive decline are vision and hearing impairments and the presence of pain. Vision and hearing impairments are often found in adults with Down syndrome and dementia (McCarron et al., 2014), as increasing age is associated with both dementia and such sensory impairments. Vision and hearing impairments may appear to cause cognitive decline, but with appropriate correction then functional abilities may improve. Pain, associated with a variety of health conditions, is also often overlooked as a treatable cause of functional decline and behavioral change and should also be considered in those with dementia (Strydom, Al-Janabi, Houston, & Ridley, 2016).

Sleep problems, including behavioral sleep disturbances and obstructive sleep apnea (a condition that affects breathing during sleep and causes frequent waking), are common among adults with Down syndrome and have been associated with the presence of dementia (Esbensen, 2016). As these problems may also exaggerate the decline among adults with Down syndrome the potential impact of these needs to be further studied. The presence of delirium or an acute confusional state can exacerbate the progression of dementia or it may be a presentation of dementia; it needs to be vigorously treated.

Although uncommon after the age of 30 years, cases of an unexplained regression in young individuals with Down syndrome have been reported (Prasher, 2002; Santoro et al., 2020). For younger adults showing decline this possibility should be considered, as this regression may occasionally be confused with dementia. The key differences are that regressions tend to present during adolescence or early adulthood, these reach a plateau, and some recovery can be expected, although not always back to the premorbid levels.

Symptoms Associated With Progression of Dementia

In addition to the importance of considering potential comorbidities during the assessment and diagnosis of dementia in people with Down syndrome, a number of comorbid conditions may develop as the dementia progresses. For example, dysphagia (swallowing difficulties) is a common complication that develops with the progression of dementia in people with Down syndrome, and may lead to aspiration pneumonia (Dodd, 2015). A dementia care pathway should therefore include regular assessments of dysphagia, as well as providing appropriate eating and drinking guidance to carers once swallowing becomes a concern (Strydom et al., 2016).

The development of neurological complications is also common in people with Down syndrome and dementia. Up to half of adults with dementia have neurological symptoms, including seizures and incontinence at initial presentation. This may pose further diagnostic difficulties, particularly in those with more severe intellectual disability (Strydom et al., 2010). Extrapyramidal signs such as rigidity, bradykinesia, and an atypical posture and gait have also been noted (Margallo-Lana et al., 2007). Neurological symptoms become more prominent as the dementia progresses, and by the end stage, individuals are often unable to walk, are incontinent, and almost always have seizures (McCarron et al., 2014; Strydom et al., 2010).

Current Treatment

Following a dementia diagnosis for individuals with Down syndrome, clinicians should carefully consider the available treatment options. Available treatments for dementia in adults with Down syndrome are similar to those for adults in the typically developing population. No drugs have yet been developed to prevent or reverse the effects of dementia, although there are treatments to slow its progression. Individuals with Down syndrome and dementia who are taking dementia medication, particularly acetylcholinesterase inhibitors, appear to have longer survival times than those who are not medicated (Eady et al., 2018), emphasizing the importance of providing appropriate treatment for those with Down syndrome and dementia. A recent Cochrane review reported that medications including donepezil, memantine, simvastatin, and antioxidants have all been studied for an effect on dementia progression in adults with Down syndrome but, because most trials were small and preliminary, the evidence base remains limited (Livingstone, Hanratty, McShane, & Macdonald, 2015).

The most commonly used drugs for Alzheimer's disease for adults in the typically developing population are acetylcholinesterase inhibitors such as donepezil, galantamine, and rivastigmine. These drugs may be of particular use in early Alzheimer's disease. The loss of basal forebrain cholinergic neurons is implicated early in the development of Alzheimer's disease, and acetylcholinesterase inhibitors prevent the breakdown of acetylcholine thus increasing its synaptic levels and boosting cholinergic function. Previous small studies have suggested donepezil may offer some benefit to adults with Down syndrome and dementia. Lott, Osann, Doran, and Nelson (2002) treated nine patients with Down syndrome and dementia with donepezil for 3 to 6 months and found that these adults showed an improvement in informant-reported changes related to dementia compared to six untreated individuals with Down syndrome and dementia. In comparison, Prasher, Huxley, Haque, and the Down syndrome Ageing Study Group (2002) conducted a double-blind trial over 24 weeks with 27 adults with Down syndrome and dementia, and found that the donepezil group had a nonsignificant reduction in deterioration compared to the placebo group.

Despite a potential benefit of donepezil for adults with Down syndrome and dementia, some individuals are unable to take acetylcholinesterase inhibitors due to side effects or because they are at a later stage of dementia. For such individuals memantine has been suggested as an alternative treatment. Memantine is thought to act primarily as a glutamate receptor NMDA (N-methyl-D-aspartate) subtype uncompetitive antagonist. However, despite memantine having some efficacy in treating adults with Alzheimer's disease without Down syndrome (Kishi et al., 2017), this benefit may not be seen in adults with Down syndrome and dementia. A randomized controlled trial on the effect of memantine on cognitive and functional decline in adults with Down syndrome with and without dementia over a year found both groups declined, with no significant difference in rates of decline for adults taking memantine compared to those taking placebo (Hanney et al., 2012). These results therefore suggest memantine may offer little benefit for adults with Down syndrome and dementia.

The general principles of medication treatment in older individuals with Down syndrome include starting at lower doses, with cautious increases, due to increased susceptibility to side effects including bradycardia and heart block when using acetylcholinesterase inhibitors (Eady, Courtenay, & Strydom, 2015). Another concern is polypharmacy, particularly in individuals with multiple comorbidities. This can be minimized by regular medication reviews, while carefully weighing the potential benefit against risk of harm (Eady et al., 2015), and awareness of issues such as confusion and memory problems associated with anticholinergic drugs that are often prescribed for incontinence; stopping such medication may result in cognitive improvement (Hassiotis, Strydom, Allen, & Walker, 2003). The use of antipsychotic medication for the behavioral and psychiatric symptoms of dementia should be minimized, as there is limited evidence for benefit and significant risk of side effects in elderly individuals, particularly those with intellectual disabilities (Sheehan et al., 2017).

In addition to pharmacological management, strategies to support the individual with dementia in maintaining independence for as long as possible are very important.

Such modifications may include adapting the living environment and care given to the individual (BPS, 2015; Courtenay, Jokinen, & Strydom, 2010; Dodd, 2015; Moran et al., 2013; Strydom et al., 2016). Essential components of postdiagnostic care include:

- Postdiagnostic counselling, support, and education offered to the person and carers or support staff to assist with dealing with the diagnosis, its implications, and the probable course at key stages of the disease.
- A comprehensive assessment of the needs of the person that takes into account premorbid abilities.
- Medical and psychological surveillance throughout the course of disease to address dementia-related needs and conditions (including myoclonus and epilepsy, dysphagia, and mobility issues), and other comorbidities.
- Regular reviews of the person's program and care plan to make appropriate adjustments in support.
- Regular medication reviews.
- Early identification of behavioral and psychological symptoms of dementia, and providing appropriate psychological interventions and environmental adaptations to address these.
- Provision of support and training to carers or support staff throughout the course of the condition.
- Considering a palliative care pathway at an appropriate time to ensure ongoing quality of life as end of life approaches.

Risk Factors for Age at Dementia Onset

In addition to considering the clinical aspects relating to the assessment, diagnosis, and treatment of dementia in people with Down syndrome, it is important to consider how those who are developing dementia can be identified at the earliest stage of cognitive decline. Such a consideration will take into account both identifying those who are at an increased risk of developing dementia, as well as identifying the earliest changes that occur as dementia develops.

As previously discussed, while all individuals with Down syndrome over the age of 30 years have amyloid-beta plaques in their brains, there is great variability in the age of dementia onset for adults with Down syndrome. This suggests the existence of risk and protective factors that affect the development of dementia. This individual variability is important to consider when assessing individuals for potential dementia and when monitoring decline in those with a diagnosis of dementia. As in the typically developing population, results from epidemiological studies show that increasing age is the greatest risk factor for dementia (Coppus et al., 2006). Understanding which other factors increase the risk of or protect against the development of dementia will allow for better identification of individuals at increased risk to improve their care, for example those individuals with specific comorbidities associated with an increased risk of dementia, and also to help identify novel treatment targets, for example through identifying genetic associations and determining relevant pathways involved in the development of dementia.

Demographic and Medical Factors

Factors that have previously been investigated for an association with age at dementia onset in people with Down syndrome include sex, age at menopause for women, level of premorbid intellectual disability, and the presence of epilepsy before the age of 20 years. Previous findings have been mixed regarding the relationship between sex and dementia development. In some studies, women show an increased risk of dementia (Lai et al., 1999) with an earlier onset compared to men (Raghavan et al., 1994), whereas in others men showed an earlier onset (Schupf et al., 1998). Among women with Down syndrome, an earlier menopause is associated with an increased risk of dementia, an earlier onset of dementia, and an earlier death (Coppus et al., 2010; Cosgrave, Tyrrell, McCarron, Gill, & Lawlor, 1999; Schupf et al., 2003). The relationship between menopause and dementia may occur through reduced brain estrogen levels as a result of the menopause, with estrogen thought to have a neuroprotective effect (Schupf et al., 2003). Adults with poorer baseline or premorbid cognitive functioning, such as those with a more severe intellectual disability, may show an increased risk of developing dementia (Temple, Jozsvai, Konstantareas, & Hewitt, 2001) and shorter survival times following dementia diagnosis (Sinai et al., 2018). This is in keeping with the cognitive reserve hypothesis, whereby adults with higher cognitive functioning at baseline have a higher cognitive reserve, and so can tolerate a higher level of cell or synaptic loss before the number of neurons and/or synapses reaches a threshold level and cognitive decline starts (Strydom, Hassiotis, King, & Livingston, 2009). However, a strong relationship between premorbid intellectual ability and the development of dementia in individuals with Down syndrome has not consistently been found (Hithersay et al., 2019). Finally, the presence of epilepsy before the age of 20 years has been associated with an earlier dementia diagnosis (Hithersay et al., 2019).

Genetic Variations

Genetic variations have also been associated with modifying the risk of dementia development in Down syndrome. There are likely a number of genetic variations that may influence an individual's risk of developing dementia, with both variations on chromosome 21 and on other chromosomes being important. In people with Down syndrome, *APP* variants (intronic polymorphisms) have been associated with the onset of dementia (Jones et al., 2010; Lee et al., 2017; Margallo-Lana et al., 2004). Aside from these variants, the greatest risk gene for developing late onset Alzheimer's disease in the typically developing population is the apolipoprotein E 4 (*APOE4*) allele, with the apolipoprotein E 2 (*APOE2*) allele "protecting" individuals against the development of Alzheimer's disease. A similar pattern is found in people with Down syndrome, as individuals possessing the

APOE4 allele show an increased risk and earlier onset of dementia (Coppus, Evenhuis, Verberne, Visser, Arias-Vasquez, et al., 2008; Hardy, Crook, Perry, Raghavan, & Roberts, 1994; Jones et al., 2013; Patel et al., 2011; Prasher et al., 2008; Schupf et al., 1996; Sekijima et al., 1998), with an increased risk of mortality in the presence of dementia (Hithersay et al., 2019). In contrast, those possessing the *APOE2* allele show protection against the development of dementia or at least a later onset (Lai et al., 1999; Royston et al., 1996).

Additional genes associated with the age of dementia onset in adults with Down syndrome have been identified, including *PICALM* (Jones et al., 2013) and *SORL1* (Lee et al., 2007; Patel et al., 2011), both of which have been associated with late-onset Alzheimer's disease in the typically developing population and are thought to be involved in amyloid processing and endocytosis. Variations in *BACE2*, which is found on chromosome 21 and is implicated in amyloid processing, have also been associated with the age of dementia onset in people with Down syndrome (Mok et al., 2014), as have variations in the tau haplotype, with a buildup of phosphorylated tau being found in the brains of individuals with Alzheimer's disease (Jones, Margallo-Lana, Prasher, & Ballard, 2008; Raha-Chowdhury et al., 2019). While these individual genes have much smaller effects on the development of dementia compared to the *APOE4* allele, considering an individual's overall genetic risk for developing Alzheimer's disease through the use of polygenic risk scores across multiple genetic loci weighted by their individual effect sizes is an approach that has recently gained attention (Chasioti, Yan, Nho, & Saykin, 2019). Such an approach may help to better identify those with Down syndrome at increased risk of developing dementia. Further, understanding the molecular pathways in which the protein products of these genes are involved may help to identify new potential treatment targets for Alzheimer's disease. For example, supporting the association between dementia onset and menopause in women with Down syndrome, variants in several genes implicated in estrogen synthesis, processing, and activity have been associated with age at dementia onset (Lee et al., 2012; Schupf et al., 2008). Findings from these genetic association studies alongside results from epidemiological studies therefore indicate that improved estrogen function may protect against the development of dementia, at least in women with Down syndrome.

Neuropsychological Changes Associated With Dementia

Understanding the time course of cognitive decline in people with Down syndrome is important to aid in the early identification of dementia, and may also provide us with information relating to the sequence of underlying neuropathological changes as dementia develops. Identifying the earliest markers of dementia development is also essential to assess the effects of potential treatments to slow the progression of dementia in clinical trials (Hithersay et al., 2021; Startin, Hamburg, et al., 2019).

As with dementia in the typically developing population, dementia in adults with Down syndrome is associated with impairments in cognitive and functional ability.

In a longitudinal study over 50 months of adults with Down syndrome aged 30 years and above, approximately 30% showed severe cognitive deterioration (Oliver, Crayton, Holland, Hall, & Bradbury, 1998), emphasizing the high prevalence of cognitive decline in this population. However, in some individuals the observed decline could have been complicated by several factors including aging, hypothyroidism, sleep apnea, or depression, as well as dementia.

Cognitive Impairments in Adults With Dementia

Cognitive decline and dementia in people with Down syndrome develops on top of an intellectual disability and multiple cognitive impairments, and so it is important to consider such premorbid cognitive differences when interpreting results. Similar to findings in the typically developing population with dementia, adults with Down syndrome and dementia show poorer performance on a variety of memory tasks compared to those without dementia (Ball, Holland, Treppner, Watson, & Huppert, 2008; Benejam, Fortea, Molina-Lopez, & Videla, 2015; Krinsky-McHale, Devenny, & Silverman, 2002; Oliver et al., 1998; Sinai, Hassiotis, Rantell, & Strydom, 2016). Similarly, carers report that adults with Down syndrome and dementia show short-term memory problems and confusion with intact long-term memory (Deb, Hare, & Prior, 2007). Poorer performance among adults with Down syndrome and dementia as compared to those without dementia has also been reported for tasks of attention and executive functioning (Adams & Oliver, 2010; Ball et al., 2006; Ball et al., 2008; Krinsky-McHale, Devenny, Kittler, & Silverman, 2008; Sinai et al., 2016). In addition to the poorer performance of adults with Down syndrome and dementia as compared to those without dementia, the suitability of tests to assess cognitive functioning also changes with the development of dementia. Dementia is associated with an increased number of individuals performing at floor levels and an increased number of individuals who are unable to undertake cognitive testing (Startin et al., 2016). Tests may therefore become unsuitable to assess the cognitive abilities of adults with Down syndrome as they develop dementia. Further, the inability of some people with Down syndrome and dementia to take part in cognitive tasks will lead to a selection bias for studies of cognitive abilities of those with dementia.

Prefrontal Lobe Dysfunction Hypothesis of Dementia in Down syndrome

In addition to the early memory impairments observed in people with Down syndrome and dementia that are characteristic of Alzheimer's disease in the typically developing population, dementia in adults with Down syndrome may be associated with changes in the behavioral functions associated with the prefrontal lobes. For example, Holland, Hon, Huppert, and Stevens (2000) found that early changes in behavior and personality were often reported in adults with Down syndrome, with these changes resulting in many adults meeting the criteria for frontal-type dementia prior to meeting the criteria for Alzheimer's disease. Following these adults longitudinally over 18 months, Holland et al. found that adults who showed early changes in behavior and personality progressed to showing an increase in the number of characteristics associated with frontal lobe (executive) dysfunction and/or memory deterioration, before progressing to the full development of Alzheimer's disease as evaluated by the fulfilment of the diagnostic criteria for dementia of the Alzheimer's disease type (*ICD–10*). These findings suggested a progression of cognitive decline, starting with behavioral and personality changes in some individuals. Ball et al. (2006) further followed this cohort over 5 years. They found that those adults who showed behavioral and personality changes or a "frontal-type" dementia at the start of the study had an increased risk of being diagnosed with Alzheimer's disease over the following 5 years, and these adults had a decline in executive functioning abilities but not episodic memory. In contrast, the group who were diagnosed with Alzheimer's disease at the start of the study showed a decline in both executive function and memory abilities over the same time period, with greater impairments in memory. Also indicating early changes in frontal lobe function with dementia development in Down syndrome, in a different sample, early cognitive decline with decreased performance for memory measures has been associated with decreased performance for measures of executive functioning and changes in behavior alongside these memory changes (Adams & Oliver, 2010).

Further demonstrating a difference in the development of dementia in people with Down syndrome as compared to the typically developing population, recent reviews of early behavioral and personality changes associated with dementia in adults with Down syndrome have concluded that these symptoms may occur before a clinical dementia diagnosis in some individuals, and monitoring these symptoms may assist in offering an early indicator of risk of cognitive decline or in monitoring the progress of decline (Dekker, Strydom, et al., 2015; Lautarescu, Holland, & Zaman, 2017). Other behavioral changes reported to be associated with the development of cognitive decline and dementia in adults with Down syndrome are mood changes, aggression, apathy, sleep disturbances, and psychiatric symptoms, specifically delusions, behavioral disturbances, symptoms of depression, and anxiety (Deb, Hare, & Prior, 2007; Dekker et al., 2018; Urv, Zigman, & Silverman, 2008, 2010). The development of specific emotional changes such as indifference and depression have been shown to be associated with brain atrophy and atypical neurological reflexes indicative of frontal lobe dysfunction (Nelson, Orme, Osann, & Lott, 2001). When considering whether an individual with Down syndrome is developing dementia, all behavioral changes should be considered. Referrals for dementia assessment are more likely to be triggered by behavioral excesses (such as aggression and restlessness) and poorer socialization skills, while those with behavioral deficits, such as social withdrawal and indifference, may be overlooked (Adams et al., 2008).

The prominence of early prefrontal presentations in Down syndrome is most likely related to the presence of premorbid deficiencies in executive functions (Lanfranchi, Jerman, Dal Pont, Alberti, & Vianello, 2010; Rowe, Lavender, & Turk, 2006). These impairments, with the associated relatively small frontal lobes (Beacher et al., 2010;

Carducci et al., 2013), may mean that adults with Down syndrome show a decreased prefrontal cognitive reserve and an increased vulnerability of the prefrontal regions to neuronal damage or a reduction in prefrontal functional compensation. It is also possible the observation of early behavioral and personality changes may be due to these being the changes that carers are particularly likely to observe and take note of, as many adults with Down syndrome have support in daily tasks that rely on memory, especially given the frequent pre-existing memory deficits.

Regardless of the cause of these early changes in behavior and personality, clinicians should be aware that these may occur with the development of dementia in people with Down syndrome. Clinical assessments should therefore include informant report of such changes to ensure the effective monitoring of changes potentially related to dementia in those with Down syndrome.

Sequence of Neuropsychological Changes Associated With Dementia

In addition to understanding which cognitive changes occur with the development of dementia in adults with Down syndrome, researchers and clinicians need to understand the time course of these cognitive changes and how these changes occur in relation to the onset of dementia. Researchers have suggested that memory impairments (Cosgrave, Tyrrell, McCarron, Gill, & Lawlor, 2000; Krinsky-McHale et al., 2002) and poorer performance on a selective attention cancellation task (Krinsky-McHale et al., 2008) may precede other changes related to dementia, potentially by up to 3 years. Similarly, an increased number of verbal intrusions during tests may predict later memory decline (Kittler, Krinsky-McHale, & Devenny, 2006), with increased intrusions potentially being an indicator of decreased inhibition. In a more recent large cross-sectional study, Startin, Hamburg, et al. (2019) found that the earliest changes in the time course of dementia development are in memory and sustained attention. This finding has been confirmed with the same participant sample through the use of data-driven methods for both cross-sectional and longitudinal data to estimate the sequence of cognitive changes with the development of dementia (Firth et al., 2018; Hithersay et al., 2021).

In adults showing early impairments in cognitive abilities, informant-reported behavioral and personality changes have been associated with poorer performance on tasks of executive function and executive memory, but not episodic memory, while informant-reported memory changes have been associated with impaired memory abilities (Ball et al., 2008; Ball, Holland, Watson, & Huppert, 2010; Fonseca et al., 2019). Further, the degree of behavioral disinhibition has been associated with performance on tasks of executive function and memory, while the degree of apathy has been associated with performance on working memory tasks (Ball et al., 2010). Increased disinhibition and executive dysfunction have been reported as dementia progresses (Fonseca et al., 2019).

In order to fully establish the time course of cognitive changes associated with the development of dementia in adults with Down syndrome, larger longitudinal studies are needed to cover a spectrum of cognitive abilities with reliable measures to determine the sequence of decline, particularly in the prodromal stage of dementia when cognitive decline has started but has not yet reached the threshold for dementia diagnosis. Several large cross-sectional studies have been performed to date to assess changes associated with aging in adults with Down syndrome, and given that the development of dementia appears to be an almost universal part of aging in adults with Down syndrome, the findings from these studies may indicate early changes in cognition as dementia develops. The evidence from cross-sectional studies indicates decline in cognitive and adaptive abilities across the lifespan of adults with Down syndrome (Ghezzo et al., 2014; Startin et al., 2016; Startin, Hamburg, et al., 2019; Tsao, Kindelberger, Freminville, Touraine, & Gerald, 2015), and it has been reported that episodic memory changes occur prior to temperament and adaptive behavior changes (Blok, Scheirs, & Thijm, 2017). Across the lifespan of adults with Down syndrome it is also clear that an increasing number of individuals perform at floor levels in older age groups, as seen in our previous work where we found higher floor effects in those aged 36 and over compared to those aged 35 and under (Startin et al., 2016).

While cross-sectional studies offer a useful way to easily assess changes across large age ranges, these studies do not take account of potential cohort effects, with changes in health and social care across time affecting adults of different ages in different ways. As longitudinal studies are not affected by cohort effects, due to the same participants being assessed at each age, these may therefore be a better design to assess the sequence of cognitive decline. The findings from Janet Carr's classic longitudinal study of individuals with Down syndrome indicate some adults who do not have clinically diagnosed dementia show a decrease in memory in their mid 40s (Carr, 2012; Carr & Collins, 2014, 2018). Due to the buildup of amyloid-beta deposits in the brains of all adults with Down syndrome from their mid-30s and the exceptionally high prevalence of dementia in people with Down syndrome (Wiseman et al., 2015), adults over the age of 35 years may be considered to be in a preclinical state of dementia even in the absence of noticeable cognitive decline. These memory decreases in adults with Down syndrome in their mid-40s in the absence of a diagnosis of dementia may therefore represent early cognitive decline due to the development of dementia, suggesting memory changes may be an early sign of dementia-related decline. Alternatively, these changes may reflect cognitive decline due to aging that is separate from dementia-related decline, though ultimately impossible to distinguish from the universal development of AD pathology in Down syndrome. Additional changes in adaptive abilities have also been observed with aging in longitudinal studies (Carr & Collins, 2014; Makary et al., 2015), with Arvio and Luostarinen (2016) suggesting that adaptive abilities start to decline from the age of 35 years. These findings of cognitive and functional decline in many adults with Down syndrome in their 30s and 40s indicate that such decline appears 10–15 years before the mean age of dementia diagnosis of 55 (McCarron et al., 2014). This observation emphasizes the importance of a baseline assessment before the age of 30 and regular follow-up assessments to detect early cognitive changes (BPS, 2015).

Neuroimaging

The use of neuroimaging to assess changes within the brain associated with the development of dementia allows us to better understand the time course of dementia development in people with Down syndrome. In particular, advances in amyloid imaging have allowed the sequence of amyloid-beta buildup to be better characterized, while studies of brain volumes, metabolism, and electrophysiological activity allow us to assess changes within the brain associated with dementia. Such changes may be of potential use as biomarkers for dementia in people with Down syndrome.

Positron Emission Tomography

Recent advances in positron emission tomography (PET) technology have resulted in the ability to visualize and quantify the amount of disease-associated amyloid-beta, and more recently tau, deposits in vivo in the brain of individuals; previous studies assessing amyloid-beta and tau buildup had relied on postmortem samples. For PET scans to image amyloid-beta buildup for example, a radioactive ligand which acts as a specific tracer—such as [11-C]-Pittsburgh compound-B (PiB) or florbetapir—is injected into the bloodstream. This then binds to the specific form of amyloid-beta in the brain associated with senile or neuritic plaques. The degree of amyloid binding can then be quantified, and its anatomical distribution identified using a PET scanner in conjunction with brain magnetic resonance imaging. The degree of amyloid binding in a PET scan has been shown to be closely related to the amount of amyloid-beta found postmortem in an individual with Down syndrome, suggesting that this technique offers a good indication of what is occurring in the brain (Sabbagh et al., 2011).

Researchers using PET scans in adults with Down syndrome have consistently found that the degree of amyloid-beta present in the brain increases with age (Annus et al., 2016; Fortea et al., 2020; Hartley et al., 2014; Jennings et al., 2015; Lao et al., 2018; Nelson et al., 2011; Rafii et al., 2015, 2017; Sabbagh et al., 2015). Jennings et al. (2015) reported the presence of amyloid binding in 7% of adults aged 40–44 years, in 53% of adults aged 45–49 years, and in 90% of adults aged 50 or older. Annus et al. (2016) reported that PiB binding started in the brains of adults with Down syndrome from age 39, with amyloid-beta buildup starting in the striatum. These findings have been supported by other recent studies; firstly results of a longitudinal PET study confirmed the early buildup of amyloid-beta in the striatum of the brains of people with Down syndrome (Lao et al., 2017), and secondly results of a neuropathological study found a dramatic increase in the presence of fibrillar amyloid after the age of 40 in adults with Down syndrome (LeVine et al., 2017).

In addition to the relationship between PET amyloid binding and age, the relationships between amyloid binding and the presence of dementia and cognitive decline are important to determine for understanding the progression of dementia. Researchers investigating the relationship between amyloid binding and dementia have found increased amyloid binding in adults with dementia compared to those without dementia (Annus et al., 2016; Fortea et al., 2020; Sabbagh et al., 2015), and this increase in amyloid binding can be seen in adults with cognitive decline not meeting the threshold for dementia as compared to adults with no observable cognitive decline (Keator et al., 2020). Findings of analyses regarding the relationship between amyloid binding and cognitive abilities have been less consistent. Although increased amyloid binding may be associated with poorer cognitive functioning (Annus et al., 2016; Nelson et al., 2011), another, albeit smaller, study found no relationship (Rafii et al., 2015). These differences in results may be due to the differences in sample sizes between these studies, with the latter study being underpowered to detect relationships between cognitive decline and amyloid binding. Alternatively, differences concerning the severity of cognitive decline between the participants in these different studies may help to explain these differences; for example, if the participants in the studies of Annus et al. (2016) and Nelson et al. (2011) had a more severe cognitive decline than the participants in Rafii et al. (2015), this may result in a significant relationship between cognitive decline and amyloid binding in the former two studies but not the latter study.

When controlling for chronological and mental age for adults with no signs of cognitive decline, Hartley et al. (2014) found limited associations between amyloid binding and cognitive ability, suggesting that adults with Down syndrome can tolerate the buildup of amyloid-beta for some time without any effects on cognitive functioning. While the results of several longitudinal studies with small samples indicate that increased amyloid-beta accumulation is associated with cognitive decline in tasks assessing memory, executive functioning, and processing speed (Hartley et al., 2017), and amyloid-beta accumulation precedes the development of cognitive decline and dementia (Mak, Bickerton, et al., 2019), further longitudinal studies with larger sample sizes are needed to better understand the relationship between amyloid-beta build-up and cognitive decline.

In addition to amyloid-beta neuropathology, Alzheimer's disease is also associated with tau neuropathology. PET studies in the typically developing population have shown a relationship between tau binding and cognitive decline (Brier et al., 2016), with a similar relationship between clinical dementia and tau pathology having being reported in postmortem brains of adults with Down syndrome (Margallo-Lana et al., 2007). PET studies of tau binding in Down syndrome and the relationships between tau binding and both dementia and cognitive decline are in their infancy, though initial reports have indicated that tau binding increases with age and better associates with cognitive decline than amyloid binding (Rafii et al., 2017). These results indicate that PET tau binding may be more useful than PET amyloid binding for researchers to assess the progression of dementia neuropathology that has a clear link to the symptoms of dementia in adults with

Down syndrome, and as a result PET tau binding may be a useful biomarker to measure the progression of dementia in clinical trials of treatments to prevent cognitive decline.

Magnetic Resonance Imaging

While PET scans allow researchers to investigate the molecular neuropathological changes that occur with the development of dementia in people with Down syndrome, such scans are expensive and require participants to undergo an injection of a radioactive tracer. Both of these factors limit the potential use of PET scans for the diagnosis and monitoring of dementia in people with Down syndrome. Instead, magnetic resonance imaging (MRI) offers a lower cost and more acceptable alternative, through determining the volumes of different brain structures in adults with Down syndrome and the changes in these with the development of dementia.

Consistent with the atrophy associated with dementia, results of studies investigating structural brain volumes in adults with Down syndrome using MRI have shown smaller volumes associated with the presence of dementia. Adults with Down syndrome and dementia show smaller brain volumes in the hippocampi, amygdalae, caudate, and putamen (Aylward et al., 1999; Beacher et al., 2009; Pearlson et al., 1998; Sabbagh et al., 2015), decreased cortical thickness in the temporoparietal, precuneus-posterior cingulate, and frontal areas (Fortea et al., 2020), and greater volumes of cerebrospinal fluid (Beacher et al., 2009) compared to adults without dementia. Results of a longitudinal MRI study show that hippocampal volume reduction is associated with the development of cognitive decline and memory changes (Pujol et al., 2018). Increasing age in adults with Down syndrome has also been associated with decreased brain volumes in a number of regions, including in the hippocampus and corpus callosum (Fortea et al., 2020; Teipel et al., 2003); in frontal, temporal, parietal, and occipital gray matter (Teipel et al., 2004); and in frontal and insular gray matter (Lao et al., 2018). Researchers comparing structural brain volumes of adults with and without amyloid binding as assessed using PET studies have found that adults with amyloid binding show posterior dominant cortical thinning and subcortical atrophy in the hippocampus, thalamus, and striatum (Annus et al., 2017; Rafii et al., 2015), and the degree of amyloid binding has been negatively correlated with cortical thickness, in particular in temporoparietal regions (Mak, Padilla, et al., 2019). These results support a contribution of amyloid-beta buildup leading to cortical atrophy. The white matter integrity of frontal tracts has further been suggested to be reduced in adults with Down syndrome and dementia compared to those without dementia (Powell et al., 2014).

These findings of hippocampal and frontal changes in adults with Down syndrome following the development of dementia relate to the developmental brain atypicalities associated with Down syndrome being further compromised with the development of dementia. As dementia in people with Down syndrome develops on an altered cognitive profile with associated differences in brain volumes, it is important to consider these premorbid differences compared to adults without Down syndrome and how this may affect the development of the symptoms of dementia. In addition, such premorbid differences in the brains and cognitive abilities of people with Down syndrome may help to explain differences in symptom progression compared to that in the typically developing population. For example, as discussed earlier, the prefrontal lobe dysfunction hypothesis states that early changes in behavior and personality are common with the development of dementia in people with Down syndrome. This prominence of frontal-like symptoms may be due to a loss of frontal white matter tract integrity, which develops on top of the altered development of the frontal lobes. Understanding the sequence of atrophy that occurs due to dementia in adults with Down syndrome and how this relates to the cognitive changes observed will require taking such premorbid differences in brain development into account.

Metabolic Rate

In addition to the changes in the brain relating to amyloid-beta and tau buildup and atrophy due to the development of dementia, the neuropathological changes that occur due to dementia result in changes in glucose metabolism due to altered levels of neuronal activity. Researchers assessing the rate of glucose metabolism using FDG (^{18}fluorodexyglucose) PET in adults with Down syndrome as a measure of neuronal activity have reported a lower metabolic rate in adults with dementia compared to those without dementia (Fortea et al., 2020; Sabbagh et al., 2015), and in adults with a higher amyloid-beta load (Rafii et al., 2015). Glucose metabolism in the frontal, parietal, and temporal cortices has further been reported to decrease with age in adults with Down syndrome (Lao et al., 2018). In addition, the levels of neurotransmitter metabolites present in the brain have also been reported to be altered in adults with dementia and Down syndrome, suggesting a difference in their metabolism (Lamar et al., 2011; Lin et al., 2016).

Electrophysiological Markers

A less invasive method to assess neurological changes with the development of dementia compared to PET and MRI comes from the use of EEG to assess electrophysiological activity. Studies assessing electrophysiological measures have reported neurological changes related to the presence of dementia in adults with Down syndrome. In particular, a slowing of the brain's natural oscillations while not doing a specific task has been consistently reported in individuals with Down syndrome and dementia during baseline EEG studies, specifically a decrease in alpha power and an increase in theta and delta (Locatelli et al., 1996; Medaglini et al., 1997; Musaeus, Salem, Sabers, Kjaer, & Waldemar, 2019; Salem et al., 2015; Visser et al., 1996). The use of magnetoencephalography (MEG) produces similar results, with the changes in activity observed also relating to cognitive performance (Garcia-Alba et al., 2019). Event-related potential (ERP) components, electrophysiological activity that is time-locked to the onset of a stimulus, have also been reported to show longer P300 latencies to their peak in adults with Down syndrome and dementia compared to those without dementia (Blackwood, St Clair, Muir, Oliver, & Dickens, 1988). Again, additional studies are needed to determine whether such changes may offer a useful biomarker to improve the diagnosis of dementia and monitoring of cognitive decline in people with Down syndrome.

Fluid Biomarkers

Clinical trials to assess potential new treatments for dementia in adults with Down syndrome require accurate markers to measure the progression of dementia. Such biomarkers would also be of use on a wider scale to monitor the progression of dementia in clinical settings. While some neuroimaging measures may be suitable for use in clinical trials, brain scans are relatively expensive and may not be tolerable for all adults with Down syndrome. The identification of alternative biomarkers as potential indicators of early cognitive decline or to monitor the progression of dementia in people with Down syndrome has therefore received great interest, in particular peripheral molecular changes in the blood or cerebrospinal fluid.

Levels of peripheral amyloid-beta peptides have been of particular interest as a biomarker for dementia, specifically levels of amyloid-beta 40 (Aβ40), amyloid-beta 42 (Aβ42), and the Aβ42/Aβ40 ratio in blood plasma, although results have been mixed as to how levels change with the development of dementia (Coppus et al., 2012; Fang et al., 2020; Fortea et al., 2020; Head et al., 2011; Jones, Hanney, Francis, & Ballard, 2009; Lee et al., 2016; Prasher, Sajith, Mehta, Zigman, & Schupf, 2010; Schupf et al., 2007, 2010). It has therefore been suggested that composite biomarker scores taking levels of both plasma amyloid-beta peptides and tau into account may better predict dementia status compared to levels of individual markers (Fang et al., 2020). As an alternative to plasma amyloid-beta levels, cerebrospinal fluid (CSF) obtained by lumbar puncture may aid in better understanding how peripheral amyloid-beta levels change with the development of dementia, as these likely better reflect levels of amyloid-beta in the brain compared to plasma levels. Although there may be concerns for the tolerability of lumbar punctures for adults with Down syndrome, there is recent evidence that it is feasible to take such measures (Carmona-Iragui et al., 2017). CSF concentrations of amyloid-beta and tau have been reported to be associated with dementia status in adults with Down syndrome, though CSF concentrations only showed very weak correlations with plasma concentrations, and plasma concentrations were not associated with dementia status (Fortea et al., 2018). These results indicate that CSF concentrations of amyloid-beta and tau may be more useful clinically than plasma concentrations, although more recent methods of quantification in blood using mass spectrometry are very promising (Nakamura et al., 2018; Schindler et al., 2019).

Several other markers have been proposed as biomarkers for dementia in people with Down syndrome. Concentration of plasma neurofilament light, a marker of neurodegeneration, has been shown to be higher in adults with Down syndrome and dementia as compared to those without dementia, and the concentration of this increases with age (Fortea et al., 2020; Strydom et al., 2018). Plasma neurofilament light concentration has further been positively associated with brain amyloid-beta pathology, and negatively associated with brain glucose metabolism, hippocampal volume, and cognitive performance (Rafii et al., 2019; Shinomoto et al., 2019). Exploring the use of neurofilament light concentration to predict dementia status, Fortea et al. (2018) reported that both plasma and CSF neurofilament light concentrations could differentiate groups of adults with Down syndrome who had no cognitive decline, cognitive decline not yet meeting the threshold for dementia diagnosis, and diagnosed dementia better than plasma markers of amyloid-beta or tau; in addition, plasma concentration of neurofilament light strongly correlated with CSF concentration. These findings indicate that neurofilament light may be an ideal plasma biomarker for dementia progression in adults with Down syndrome (Startin, Ashton, et al., 2019).

Increased levels of plasma and urine neopterin, a marker for activated cellular immunity and inflammation, have also been associated with dementia in adults with Down syndrome, and may also predict the development of subsequent dementia or decline (Coppus, Fekkes, Verhoeven, Evenhuis, & van Duijn, 2009; Zis, Strydom, Buckley, Adekitan, & McHugh, 2017). Further, a combination of amyloid-beta and inflammation markers may be predictive of cognitive decline in adults with Down syndrome (Iulita et al., 2016). Other potential biomarkers for dementia among people with Down syndrome include serum MHPG, a noradrenergic metabolite (Dekker, Coppus, et al., 2015); DHEA, a steroid hormone (Landt et al., 2011); and markers associated with oxidative stress, specifically superoxide dismutase (Zis, Dickinson, Shende, Walker, & Strydom, 2012) and iPF2alpha (Zis et al., 2014).

Summary and Future Directions

There is a very high risk of developing dementia among adults with Down syndrome, with the risk of developing dementia increasing as age increases. The variability in age of dementia onset between individuals suggests the potential presence of risk and protective factors that modify the risk of dementia, and future studies aimed at identifying these factors will aid in identifying individuals at increased risk and in allowing improved monitoring and detection of early decline. To identify genetic factors in particular larger studies will be needed and study groups will need to combine samples. Such consortia are currently being set up.

These studies of biomarkers and genetic variations associated with the development of dementia will hopefully allow potential new therapeutic targets to be identified. There is little evidence for the effectiveness of existing pharmacological interventions to slow the progression of dementia in adults with Down syndrome. As effective treatments will likely need to be used prior to the start of cognitive decline, a thorough understanding of the progression of dementia is necessary (Hithersay, Hamburg, Knight, & Strydom, 2017). Large longitudinal studies will be vital to identify the earliest neuropsychological changes associated with cognitive decline in adults, with previous studies suggesting an early involvement of behavioral and personality changes in addition to memory impairments. In addition, recent advances in neuroimaging and identifying biomarkers are promising in informing us about the development of dementia, and future studies using PET imaging for tau will be of great interest for researchers.

Such neuroimaging and biomarker tools are currently unsuitable for clinical use, however, with informed clinical assessment being vital for the identification of dementia in Down syndrome. For accurate clinical diagnosis, it is essential to establish baseline functions and to conduct regular assessments to detect cognitive or functional decline. Alternative explanations for declines must be considered, with dementia only being diagnosed if there is no alternative cause (for example, depression or sleep apnea). Postdiagnostic care is important to consider, with regular reviews and support adapted as necessary.

The high incidence of dementia in adults with Down syndrome will continue to be a major health consideration, and advances in understanding the progression of dementia and factors modifying the risk of developing dementia will improve the care available. These advances may allow for the identification of novel treatment targets to delay dementia onset or aid in the earlier detection or monitoring of individuals at increased risk of developing dementia as well as those showing signs of cognitive decline.

References

Adams, D., & Oliver, C. (2010). The relationship between acquired impairments of executive function and behaviour change in adults with Down syndrome. *J Intellect Disabil Res*, *54*, 393–405. doi:10.1111/j.1365-2788.2010.01271.x

Adams, D., Oliver, C., Kalsy, S., Peters, S., Broquard, M., Basra, T., . . . McQuillan, S. (2008). Behavioural characteristics associated with dementia assessment referrals in adults with Down syndrome. *J Intellect Disabil Res*, *52*, 358–368. doi:10.1111/j.1365-2788.2007.01036.x

Alexander, M., Ding, Y., Foskett, N., Petri, H., Wandel, C., & Khwaja, O. (2016). Population prevalence of Down's syndrome in the United Kingdom. *J Intellect Disabil Res*, *60*, 874–878. doi:10.1111/jir.12277

American Psychiatric Association. (1994). *Diagnostic and statistical manual of mental disorders* (4th ed.). Washington DC: American Psychiatric Association.

American Psychiatric Association. (2013). *Diagnostic and statistical manual of mental disorders* (5th ed.). Washington DC: American Psychiatric Association.

Annus, T., Wilson, L. R., Acosta-Cabronero, J., Cardenas-Blanco, A., Hong, Y. T., Fryer, T. D., . . . Nestor, P. J. (2017). The Down syndrome brain in the presence and absence of fibrillar beta-amyloidosis. *Neurobiol Aging*, *53*, 11–19. doi:10.1016/j.neurobiolaging.2017.01.009

Annus, T., Wilson, L. R., Hong, Y. T., Acosta-Cabronero, J., Fryer, T. D., Cardenas-Blanco, A., . . . Holland, A. J. (2016). The pattern of amyloid accumulation in the brains of adults with Down syndrome. *Alzheimers Dement*, *12*, 538–545. doi:10.1016/j.jalz.2015.07.490

Arvio, M., & Luostarinen, L. (2016). Down syndrome in adults: A 27-year follow-up of adaptive skills. *Clin Genet*, *90*, 456–460. doi:10.1111/cge.12787

Aylward, E. H., Li, Q., Honeycutt, N. A., Warren, A. C., Pulsifer, M. B., Barta, P. E., . . . Pearlson, G. D. (1999). MRI volumes of the hippocampus and amygdala in adults with Down's syndrome with and without dementia. *Am J Psychiatry*, *156*, 564–568.

Ball, S. L., Holland, A. J., Hon, J., Huppert, F. A., Treppner, P., & Watson, P. C. (2006). Personality and behaviour changes mark the early stages of Alzheimer's disease in adults with Down's syndrome: Findings from a prospective population-based study. *Int J Geriatr Psychiatry, 21*, 661–673. doi:10.1002/gps.1545

Ball, S. L., Holland, A. J., Huppert, F. A., Treppner, P., Watson, P., & Hon, J. (2004). The modified CAMDEX informant interview is a valid and reliable tool for use in the diagnosis of dementia in adults with Down's syndrome. *J Intellect Disabil Res, 48*, 611–620. doi:10.1111/j.1365-2788.2004.00630.x

Ball, S. L., Holland, A. J., Treppner, P., Watson, P. C., & Huppert, F. A. (2008). Executive dysfunction and its association with personality and behaviour changes in the development of Alzheimer's disease in adults with Down syndrome and mild to moderate learning disabilities. *Br J Clin Psychol, 47*, 1–29. doi:10.1348/014466507X230967

Ball, S. L., Holland, A. J., Watson, P. C., & Huppert, F. A. (2010). Theoretical exploration of the neural bases of behavioural disinhibition, apathy and executive dysfunction in preclinical Alzheimer's disease in people with Down's syndrome: Potential involvement of multiple frontal-subcortical neuronal circuits. *J Intellect Disabil Res, 54*, 320–336. doi:10.1111/j.1365-2788.2010.01261.x

Beacher, F., Daly, E., Simmons, A., Prasher, V., Morris, R., Robinson, C., . . . Murphy, D. G. (2009). Alzheimer's disease and Down's syndrome: An in vivo MRI study. *Psychol Med, 39*, 675–684. doi:10.1017/S0033291708004054

Beacher, F., Daly, E., Simmons, A., Prasher, V., Morris, R., Robinson, C., . . . Murphy, D. G. (2010). Brain anatomy and ageing in non-demented adults with Down's syndrome: An in vivo MRI study. *Psychol Med, 40*, 611–619. doi:10.1017/S0033291709990985

Benejam, B., Fortea, J., Molina-Lopez, R., & Videla, S. (2015). Patterns of performance on the modified cued recall test in Spanish adults with Down syndrome with and without dementia. *Am J Intellect Dev Disabil, 120*, 481–489. doi:10.1352/1944-7558-120.6.481

Blackwood, D. H., St Clair, D. M., Muir, W. J., Oliver, C. J., & Dickens, P. (1988). The development of Alzheimer's disease in Down's syndrome assessed by auditory event-related potentials. *J Ment Defic Res, 32*, 439–453.

Blok, J. B., Scheirs, J. G., & Thijm, N. S. (2017). Personality and behavioural changes do not precede memory problems as possible signs of dementia in ageing people with Down syndrome. *Int J Geriatr Psychiatry, 32*, 1257–1263. doi:10.1002/gps.4606

Brier, M. R., Gordon, B., Friedrichsen, K., McCarthy, J., Stern, A., Christensen, J., . . . Ances, B. M. (2016). Tau and Abeta imaging, CSF measures, and cognition in Alzheimer's disease. *Sci Transl Med, 8*, 338ra366. doi:10.1126/scitranslmed.aaf2362

British Psychological Society. (2015). *Dementia and people with intellectual disabilities*. Leicester, UK: The British Psychological Society.

Carducci, F., Onorati, P., Condoluci, C., Di Gennaro, G., Quarato, P. P., Pierallini, A., . . . Albertini, G. (2013). Whole-brain voxel-based morphometry study of children and adolescents with Down syndrome. *Funct Neurol, 28*, 19–28.

Carmona-Iragui, M., Santos, T., Videla, S., Fernandez, S., Benejam, B., Videla, L., . . . Fortea, J. (2017). Feasibility of lumbar puncture in the study of cerebrospinal fluid biomarkers for Alzheimer's disease in subjects with Down syndrome. *J Alzheimers Dis, 55*, 1489–1496. doi:10.3233/JAD-160827

Carr, J. (2012). Six weeks to 45 years: A longitudinal study of a population with Down syndrome. *J Appl Res Intellect Disabil, 25*, 414–422. doi:10.1111/j.1468-3148.2011.00676.x

Carr, J., & Collins, S. (2014). Ageing and dementia in a longitudinal study of a cohort with Down syndrome. *J Appl Res Intellect Disabil, 27*, 555–563. doi:10.1111/jar.12093

Carr, J., & Collins, S. (2018). 50 years with Down syndrome: A longitudinal study. *J Appl Res Intellect Disabil, 31*, 743–750. doi:10.1111/jar.12438

Chasioti, D., Yan, J., Nho, K., & Saykin, A. J. (2019). Progress in polygenic composite scores in Alzheimer's and other complex diseases. *Trends Genet, 35*, 371–382. doi:10.1016/j.tig.2019.02.005

Coppus, A., Evenhuis, H., Verberne, G. J., Visser, F., van Gool, P., Eikelenboom, P., & van Duijin, C. (2006). Dementia and mortality in persons with Down's syndrome. *J Intellect Disabil Res, 50*, 768–777. doi:10.1111/j.1365-2788.2006.00842.x

Coppus, A. M., Evenhuis, H. M., Verberne, G. J., Visser, F. E., Arias-Vasquez, A., Sayed-Tabatabaei, F. A., . . . van Duijn, C. M. (2008). The impact of apolipoprotein E on dementia in persons with Down's syndrome. *Neurobiol Aging, 29*, 828–835. doi:10.1016/j.neurobiolaging.2006.12.013

Coppus, A. M., Evenhuis, H. M., Verberne, G. J., Visser, F. E., Eikelenboom, P., van Gool, W. A., . . . van Duijn, C. M. (2010). Early age at menopause is associated with increased risk of dementia and mortality in women with Down syndrome. *J Alzheimers Dis, 19*, 545–550. doi:10.3233/JAD-2010-1247

Coppus, A. M., Evenhuis, H. M., Verberne, G. J., Visser, F. E., Oostra, B. A., Eikelenboom, P., . . . van Duijn, C. M. (2008). Survival in elderly persons with Down syndrome. *J Am Geriatr Soc, 56*, 2311–2316. doi:10.1111/j.1532-5415.2008.01999.x

Coppus, A. M., Fekkes, D., Verhoeven, W. M., Evenhuis, H. M., & van Duijn, C. M. (2009). Neopterin and the risk of dementia in persons with Down syndrome. *Neurosci Lett, 458*, 60–64. doi:10.1016/j.neulet.2009.04.020

Coppus, A. M., Schuur, M., Vergeer, J., Janssens, A. C., Oostra, B. A., Verbeek, M. M., & van Duijn, C. M. (2012). Plasma beta amyloid and the risk of Alzheimer's disease in Down syndrome. *Neurobiol Aging, 33*, 1988–1994. doi:10.1016/j.neurobiolaging.2011.08.007

Cosgrave, M. P., Tyrrell, J., McCarron, M., Gill, M., & Lawlor, B. A. (1999). Age at onset of dementia and age of menopause in women with Down's syndrome. *J Intellect Disabil Res, 43*, 461–465.

Cosgrave, M. P., Tyrrell, J., McCarron, M., Gill, M., & Lawlor, B. A. (2000). A five year follow-up study of dementia in persons with Down's syndrome: Early symptoms and patterns of deterioration. *Ir J Psych Med, 17*, 5–11.

Courtenay, K., Jokinen, N. S., & Strydom, A. (2010). Caregiving and adults with intellectual disabilities affected by dementia. *J Policy Pract Intellect Disabil, 7*, 26–33.

Crayton, L., Oliver, C., Holland, A., Bradbury, J., & Hall, S. (1998). The neuropsychological assessment of age related cognitive deficits in adults with Down's syndrome. *J Appl Res Intellect Disabil, 11*, 255–272.

Davidson, Y. S., Robinson, A., Prasher, V. P., & Mann, D. M. A. (2018). The age of onset and evolution of Braak tangle stage and Thal amyloid pathology of Alzheimer's disease in individuals with Down syndrome. *Acta Neuropathol Commun, 6*, 56. doi:10.1186/s40478-018-0559-4

De Simone, R., Puig, X. S., Gelisse, P., Crespel, A., & Genton, P. (2010). Senile myoclonic epilepsy: Delineation of a common condition associated with Alzheimer's disease in Down syndrome. *Seizure, 19*, 383–389. doi:10.1016/j.seizure.2010.04.008

Deb, S., & Braganza, J. (1999). Comparison of rating scales for the diagnosis of dementia in adults with Down's syndrome. *J Intellect Disabil Res, 43*, 400–407.

Deb, S., Hare, M., & Prior, L. (2007). Symptoms of dementia among adults with Down's syndrome: A qualitative study. *J Intellect Disabil Res, 51*, 726–739. doi:10.1111/j.1365-2788.2007.00956.x

Deb, S., Hare, M., Prior, L., & Bhaumik, S. (2007). Dementia screening questionnaire for individuals with intellectual disabilities. *Br J Psychiatry, 190*, 440–444. doi:10.1192/bjp.bp.106.024984

Dekker, A. D., Coppus, A. M., Vermeiren, Y., Aerts, T., van Duijn, C. M., Kremer, B. P., . . . De Deyn, P. P. (2015). Serum MHPG strongly predicts conversion to Alzheimer's disease in behaviorally characterized subjects with Down syndrome. *J Alzheimers Dis, 43*, 871–891. doi:10.3233/JAD-140783

Dekker, A. D., Sacco, S., Carfi, A., Benejam, B., Vermeiren, Y., Beugelsdijk, G., . . . De Deyn, P. P. (2018). The Behavioral and Psychological Symptoms of Dementia in Down Syndrome (BPSD-DS) Scale: Comprehensive assessment of psychopathology in Down syndrome. *J Alzheimers Dis, 63*, 797–819. doi:10.3233/JAD-170920

Dekker, A. D., Strydom, A., Coppus, A. M., Nizetic, D., Vermeiren, Y., Naude, P. J., . . . De Deyn, P. P. (2015). Behavioural and psychological symptoms of dementia in Down syndrome: Early indicators of clinical Alzheimer's disease? *Cortex, 73*, 36–61. doi:10.1016/j.cortex.2015.07.032

Dodd, K. D. (2015). Care considerations for dementia in people with Down's syndrome: A management perspective. *Neurodegener Dis Manag, 5*, 293–304. doi:10.2217/nmt.15.28

d'Orsi, G., Specchio, L. M., & Apulian Study Group on Senile Myoclonic, E. (2014). Progressive myoclonus epilepsy in Down syndrome patients with dementia. *J Neurol, 261*, 1584–1597. doi:10.1007/s00415-014-7376-x

Eady, N., Courtenay, K., & Strydom, A. (2015). Pharmacological management of behavioral and psychiatric symptoms in older adults with intellectual disability. *Drugs Aging, 32*, 95–102. doi:10.1007/s40266-014-0236-7

Eady, N., Sheehan, R., Rantell, K., Sinai, A., Bernal, J., Bohnen, I., . . . Strydom, A. (2018) Impact of cholinesterase inhibitors or memantine on survival in adults with Down syndrome and dementia: clinical cohort study. *Br J Psychiatry, 212*, 155–160. doi:10.1192/bjp.2017.21

Englund, A., Jonsson, B., Zander, C. S., Gustafsson, J., & Anneren, G. (2013). Changes in mortality and causes of death in the Swedish Down syndrome population. *Am J Med Genet A, 161A*, 642–649. doi:10.1002/ajmg.a.35706

Esbensen, A. J. (2010). Health conditions associated with aging and end of life of adults with Down syndrome. *Int Rev Res Ment Retard, 39*, 107–126. doi:10.1016/S0074-7750(10)39004-5

Esbensen, A. J. (2016). Sleep problems and associated comorbidities among adults with Down syndrome. *J Intellect Disabil Res, 60*, 68–79. doi:10.1111/jir.12236

Evenhuis, H. M. (1996). Further evaluation of the Dementia Questionnaire for Persons with Mental Retardation (DMR). *J Intellect Disabil Res, 40*, 369–373.

Fang, W. Q., Hwu, W. L., Chien, Y. H., Yang, S. Y., Chieh, J. J., Chang, L. M., . . . Chiu, M. J. (2020). Composite scores of plasma tau and beta-amyloids correlate with dementia in Down syndrome. *ACS Chem Neurosci, 11*, 191–196. doi:10.1021/acschemneuro.9b00585

Firth, N. C., Startin, C. M., Hithersay, R., Hamburg, S., Wijeratne, P. A., Mok, K. Y., . . . Strydom, A. (2018). Aging related cognitive changes associated with Alzheimer's disease in Down syndrome. *Ann Clin Transl Neurol, 5*, 741–751. doi:10.1002/acn3.571

Fletcher, R. J., Barnhill, J., McCarthy, J., & Strydom, A. (2016). From DSM to DM-ID. *J Ment Health Res Intellect Disabil, 9*, 189–204.

Fonseca, L. M., Mattar, G. P., Haddad, G. G., Goncalves, A. S., Miguel, A. Q. C., Guilhoto, L. M., . . . Hoexter, M. Q. (2019). Frontal-subcortical behaviors during Alzheimer's disease in individuals with Down syndrome. *Neurobiol Aging, 78*, 186–194. doi:10.1016/j.neurobiolaging.2019.02.028

Fortea, J., Carmona-Iragui, M., Benejam, B., Fernandez, S., Videla, L., Barroeta, I., . . . Lleo, A. (2018). Plasma and CSF biomarkers for the diagnosis of Alzheimer's disease in adults with Down syndrome: A cross-sectional study. *Lancet Neurol, 17*, 860–869. doi:10.1016/S1474-4422(18)30285-0

Fortea, J., Vilaplana, E., Carmona-Iragui, M., Benejam, B., Videla, L., Barroeta, I., . . . Lleo, A. (2020). Clinical and biomarker changes of Alzheimer's disease in adults with Down syndrome: A cross-sectional study. *Lancet, 395*, 1988–1997. doi:10.1016/S0140-6736(20)30689-9

Garcia-Alba, J., Ramirez-Torano, F., Esteba-Castillo, S., Bruna, R., Moldenhauer, F., Novell, R., . . . Fernandez, A. (2019). Neuropsychological and neurophysiological characterization of mild cognitive impairment and Alzheimer's disease in Down syndrome. *Neurobiol Aging, 84*, 70–79. doi:10.1016/j.neurobiolaging.2019.07.017

Gedye, A. (1995). *Dementia Scale for Down Syndrome*. Gedye Research & Consulting.

Ghezzo, A., Salvioli, S., Solimando, M. C., Palmieri, A., Chiostergi, C., Scurti, M., . . . Franceschi, C. (2014). Age-related changes of adaptive and neuropsychological features in persons with Down syndrome. *PLoS One, 9*, e113111. doi:10.1371/journal.pone.0113111

Gholipour, T., Mitchell, S., Sarkis, R. A., & Chemali, Z. (2017). The clinical and neurobehavioral course of Down syndrome and dementia with or without new-onset epilepsy. *Epilepsy Behav, 68*, 11–16. doi:10.1016/j.yebeh.2016.12.014

Hanney, M., Prasher, V., Williams, N., Jones, E. L., Aarsland, D., Corbett, A., . . . MEADOWS trial researchers. (2012). Memantine for dementia in adults older than 40 years with Down's syndrome (MEADOWS): A randomised, double-blind, placebo-controlled trial. *Lancet, 379*, 528–536. doi:10.1016/S0140-6736(11)61676-0

Hardy, J., Crook, R., Perry, R., Raghavan, R., & Roberts, G. (1994). ApoE genotype and Down's syndrome. *Lancet, 343*, 979–980.

Hartley, S. L., Handen, B. L., Devenny, D. A., Hardison, R., Mihaila, I., Price, J. C., . . . Christian, B. T. (2014). Cognitive functioning in relation to brain amyloid-beta in healthy adults with Down syndrome. *Brain, 137*, 2556–2563. doi:10.1093/brain/awu173

Hartley, S. L., Handen, B. L., Devenny, D., Mihaila, I., Hardison, R., Lao, P. J., . . . Christian, B. T. (2017). Cognitive decline and brain amyloid-beta accumulation across 3 years in adults with Down syndrome. *Neurobiol Aging, 58*, 68–76. doi:10.1016/j.neurobiolaging.2017.05.019

Hassiotis, A., Strydom, A., Allen, K., & Walker, Z. (2003). A memory clinic for older people with intellectual disabilities. *Aging Ment Health, 7*, 418–423. doi:10.1080/13607860310001594664

Head, E., Doran, E., Nistor, M., Hill, M., Schmitt, F. A., Haier, R. J., & Lott, I. T. (2011). Plasma amyloid-beta as a function of age, level of intellectual disability, and presence of dementia in Down syndrome. *J Alzheimers Dis, 23*, 399–409. doi:10.3233/JAD-2010-101335

Hithersay, R., Hamburg, S., Knight, B., & Strydom, A. (2017). Cognitive decline and dementia in Down syndrome. *Curr Opin Psychiatry, 30*, 102–107. doi:10.1097/YCO.0000000000000307

Hithersay, R., Startin, C. M., Hamburg, S., Mok, K. Y., Hardy, J., Fisher, E. M. C., . . . Strydom, A. (2019). Association of dementia with mortality among adults with Down syndrome older than 35 years. *JAMA Neurol, 76*, 152–160. doi:10.1001/jamaneurol.2018.3616

Hithersay, R., Baksh, R. A., Startin, C. M., Wijeratne, P., Hamburg, S., Carter, B., . . . Strydom, A. (2021). Optimal age and outcome measures for Alzheimer's disease prevention trials in people with Down syndrome. *Alzheimers Dement, 17*, 595–604. doi:10.1002/alz.12222

Holland, A. J., Hon, J., Huppert, F. A., & Stevens, F. (2000). Incidence and course of dementia in people with Down's syndrome: Findings from a population-based study. *J Intellect Disabil Res, 44*, 138–146.

Holland, A. J., Hon, J., Huppert, F. A., Stevens, F., & Watson, P. (1998). Population-based study of the prevalence and presentation of dementia in adults with Down's syndrome. *Br J Psychiatry, 172*, 493–498.

Hon, J., Huppert, F. A., Holland, A. J., & Watson, P. (1999). Neuropsychological assessment of older adults with Down's syndrome: An epidemiological study using the Cambridge Cognitive Examination (CAMCOG). *Br J Clin Psychol, 38*, 155–165.

Huxley, A., Prasher, V. P., & Haque, M. S. (2000). The dementia scale for Down's syndrome. *J Intellect Disabil Res, 44*, 697–698.

Iulita, M. F., Ower, A., Barone, C., Pentz, R., Gubert, P., Romano, C., . . . Cuello, A. C. (2016). An inflammatory and trophic disconnect biomarker profile revealed in Down syndrome plasma: Relation to cognitive decline and longitudinal evaluation. *Alzheimers Dement, 12*, 1132–1148. doi:10.1016/j.jalz.2016.05.001

Jamieson-Craig, R., Scior, K., Chan, T., Fenton, C., & Strydom, A. (2010). Reliance on carer reports of early symptoms of dementia among adults with intellectual disabilities. *J Policy Pract Intellect Disabil, 7*, 34–41.

Jennings, D., Seibyl, J., Sabbagh, M., Lai, F., Hopkins, W., Bullich, S., . . . Marek, K. (2015). Age dependence of brain beta-amyloid deposition in Down syndrome: An [18F]florbetaben PET study. *Neurology, 84*, 500–507. doi:10.1212/WNL.0000000000001212

Jones, E. L., Ballard, C. G., Prasher, V. P., Arno, M., Tyrer, S., Moore, B., & Hanney, M. L. (2010). An intron 7 polymorphism in APP affects the age of onset of dementia in Down syndrome. *Int J Alzheimers Dis, 2011*, 929102. doi:10.4061/2011/929102

Jones, E. L., Hanney, M., Francis, P. T., & Ballard, C. G. (2009). Amyloid beta concentrations in older people with Down syndrome and dementia. *Neurosci Lett, 451*, 162–164. doi:10.1016/j.neulet.2008.12.030

Jones, E. L., Margallo-Lana, M., Prasher, V. P., & Ballard, C. G. (2008). The extended tau haplotype and the age of onset of dementia in Down syndrome. *Dement Geriatr Cogn Disord, 26*, 199–202. doi:10.1159/000152044

Jones, E. L., Mok, K., Hanney, M., Harold, D., Sims, R., Williams, J., & Ballard, C. (2013). Evidence that PICALM affects age at onset of Alzheimer's dementia in Down syndrome. *Neurobiol Aging, 34*, 2441 e2441–2445. doi:10.1016/j.neurobiolaging.2013.03.018

Keator, D. B., Phelan, M. J., Taylor, L., Doran, E., Krinsky-McHale, S., Price, J., . . . Lott, I. T. (2020). Down syndrome: Distribution of brain amyloid in mild cognitive impairment. *Alzheimers Dement (Amst), 12*, e12013. doi:10.1002/dad2.12013

Kishi, T., Matsunaga, S., Oya, K., Nomura, I., Ikuta, T., & Iwata, N. (2017). Memantine for Alzheimer's disease: An updated systematic review and meta-analysis. *J Alzheimers Dis, 60*, 401–425. doi:10.3233/JAD-170424

Kittler, P., Krinsky-McHale, S. J., & Devenny, D. A. (2006). Verbal intrusions precede memory decline in adults with Down syndrome. *J Intellect Disabil Res, 50*, 1–10. doi:10.1111/j.1365-2788.2005.00715.x

Krinsky-McHale, S. J., Devenny, D. A., Kittler, P., & Silverman, W. (2008). Selective attention deficits associated with mild cognitive impairment and early stage Alzheimer's disease in adults with Down syndrome. *Am J Ment Retard, 113*, 369–386. doi:10.1352/2008.113:369-386

Krinsky-McHale, S. J., Devenny, D. A., & Silverman, W. P. (2002). Changes in explicit memory associated with early dementia in adults with Down's syndrome. *J Intellect Disabil Res, 46*, 198–208.

Lai, F., Kammann, E., Rebeck, G. W., Anderson, A., Chen, Y., & Nixon, R. A. (1999). APOE genotype and gender effects on Alzheimer disease in 100 adults with Down syndrome. *Neurology, 53*, 331–336.

Lamar, M., Foy, C. M., Beacher, F., Daly, E., Poppe, M., Archer, N., . . . Murphy, D. G. (2011). Down syndrome with and without dementia: An in vivo proton magnetic resonance spectroscopy study with implications for Alzheimer's disease. *NeuroImage, 57*, 63–68. doi:10.1016/j.neuroimage.2011.03.073

Landt, J., Ball, S. L., Holland, A. J., Hon, J., Owen, A., Treppner, P., & Herbert, J. (2011). Age-related changes in plasma dehydroepiandrosterone levels in adults with Down's syndrome and the risk of dementia. *J Neuroendocrinol, 23*, 450–455. doi:10.1111/j.1365-2826.2011.02118.x

Lanfranchi, S., Jerman, O., Dal Pont, E., Alberti, A., & Vianello, R. (2010). Executive function in adolescents with Down syndrome. *J Intellect Disabil Res, 54*, 308–319. doi:10.1111/j.1365-2788.2010.01262.x

Lao, P. J., Handen, B. L., Betthauser, T. J., Mihaila, I., Hartley, S. L., Cohen, A. D., . . . Christian, B. T. (2018). Alzheimer-like pattern of hypometabolism emerges with elevated amyloid-beta burden in Down syndrome. *J Alzheimers Dis, 61*, 631–644. doi:10.3233/JAD-170720

Lao, P. J., Handen, B. L., Betthauser, T. J., Mihaila, I., Hartley, S. L., Cohen, A. D., . . . Christian, B. T. (2017). Longitudinal changes in amyloid positron emission tomography and volumetric magnetic resonance imaging in the nondemented Down syndrome population. *Alzheimers Dement (Amst), 9*, 1–9. doi:10.1016/j.dadm.2017.05.001

Lautarescu, B. A., Holland, A. J., & Zaman, S. H. (2017). The early presentation of dementia in people with Down syndrome: A systematic review of longitudinal studies. *Neuropsychol Rev, 27*, 31–45. doi:10.1007/s11065-017-9341-9

Lee, J. H., Chulikavit, M., Pang, D., Zigman, W. B., Silverman, W., & Schupf, N. (2007). Association between genetic variants in sortilin-related receptor 1 (SORL1) and Alzheimer's disease in adults with Down syndrome. *Neurosci Lett, 425*, 105–109. doi:10.1016/j.neulet.2007.08.042

Lee, J. H., Gurney, S., Pang, D., Temkin, A., Park, N., Janicki, S. C., . . . Schupf, N. (2012). Polymorphisms in HSD17B1: Early onset and increased risk of Alzheimer's disease in women with Down syndrome. *Curr Gerontol Geriatr Res, 2012*, 361218. doi:10.1155/2012/361218

Lee, J. H., Lee, A. J., Dang, L. H., Pang, D., Kisselev, S., Krinsky-McHale, S. J., . . . Schupf, N. (2017). Candidate gene analysis for Alzheimer's disease in adults with Down syndrome. *Neurobiol Aging, 56*, 150–158. doi:10.1016/j.neurobiolaging.2017.04.018

Lee, N. C., Yang, S. Y., Chieh, J. J., Huang, P. T., Chang, L. M., Chiu, Y. N., . . . Chiu, M. J. (2016). Blood beta-amyloid and tau in Down syndrome: A comparison with Alzheimer's disease. *Front Aging Neurosci, 8*, 316. doi:10.3389/fnagi.2016.00316

LeVine, H., 3rd, Spielmann, H. P., Matveev, S., Cauvi, F. M., Murphy, M. P., Beckett, T. L., . . . Head, E. (2017). Down syndrome: Age-dependence of PiB binding in postmortem frontal cortex across the lifespan. *Neurobiol Aging, 54*, 163–169. doi:10.1016/j.neurobiolaging.2017.03.005

Lin, A. L., Powell, D., Caban-Holt, A., Jicha, G., Robertson, W., Gold, B. T., . . . Head, E. (2016). ^{1}H-MRS metabolites in adults with Down syndrome: Effects of dementia. *Neuroimage Clin, 11*, 728–735. doi:10.1016/j.nicl.2016.06.001

Livingstone, N., Hanratty, J., McShane, R., & Macdonald, G. (2015). Pharmacological interventions for cognitive decline in people with Down syndrome. *Cochrane Database Syst Rev*CD011546. doi:10.1002/14651858.CD011546.pub2

Locatelli, T., Fornara, C., Medaglini, S., Alberoni, M., Franceschi, M., Rinaldi, L., . . . Comi, G. (1996). Quantified electroencephalogram in adult patients with Down's syndrome. *Dev Brain Dysfunc, 9*, 215–223.

Lott, I. T., Doran, E., Nguyen, V. Q., Tournay, A., Movsesyan, N., & Gillen, D. L. (2012). Down syndrome and dementia: Seizures and cognitive decline. *J Alzheimers Dis, 29*, 177–185. doi:10.3233/JAD-2012-111613

Lott, I. T., Osann, K., Doran, E., & Nelson, L. (2002). Down syndrome and Alzheimer disease: Response to donepezil. *Arch Neurol, 59*, 1133–1136.

Mak, E., Bickerton, A., Padilla, C., Walpert, M. J., Annus, T., Wilson, L. R., . . . Holland, A. J. (2019). Longitudinal trajectories of amyloid deposition, cortical thickness, and tau in Down syndrome: A deep-phenotyping case report. *Alzheimers Dement (Amst), 11*, 654–658. doi:10.1016/j.dadm.2019.04.006

Mak, E., Padilla, C., Annus, T., Wilson, L. R., Hong, Y. T., Fryer, T. D., . . . Holland, A. J. (2019). Delineating the topography of amyloid-associated cortical atrophy in Down syndrome. *Neurobiol Aging, 80*, 196–202. doi:10.1016/j.neurobiolaging.2019.02.018

Makary, A. T., Testa, R., Tonge, B. J., Einfeld, S. L., Mohr, C., & Gray, K. M. (2015). Association between adaptive behaviour and age in adults with Down syndrome without dementia: Examining the range and severity of adaptive behaviour problems. *J Intellect Disabil Res, 59*, 689–702. doi:10.1111/jir.12172

Mann, D. M. (1988). Alzheimer's disease and Down's syndrome. *Histopathology, 13*, 125–137.

Margallo-Lana, M., Morris, C. M., Gibson, A. M., Tan, A. L., Kay, D. W., Tyrer, S. P., . . . Ballard, C. G. (2004). Influence of the amyloid precursor protein locus on dementia in Down syndrome. *Neurology, 62*, 1996–1998.

Margallo-Lana, M. L., Moore, P. B., Kay, D. W., Perry, R. H., Reid, B. E., Berney, T. P., & Tyrer, S. P. (2007). Fifteen-year follow-up of 92 hospitalized adults with Down's syndrome: Incidence of cognitive decline, its relationship to age and neuropathology. *J Intellect Disabil Res*, *51*, 463–477. doi:10.1111/j.1365-2788.2006.00902.x

McCarron, M., Gill, M., McCallion, P., & Begley, C. (2005). Health co-morbidities in ageing persons with Down syndrome and Alzheimer's dementia. *J Intellect Disabil Res*, *49*, 560–566. doi:10.1111/j.1365-2788.2005.00704.x

McCarron, M., McCallion, P., Reilly, E., & Mulryan, N. (2014). A prospective 14-year longitudinal follow-up of dementia in persons with Down syndrome. *J Intellect Disabil Res*, *58*, 61–70. doi:10.1111/jir.12074

Medaglini, S., Locatelli, T., Fornara, C., Alberoni, M., Comola, M., Franceschi, M., . . . Comi, G. (1997). P300 and EEG mapping in Down's syndrome. *J Psychophysiol*, *11*, 48–58.

Mok, K. Y., Jones, E. L., Hanney, M., Harold, D., Sims, R., Williams, J., . . . Hardy, J. (2014). Polymorphisms in BACE2 may affect the age of onset Alzheimer's dementia in Down syndrome. *Neurobiol Aging*, *35*, 1513 e1511–1515. doi:10.1016/j.neurobiolaging.2013.12.022

Moran, J. A., Rafii, M. S., Keller, S. M., Singh, B. K., Janicki, M. P., American Academy of Developmental Medicine and Dentistry, . . . American Association on Intellectual and Developmental Disabilities. (2013). The National Task Group on Intellectual Disabilities and Dementia Practices consensus recommendations for the evaluation and management of dementia in adults with intellectual disabilities. *Mayo Clin Proc*, *88*, 831–840. doi:10.1016/j.mayocp.2013.04.024

Musaeus, C. S., Salem, L. C., Sabers, A., Kjaer, T. W., & Waldemar, G. (2019). Associations between electroencephalography power and Alzheimer's disease in persons with Down syndrome. *J Intellect Disabil Res*, *63*, 1151–1157. doi:10.1111/jir.12627

Nakamura, A., Kaneko, N., Villemagne, V. L., Kato, T., Doecke, J., Dore, V., . . . Yanagisawa, K. (2018). High performance plasma amyloid-beta biomarkers for Alzheimer's disease. *Nature*, *554*, 249–254. doi:10.1038/nature25456

Nelson, L. D., Orme, D., Osann, K., & Lott, I. T. (2001). Neurological changes and emotional functioning in adults with Down syndrome. *J Intellect Disabil Res*, *45*, 450–456.

Nelson, L. D., Siddarth, P., Kepe, V., Scheibel, K. E., Huang, S. C., Barrio, J. R., & Small, G. W. (2011). Positron emission tomography of brain beta-amyloid and tau levels in adults with Down syndrome. *Arch Neurol*, *68*, 768–774. doi:10.1001/archneurol.2011.104

Oliver, C., Crayton, L., Holland, A., Hall, S., & Bradbury, J. (1998). A four year prospective study of age-related cognitive change in adults with Down's syndrome. *Psychol Med*, *28*, 1365–1377.

Patel, A., Rees, S. D., Kelly, M. A., Bain, S. C., Barnett, A. H., Thalitaya, D., & Prasher, V. P. (2011). Association of variants within APOE, SORL1, RUNX1, BACE1 and ALDH18A1 with dementia in Alzheimer's disease in subjects with Down syndrome. *Neurosci Lett*, *487*, 144–148. doi:10.1016/j.neulet.2010.10.010

Pearlson, G. D., Breiter, S. N., Aylward, E. H., Warren, A. C., Grygorcewicz, M., Frangou, S., . . . Pulsifer, M. B. (1998). MRI brain changes in subjects with Down syndrome with and without dementia. *Dev Med Child Neurol*, *40*, 326–334.

Powell, D., Caban-Holt, A., Jicha, G., Robertson, W., Davis, R., Gold, B. T., . . . Head, E. (2014). Frontal white matter integrity in adults with Down syndrome with and without dementia. *Neurobiol Aging*, *35*, 1562–1569. doi:10.1016/j.neurobiolaging.2014.01.137

Prasher, V. (2002). Disintegrative syndrome in young adults. *Ir J Psychol Med*, *19*, 101. doi:10.1017/S0790966700007205

Prasher, V. P., Huxley, A., Haque, M. S., & Down syndrome Ageing Study, G. (2002). A 24-week, double-blind, placebo-controlled trial of donepezil in patients with Down syndrome and Alzheimer's disease—Pilot study. *Int J Geriatr Psychiatry*, *17*, 270–278.

Prasher, V. P., Sajith, S. G., Mehta, P., Zigman, W. B., & Schupf, N. (2010). Plasma beta-amyloid and duration of Alzheimer's disease in adults with Down syndrome. *Int J Geriatr Psychiatry*, *25*, 202–207. doi:10.1002/gps.2321

Prasher, V. P., Sajith, S. G., Rees, S. D., Patel, A., Tewari, S., Schupf, N., & Zigman, W. B. (2008). Significant effect of APOE epsilon 4 genotype on the risk of dementia in Alzheimer's disease and mortality in persons with Down syndrome. *Int J Geriatr Psychiatry*, *23*, 1134–1140. doi:10.1002/gps.2039

Presson, A. P., Partyka, G., Jensen, K. M., Devine, O. J., Rasmussen, S. A., McCabe, L. L., & McCabe, E. R. (2013). Current estimate of Down syndrome population prevalence in the United States. *J Pediatr*, *163*, 1163–1168. doi:10.1016/j.jpeds.2013.06.013

Pujol, J., Fenoll, R., Ribas-Vidal, N., Martinez-Vilavella, G., Blanco-Hinojo, L., Garcia-Alba, J., . . . Esteba-Castillo, S. (2018). A longitudinal study of brain anatomy changes preceding dementia in Down syndrome. *Neuroimage Clin, 18*, 160–166. doi:10.1016/j.nicl.2018.01.024

Rafii, M. S., Donohue, M. C., Matthews, D. C., Muranevici, G., Ness, S., O'Bryant, S. E., & Rissman, R. A. (2019). Plasma neurofilament light and Alzheimer's disease biomarkers in Down syndrome: Results from the Down Syndrome Biomarker Initiative (DSBI). *J Alzheimers Dis, 70*, 131–138. doi:10.3233/JAD-190322

Rafii, M. S., Lukic, A. S., Andrews, R. D., Brewer, J., Rissman, R. A., Strother, S. C., . . . Alzheimer's Disease Neuroimaging Institute. (2017). PET imaging of tau pathology and relationship to amyloid, longitudinal MRI, and cognitive change in Down syndrome: Results from the Down Syndrome Biomarker Initiative (DSBI). *J Alzheimers Dis, 60*, 439–450. doi:10.3233/JAD-170390

Rafii, M. S., Wishnek, H., Brewer, J. B., Donohue, M. C., Ness, S., Mobley, W. C., . . . Rissman, R. A. (2015). The Down syndrome biomarker initiative (DSBI) pilot: Proof of concept for deep phenotyping of Alzheimer's disease biomarkers in Down syndrome. *Front Behav Neurosci, 9*, 239. doi:10.3389/fnbeh.2015.00239

Raghavan, R., Khin-Nu, C., Brown, A. G., Day, K. A., Tyrer, S. P., Ince, P. G., . . . Perry, R. H. (1994). Gender differences in the phenotypic expression of Alzheimer's disease in Down's syndrome (trisomy 21). *Neuroreport, 5*, 1393–1396.

Raha-Chowdhury, R., Henderson, J. W., Raha, A. A., Vuono, R., Bickerton, A., Jones, E., . . . Zaman, S. H. (2019). Choroid plexus acts as gatekeeper for TREM2, abnormal accumulation of ApoE, and fibrillary tau in Alzheimer's disease and in Down syndrome dementia. *J Alzheimers Dis, 69*, 91–109. doi:10.3233/JAD-181179

Rovelet-Lecrux, A., Hannequin, D., Raux, G., Le Meur, N., Laquerriere, A., Vital, A., . . . Campion, D. (2006). APP locus duplication causes autosomal dominant early-onset Alzheimer disease with cerebral amyloid angiopathy. *Nat Genet, 38*, 24–26. doi:10.1038/ng1718

Rowe, J., Lavender, A., & Turk, V. (2006). Cognitive executive function in Down's syndrome. *Br J Clin Psychol, 45*, 5–17. doi:10.1348/014466505X29594

Royston, M. C., Mann, D., Pickering-Brown, S., Owen, F., Perry, R., Ragbavan, R., . . . Roberts, G. W. (1996). ApoE2 allele, Down's syndrome, and dementia. *Ann N Y Acad Sci, 777*, 255–259.

Ryan, N. S., Nicholas, J. M., Weston, P. S., Liang, Y., Lashley, T., Guerreiro, R., . . . Fox, N. C. (2016). Clinical phenotype and genetic associations in autosomal dominant familial Alzheimer's disease: A case series. *Lancet Neurol, 15*, 1326–1335. doi:10.1016/S1474-4422(16)30193-4

Sabbagh, M. N., Chen, K., Rogers, J., Fleisher, A. S., Liebsack, C., Bandy, D., . . . Reiman, E. M. (2015). Florbetapir PET, FDG PET, and MRI in Down syndrome individuals with and without Alzheimer's dementia. *Alzheimers Dement, 11*, 994–1004. doi:10.1016/j.jalz.2015.01.006

Sabbagh, M. N., Fleisher, A., Chen, K., Rogers, J., Berk, C., Reiman, E., . . . Beach, T. G. (2011). Positron emission tomography and neuropathologic estimates of fibrillar amyloid-beta in a patient with Down syndrome and Alzheimer disease. *Arch Neurol, 68*, 1461–1466. doi:10.1001/archneurol.2011.535

Salem, L. C., Sabers, A., Kjaer, T. W., Musaeus, C., Nielsen, M. N., Nielsen, A. G., & Waldemar, G. (2015). Quantitative electroencephalography as a diagnostic Tool for Alzheimer's dementia in adults with Down syndrome. *Dement Geriatr Cogn Dis Extra, 5*, 404–413.

Santoro, S. L., Cannon, S., Capone, G., Franklin, C., Hart, S. J., Hobensack, V., . . . Skotko, B. G. (2020). Unexplained regression in Down syndrome: 35 cases from an international Down syndrome database. *Genet Med, 22*, 767–776. doi:10.1038/s41436-019-0706-8

Schindler, S. E., Bollinger, J. G., Ovod, V., Mawuenyega, K. G., Li, Y., Gordon, B. A., . . . Bateman, R. J. (2019). High-precision plasma beta-amyloid 42/40 predicts current and future brain amyloidosis. *Neurology, 93*, e1647–e1659. doi:10.1212/WNL.0000000000008081

Schupf, N., Kapell, D., Lee, J. H., Zigman, W., Canto, B., Tycko, B., & Mayeux, R. (1996). Onset of dementia is associated with apolipoprotein E epsilon4 in Down's syndrome. *Ann Neurol, 40*, 799–801. doi:10.1002/ana.410400518

Schupf, N., Kapell, D., Nightingale, B., Rodriguez, A., Tycko, B., & Mayeux, R. (1998). Earlier onset of Alzheimer's disease in men with Down syndrome. *Neurology, 50*, 991–995.

Schupf, N., Lee, J. H., Wei, M., Pang, D., Chace, C., Cheng, R., . . . Silverman, W. (2008). Estrogen receptor-alpha variants increase risk of Alzheimer's disease in women with Down syndrome. *Dement Geriatr Cogn Disord, 25*, 476–482. doi:10.1159/000126495

Schupf, N., Pang, D., Patel, B. N., Silverman, W., Schubert, R., Lai, F., . . . Mayeux, R. (2003). Onset of dementia is associated with age at menopause in women with Down's syndrome. *Ann Neurol, 54*, 433–438. doi:10.1002/ana.10677

Schupf, N., Patel, B., Pang, D., Zigman, W. B., Silverman, W., Mehta, P. D., & Mayeux, R. (2007). Elevated plasma beta-amyloid peptide Abeta(42) levels, incident dementia, and mortality in Down syndrome. *Arch Neurol, 64*, 1007–1013. doi:10.1001/archneur.64.7.1007

Schupf, N., Zigman, W. B., Tang, M. X., Pang, D., Mayeux, R., Mehta, P., & Silverman, W. (2010). Change in plasma AB peptides and onset of dementia in adults with Down syndrome. *Neurology, 75*, 1639–1644. doi:10.1212/WNL.0b013e3181fb448b

Sekijima, Y., Ikeda, S., Tokuda, T., Satoh, S., Hidaka, H., Hidaka, E., . . . Yanagisawa, N. (1998). Prevalence of dementia of Alzheimer type and apolipoprotein E phenotypes in aged patients with Down's syndrome. *Eur Neurol, 39*, 234–237.

Sheehan, R., Horsfall, L., Strydom, A., Osborn, D., Walters, K., & Hassiotis, A. (2017). Movement side effects of antipsychotic drugs in adults with and without intellectual disability: UK population-based cohort study. *BMJ Open, 7*, e017406. doi:10.1136/bmjopen-2017-017406

Sheehan, R., Sinai, A., Bass, N., Blatchford, P., Bohnen, I., Bonell, S., . . . Strydom, A. (2015). Dementia diagnostic criteria in Down syndrome. *Int J Geriatr Psychiatry, 30*, 857–863. doi:10.1002/gps.4228

Shinomoto, M., Kasai, T., Tatebe, H., Kondo, M., Ohmichi, T., Morimoto, M., . . . Tokuda, T. (2019). Plasma neurofilament light chain: A potential prognostic biomarker of dementia in adult Down syndrome patients. *PLoS One, 14*, e0211575. doi:10.1371/journal.pone.0211575

Sinai, A., Hassiotis, A., Rantell, K., & Strydom, A. (2016). Assessing specific cognitive deficits associated with dementia in older adults with Down syndrome: Use and validity of the Arizona Cognitive Test Battery (ACTB). *PLoS One, 11*, e0153917. doi:10.1371/journal.pone.0153917

Sinai, A., Mokrysz, C., Bernal, J., Bohnen, I., Bonell, S., Courtenay, K., . . . Strydom, A. (2018). Predictors of age of diagnosis and survival of Alzheimer's disease in Down syndrome. *J Alzheimers Dis, 61*, 717–728. doi:10.3233/JAD-170624

Startin, C. M., Ashton, N. J., Hamburg, S., Hithersay, R., Wiseman, F. K., Mok, K. Y., . . . Strydom, A. (2019). Plasma biomarkers for amyloid, tau, and cytokines in Down syndrome and sporadic Alzheimer's disease. *Alzheimers Res Ther, 11*, 26. doi:10.1186/s13195-019-0477-0

Startin, C. M., Hamburg, S., Hithersay, R., Al-Janabi, T., Mok, K. Y., Hardy, J., . . . Strydom, A. (2019). Cognitive markers of preclinical and prodromal Alzheimer's disease in Down syndrome. *Alzheimers Dement, 15*, 245–257. doi:10.1016/j.jalz.2018.08.009

Startin, C. M., Hamburg, S., Hithersay, R., Davies, A., Rodger, E., Aggarwal, N., . . . Strydom, A. (2016). The LonDownS adult cognitive assessment to study cognitive abilities and decline in Down syndrome. *Wellcome Open Res, 1*, 11. doi:10.12688/wellcomeopenres.9961.1

Strydom, A., Al-Janabi, T., Houston, M., & Ridley, J. (2016). Best practice in caring for adults with dementia and learning disabilities. *Nurs Stand, 31*, 42–51. doi:10.7748/ns.2016.e10524

Strydom, A., Chan, T., Fenton, C., Jamieson-Craig, R., Livingston, G., & Hassiotis, A. (2013). Validity of criteria for dementia in older people with intellectual disability. *Am J Geriatr Psychiatry, 21*, 279–288. doi:10.1016/j.jagp.2012.11.017

Strydom, A., Hassiotis, A., King, M., & Livingston, G. (2009). The relationship of dementia prevalence in older adults with intellectual disability (ID) to age and severity of ID. *Psychol Med, 39*, 13–21. doi:10.1017/S0033291708003334

Strydom, A., Heslegrave, A., Startin, C. M., Mok, K. Y., Hardy, J., Groet, J., . . . Consortium, L. (2018). Neurofilament light as a blood biomarker for neurodegeneration in Down syndrome. *Alzheimers Res Ther, 10*, 39. doi:10.1186/s13195-018-0367-x

Strydom, A., Shooshtari, S., Lee, L., Raykar, V., Torr, J., Tsiouris, J., . . . Maaskant, M. (2010). Dementia in older adults with intellectual disabilities—epidemiology, presentation, and diagnosis. *J Policy Pract Intellect Disabil, 7*, 96–110.

Teipel, S. J., Alexander, G. E., Schapiro, M. B., Moller, H. J., Rapoport, S. I., & Hampel, H. (2004). Age-related cortical grey matter reductions in non-demented Down's syndrome adults determined by MRI with voxel-based morphometry. *Brain, 127*, 811–824. doi:10.1093/brain/awh101

Teipel, S. J., Schapiro, M. B., Alexander, G. E., Krasuski, J. S., Horwitz, B., Hoehne, C., . . . Hampel, H. (2003). Relation of corpus callosum and hippocampal size to age in nondemented adults with Down's syndrome. *Am J Psychiatry, 160*, 1870–1878.

Temple, V., Jozsvai, E., Konstantareas, M. M., & Hewitt, T. A. (2001). Alzheimer dementia in Down's syndrome: The relevance of cognitive ability. *J Intellect Disabil Res, 45*, 47–55.

Tsao, R., Kindelberger, C., Freminville, B., Touraine, R., & Gerald, B. (2015). Variability of the aging process in dementia-free adults with Down syndrome. *Am J Intellect Dev Disabil, 120*, 3–15. doi:10.1352/1944-7558-120.1.3

Tsiouris, J. A., Patti, P. J., & Flory, M. J. (2014). Effects of antidepressants on longevity and dementia onset among adults with Down syndrome: A retrospective study. *J Clin Psychiatry, 75*, 731–737. doi:10.4088/JCP.13m08562

Tyrrell, J., Cosgrave, M., McCarron, M., McPherson, J., Calvert, J., Kelly, A., . . . Lawlor, B. A. (2001). Dementia in people with Down's syndrome. *Int J Geriatr Psychiatry, 16*, 1168–1174.

Uppal, H., Chandran, S., & Potluri, R. (2015). Risk factors for mortality in Down syndrome. *J Intellect Disabil Res, 59*, 873–881. doi:10.1111/jir.12196

Urv, T. K., Zigman, W. B., & Silverman, W. (2008). Maladaptive behaviors related to dementia status in adults with Down syndrome. *Am J Ment Retard, 113*, 73–86. doi:10.1352/0895-8017(2008)113[73:MBRTDS]2.0.CO;2

Urv, T. K., Zigman, W. B., & Silverman, W. (2010). Psychiatric symptoms in adults with Down syndrome and Alzheimer's disease. *Am J Intellect Dev Disabil, 115*, 265–276. doi:10.1352/1944-7558-115.4.265

Van Buggenhout, G. J., Trommelen, J. C., Schoenmaker, A., De Bal, C., Verbeek, J. J., Smeets, D. F., . . . Fryns, J. P. (1999). Down syndrome in a population of elderly mentally retarded patients: Genetic-diagnostic survey and implications for medical care. *Am J Med Genet, 85*, 376–384.

Visser, F. E., Aldenkamp, A. P., van Huffelen, A. C., Kuilman, M., Overweg, J., & van Wijk, J. (1997). Prospective study of the prevalence of Alzheimer-type dementia in institutionalized individuals with Down syndrome. *Am J Ment Retard, 101*, 400–412.

Visser, F. E., Kuilman, M., Oosting, J., Overweg, J., van Wijk, J., & van Huffelen, A. C. (1996). Use of electroencephalography to detect Alzheimer's disease in Down's syndrome. *Acta Neurol Scand, 94*, 97–103.

Walsh, D. M., Doran, E., Silverman, W., Tournay, A., Movsesyan, N., & Lott, I. T. (2015). Rapid assessment of cognitive function in Down syndrome across intellectual level and dementia status. *J Intellect Disabil Res, 59*, 1071–1079. doi:10.1111/jir.12200

Wark, S., Hussain, R., & Parmenter, T. (2014). Down syndrome and dementia: Is depression a confounder for accurate diagnosis and treatment? *J Intellect Disabil, 18*, 305–314. doi:10.1177/1744629514552152

World Health Organization. (1992). *The ICD–10 classification of mental and behavioural disorders: Clinical.* Geneva, Switzerland: World Health Organization.

Wiseman, F. K., Al-Janabi, T., Hardy, J., Karmiloff-Smith, A., Nizetic, D., Tybulewicz, V. L., . . . Strydom, A. (2015). A genetic cause of Alzheimer disease: Mechanistic insights from Down syndrome. *Nat Rev Neurosci, 16*, 564–574. doi:10.1038/nrn3983

Wisniewski, K. E., Wisniewski, H. M., & Wen, G. Y. (1985). Occurrence of neuropathological changes and dementia of Alzheimer's disease in Down's syndrome. *Ann Neurol, 17*, 278–282. doi:10.1002/ana.410170310

Wu, J., & Morris, J. K. (2013). The population prevalence of Down's syndrome in England and Wales in 2011. *Eur J Hum Genet, 21*, 1016–1019. doi:10.1038/ejhg.2012.294

Zis, P., Dickinson, M., Shende, S., Walker, Z., & Strydom, A. (2012). Oxidative stress and memory decline in adults with Down syndrome: Longitudinal study. *J Alzheimers Dis, 31*, 277–283. doi:10.3233/JAD-2012-120073

Zis, P., McHugh, P., McQuillin, A., Pratico, D., Dickinson, M., Shende, S., . . . Strydom, A. (2014). Memory decline in Down syndrome and its relationship to iPF2alpha, a urinary marker of oxidative stress. *PLoS One, 9*, e97709. doi:10.1371/journal.pone.0097709

Zis, P., & Strydom, A. (2018). Clinical aspects and biomarkers of Alzheimer's disease in Down syndrome. *Free Radic Biol Med, 114*, 3–9. doi:10.1016/j.freeradbiomed.2017.08.024

Zis, P., Strydom, A., Buckley, D., Adekitan, D., & McHugh, P. C. (2017). Cognitive ability in Down syndrome and its relationship to urinary neopterin, a marker of activated cellular immunity. *Neurosci Lett, 636*, 254–257. doi:10.1016/j.neulet.2016.11.023

CHAPTER

21 Cellular and Molecular Brain Development in Down Syndrome

Nadine M. Aziz *and* Tarik F. Haydar

Abstract

One of the major tenets of neuroscience is that early development sets the playing field and provides the building blocks for the intricate connections and functions of the mature nervous system. This critical dependence on neurodevelopment has been studied in many model organisms and can be seen most acutely in the human disorders with prenatal or early postnatal onset. The most common genetically determined neurodevelopmental disorder is trisomy 21, or Down syndrome (DS), and changes in early brain development are known to impact the course of life for people with DS. In this chapter, the authors present current knowledge regarding the brain systems that are affected during development in DS and how these early changes are followed by longer-lasting alterations in the neurons and glia that populate the developing brain. The authors focus on the mouse models and human studies that have characterized the genetic and cellular changes to the nervous system, and they discuss how this knowledge can be used to develop rational approaches to helping people with DS achieve greater independence and quality of life.

Key Words: Neurodevelopment, mouse models, biomarkers, brain phenotypes, cellular hallmarks, therapeutic development

Concerted efforts have been made in Down syndrome (DS) research to develop therapies specifically aimed at the cognitive component of DS. Intellectual disability is fully penetrant in individuals with DS but, for reasons not yet fully understood, it can present on a scale from minor to profound depending on the person, creating a pressing need for "personalized" treatments designed for individuals. To do this, scientists studying DS must not only detail the full list of nervous system changes associated with the syndrome, but must also identify the early biomarkers that can predict the needs of each person.

Brain Phenotypes Across the Lifespan of Individuals With DS

The neuropathological consequences of trisomy 21 begin during fetal development and the resulting cognitive ramifications evolve throughout life. Changes to brain structure are detectable as early as 20 weeks of gestation in postmortem fetal brains, characterized by an increase in apoptosis, or programmed cell death, in the stem and progenitor cells of the neocortex and hippocampus and within the maturing cells of the neocortical white and gray matter (Guidi, Ciani, Bonasoni, Santini, & Bartesaghi, 2011; Wisniewski & Kida, 1994). This is accompanied by a decrease in prenatal neurogenesis and synaptogenesis, as well as reduced expansion of the frontal lobe and cerebellum (Bahado-Singh et al., 1992; Guihard-Costa, Khung, Delbecque, Menez, & Delezoide, 2006; Larsen et al., 2008; Petit, LeBoutillier, Alfano, & Becker, 1984; Weitzdoerfer, Dierssen, Fountoulakis, & Lubec, 2001; Winter et al., 1998; Wisniewski, Laure-Kamionowska, & Wisniewski, 1984). Decreases in cellular migration and neurotransmitter levels have also been observed in fetal brains with DS (Contestabile et al., 2007; Guidi et al., 2008; Whittle, Sartori, Dierssen, Lubec, & Singewald, 2007), both of which are consistent with decreased neuron production early in development.

The early decreases in neuron formation have lasting effects. For example, infants with DS have decreased overall brain weight caused by cortical and hippocampal hypoplasia, decreased synapse formation and dendritic branching, and reduced cerebellar and brainstem volumes (L. Becker, Mito, Takashima, & Onodera, 1991; Becker, Armstrong, & Chan, 1986; Golden & Hyman, 1994; Ross, Galaburda, & Kemper, 1984; Schmidt-Sidor, Wisniewski, Shepard, & Sersen, 1990; Takashima, Becker, Armstrong, & Chan, 1981; Wisniewski, 1990; Wisniewski et al., 1984). Delayed myelination and alterations in various white matter tracts have also been reported (Becker et al., 1991; Olmos-Serrano, Kang, et al., 2016; Wisniewski & Schmidt-Sidor, 1989). Throughout adolescence and into adulthood, morphological, cellular, and subcellular parameters of brain structure and function continue to diverge in individuals with DS compared to typically developing people (Lott, 2012). By adulthood, the brains of individuals with DS show simplified gyrification and a 24% reduction in size, with decreases in volume of the cerebellum (33%), hippocampus (27%), frontal cortex (17%), dorsolateral prefrontal cortex, anterior cingulate gyrus, and inferior temporal and parietal cortex, as well as changes to parietal white matter (Coyle, Oster-Granite, & Gearhart, 1986; Jernigan, Bellugi, Sowell, Doherty, & Hesselink, 1993; Pinter, Brown, et al., 2001; Pinter, Eliez, Schmitt, Capone, & Reiss, 2001; Raz et al., 1995; Teipel et al., 2003, 2004; White, Alkire, & Haier, 2003; Wisniewski, 1990). Increases in volume of the parahippocampal gyrus have been observed as well (White et al., 2003).

Along with, and perhaps directly related to these neuroanatomical alterations, atypical cognition begins during infancy and childhood and is a hallmark of persons with DS. Aside from motor deficits at birth, early learning impairments lead to a progressive decline in intellectual quotient after the first year of life, delayed language acquisition, and altered hippocampal-dependent explicit and spatial memory (Fidler & Nadel, 2007; Gibson, Groeneweg, Jerry, & Harris, 1988; Nadel, 2003; Ohr & Fagen, 1994; Pennington, Moon, Edgin, Stedron, & Nadel, 2003; Vicari, 2004; Vicari, Marotta, & Carlesimo, 2004; Vicari, Pontillo, & Armando, 2013; Wishart, 1993). More contemporary neurocognitive assessments have allowed for further subdivisions of the learning and memory phenotype into particular memory modalities and have pointed to areas of the brain that control those functions (Bostelmann et al., 2018; Farran et al., 2019; Foti et al., 2018; Purser et al., 2015; Shalev et al., 2019). Later in life, by approximately 40 years of age, almost all adults with DS will exhibit Alzheimer's neuropathology; however, not all will display clinical signs of Alzheimer's dementia (Head, Lott, Wilcock, & Lemere, 2016; Wilcock et al., 2015). Other identified changes in late adulthood include altered neurotransmission in cholinergic, noradrenergic, and GABAergic systems (Araujo, Torres, & Guilhoto, 2015; Coyle et al., 1986).

Due to these distinct spatiotemporal changes in the brains of individuals with DS, interventional therapies must be tailored to specific targets and life stages in order to maximize their efficacy (Haydar, 2020). For example, although early progression of brain development may influence later stages of growth and function, treatments designed to be advantageous during embryonic brain development likely need to be distinct from those targeting the early onset Alzheimer's pathology. Despite our rich understanding of the neuroanatomical changes associated with DS, neurocognitive interventions have been hampered by the fact that postmortem human studies alone cannot elucidate the specific, targetable mechanisms underlying DS phenotypes over the lifespan of affected individuals (de Wert, Dondorp, & Bianchi, 2016). This is because postmortem tissue cannot provide in vivo functional endpoints or real-time physiological responses to treatment.

State of Neurocognitive Therapies in DS

While several preclinical trials of potential neuropharmacotherapies have been conducted in mouse models of DS, none have successfully shown comprehensive and reproducible amelioration of brain defects in the mice and, to date, no resultant clinical trials have been successful (Gardiner, 2015; Herault et al., 2017; Stagni, Giacomini, Guidi, Ciani, & Bartesaghi, 2015). As mentioned above, because DS-related neuropathology develops in a spatiotemporal manner, therapies or a combination of therapies that target distinct periods over the lifespan are necessary to address the varied etiologies of the associated intellectual disability (Bartesaghi et al., 2015; Lott & Dierssen, 2010). A notable exception would be treatment that can fully silence the extra chromosome very soon after conception (Jiang et al., 2013).

Notably, because brain changes during fetal development may relate to the brain defects observed later in life, interest in prenatal therapy has been growing within the DS research community (Guedj, Bianchi, & Delabar, 2014; Guidi et al., 2014; Stagni et al., 2016). Evidence from mouse studies suggests that neuropharmacotherapies are more restorative and have longer lasting effects when administered during phases of neural development than when given to adult mice (Bartesaghi et al., 2015; Das et al., 2013; Guidi et al., 2014). With the advent of highly accurate noninvasive prenatal testing as early as 10 weeks of gestation and rapid developments in personalized medicine, clinicians are now for the first time uniquely positioned to therapeutically target this early prenatal window when the central nervous system (CNS) is experiencing dynamic changes and rapid growth (Gil, Quezada, Revello, Akolekar, & Nicolaides, 2015; Taylor-Phillips et al., 2016). Thus, a combinatorial therapeutic strategy based on a personalized prenatal and postnatal administration schedule has tremendous potential for alleviating the brain changes associated with DS and their resultant intellectual disability. This ambitious goal requires attention to moral and ethical constraints as well as confirmation of the linkage between prenatal and postnatal brain dynamics in DS. Until these necessary requirements can be achieved, current efforts at therapy are focused on the postnatal and adult brain. Unfortunately, postmortem human tissue and vital imaging procedures such as magnetic resonance imaging (MRI) and positron emission tomography (PET) scanning do not provide sufficient resolution of the mechanisms leading to brain changes in DS. This has led to a greater emphasis on mouse models of DS since multiple animals can be compared together and because advanced molecular and cellular techniques can be employed.

Mouse Models of DS

To delineate the emergence and the underlying cause(s) of brain alterations in DS, much work in the past 4 decades has relied on mouse models of the disorder. Comparisons of DNA sequences between the mouse and human genomes identified approximately 175 genes on human chromosome 21 (Hsa21) that are conserved in mice (Das & Reeves, 2011). Mouse genes that are orthologous (have conserved function) to those on Hsa21 can be found in clusters on mouse chromosomes (Mmu) 16, 17, and 10. This similarity between Hsa21 and Mmu10, Mmu16, and Mmu17 has allowed for the generation of a wide array of mouse models to better characterize the relationships between gene triplication and the cellular, subcellular, and molecular determinants of brain development and function in people with DS. There are three broad groups of DS mouse models: mice with a full chromosomal triplication (such as that found in 95% of people with DS), those with partial trisomy caused by translocation (found in 5% of human cases), and those with single-gene triplications geared towards understanding the role of that gene in isolation. These mouse models have been integral in identifying dosage-dependent single genes or gene clusters, elucidating genome-wide perturbations, and identifying targetable mechanisms for therapeutic intervention. However, a lack of standardized testing paradigms has generated conflicting reports and hindered direct comparisons of DS phenotypes among the different models (Das & Reeves, 2011; Gupta, Dhanasekaran, & Gardiner, 2016; Haydar & Reeves, 2012; Herault et al., 2017; Moore & Roper, 2007; Starbuck, Dutka, Ratliff, Reeves, & Richtsmeier, 2014). Thus, there is a large unmet need for an intraspecies screen that confirms links between the triplicated orthologous genes in various trisomy models with DS phenotypes. Next, we will briefly discuss the three broad groups of mouse models used to study DS as an additional resource to the chapter on mouse models (see Moyer & Reeves, this volume).

Whole Chromosome Triplication Models

Ts16

The first model designed to study the consequences of trisomy 21 was the trisomy 16 (Ts16) mouse (Gropp, Kolbus, & Giers, 1975). Ts16 mice contain a full triplication of Mmu16 which, along with many Hsa21 orthologues, also includes genes that are found on Hsa3 and Hsa22. Ts16 mice are trisomic for many DS-irrelevant genes and therefore have significant genetic dissimilarity to people with DS. However, analyses of these mice yielded valuable information about brain development, which helped identify key developmental processes for future assessment in more contemporary mouse models of DS and in the brains of people with DS. Specifically, Ts16 embryos show a diminished brain size characterized by a decrease in radial thickness of the pallium as well as altered tangential growth (Haydar, Blue, Molliver, Krueger, & Yarowsky, 1996; Haydar, Nowakowski, Yarowsky, & Krueger, 2000). Concomitant with this observed microcephaly is a lengthened cell cycle, increased apoptosis, and a decreased number of cortical progenitor cells, suggesting that neurogenesis deficits and increased cell death underlie the changes in embryonic brain growth (Haydar et al., 1996, 2000). Furthermore, these mice also express some phenotypes that are often seen in individuals with DS, such as craniofacial, immunological, and congenital heart abnormalities (Gearhart, Davisson, & Oster-Granite, 1986) as well as age-dependent deficits in cholinergic systems within the basal forebrain (Holtzman et al., 1992). Notwithstanding these early findings, the many genes unrelated to DS and the perinatal lethality of Ts16 mice have led to the disuse of this model.

Tc1

Another mouse model with a full chromosomal triplication is the Tc1 (MGI symbol: Tc[Hsa21]1TybEmcf) mouse which carries an exogenous copy of ~90% of Hsa21, including all regulatory elements. In theory, the study of this mouse is advantageous for three reasons: (a) epigenetic modifications and transcriptional regulators affecting Hsa21 genes are maintained, (b) random integration of transgenic material into the mouse genome is avoided, and (c) the need for triplication of the three distinct mouse chromosomal regions that contain Hsa21 orthologues is bypassed (O'Doherty et al., 2005). However, the Tc1 mouse line also exhibits some limitations, including a low transmission frequency of the human transchromosome, mosaic expression of the Hsa21 genetic material in different tissues, and the lack of functional trisomy of an important DS-related gene, *Amyloid precursor protein (APP)*, that may play a role in the early-onset Alzheimer's pathology seen in individuals with DS. Nonetheless, similar to what is seen in humans with DS, these mice show deficits in hippocampal long-term potentiation (LTP) and hippocampal circuitry, novel-object recognition abnormalities, hypocellularity and dysgenesis of the cerebellum, altered spine morphology, congenital heart defects, and a decrease in T-lymphocyte activation in response to stimulation (Haas et al., 2013; O'Doherty et al., 2005; Powell et al., 2016; Witton et al., 2015). In addition, recent work has shown that these mice also exhibit dysregulation of the major hippocampal signaling protein Wnt caused by triplication of the *DYRK1A* gene (Granno et al., 2019).

Segmental Trisomy Models

Unlike the full chromosomal trisomy models, segmental trisomy models contain triplications of subregions of Mmu16, 10, and 17. Because Mmu16 contains the largest number of DS-relevant genes, classical models including the Ts65Dn, Ts1Cje, Ts2Cje, and Ts1Rhr all contain segmental trisomy of various subparts of this mouse chromosome. More contemporary models contain larger numbers of DS-relevant genes while some contain smaller subsets of Mmu16 genes to identify the minimum essential dosage-sensitive genes giving rise to a specific phenotype.

Ts65Dn

The first segmental trisomy model was the Ts65Dn mouse (MGI symbol: Ts[17^{16}]65Dn; Davisson, Schmidt, & Akeson, 1990), generated almost three decades ago by cesium irradiation that induced a reciprocal translocation of Mmu16 onto a marker chromosome containing the centromeric portion of Mmu17. Since this triplication is carried as an additional chromosome, it mirrors the aneuploidy observed in 95% of DS cases (Shin et al., 2010). The triplicated segment consists of 104 Hsa21 orthologous genes and 60 nonorthologous genes on the Mmu17 centromere that are not triplicated in DS (Duchon et al., 2011). Of these 60 unrelated genes, ~35 are protein coding. Despite this genetic flaw, Ts65Dn has been the most widely used mouse model of DS, and fine details of brain growth and function have been discerned in these mice.

Ts65Dn mice exhibit many DS-related brain phenotypes, including elongated cell cycle, decreased neurogenesis, altered cortical lamination, frontal lobe and cerebellar hypoplasia, and microcephaly during embryonic development (Chakrabarti, Galdzicki, & Haydar, 2007; Contestabile, Fila, Bartesaghi, & Ciani, 2009; Contestabile, Fila, Cappellini, Bartesaghi, & Ciani, 2009; Contestabile et al., 2007). Upon birth and until weaning, Ts65Dn mice show a consistent decrease in body length and body weight compared to their control euploid littermates that do not have triplication (Olmos-Serrano, Tyler, Cabral, & Haydar, 2016). After birth, Ts65Dn animals continue to display delays in achieving both early and late developmental milestones with a concomitant misallocation of excitatory and inhibitory neurons in the cortex and hippocampus (Chakrabarti et al., 2010; Olmos-Serrano, Tyler, et al., 2016). These changes are associated with severe consequences to neuronal communication in the neocortex, hippocampus, and cerebellum (Belichenko et al., 2004). Subcellularly, Ts65Dn mice have a decreased number of excitatory synapses, alterations in presynaptic boutons, abnormal dendritic morphology, region-specific changes in density and size of spines, increased number of GABAergic interneurons and inhibitory synapses, increased size of the synaptic cleft, and altered LTP in the hippocampus. In fact, overinhibition in the hippocampus is so profound that the

LTP could not be induced *ex vivo* in Ts65Dn hippocampal slices without the use of the GABA receptor antagonist pricrotoxin (Belichenko, Kleschevnikov, Salehi, Epstein, & Mobley, 2007). Additionally, the Ts65Dn hippocampus is also characterized by abnormal morphology, reduced cell proliferation, increased apoptosis, hypoplasia of the granular and subgranular cell layers, and a decrease in the volume of the dentate gyrus (Contestabile et al., 2007; Lorenzi & Reeves, 2006). In the cerebellum, adult Ts65Dn mice exhibit abnormal cerebellar granule cell morphology and a 76% decrease in granule cell density compared to euploid mice (Baxter, Moran, Richtsmeier, Troncoso, & Reeves, 2000; Olson, Roper, et al., 2004). Cerebellar deficits are not limited to the granule cell layer, as Purkinje cell density is also reduced by 10% and overall cerebellar volume is reduced by 12% compared to age-matched euploid control animals (Olson et al., 2007). While the degree of understanding of Ts65Dn brain development and function far outstrips the corresponding knowledge in the human brain, several changes first found in Ts65Dn have been confirmed in human samples. Regarding the brain alterations found later in life, Ts65Dn mice also display signs of Alzheimer's-like pathology that seem related to the gene dosage of *APP*. These include an increase in beta-amyloid in the brain and degeneration in cholinergic neurons of the basal forebrain. Despite these signs of neurodegeneration, no plaques or tangles are seen in the brains of older Ts65Dn mice, a disconnect with the human brain that is likely due to small changes in the sequence of mouse *APP* (see the section "Aging Phenotypes").

Since its generation, the Ts65Dn mouse model has been the workhorse of the DS research community, and many of its neurological phenotypes have been discovered and refined over the past two decades. In fact, newly emerging technologies are still allowing for novel discoveries in the Ts65Dn brain and the spinal cord. Chief among those are the white matter defects, proteomic abnormalities, and inflammation phenotypes. The white matter phenotype was discovered in a global gene expression analysis of human brains from individuals with DS, starting during mid-fetal development and extending to adulthood (Olmos-Serrano, Kang, et al., 2016). This brain transcriptome study helped identify dysregulated gene networks governing oligodendrocyte maturation and myelination and indicated that immature oligodendrocytes may be enriched at the expense of mature oligodendrocytes. Expression levels of genes related to myelination were then found to be decreased in mouse and human brain samples. Following these discoveries, Ts65Dn mice were used to further investigate the temporal, spatial, and molecular profiles of this dysmyelination phenotype, further identifying decreases in gene and protein expression of myelin components and significant reductions in myelination of the anterior cingulate cortex. As found in human brains, myelination defects in Ts65Dn are concomitant with an increase in the number of oligodendrocyte precursor cells and a decrease in mature oligodendrocytes within major brain white matter tracts. The myelin organization is itself compromised in Ts65Dn with decreases in the number of nodes of Ranvier, which are sites for electrical conduction along the neuronal axons. Reduced expression of key nodal proteins is evident in the brain samples as well. All of these changes to the cells and proteins that form the brain myelin combine to significantly change brain connectivity: the speed of action potentials down the myelinated fibers connecting the two brain hemispheres is reduced in Ts65Dn brains (Olmos-Serrano, Kang, et al., 2016).

Olmos-Serrano, Kang, et al. (2016) also identified several other functional gene pathways that are perturbed in brains of people with DS. One of these pathways relates to the immune response. Throughout life, there is an upregulation in interferon signaling in the frontal cortex of people with DS (Olmos-Serrano, Kang, et al., 2016). This phenotype has been recapitulated in a proteomic study of peripheral blood from people with DS, in embryonic and adult Ts65Dn brains, and in two other segmental trisomy mouse models: Ts1Cje and Dp(16)1/Yey mice (Aziz et al., 2018; Ling et al., 2014; Sullivan et al., 2017). This connection to the immune system is now under active study for future cognitive therapies.

Careful study of Ts65Dn has identified certain aspects of intellectual and motor function that may be altered in DS. Extensive behavioral profiling of Ts65Dn mice has identified impairments in learning and memory using a multitude of cued learning and spatial learning paradigms, such as the Morris water maze (spatial memory/cognitive flexibility involving the hippocampus, striatum, cerebellum, and cortex), contextual fear conditioning (associative memory involving the hippocampus, frontal cortex, cingulate cortex, amygdala, and mediodorsal nucleus of the thalamus), novel object recognition (episodic memory involving the perirhinal cortex and hippocampus), T-Maze, and Y-Maze (short-term working memory; Herault et al., 2017). In addition, motor strength, motor coordination, locomotion, and exploration have been studied using tests such as the Rotarod, grip strength, and open field. Ts65Dn performance has historically varied on Rotarod tests, but these animals display a consistent deficit in all other learning/memory and motor tasks (Aziz et al., 2018; Costa, Stasko, Schmidt, & Davisson, 2010; Costa, Walsh, & Davisson, 1999; Hampton, Stasko, Kale, Amende, & Costa, 2004; Klein et al., 1996; Olmos-Serrano, Tyler, et al., 2016). Recent work has elucidated the cellular underpinning of the motor dysfunction observed in Ts65Dn and identified a developmental and postnatal time course for various neuroanatomical changes within the spinal cord (Aziz et al., 2019). Lastly, Ts65Dn mice show an age-related decline in Morris water maze performance when the same animals were assessed at 2 and at 11 months, indicating that worsening of brain function over the lifespan can be measured in individual animals (Olmos-Serrano, Tyler, et al., 2016). These studies may be useful in understanding which brain functions are altered during life in people with DS, narrowing down the brain areas involved, and providing increased resolution for future cognitive therapies.

Ts1Cje and Ts2Cje

In 1998, approximately a decade after the generation of the Ts65Dn mouse, Sago et al. described the Ts1Cje mouse model of DS (MGI symbol: Ts[16C-tel]1Cje) containing a subset of genes compared to Ts65Dn (Sago et al., 1998). It was generated via reciprocal translocation of the distal portion of Mmu16 onto the telomeric region of Mmu12. This created an elongated Mmu12 carrying an additional dose of 71 Hsa21 genes, but this fusion of Mmu16 genes onto Mmu12 led to the deletion of one copy each of seven telomeric genes (A. Duchon et al., 2011). Ts1Cje mice show no appreciable DS-related brain phenotypes during pre- and perinatal development (Aziz et al., 2018). However, these mice do show defects in both early and late developmental milestones and in motor and cognitive behaviors as adults (Aziz et al., 2018). Although Ts1Cje animals do not contain the nonorthologous triplicated genes found in Ts65Dn, the smaller triplicated segment and loss of a functional copy of *Superoxide dismutase 1* in Ts1Cje led to the scarce use of this model. Nevertheless, comparative analysis of differential gene expression in Ts1Cje, Ts65Dn, and Dp(16)1/Yey brains identify a common dysregulation in interferon-based signaling and immune response both during embryonic development and adulthood (Aziz et al., 2018; Ling et al., 2014). Ts1Cje may therefore be useful for preclinical studies investigating immune regulation.

Similar to the Ts1Cje mouse, the Ts2Cje mouse (MGI symbol: Rb[12.Ts17^{16}65Dn]2Cje) was created by translocation of the Ts65Dn triplicated region onto Mmu12 (Villar et al., 2005). Therefore, the Ts2Cje mouse is a genocopy of the Ts65Dn mouse, but its triplicated region is expressed as an elongation on chromosome 12 rather than a freely segregating chromosome. It remains unknown whether a freely segregating chromosome is necessary for some of the neurological symptoms in the 95% of people with DS who have such a triplication, but comparisons between Ts65Dn and Ts2Cje animals may help resolve this question.

Ts1Rhr and DSCR

To further characterize the genetic basis of the phenotypes observed in the Ts65Dn mice, a new mouse model known as the Ts1Rhr was developed in 2004 by Olsen and colleagues (Olson, Richtsmeier, Leszl, & Reeves, 2004). This mouse was trisomic for a 33-gene subset of the genes triplicated in Ts65Dn and Ts1Cje mice. This subset of genes came to be known as the "DS critical region" (DSCR), which had once been predicted to be sufficient to produce most DS phenotypes. These mice exhibited significant changes in certain learning and memory tasks, including the open field test, the novel object recognition test, and the T-maze. Ts1Rhr mice also showed defects in LTP. However, Ts1Rhr mice did not recapitulate the deficits in overall brain volume, in cerebellar volume, and in the cerebellar granular and Purkinje cell densities seen in Ts65Dn. In addition, Ts1Rhr performance on the Morris water maze, a gold standard learning and memory task, was intact, as were some aspects of hippocampal physiology. Overall, only a subset of phenotypes first found in Ts65Dn showed significant differences between Ts1Rhr and their euploid controls, indicating that the DSCR alone is not sufficient to produce the histopathogenesis seen in Ts65Dn mice. Conversely, normalizing the dosage of the so-called DSCR in Ts65Dn also normalized Morris water maze performance. This led to the final conclusion that the DSCR alone is not sufficient to produce the canonical brain phenotypes associated with DS, but that dosage-sensitive genes within this region clearly subserve learning and memory function in the Ts65Dn mice (N. P. Belichenko et al., 2009; Olson et al., 2007).

Dp(16)1/Yey, Dp(10)2/Yey, and Dp(17)3/Yey Mice and Their Derivatives

To address the issues of DS-irrelevant gene triplication and low numbers of Hsa21 genes in the many mouse models, Li et al. created the Dp(16)1/Yey (MGI symbol: Dp[16Lipi-Zbtb21]1Yey) mouse model of DS in 2007 using Cre-mediated recombination of the entire Hsa21 syntenic region on Mmu16 (Li et al., 2007). This allowed the addition of the entire 23.3Mb segment of Hsa21 orthologues onto the distal portion of Mmu16. Similar to the Ts1Cje, the additional genetic material is carried as an elongation of Mmu16 and not as an additional freely segregating chromosome (Z. Li et al., 2007). Along with the Dp(16)1/Yey mouse model, Li et al. generated two other mouse models using Cre-mediated recombination to triplicate the Hsa21 syntenic regions of Mmu10 and Mmu17. These mice are known as Dp(10)2/Yey (MGI symbol: Dp[10Prmt2-Pdxk]2Yey) and Dp(17)3/Yey (MGI symbol: Dp[17Abcg1-Rrp1b]3Yey), respectively. These three duplication mice can be interbred to generate a compound trisomic mouse containing a triplication of all syntenic regions of Hsa21. While this model may be the most genetically similar to the genetic makeup of individuals with DS, it has two major disadvantages: (a) the cost and difficulty of its breeding is prohibitive, and (b) the trisomy is expressed as an elongation of each duplicated chromosome, unlike the extra freely segregating chromosome in most cases of human DS. Despite its improved genetic similarity to human DS, this compound model was only found to exhibit minor changes such as impaired grip strength, altered contextual fear conditioning, slight dysfunction in hippocampal physiology, and changes in body weight and length (Yu, Li, et al., 2010).

Similar to the compound model, the Dp(16)1/Yey mouse was expected to recapitulate and extend the phenotypes observed in the Ts65Dn mouse. Instead, it showed a unique phenotypic profile. Most strikingly, Dp(16)1/Yey embryonic brains showed none of the anatomical or cytoarchitectural deficits found in the Ts65Dn mice. Instead, the Dp(16)1/Yey mice showed appreciable neuroanatomical defects only around postnatal day 15, in later-acquired developmental milestones, and in adult motor and learning/memory tasks, such as the hindlimb reflex, rotarod, and Morris water maze (Aziz et al., 2018; Goodliffe et al., 2016). These findings challenged a long-held belief that most neurological sequelae of DS, at least those modeled by trisomic mice, originate during embryonic development. In addition, the lack of prenatal brain phenotypes in Dp(16)1/Yey is concomitant with a relatively low number of differentially regulated genes in both the embryonic and adult brain compared to Ts1Cje and Ts65Dn. In theory, the increase in number of triplicated Hsa21 orthologues should drive more exacerbated genomic disruptions. Since this appears not to be the case, new hypotheses have proposed that the additional genes triplicated in

Dp(16)1/Yey may compensate for (or buffer) the deleterious effects of the smaller number of genes in Ts1Cje and Ts65Dn. Alternatively, the mechanism of the triplication is also different (elongation of an existing chromosome versus a freely segregating additional chromosome) and this difference may have an effect on brain development. These potential compensatory mechanisms and/or specific contributions arising from aneuploidy still need to be tested.

An important contribution of studies on the Dp(16)1/Yey, Dp(10)2/Yey, and Dp(17)3/Yey models has been the characterization of the effect of the Mmu17 and Mmu10 syntenic genes on specific DS-related phenotypes. For example, Zhang et al. (2013) showed that some aspects of the learning and memory dysfunction and its underlying anatomical basis may be due to specific combinations of Hsa21 orthologues on Mmu16 and Mmu17 (Zhang et al., 2013), and other studies correlated this combinatorial effect to synaptic physiology as well (Jiang et al., 2015; Yu, Liu, et al., 2010). These studies illustrate the complex relationships between genes on Hsa21 that are at least somewhat preserved among their murine orthologues. To better study gene-phenotype relationships, several mouse lines were derived with consecutively smaller segmental trisomies. These included the Dp1Tyb (MGI symbol: Dp[16Lipi-Zbtb21]1TybEmcf) mice and their derived segmental trisomy models, as well as the group of Dp/DfYah mice, which were constructed using CRISPR/Cas-mediated systems by the Tybuleiwicz/Fisher and Herault laboratories, respectively (Besson et al., 2007; Brault et al., 2015; Duchon, Besson, Pereira, Magnol, & Hérault, 2008; Pereira et al., 2009). These models contain sequentially smaller segments of triplicated or deleted genes and were developed in an attempt to identify the minimal essential genes underlying various DS-related phenotypes in the mouse. Their use led to important discoveries, predominantly about genes that are relevant in congenital heart defects (Lana-Elola et al., 2016; Liu et al., 2014; Raveau et al., 2012).

Single-Gene Models

Prior to the development of suitable DS mouse models, information regarding the role of specific Hsa21 genes came from gene function studies in other fields. Examples of this are *SOD1* and *APP*, which were identified in patient populations with amyotrophic lateral sclerosis and Alzheimer's disease (AD), respectively. However, while gene function has been classically studied with deletion, inactivation, or overexpression approaches, these strategies on their own are not directly applicable to DS. This is because trisomy 21 is not a single-gene disorder, but rather a gene population abnormality. Modern genetic evidence shows that genes operate in networks that are expressed in different tissues of the body (and in different parts of the brain) at different times in development. The triplication of multiple genes in DS therefore alters many different gene networks and can impact different body structures at different times during life. Thus, the study of any single gene should be carried out against this genetic backdrop in order to best replicate the widespread interactions that exist between genes and gene groups in DS. Single-gene models can therefore not be models of DS per se, but some information from these mice has contributed to our understanding of specific gene functions and the networks they operate within. Moreover, knowledge of the action and sequence of single genes that are triplicated in DS allows for gene dosage normalization within the triplicated segments in model mice. These studies are described below for several genes known to play important roles in the pathophysiology of DS.

DYRK1A

The gene encoding the Dual-specificity tyrosine-phosphorylated regulated kinase 1A, or DYRK1A, plays an important role in brain development and brain function in mice and humans and is therefore an attractive candidate to investigate in DS (Moller et al., 2008). DYRK1A has also been implicated in the pathophysiology of AD due to its role in Tau phosphorylation, a hallmark pathological finding in AD. Many researchers have used transgenic mice to study the function of DYRK1A and how its dosage imbalance may affect neurocognition in mice (Altafaj et al., 2001; Dierssen & de Lagrán, 2006; Fotaki et al., 2002; Ruiz-Mejias et al., 2016). However, the most relevant findings come from studies in which the gene dosage or activity of DYRK1A was normalized in trisomic mice. While Ts65Dn mice with a normalized *Dyrk1a* gene dosage still exhibit neuroanatomical abnormalities such as reduced cerebellar volume, these mice show rescues of cell types in the cerebellum, hippocampus, medial septum, and cingulate cortex. They also exhibit decreases in cholinergic degeneration, levels of APP and tau, and tau hyperphosphorylation in select regions of the brain (Garcia-Cerro et al., 2018; García-Cerro, Rueda, Vidal, Lantigua, & Martínez-Cué, 2017). Supporting these gene-dosage correction studies, inhibition of brain DYRK1A with small molecules leads to improved performance on select neurocognitive assessments in both Ts65Dn and Dp16 mice (Nguyen et al., 2018). One prominent DYRK1A inhibitor is epigallocatechine gallate (EGCG). While some evidence indicates that EGCG has beneficial effects in trisomic mouse models (De la Torre et al., 2014; de la Torre & Dierssen, 2012; Duchon & Herault, 2016), evidence that observed cognitive improvements are due to EGCG's direct effect on DYRK1A remains to be confirmed (Stringer, Abeysekera, Dria, Roper, & Goodlett, 2015; Stringer, Goodlett, & Roper, 2017).

RCAN1

RCAN1, also known as *DSCR1*, is another gene of interest in DS, largely due to its role in the regulation of the intracellular calcium sensor calcineurin, vesicular trafficking, oxidative stress, angiogenesis, mitochondrial function, and inflammation (Pritchard & Martin, 2013). *Rcan1* is highly expressed in mouse brains both during embryonic development and postnatally, so it may indeed play a role in various aspects of brain development and function. Mice with *Rcan1* overexpression have multiple neuroanatomical abnormalities, including a reduction in the volume and cell number of the hippocampus as well as in hippocampal neurogenesis and LTP (Martin et al., 2012; Xing et al., 2013). Supporting its role in brain function, *Rcan1* knock-out mice also exhibit deficits in LTP as well as in spatial learning and memory tasks (Hoeffer et al., 2007) and both overexpression and ablation of *Rcan1* in mice decreases exocytosis and affects vesicle fusion and quantal release (Zanin, Mackenzie, Peiris, Pritchard, & Keating, 2013). RCAN1 has also been shown to play a role in tumor growth during cancer. In fact, when mice that model human lung adenocarcinoma were bred with *Rcan1* knock-out mice, tumor growth was decreased and survival rates improved (M. Shin, Siffel, & Correa, 2010). Similar findings were obtained from a study on mice modeling pancreatic cancer (Lee, Shin, & Baek, 2013). These observations suggest that RCAN1 may play a protective role in people with DS, since the incidence of most solid tumors is significantly reduced in the DS population. Using a gene-dosage normalization strategy to normalize *Rcan1* triplication in Ts65Dn mice, Baek and colleagues showed that *Rcan1* triplication is necessary for tumor size reduction but did not determine whether this affected the neurological phenotypes in this mouse (Baek et al., 2009). Together, the evidence from these studies identify *Rcan1* as a potential major player in DS phenotypes and set the stage for more in-depth studies within DS mouse models.

OLIG1/2

Oligodendrocyte transcription factors (*Olig*) *1* and *2* are also found on Hsa21 and are typically triplicated in mouse models of DS. Several studies in the early 2000s identified the role of these transcription factors in the developing CNS, demonstrating the expression pattern and some unique roles of OLIG1/2 in oligodendrocyte lineage specification in brain and spinal cord (Lu et al., 2000; Takebayashi et al., 2000; Zhou & Anderson, 2002). Prior to their expression in oligodendrocyte precursors, OLIG1/2 are also expressed in other cell types affected in DS, including the neurogenic populations giving rise to either inhibitory cortical interneurons or spinal motor neurons during early embryogenesis (Lu et al., 2002; Mizuguchi et al., 2001; Novitch, Chen, & Jessell, 2001). This discovery of bipotential *Olig1/2*-expressing progenitors cemented the importance of these two genes in the specification and differentiation of not only oligodendrocytes, but principle neuronal populations within both the brain and spinal cord. Since then, several researchers have focused on the mechanisms of action of OLIG1/2 in these distinct cell types using a variety of animal models. One tool that was developed to further characterize the importance of OLIG1/2 in CNS development was the *Olig1/2* knock-out mouse model. Studies in the spinal cords of these mutant mice showed an ablation in the motor neuron population as well as a block in the differentiation of spinal oligodendrocytes (Zhou & Anderson, 2002). In addition, because these two genes are expressed on Hsa21, their role in DS-related CNS phenotypes has been of great interest. For example, Chakrabarti et al. (2010) identified several developmental brain phenotypes in Ts65Dn mice that correlated with the triplication of the *Olig1/2* genes. Specifically, perinatal Ts65Dn mice were found to have an overproduction of a subset of inhibitory interneurons in the forebrain coupled with an increase in proliferation and shifts in gene expression in the progenitors of these interneurons during embryogenesis (Chakrabarti et al., 2010). Normalization of the gene dosage of just *Olig1/2* in these Ts65Dn mice rescued these phenotypes. This work, which was the first to show a misallocation of neuronal subtypes in the Ts65Dn cortex and hippocampus and to identify the developmental changes giving rise to these postnatal brain phenotypes, was recently reproduced in a study utilizing human induced pluripotent stem cells and chimeric mouse brains (Xu, Roby, & Callaway, 2010). In additional study with *Olig2*-overexpressing transgenic line, Liu et al. (2015) showed that *Olig2* upregulation in cortical progenitors led to early cell cycle exit, widespread cell death, microcephaly, cortical dyslamination, hippocampus malformation, and profound motor deficits. Ectopic misexpression of *Olig2* impaired cortical progenitor proliferation and caused precocious cell cycle exit (Liu et al., 2015). This study also showed that *Olig2* is a negative regulator of *Nfatc4*, *Dscr1/Rcan1*, and *Dyrk1a*, other critical neurogenic genes present on Hsa21. How these interactions are affected when those genes, as well as all other Hsa21 genes, are triplicated is still under investigation.

Aging Phenotypes

Several main findings in people aging with DS have either been discovered or recapitulated in mouse models, in particular in the Ts65Dn mouse. The Ts65Dn mice exhibit an array of phenotypes suggestive of an early-aging phenotype. These include a progressive degeneration of cholinergic neurons in the basal forebrain, increases in APP levels in the hippocampus and striatum, changes in synapses and synaptic plasticity, loss in neurotrophic signaling, changes in monoamine neurotransmitter levels, deterioration in spatial learning and memory, and decreased cognitive flexibility (Cooper et al., 2001; Dekker et al., 2017; Granholm, Sanders, & Crnic, 2000; Hunter, Bimonte, & Granholm, 2003; Hunter, Isacson, et al., 2003; Hyde & Crnic, 2001; Olmos-Serrano, Tyler, et al., 2016). Linking the gene triplication in DS to aging phenotypes, some of these changes were not observed in mouse models of DS where *App* is not triplicated. Specifically, changes in cholinergic neurons and neurotrophic signaling were not seen in Ts1Cje mice that contain only two copies of *App*, in contrast to the Ts65Dn mice which contain three copies (Salehi et al., 2006). These data are notable because they implicate the gene dosage of *App* in these hallmark phenotypes. While *App* gene expression, APP protein levels, and amount of soluble APP protein fragments increase with age in Ts65Dn brains, levels of Abeta40 and Abeta42 do not (Choi et al., 2009). In addition, due to the difference in the amino acid sequence of the human and murine APP, Ts65Dn brains do not form or accumulate amyloid plaques (Jankowsky et al., 2007). Therefore, while APP likely plays an important role in aging in Ts65Dn mice, its differential processing in humans may be linked to additional phenotypes that are not replicated in the mice. Additional age-related phenotypes in Ts65Dn mice, perhaps unlinked to APP, include dysregulation in global brain protein expression that is exacerbated with age, particularly in the cortex (Ahmed, Block, Tong, Davisson, & Gardiner, 2017). Altered autophagy, mTOR signaling, and protein oxidation in aged Ts65Dn brains have also been reported (Tramutola et al., 2016).

Aging-related deficits were also observed in the Dp(16)1/Yey mouse model of DS. In particular, these were most pronounced in spatial memory and cognitive flexibility as assessed by an improved Morris water maze paradigm (Goodliffe et al., 2016). In addition, the degeneration of cholinergic neurons was observed in the spinal cord (Watson-Scales et al., 2018). Tc1 mice also exhibited age-related decrease in cholinergic neurons in the spinal cord (Watson-Scales et al., 2018), but due to lack of *App* triplication, this mouse model has not been extensively used for age-related studies in DS.

Other Murine Phenotypes and How They Relate to DS

Aside from the neuropathologies outlined above, mouse models of DS also recapitulate some other DS-related changes. These include craniofacial alterations, musculoskeletal abnormalities, and congenital heart defects (CHD; Billingsley et al., 2013; Blazek, Abeysekera, Li, & Roper, 2015; Blazek, Gaddy, Meyer, Roper, & Li, 2011; Richtsmeier, Zumwalt, Carlson, Epstein, & Reeves, 2002). Because 40% of newborns with DS present with CHD, this aspect of the syndrome has been the focus of many studies in the past 5 years, and CHD can be observed in Ts65Dn, Ts1Cje, Dp(16)1/Yey, Dp1Tyb, and Tc1 mice. Therefore, the reproducibility of this phenotype in multiple cytogenetically distinct models has confirmed its validity and allowed for more detailed analyses of its genetic underpinnings. For example, CRISPR/Cas-mediated chromosomal rearrangement technology has been used to generate a variety of Dp1Tyb-derived mice with sequentially smaller segments of the syntenic region on Mmu16. In this manner, these investigators are able to map the dosage-sensitive genes and the minimum required region for CHD induction (Lana-Elola et al., 2016; Li et al., 2016).

In addition, several groups have identified widespread dysregulation in the immune system of people with DS. These changes were reproduced and further investigated in several mouse models of DS. The results indicate that gene networks related to inflammation and immune responses in the brain are perturbed over the lifespan of Ts1Cje, Ts65Dn, and Dp(16)1/Yey mice. This phenotype represents a systemwide abnormality affecting brain health during important stages of development and throughout life (Aziz et al., 2018; Olmos-Serrano, Kang, et al., 2016; Sullivan et al., 2017).

Gene-Dosage Hypothesis Versus Aneuploidy—Gene/Phenotype Relationship

The assertion that gene dosage underpins DS phenotypes has long governed mechanistic studies aimed at elucidating relationships between particular genes and observed phenotypes (Chakrabarti et al., 2010; M. A. Pritchard & Kola, 1999; Rachidi & Lopes, 2008;

Roper & Reeves, 2006). Testing this hypothesis in humans has been extremely complex and impractical given the scarcity of tissue and the inability to alter single genes, or groups of genes, to test outcomes. Thus, mouse models have become once again an invaluable tool in the quest to characterize the contributions of specific genes to DS phenotypes. Tissue-specific transcriptomic analyses in human brains and in Ts65Dn and Ts1Cje mice have shed light on the fact that dysregulation in gene expression is subtle, yet not uniform, across different areas of the cerebral cortex and that widespread aberrations in regions of the genome that are not triplicated are also present. These studies have revealed complex regulation that is not solely explained by allelic number (Aziz et al., 2018; Goodliffe et al., 2016; Guedj, Pennings, Ferres, et al., 2015; Guedj, Pennings, Wick, & Bianchi, 2015; Kahlem et al., 2004; Letourneau et al., 2014; Lyle, Gehrig, Neergaard-Henrichsen, Deutsch, & Antonarakis, 2004; Olmos-Serrano, Kang, et al., 2016; Potier et al., 2006; Saran, Pletcher, Natale, Cheng, & Reeves, 2003). Other work on the DSCR in mice reinforced the fact that, unlike single-gene mutation disorders (e.g., fragile X or Tay-Sachs disease), dysregulation of single genes or even smaller subsets of genes is not sufficient to produce a DS-relevant phenotype. Rather, the unique genetic landscape arising from the additive global effect of Hsa21 syntenic gene triplication is in itself necessary to produce the common phenotypes associated with DS (Olson, Richtsmeier, et al., 2004).

The hypothesis that small cumulative genetic or epigenetic changes manifest as DS phenotypes may offer an explanation for the presence of histological phenotypes in Ts65Dn but not Ts1Cje embryonic brains, since the former has more triplicated genes. However, this is largely contradicted by the lack of phenotype in Dp(16)1/Yey embryos. Since somatic and brain-growth abnormalities are measurable during gestation in fetuses with DS, the DS phenotypes found in Ts65Dn mice would be expected to be exacerbated as the number of triplicated genes within the Mmu16 syntenic region increases (e.g., in Dp[16]1/Yey). However, this is not the case (Aziz et al., 2018; Goodliffe et al., 2016). Thus, the gene-dosage hypothesis alone is not sufficient to explain the sequelae of Hsa21 triplication. Significant factors to consider are the physical state of triplicated chromatin and the presence of an additional chromosome, or aneuploidy, in 95% of cases of DS (Shin et al., 2010). According to the amplified developmental instability hypothesis, most DS phenotypes may be a result of a non-gene-specific disturbance in chromosomal balance, leading to disrupted homeostasis (Pritchard & Kola, 1999). This hypothesis suggests a common mechanism underlying abnormal phenotypes observed in people with different aneuploidies (i.e., trisomies 21, 18, and 13), while simultaneously accounting for inter-individual variation among people with DS. Thus, aneuploidy itself may be a major determinant in the manifestation of DS phenotypes.

In-depth cellular studies in Ts65Dn mice have shown that Ts65Dn embryos and neonates exhibit decreased proliferation and elongation of the cell cycle in the brain and in peripheral tissue (Chakrabarti et al., 2007; Contestabile, Fila, Bartesaghi, et al., 2009; Contestabile, Fila, Cappellini, et al., 2009; Contestabile et al., 2007). Furthermore, gene expression analysis in these mice pinpointed a specific decrease in regulators of G(2)/M and G(1)/S cell cycle transition (Contestabile et al., 2007). Thus, we suggest that cell-cycle aberrations due to the presence of an additional chromosome in Ts65Dn mice may be necessary in conjunction with the gene-dosage imbalance for the induction of the unique abnormalities seen in embryonic brain morphogenesis in this model. This is a possible explanation for why Ts1Cje and Dp(16)1/Yey (and other) embryos show no apparent DS-related prenatal brain development deficits. Thus, the combination of abnormal gene dosage and developmental instability, resulting from the aneuploidy itself, may be a major modulator of abnormal brain phenotypes in the mouse. This theory may be further substantiated by evidence that people with a translocation of the long arm of chromosome 21, who have triplication of Hsa21 genes but no aneuploidy, exhibit less severe phenotypes compared to the 95% of people with DS who have aneuploidy (Chandra et al., 2010; Prasher, 1995). Further supporting this idea, evidence from assessments of synaptic integrity, dendritic branching, and spine morphology in adult Ts65Dn and Ts1Cje indicated that some of the Ts65Dn cellular phenotypes were present but were significantly less severe in Ts1Cje mice (P. V. Belichenko et al., 2007). Additional large-scale studies are necessary to fully characterize molecular, histological, and cognitive differences in these two affected human populations and to compare aneuploid to nonaneuploid mouse models.

A Mouse Is Not a Human

While the use of mouse models in biomedical research has been immensely fruitful, several caveats need to be noted when using mice to model brain development and function of high-ordered organisms, such as nonhuman primates and humans. Many of the findings described in this chapter are similar between mice and humans. However, detailed analyses of murine and primate brain development and cytoarchitecture uncover multiple inconsistencies that should be considered when interpreting data.

First, germinal zone complexity differs immensely between mice and human/nonhuman primates, with primates exhibiting an increase in varieties of neural progenitors and in the physical size of the germinal zone, which likely relate to the increased neuronal heterogeneity and elevated cognitive capacity in primates (Defelipe, 2011; Rakic, 1995). While the origins of certain cell types, such as interneurons (INs), are similar between mice and primates, their proportions differ greatly. For example INs make up approximately 15% of cortical neurons in mice, yet that population balloons to approximately 25%–30% in humans (Kawaguchi & Kubota, 1997; Markram et al., 2004). Second, excitatory neurons, in particular layer III pyramidal cells, also fundamentally differ in their structural and physiological properties between mice and primates (Luebke, 2017). Third, the process of myelination also differs greatly between mice and humans, as myelinogenesis begins around midgestation in humans but postnatally in mice (de Graaf-Peters & Hadders-Algra, 2006; Igor Jakovcevski; I. Jakovcevski, Filipovic, Mo, Rakic, & Zecevic,

2009). In addition, myelination is complete at approximately P21 in mice but not until the third decade of life in humans (Barrera et al., 2013; de Graaf-Peters & Hadders-Algra, 2006; Stiles & Jernigan, 2010). Lastly, spatiotemporal distribution of oligodendrocyte differentiation signals also differ between mouse and human and may in fact underlie the unique vulnerability of humans to demyelinating diseases (I. Jakovcevski et al., 2009).

Thus, while many concepts learned from mouse brain studies are generalizable to humans, careful attention should be paid when modeling development, organization, and function of human CNS in mice, especially in such a complex genetic disorder as DS.

An Expanded Preclinical Pipeline

Despite the caveats noted in the preceding section, several key biological processes in the brain (including cerebellar development, white matter formation, and establishing the ratio of excitatory and inhibitory neurons) appear to be shared between mouse models and people with DS. In fact, the slower proliferation and expansion of the precursor cells in the external granule layer of the cerebellum was first identified in the Ts65Dn mouse and then replicated in other models before being confirmed in human studies (Contestabile et al., 2007; Guidi et al., 2011; Gutierrez-Castellanos et al., 2013; Patkee et al., 2022; Roper et al., 2006). The mechanisms leading to this slower cerebellar neurogenesis appear to be due to reductions in signaling through the Sonic Hedgehog (Shh) pathway. Since alterations in the cerebellum could influence motor and cognitive function in persons with DS, researchers now aims to test whether Shh agonists may form part of a comprehensive strategy to improve these neurological aspects in people with DS. The same path to treatment (i.e., replication of a brain alteration in models and people prior to the onset of preclinical and clinical trials) is also being pursued for the white-matter defects and the excitatory/inhibitory imbalance. While the traditional clinical trial pathway would have historically moved from trisomic mice to people with DS, the advent of individual-specific pluripotent stem cells now enables preclinical testing on the exact human cell type targeted for a given treatment. These stem cells, isolated from a person while in a clinic, offer the advantage of using a person's own cells for research on their particular individual manifestation of the disorder. As this technology advances, the response of these cells to treatments will be measured within a 3D environment closely matching their in vivo niche. This will greatly improve the selectivity and efficacy of future approaches to the neurological sequelae of DS.

The Future of Mouse Models of DS

Mouse models of DS can provide tangible insights for drug discovery, and model selection is a critical first step for establishing an experimental paradigm with high translational potential (McGonigle, 2014; Perrin, 2014). These models are essential for target discovery, as well as for toxicological, pharmacological, dosage, and timing of administration studies and are thus an important step in transitioning an experimental drug from the lab to the clinic. As such, rigorous preclinical studies focusing on how phenotypes manifest in mice and human and their timing of onset are essential. These data will identify the appropriate model based on the proposed drug's mechanism of action and timing of administration. As spatiotemporal targeting of therapeutic intervention is likely to be the most effective in ameliorating life-stage specific DS phenotypes, models should be chosen carefully based on the onset and magnitude of DS-relevant phenotypes for preclinical trials. Additionally, a rigorous standardized screen of phenotypic changes should be adopted when analyzing drug efficacy; establishing proper endpoints is key when determining the translational value of a therapeutic. Recent work provides a framework for such a screen, showing combinatorial data regarding gene expression, histology, and behavior at key points over the lifespan of mice of multiple strains (Aziz et al., 2018). This minimum essential screen should be employed to ensure consistency in experimental setups, improve reproducibility of results, and provide endpoints and biomarkers in future drug screens and clinical trials. Despite their many shortcomings, mouse models of DS have aided in-depth characterization of many DS-related phenotypes over the past three decades. Their use in preclinical studies will eventually lead to successful therapeutic development that will undoubtedly greatly improve the quality of life of individuals with DS and their community of caregivers.

Conclusion

Neurological hallmarks of DS include intellectual disability, motor dysfunction, and early onset of Alzheimer's neuropathology. These postnatal phenotypes are preceded by consistent and widespread histological changes in fetal brains and delayed acquisition of developmental milestones starting at birth. Thus, current scientific evidence suggests that early changes in neural development may establish the path for the observed CNS abnormalities throughout life. However, knowledge gleaned from both DS clinical research and mouse model studies also indicates that the complex constellation of symptoms associated with DS changes in unique ways over the lifespan. Therefore, while embryogenesis my present the ideal treatment window, other periods throughout life may also represent favorable and accessible moments for age-specific therapeutic interventions. Mouse models of DS have been used as a first foray into understanding these spatiotemporal anatomical, cellular, and molecular changes. Joined together with patient-specific stem-cell systems, these tools will be critical for fully understanding the cellular and molecular time course of DS and supporting future drug development efforts aimed at providing greater quality of life and independence for people with DS

References

Ahmed, M. M., Block, A., Tong, S., Davisson, M. T., & Gardiner, K. J. (2017). Age exacerbates abnormal protein expression in a mouse model of Down syndrome. *Neurobiology of Aging*, *57*, 120–132. doi:10.1016/j.neurobiolaging.2017.05.002

Altafaj, X., Dierssen, M., Baamonde, C., Martí, E., Visa, J., Guimerà, J., . . . Estivill, X. (2001). Neurodevelopmental delay, motor abnormalities and cognitive deficits in transgenic mice overexpressing Dyrk1A (minibrain), a murine model of Down's syndrome. *Human Molecular Genetics, 10*(18), 1915–1923. doi:10.1093/hmg/10.18.1915

Araujo, B. H., Torres, L. B., & Guilhoto, L. M. (2015). Cerebal overinhibition could be the basis for the high prevalence of epilepsy in persons with Down syndrome. *Epilepsy Behav, 53*, 120–125. doi:10.1016/j.yebeh.2015.10.004

Aziz, N. M., Guedj, F., Pennings, J. L. A., Olmos-Serrano, J. L., Siegel, A., Haydar, T. F., & Bianchi, D. W. (2018). Lifespan analysis of brain development, gene expression and behavioral phenotypes in the Ts1Cje, Ts65Dn and Dp(16)1/Yey mouse models of Down syndrome. *Disease Models & Mechanisms, 11*(6). doi:10.1242/dmm.031013

Aziz, N. M., Klein, J. A., Brady, M. R., Olmos-Serrano, J. L., Gallo, V., & Haydar, T. F. (2019). Spatiotemporal development of spinal neuronal and glial populations in the Ts65Dn mouse model of Down syndrome. *Journal of Neurodevelpmental Disorders, 11*(1), 35. doi:10.1186/s11689-019-9294-9

Baek, K.–H., Zaslavsky, A., Lynch, R. C., Britt, C., Okada, Y., Siarey, R. J., . . . Ryeom, S. (2009). Down's syndrome suppression of tumour growth and the role of the calcineurin inhibitor DSCR1. *Nature, 459*(7250), 1126–1130. doi:10.1038/nature08062

Bahado–Singh, R. O., Wyse, L., Dorr, M. A., Copel, J. A., O'Connor, T., & Hobbins, J. C. (1992). Fetuses with Down syndrome have disproportionately shortened frontal lobe dimensions on ultrasonographic examination. *American Journal of Obstetrics and Gynecology, 167*(4 Pt 1), 1009–1014.

Barrera, K., Chu, P., Abramowitz, J., Steger, R., Ramos, R. L., & Brumberg, J. C. (2013). Organization of myelin in the mouse somatosensory barrel cortex and the effects of sensory deprivation. *Developmental Neurobiology, 73*(4), 297–314. doi:10.1002/dneu.22060

Bartesaghi, R., Haydar, T. F., Delabar, J. M., Dierssen, M., Martínez–Cué, C., & Bianchi, D. W. (2015). New perspectives for the rescue of cognitive disability in Down syndrome. *Journal of Neuroscience, 35*(41), 13843–13852. doi:10.1523/JNEUROSCI.2775-15.2015

Baxter, L. L., Moran, T. H., Richtsmeier, J. T., Troncoso, J., & Reeves, R. H. (2000). Discovery and genetic localization of Down syndrome cerebellar phenotypes using the Ts65Dn mouse. *Human Molecular Genetics, 9*(2), 195–202.

Becker, L. E., Armstrong, D. L., & Chan, F. (1986). Dendritic atrophy in children with Down's syndrome. *Annals of Neurology, 20*(4), 520–526.

Becker, L., Mito, T., Takashima, S., & Onodera, K. (1991). Growth and development of the brain in Down syndrome. *Progress in Clinical and Biological Research, 373*, 133–152.

Belichenko, N. P., Belichenko, P. V., Kleschevnikov, A. M., Salehi, A., Reeves, R. H., & Mobley, W. C. (2009). The "Down syndrome critical region" is sufficient in the mouse model to confer behavioral, neurophysiological, and synaptic phenotypes characteristic of Down syndrome. *Journal of Neuroscience, 29*(18), 5938–5948. doi:10.1523/jneurosci.1547-09.2009

Belichenko, P. V., Kleschevnikov, A. M., Salehi, A., Epstein, C. J., & Mobley, W. C. (2007). Synaptic and cognitive abnormalities in mouse models of Down syndrome: Exploring genotype-phenotype relationships. *The Journal of Comparative Neurology, 504*(4), 329–345. doi:10.1002/cne.21433

Belichenko, P. V., Masliah, E., Kleschevnikov, A. M., Villar, A. J., Epstein, C. J., Salehi, A., & Mobley, W. C. (2004). Synaptic structural abnormalities in the Ts65Dn mouse model of Down Syndrome. *The Journal of Comparative Neurology, 480*(3), 281–298. doi:10.1002/cne.20337

Besson, V., Brault, V., Duchon, A., Togbe, D., Bizot, J.–C., Quesniaux, V. F. J., . . . Hérault, Y. (2007). Modeling the monosomy for the telomeric part of human chromosome 21 reveals haploinsufficient genes modulating the inflammatory and airway responses. *Human Molecular Genetics, 16*(17), 2040–2052. doi:10.1093/hmg/ddm152

Billingsley, C. N., Allen, J. R., Baumann, D. D., Deitz, S. L., Blazek, J. D., Newbauer, A., . . . Roper, R. J. (2013). Non-trisomic homeobox gene expression during craniofacial development in the Ts65Dn mouse model of Down syndrome. *American Journal of Medical Genetics, Part A, 161a*(8), 1866–1874. doi:10.1002/ajmg.a.36006

Blazek, J. D., Abeysekera, I., Li, J., & Roper, R. J. (2015). Rescue of the abnormal skeletal phenotype in Ts65Dn Down syndrome mice using genetic and therapeutic modulation of trisomic Dyrk1a. *Human Molecular Genetics, 24*(20), 5687–5696. doi:10.1093/hmg/ddv284

Blazek, J. D., Gaddy, A., Meyer, R., Roper, R. J., & Li, J. (2011). Disruption of bone development and homeostasis by trisomy in Ts65Dn Down syndrome mice. *Bone, 48*(2), 275–280. doi:10.1016/j.bone.2010.09.028

Bostelmann, M., Costanzo, F., Martorana, L., Menghini, D., Vicari, S., Lavenex, P. B., & Lavenex, P. (2018). Low-resolution place and response learning capacities in Down syndrome. *Frontiers in Psychology, 9,* 2049. doi:10.3389/fpsyg.2018.02049

Brault, V., Duchon, A., Romestaing, C., Sahun, I., Pothion, S., Karout, M., . . . Hérault, Y. (2015). Opposite phenotypes of muscle strength and locomotor function in mouse models of partial trisomy and monosomy 21 for the proximal Hspa13-App region. *PLoS Genetics, 11*(3), e1005062. doi:10.1371/journal.pgen.1005062

Chakrabarti, L., Best, T. K., Cramer, N. P., Carney, R. S., Isaac, J. T., Galdzicki, Z., & Haydar, T. F. (2010). Olig1 and Olig2 triplication causes developmental brain defects in Down syndrome. *Nature Neuroscience, 13*(8), 927–934. doi:10.1038/nn.2600

Chakrabarti, L., Galdzicki, Z., & Haydar, T. F. (2007). Defects in embryonic neurogenesis and initial synapse formation in the forebrain of the Ts65Dn mouse model of Down syndrome. *Journal of Neuroscience, 27*(43), 11483–11495. doi:10.1523/jneurosci.3406-07.2007

Chandra, N., Cyril, C., Lakshminarayana, P., Nallasivam, P., Ramesh, A., Gopinath, P. M., & Marimuthu, K. M. (2010). Cytogenetic evaluation of Down syndrome: A Review of 1020 referral cases. *International Journal of Human Genetics, 10*(1–3), 87–93. doi.org/10.1080/09723757.2010.11886090

Choi, J. H. K., Berger, J. D., Mazzella, M. J., Morales-Corraliza, J., Cataldo, A. M., Nixon, R. A., . . . Mathews, P. M. (2009). Age-dependent dysregulation of brain amyloid precursor protein in the Ts65Dn Down syndrome mouse model. *Journal of Neurochemistry, 110*(6), 1818–1827. doi:10.1111/j.1471-4159.2009.06277.x

Contestabile, A., Fila, T., Bartesaghi, R., & Ciani, E. (2009). Cell cycle elongation impairs proliferation of cerebellar granule cell precursors in the Ts65Dn mouse, an animal model for Down syndrome. *Brain Pathology, 19*(2), 224–237. doi:10.1111/j.1750-3639.2008.00168.x

Contestabile, A., Fila, T., Cappellini, A., Bartesaghi, R., & Ciani, E. (2009). Widespread impairment of cell proliferation in the neonate Ts65Dn mouse, a model for Down syndrome. *Cell Proliferation, 42*(2), 171–181. doi:10.1111/j.1365-2184.2009.00587.x

Contestabile, A., Fila, T., Ceccarelli, C., Bonasoni, P., Bonapace, L., Santini, D., . . . Ciani, E. (2007). Cell cycle alteration and decreased cell proliferation in the hippocampal dentate gyrus and in the neocortical germinal matrix of fetuses with Down syndrome and in Ts65Dn mice. *Hippocampus, 17*(8), 665–678. doi:10.1002/hipo.20308

Cooper, J. D., Salehi, A., Delcroix, J. D., Howe, C. L., Belichenko, P. V., Chua-Couzens, J., . . . Mobley, W. C. (2001). Failed retrograde transport of NGF in a mouse model of Down's syndrome: Reversal of cholinergic neurodegenerative phenotypes following NGF infusion. *Proceedings of the National Academy of Sciences of the United States of America, 98*(18), 10439–10444. doi:10.1073/pnas.181219298

Costa, A. C., Stasko, M. R., Schmidt, C., & Davisson, M. T. (2010). Behavioral validation of the Ts65Dn mouse model for Down syndrome of a genetic background free of the retinal degeneration mutation Pde6b(rd1). *Behavioural Brain Research, 206*(1), 52–62. doi:10.1016/j.bbr.2009.08.034

Costa, A. C., Walsh, K., & Davisson, M. T. (1999). Motor dysfunction in a mouse model for Down syndrome. *Physiology & Behavior, 68*(1–2), 211–220. doi:10.1016/s0031-9384(99)00178-x

Coyle, J. T., Oster-Granite, M. L., & Gearhart, J. D. (1986). The neurobiologic consequences of Down syndrome. *Brain Research Bulletin, 16*(6), 773–787.

Das, I., Park, J. M., Shin, J. H., Jeon, S. K., Lorenzi, H., Linden, D. J., . . . Reeves, R. H. (2013). Hedgehog agonist therapy corrects structural and cognitive deficits in a Down syndrome mouse model. *Science Translational Medicine, 5*(201), 101–120. doi:10.1126/scitranslmed.3005983

Das, I., & Reeves, R. H. (2011). The use of mouse models to understand and improve cognitive deficits in Down syndrome. *Disease Models & Mechanisms, 4*(5), 596–606. doi:10.1242/dmm.007716

Davisson, M. T., Schmidt, C., & Akeson, E. C. (1990). Segmental trisomy of murine chromosome 16: A new model system for studying Down syndrome. *Progress in Clinical and Biological Research, 360,* 263–280.

de Graaf-Peters, V. B., & Hadders-Algra, M. (2006). Ontogeny of the human central nervous system: What is happening when? *Early Human Development, 82*(4), 257–266. doi:10.1016/j.earlhumdev.2005.10.013

De la Torre, R., De Sola, S., Pons, M., Duchon, A., de Lagran, M. M., Farré, M., . . . Dierssen, M. (2014). Epigallocatechin-3-gallate, a DYRK1A inhibitor, rescues cognitive deficits in Down syndrome mouse models and in humans. *Molecular Nutrition & Food Research, 58*(2), 278–288. doi:10.1002/mnfr.201300325 de la Torre, R., & Dierssen, M. (2012). Therapeutic approaches in the improvement of cognitive performance in Down syndrome: Past, present, and future. *Progress in Brain Research, 197*, 1–14. doi:10.1016/B978-0-444-54299-1.00001-7

de Wert, G., Dondorp, W., & Bianchi, D. W. (2016). Fetal therapy for Down syndrome: An ethical exploration. *Prenatal Diagnosis, 37*(3), 222–228. doi:10.1002/pd.4995

Defelipe, J. (2011). The evolution of the brain, the human nature of cortical circuits, and intellectual creativity. *Frontiers in Neuroanatomy, 5*, 29. doi:10.3389/fnana.2011.00029

Dekker, A. D., Vermeiren, Y., Albac, C., Lana-Elola, E., Watson-Scales, S., Gibbins, D., . . . De Deyn, P. P. (2017). Aging rather than aneuploidy affects monoamine neurotransmitters in brain regions of Down syndrome mouse models. *Neurobiology of Disease, 105*, 235–244. doi:10.1016/j.nbd.2017.06.007

Dierssen, M., & de Lagrán, M. M. (2006). DYRK1A (dual-specificity tyrosine-phosphorylated and -regulated kinase 1A): a gene with dosage effect during development and neurogenesis. *The Scientific World Journal, 6*, 1911–1922. doi:10.1100/tsw.2006.319

Duchon, A., Besson, V., Pereira, P. L., Magnol, L., & Hérault, Y. (2008). Inducing segmental aneuploid mosaicism in the mouse through targeted asymmetric sister chromatid event of recombination. *Genetics, 180*(1), 51–59. doi:10.1534/genetics.108.092312

Duchon, A., & Herault, Y. (2016). DYRK1A, a dosage-sensitive gene involved in neurodevelopmental disorders, is a target for drug development in Down syndrome. *Frontiers in Behavioral Neuroscience, 10*, 104. doi:10.3389/fnbeh.2016.00104

Duchon, A., Raveau, M., Chevalier, C., Nalesso, V., Sharp, A. J., & Herault, Y. (2011). Identification of the translocation breakpoints in the Ts65Dn and Ts1Cje mouse lines: Relevance for modeling Down syndrome. *Mammalian Genome Society, 22*(11–12), 674–684. doi:10.1007/s00335-011-9356-0

Farran, E. K., Bowler, A., Karmiloff-Smith, A., D'Souza, H., Mayall, L., & Hill, E. L. (2019). Cross-domain associations between motor ability, independent exploration, and large-scale spatial navigation; Attention deficit hyperactivity disorder, Williams syndrome, and typical development. *Frontiers in Human Neuroscience, 13*, 225. doi:10.3389/fnhum.2019.00225

Fidler, D. J., & Nadel, L. (2007). Education and children with Down syndrome: Neuroscience, development, and intervention. *Mental Retardation and Developmental Disabilities Research Reviews, 13*(3), 262–271. doi:10.1002/mrdd.20166

Fotaki, V., Dierssen, M., Alcántara, S., Martínez, S., Martí, E., Casas, C., . . . Arbonés, M. L. (2002). Dyrk1A haploinsufficiency affects viability and causes developmental delay and abnormal brain morphology in mice. *Molecular and Cellular Biology, 22*(18), 6636–6647. doi:10.1128/MCB.22.18.6636-6647.2002

Foti, F., Menghini, D., Alfieri, P., Costanzo, F., Mandolesi, L., Petrosini, L., & Vicari, S. (2018). Learning by observation and learning by doing in Down and Williams syndromes. *Developmental Science, 21*(5), e12642. doi:10.1111/desc.12642

García-Cerro, S., Rueda, N., Vidal, V., Lantigua, S., & Martínez-Cué, C. (2017). Normalizing the gene dosage of Dyrk1A in a mouse model of Down syndrome rescues several Alzheimer's disease phenotypes. *Neurobiology of Disease, 106*, 76–88. doi:10.1016/j.nbd.2017.06.010

Garcia-Cerro, S., Vidal, V., Lantigua, S., Berciano, M. T., Lafarga, M., Ramos-Cabrer, P., . . . Martinez-Cue, C. (2018). Cerebellar alterations in a model of Down syndrome: The role of the Dyrk1A gene. *Neurobiology of Disease, 110*, 206–217. doi:10.1016/j.nbd.2017.12.002

Gardiner, K. J. (2015). Pharmacological approaches to improving cognitive function in Down syndrome: Current status and considerations. *Drug Design, Development and Therapy, 9*, 103–125. doi:10.2147/dddt.s51476

Gearhart, J. D., Davisson, M. T., & Oster-Granite, M. L. (1986). Autosomal aneuploidy in mice: Generation and developmental consequences. *Brain Research Bulletin, 16*(6), 789–801.

Gibson, D., Groeneweg, G., Jerry, P., & Harris, A. (1988). Age and pattern of intellectual decline among Down syndrome and other mentally retarded adults. *International Journal of Rehabilitation Research, 11*(1), 47–55.

Gil, M. M., Quezada, M. S., Revello, R., Akolekar, R., & Nicolaides, K. H. (2015). Analysis of cell-free DNA in maternal blood in screening for fetal aneuploidies: Updated meta-analysis. *Ultrasound in Obstetrics & Gynecology, 45*(3), 249–266. doi:10.1002/uog.14791

Golden, J. A., & Hyman, B. T. (1994). Development of the superior temporal neocortex is anomalous in trisomy 21. *Journal of Neuropathology and Experimental Neurology, 53*(5), 513–520.

Goodliffe, J. W., Olmos-Serrano, J. L., Aziz, N. M., Pennings, J. L., Guedj, F., Bianchi, D. W., & Haydar, T. F. (2016). Absence of prenatal forebrain defects in the Dp(16)1Yey/+ mouse model of Down syndrome. *Journal of Neuroscience, 36*(10), 2926–2944. doi:10.1523/jneurosci.2513-15.2016

Granholm, A.-C. E., Sanders, L. A., & Crnic, L. S. (2000). Loss of cholinergic phenotype in basal forebrain coincides with cognitive decline in a mouse model of Down's syndrome. *Experimental Neurology, 161*(2), 647–663. doi:10.1006/exnr.1999.7289

Granno, S., Nixon–Abell, J., Berwick, D. C., Tosh, J., Heaton, G., Almudimeegh, S., . . . Harvey, K. (2019). Downregulated Wnt/β-catenin signalling in the Down syndrome hippocampus. *Scientific Reports, 9*(1), 7322. doi:10.1038/s41598-019-43820-4

Gropp, A., Kolbus, U., & Giers, D. (1975). Systematic approach to the study of trisomy in the mouse. II. *Cytogenetics and Cell Genetics, 14*(1), 42–62.

Guedj, F., Bianchi, D. W., & Delabar, J. M. (2014). Prenatal treatment of Down syndrome: A reality? *Current Opinion in Obstetrics & Gynecology, 26*(2), 92–103. doi:10.1097/gco.0000000000000056

Guedj, F., Pennings, J. L., Ferres, M. A., Graham, L. C., Wick, H. C., Miczek, K. A., . . . Bianchi, D. W. (2015). The fetal brain transcriptome and neonatal behavioral phenotype in the Ts1Cje mouse model of Down syndrome. *American Journal of Medical Genetics, Part A, 167A*(9), 1993–2008. doi:10.1002/ajmg.a.37156

Guedj, F., Pennings, J. L., Wick, H. C., & Bianchi, D. W. (2015). Analysis of adult cerebral cortex and hippocampus transcriptomes reveals unique molecular changes in the Ts1Cje mouse model of Down syndrome. *Brain Pathology, 25*(1), 11–23. doi:10.1111/bpa.12151

Guidi, S., Bonasoni, P., Ceccarelli, C., Santini, D., Gualtieri, F., Ciani, E., & Bartesaghi, R. (2008). Neurogenesis impairment and increased cell death reduce total neuron number in the hippocampal region of fetuses with Down syndrome. *Brain Pathology, 18*(2), 180–197. doi:BPA113 [pii]10.1111/j.1750-3639.2007.00113.x

Guidi, S., Ciani, E., Bonasoni, P., Santini, D., & Bartesaghi, R. (2011). Widespread proliferation impairment and hypocellularity in the cerebellum of fetuses with Down syndrome. *Brain Pathology, 21*(4), 361–373. doi:10.1111/j.1750-3639.2010.00459.x

Guidi, S., Stagni, F., Bianchi, P., Ciani, E., Giacomini, A., De Franceschi, M., . . . Bartesaghi, R. (2014). Prenatal pharmacotherapy rescues brain development in a Down's syndrome mouse model. *Brain, 137*(Pt 2), 380–401. doi:10.1093/brain/awt340

Guihard-Costa, A. M., Khung, S., Delbecque, K., Menez, F., & Delezoide, A. L. (2006). Biometry of face and brain in fetuses with trisomy 21. *Pediatric Research, 59*(1), 33–38. doi:10.1203/01.pdr.0000190580.88391.9a

Gupta, M., Dhanasekaran, A. R., & Gardiner, K. J. (2016). Mouse models of Down syndrome: Gene content and consequences. *Mammalian Genome Society, 27*, 538–555. doi:10.1007/s00335-016-9661-8

Gutierrez-Castellanos, N., Winkelman, B. H., Tolosa-Rodriguez, L., Devenney, B., Reeves, R. H., & De Zeeuw, C. I. (2013). Size does not always matter: Ts65Dn Down syndrome mice show cerebellum-dependent motor learning deficits that cannot be rescued by postnatal SAG treatment. *Journal of Neuroscience, 33*(39), 15408–15413. doi:10.1523/jneurosci.2198-13.2013

Haas, M. A., Bell, D., Slender, A., Lana-Elola, E., Watson-Scales, S., Fisher, E. M., . . . Guillemot, F. (2013). Alterations to dendritic spine morphology, but not dendrite patterning, of cortical projection neurons in Tc1 and Ts1Rhr mouse models of Down syndrome. *PLoS ONE, 8*(10), e78561. doi:10.1371/journal.pone.0078561

Hampton, T. G., Stasko, M. R., Kale, A., Amende, I., & Costa, A. C. (2004). Gait dynamics in trisomic mice: Quantitative neurological traits of Down syndrome. *Physiology & Behavior, 82*(2–3), 381–389. doi:10.1016/j.physbeh.2004.04.006

Haydar, T. F. (2020). Neurogenesis, myelination, and circuitry: The case for a distributed therapeutic regimen in Down syndrome. *American Journal on Intellectual and Developmental Disabilities, 125*(2), 100–102. doi:10.1352/1944-7558-125.2.100

Haydar, T. F., Blue, M. E., Molliver, M. E., Krueger, B. K., & Yarowsky, P. J. (1996). Consequences of trisomy 16 for mouse brain development: Corticogenesis in a model of Down syndrome. *Journal of Neuroscience, 16*(19), 6175–6182.

Haydar, T. F., Nowakowski, R. S., Yarowsky, P. J., & Krueger, B. K. (2000). Role of founder cell deficit and delayed neuronogenesis in microencephaly of the trisomy 16 mouse. *Journal of Neuroscience, 20*(11), 4156–4164.

Haydar, T. F., & Reeves, R. H. (2012). Trisomy 21 and early brain development. *Trends in Neurosciences, 35*(2), 81–91. doi:10.1016/j.tins.2011.11.001

Head, E., Lott, I. T., Wilcock, D. M., & Lemere, C. A. (2016). Aging in Down syndrome and the development of Alzheimer's disease neuropathology. *Current Alzheimer Research, 13*(1), 18–29.

Herault, Y., Delabar, J. M., Fisher, E. M. C., Tybulewicz, V. L. J., Yu, E., & Brault, V. (2017). Rodent models in Down syndrome research: Impact and future opportunities. *Disease Models & Mechanisms, 10*(10), 1165–1186. doi:10.1242/dmm.029728

Hoeffer, C. A., Dey, A., Sachan, N., Wong, H., Patterson, R. J., Shelton, J. M., . . . Rothermel, B. A. (2007). The Down syndrome critical region protein RCAN1 regulates long-term potentiation and memory via inhibition of phosphatase signaling. *The Journal of Neuroscience: The Official Journal of the Society for Neuroscience, 27*(48), 13161–13172. doi:10.1523/JNEUROSCI.3974-07.2007

Holtzman, D. M., Li, Y. W., DeArmond, S. J., McKinley, M. P., Gage, F. H., Epstein, C. J., & Mobley, W. C. (1992). Mouse model of neurodegeneration: Atrophy of basal forebrain cholinergic neurons in trisomy 16 transplants. *Proceedings of the National Academy of Sciences of the United States of America, 89*(4), 1383–1387.

Hunter, C. L., Bimonte, H. A., & Granholm, A. C. E. (2003). Behavioral comparison of 4 and 6 month-old Ts65Dn mice: Age-related impairments in working and reference memory. *Behavioural Brain Research, 138*(2), 121–131.

Hunter, C. L., Isacson, O., Nelson, M., Bimonte-Nelson, H., Seo, H., Lin, L., . . . Granholm, A.-C. (2003). Regional alterations in amyloid precursor protein and nerve growth factor across age in a mouse model of Down's syndrome. *Neuroscience Research, 45*(4), 437–445.

Hyde, L. A., & Crnic, L. S. (2001). Age-related deficits in context discrimination learning in Ts65Dn mice that model Down syndrome and Alzheimer's disease. *Behavioral Neuroscience, 115*(6), 1239–1246.

Jakovcevski, I., Filipovic, R., Mo, Z., Rakic, S., & Zecevic, N. (2009). Oligodendrocyte development and the onset of myelination in the human fetal brain. *Frontiers in Neuroanatomy, 3*, 5. doi:10.3389/neuro.05.005.2009

Jankowsky, J. L., Younkin, L. H., Gonzales, V., Fadale, D. J., Slunt, H. H., Lester, H. A., . . . Borchelt, D. R. (2007). Rodent A beta modulates the solubility and distribution of amyloid deposits in transgenic mice. *The Journal of Biological Chemistry, 282*(31), 22707–22720. doi:10.1074/jbc.M611050200

Jernigan, T. L., Bellugi, U., Sowell, E., Doherty, S., & Hesselink, J. R. (1993). Cerebral morphologic distinctions between Williams and Down syndromes. *Archives of Neurology, 50*(2), 186–191.

Jiang, J., Jing, Y., Cost, G. J., Chiang, J. C., Kolpa, H. J., Cotton, A. M., . . . Lawrence, J. B. (2013). Translating dosage compensation to trisomy 21. *Nature, 500*(7462), 296–300. doi:10.1038/nature12394

Jiang, X., Liu, C., Yu, T., Zhang, L., Meng, K., Xing, Z., . . . Yu, Y. E. (2015). Genetic dissection of the Down syndrome critical region. *Human Molecular Genetics, 24*(22), 6540–6551. doi:10.1093/hmg/ddv364

Kahlem, P., Sultan, M., Herwig, R., Steinfath, M., Balzereit, D., Eppens, B., . . . Yaspo, M. L. (2004). Transcript level alterations reflect gene dosage effects across multiple tissues in a mouse model of Down syndrome. *Genome Research, 14*(7), 1258–1267. doi:10.1101/gr.1951304

Kawaguchi, Y., & Kubota, Y. (1997). GABAergic cell subtypes and their synaptic connections in rat frontal cortex. *Cerebral Cortex, 7*(6), 476–486.

Klein, S. L., Kriegsfeld, L. J., Hairston, J. E., Rau, V., Nelson, R. J., & Yarowsky, P. J. (1996). Characterization of sensorimotor performance, reproductive and aggressive behaviors in segmental trisomic 16 (Ts65Dn) mice. *Physiology & Behavior, 60*(4), 1159–1164. doi:10.1016/0031-9384(96)00218-1

Lana-Elola, E., Watson-Scales, S., Slender, A., Gibbins, D., Martineau, A., Douglas, C., . . . Tybulewicz, V. L. (2016). Genetic dissection of Down syndrome-associated congenital heart defects using a new mouse mapping panel. *Elife, 5* e11614. doi:10.7554/eLife.11614

Larsen, K. B., Laursen, H., Graem, N., Samuelsen, G. B., Bogdanovic, N., & Pakkenberg, B. (2008). Reduced cell number in the neocortical part of the human fetal brain in Down syndrome. *Annals of Anatomy, 190*(5), 421–427. doi:10.1016/j.aanat.2008.05.007

Lee, J. C., Shin, J., & Baek, K.-H. (2013). Trisomy of the Dscr1 gene suppresses early progression of pancreatic intraepithelial neoplasia driven by oncogenic Kras. *Biochemical and Biophysical Research Communications, 440*(1), 50–55. doi:10.1016/j.bbrc.2013.09.033

Letourneau, A., Santoni, F. A., Bonilla, X., Sailani, M. R., Gonzalez, D., Kind, J., . . . Antonarakis, S. E. (2014). Domains of genome-wide gene expression dysregulation in Down's syndrome. *Nature, 508*(7496), 345–350. doi:10.1038/nature13200

Li, H., Edie, S., Klinedinst, D., Jeong, J. S., Blackshaw, S., Maslen, C. L., & Reeves, R. H. (2016). Penetrance of congenital heart disease in a mouse model of Down syndrome depends on a trisomic potentiator of a disomic modifier. *Genetics, 203*(2), 763–770. doi:10.1534/genetics.116.188045

Li, Z., Yu, T., Morishima, M., Pao, A., LaDuca, J., Conroy, J., . . . Yu, Y. E. (2007). Duplication of the entire 22.9 Mb human chromosome 21 syntenic region on mouse chromosome 16 causes cardiovascular and gastrointestinal abnormalities. *Human Molecular Genetics*, *16*(11), 1359–1366. doi:10.1093/hmg/ddm086

Ling, K. H., Hewitt, C. A., Tan, K. L., Cheah, P. S., Vidyadaran, S., Lai, M. I., . . . Scott, H. S. (2014). Functional transcriptome analysis of the postnatal brain of the Ts1Cje mouse model for Down syndrome reveals global disruption of interferon-related molecular networks. *BMC Genomics*, *15*, 624. doi:10.1186/1471-2164-15-624

Liu, C., Morishima, M., Jiang, X., Yu, T., Meng, K., Ray, D., . . . Yu, Y. E. (2014). Engineered chromosome-based genetic mapping establishes a 3.7 Mb critical genomic region for Down syndrome-associated heart defects in mice. *Human Genetics*, *133*(6), 743–753. doi:10.1007/s00439-013-1407-z

Liu, W., Zhou, H., Liu, L., Zhao, C., Deng, Y., Chen, L., . . . Richard Lu, Q. (2015). Disruption of neurogenesis and cortical development in transgenic mice misexpressing Olig2, a gene in the Down syndrome critical region. *Neurobiology of Disease*, *77*, 106–116. doi:10.1016/j.nbd.2015.02.021

Lorenzi, H. A., & Reeves, R. H. (2006). Hippocampal hypocellularity in the Ts65Dn mouse originates early in development. *Brain Research*, *1104*(1), 153–159. doi:10.1016/j.brainres.2006.05.022

Lott, I. T. (2012). Neurological phenotypes for Down syndrome across the life span. *Progress in Brain Research*, *197*, 101–121. doi:10.1016/b978-0-444-54299-1.00006-6

Lott, I. T., & Dierssen, M. (2010). Cognitive deficits and associated neurological complications in individuals with Down's syndrome. *The Lancet. Neurology*, *9*(6), 623–633. doi:10.1016/s1474-4422(10)70112-5

Lu, Q. R., Sun, T., Zhu, Z., Ma, N., Garcia, M., Stiles, C. D., & Rowitch, D. H. (2002). Common developmental requirement for Olig function indicates a motor neuron/oligodendrocyte connection. *Cell*, *109*(1), 75–86.

Lu, Q. R., Yuk, D., Alberta, J. A., Zhu, Z., Pawlitzky, I., Chan, J., . . . Rowitch, D. H. (2000). Sonic hedgehog–regulated oligodendrocyte lineage genes encoding bHLH proteins in the mammalian central nervous system. *Neuron*, *25*(2), 317–329.

Luebke, J. I. (2017). Pyramidal neurons are not generalizable building blocks of cortical networks. *Frontiers in Neuroanatomy*, *11*, 11. doi:doi:10.3389/fnana.2017.00011

Lyle, R., Gehrig, C., Neergaard-Henrichsen, C., Deutsch, S., & Antonarakis, S. E. (2004). Gene expression from the aneuploid chromosome in a trisomy mouse model of Down syndrome. *Genome Research*, *14*(7), 1268–1274. doi:10.1101/gr.2090904

Markram, H., Toledo-Rodriguez, M., Wang, Y., Gupta, A., Silberberg, G., & Wu, C. (2004). Interneurons of the neocortical inhibitory system. *Nature Reviews: Neuroscience*, *5*(10), 793–807. doi:10.1038/nrn1519

Martin, K. R., Corlett, A., Dubach, D., Mustafa, T., Coleman, H. A., Parkington, H. C., . . . Pritchard, M. A. (2012). Over-expression of RCAN1 causes Down syndrome-like hippocampal deficits that alter learning and memory. *Human Molecular Genetics*, *21*(13), 3025–3041. doi:10.1093/hmg/dds134

McGonigle, P. (2014). Animal models of CNS disorders. *Biochemical Pharmacology*, *87*(1), 140–149. doi:10.1016/j.bcp.2013.06.016

Mizuguchi, R., Sugimori, M., Takebayashi, H., Kosako, H., Nagao, M., Yoshida, S., . . . Nakafuku, M. (2001). Combinatorial roles of olig2 and neurogenin2 in the coordinated induction of pan-neuronal and subtype-specific properties of motoneurons. *Neuron*, *31*(5), 757–771.

Moller, R. S., Kubart, S., Hoeltzenbein, M., Heye, B., Vogel, I., Hansen, C. P., . . . Kalscheuer, V. M. (2008). Truncation of the Down syndrome candidate gene DYRK1A in two unrelated patients with microcephaly. *American Journal of Human Genetics*, *82*(5), 1165–1170. doi:10.1016/j.ajhg.2008.03.001

Moore, C. S., & Roper, R. J. (2007). The power of comparative and developmental studies for mouse models of Down syndrome. *Mammalian Genome Society*, *18*(6–7), 431–443. doi:10.1007/s00335-007-9030-8

Nadel, L. (2003). Down's syndrome: A genetic disorder in biobehavioral perspective. *Genes, Brain, and Behavior*, *2*(3), 156–166.

Nguyen, T. L., Duchon, A., Manousopoulou, A., Loaëc, N., Villiers, B., Pani, G., . . . Herault, Y. (2018). Correction of cognitive deficits in mouse models of Down syndrome by a pharmacological inhibitor of DYRK1A. *Disease Models & Mechanisms*, *11*(9), dmm035634. doi:10.1242/dmm.035634

Novitch, B. G., Chen, A. I., & Jessell, T. M. (2001). Coordinate regulation of motor neuron subtype identity and pan-neuronal properties by the bHLH repressor Olig2. *Neuron*, *31*(5), 773–789.

O'Doherty, A., Ruf, S., Mulligan, C., Hildreth, V., Errington, M. L., Cooke, S., . . . Fisher, E. M. (2005). An aneuploid mouse strain carrying human chromosome 21 with Down syndrome phenotypes. *Science*, *309*(5743), 2033–2037. doi:10.1126/science.1114535

Ohr, P. S., & Fagen, J. W. (1994). Contingency learning in 9-month-old infants with Down syndrome. *American Journal of Mental Retardation, 99*(1), 74–84.

Olmos-Serrano, J. L., Kang, H. J., Tyler, W. A., Silbereis, J. C., Cheng, F., Zhu, Y., . . . Sestan, N. (2016). Down syndrome developmental brain transcriptome reveals defective oligodendrocyte differentiation and myelination. *Neuron, 89*(6), 1208–1222. doi:10.1016/j.neuron.2016.01.042

Olmos-Serrano, J. L., Tyler, W. A., Cabral, H. J., & Haydar, T. F. (2016). Longitudinal measures of cognition in the Ts65Dn mouse: Refining windows and defining modalities for therapeutic intervention in Down syndrome. *Experimental Neurology, 279*, 40–56. doi:10.1016/j.expneurol.2016.02.005

Olson, L. E., Richtsmeier, J. T., Leszl, J., & Reeves, R. H. (2004). A chromosome 21 critical region does not cause specific Down syndrome phenotypes. *Science, 306*(5696), 687–690. doi:10.1126/science.1098992

Olson, L. E., Roper, R. J., Baxter, L. L., Carlson, E. J., Epstein, C. J., & Reeves, R. H. (2004). Down syndrome mouse models Ts65Dn, Ts1Cje, and Ms1Cje/Ts65Dn exhibit variable severity of cerebellar phenotypes. *Developmental Dynamics, 230*(3), 581–589. doi:10.1002/dvdy.20079

Olson, L. E., Roper, R. J., Sengstaken, C. L., Peterson, E. A., Aquino, V., Galdzicki, Z., . . . Reeves, R. H. (2007). Trisomy for the Down syndrome "critical region" is necessary but not sufficient for brain phenotypes of trisomic mice. *Human Molecular Genetics, 16*(7), 774–782. doi:10.1093/hmg/ddm022

Patkee, P. A., Baburamani, A. A., Kyriakopoulou, V., Davidson, A., Avini, E., Dimitrova, R., . . . Rutherford, M. A. (2022). Early alterations in cortical and cerebellar regional brain growth in Down Syndrome: An in-vivo fetal and neonatal MRI assessment. *bioRxiv, 35*. doi: 10.1016/j.nicl.2019.102139

Pennington, B. F., Moon, J., Edgin, J., Stedron, J., & Nadel, L. (2003). The neuropsychology of Down syndrome: Evidence for hippocampal dysfunction. *Child Development, 74*(1), 75–93.

Pereira, P. L., Magnol, L., Sahún, I., Brault, V., Duchon, A., Prandini, P., . . . Herault, Y. (2009). A new mouse model for the trisomy of the Abcg1-U2af1 region reveals the complexity of the combinatorial genetic code of down syndrome. *Human Molecular Genetics, 18*(24), 4756–4769. doi:10.1093/hmg/ddp438

Perrin, S. (2014). Preclinical research: Make mouse studies work. *Nature, 507*(7493), 423–425. doi:10.1038/507423a

Petit, T. L., LeBoutillier, J. C., Alfano, D. P., & Becker, L. E. (1984). Synaptic development in the human fetus: A morphometric analysis of normal and Down's syndrome neocortex. *Experimental Neurology, 83*(1), 13–23.

Pinter, J. D., Brown, W. E., Eliez, S., Schmitt, J. E., Capone, G. T., & Reiss, A. L. (2001). Amygdala and hippocampal volumes in children with Down syndrome: A high-resolution MRI study. *Neurology, 56*(7), 972–974.

Pinter, J. D., Eliez, S., Schmitt, J. E., Capone, G. T., & Reiss, A. L. (2001). Neuroanatomy of Down's syndrome: A high-resolution MRI study. *The American Journal of Psychiatry, 158*(10), 1659–1665.

Potier, M. C., Rivals, I., Mercier, G., Ettwiller, L., Moldrich, R. X., Laffaire, J., . . . Dauphinot, L. (2006). Transcriptional disruptions in Down syndrome: A case study in the Ts1Cje mouse cerebellum during postnatal development. *Journal of Neurochemistry, 97 Suppl 1*, 104–109. doi:10.1111/j.1471-4159.2005.03624.x

Powell, N. M., Modat, M., Cardoso, M. J., Ma, D., Holmes, H. E., Yu, Y., . . . Ourselin, S. (2016). Fully-automated muMRI morphometric phenotyping of the Tc1 Mouse model of Down syndrome. *PLoS ONE, 11*(9), e0162974. doi:10.1371/journal.pone.0162974

Prasher, V. (1995). Comparison of physical and psychiatric status in individuals with translocation and trisomy 21 Down syndrome. *Down Syndrome Research and Practice, 3*(1), 9–13.

Pritchard, M. A., & Kola, I. (1999). The "gene dosage effect" hypothesis versus the "amplified developmental instability" hypothesis in Down syndrome. *Journal of Neural Transmission Suppl, 57*, 293–303.

Pritchard, M. A., & Martin, K. R. (2013). RCAN1 and its potential contribution to the Down syndrome phenotype. In Subrata K. Dey (Ed.), *Down syndrome*. London: IntechOpen. doi: 10.5772/46009

Purser, H. R. M., Farran, E. K., Courbois, Y., Lemahieu, A., Sockeel, P., Mellier, D., & Blades, M. (2015). The development of route learning in Down syndrome, Williams syndrome and typical development: Investigations with virtual environments. *Developmental Science, 18*(4), 599–613. doi:10.1111/desc.12236

Rachidi, M., & Lopes, C. (2008). Mental retardation and associated neurological dysfunctions in Down syndrome: A consequence of dysregulation in critical chromosome 21 genes and associated molecular pathways. *European Journal of Paediatric Neurology, 12*(3), 168–182. doi:10.1016/j.ejpn.2007.08.010

Rakic, P. (1995). A small step for the cell, a giant leap for mankind: A hypothesis of neocortical expansion during evolution. *Trends in Neurosciences, 18*(9), 383–388.

Raveau, M., Lignon, J. M., Nalesso, V., Duchon, A., Groner, Y., Sharp, A. J., . . . Hérault, Y. (2012). The App-Runx1 region is critical for birth defects and electrocardiographic dysfunctions observed in a Down syndrome mouse model. *PLoS Genetics, 8*(5), e1002724. doi:10.1371/journal.pgen.1002724

Raz, N., Torres, I. J., Briggs, S. D., Spencer, W. D., Thornton, A. E., Loken, W. J., . . . Acker, J. D. (1995). Selective neuroanatomic abnormalities in Down's syndrome and their cognitive correlates: Evidence from MRI morphometry. *Neurology, 45*(2), 356–366.

Richtsmeier, J. T., Zumwalt, A., Carlson, E. J., Epstein, C. J., & Reeves, R. H. (2002). Craniofacial phenotypes in segmentally trisomic mouse models for Down syndrome. *American Journal of Medical Genetics, 107*(4), 317–324.

Roper, R. J., Baxter, L. L., Saran, N. G., Klinedinst, D. K., Beachy, P. A., & Reeves, R. H. (2006). Defective cerebellar response to mitogenic Hedgehog signaling in Down [corrected] syndrome mice. *Proceedings of the National Academy of Sciences of the United States of America, 103*(5), 1452–1456. doi:10.1073/pnas.0510750103

Roper, R. J., & Reeves, R. H. (2006). Understanding the basis for Down syndrome phenotypes. *PLoS Genetics, 2*(3), e50. doi:10.1371/journal.pgen.0020050

Ross, M. H., Galaburda, A. M., & Kemper, T. L. (1984). Down's syndrome: Is there a decreased population of neurons? *Neurology, 34*(7), 909–916.

Ruiz-Mejias, M., Martinez de Lagran, M., Mattia, M., Castano-Prat, P., Perez-Mendez, L., Ciria-Suarez, L., . . . Dierssen, M. (2016). Overexpression of Dyrk1A, a Down syndrome candidate, decreases excitability and impairs gamma oscillations in the prefrontal cortex. *The Journal of Neuroscience, 36*(13), 3648–3659. doi:10.1523/JNEUROSCI.2517-15.2016

Sago, H., Carlson, E. J., Smith, D. J., Kilbridge, J., Rubin, E. M., Mobley, W. C., . . . Huang, T. T. (1998). Ts1Cje, a partial trisomy 16 mouse model for Down syndrome, exhibits learning and behavioral abnormalities. *Proceedings of the National Academy of Sciences of the United States of America, 95*(11), 6256–6261.

Salehi, A., Delcroix, J.-D., Belichenko, P. V., Zhan, K., Wu, C., Valletta, J. S., . . . Mobley, W. C. (2006). Increased app expression in a mouse model of Down's syndrome disrupts NGF transport and causes cholinergic neuron degeneration. *Neuron, 51*(1), 29–42. doi:10.1016/j.neuron.2006.05.022

Saran, N. G., Pletcher, M. T., Natale, J. E., Cheng, Y., & Reeves, R. H. (2003). Global disruption of the cerebellar transcriptome in a Down syndrome mouse model. *Human Molecular Genetics, 12*(16), 2013–2019.

Schmidt-Sidor, B., Wisniewski, K. E., Shepard, T. H., & Sersen, E. A. (1990). Brain growth in Down syndrome subjects 15 to 22 weeks of gestational age and birth to 60 months. *Clinical Neuropathology, 9*(4), 181–190.

Shalev, N., Steele, A., Nobre, A. C., Karmiloff-Smith, A., Cornish, K., & Scerif, G. (2019). Dynamic sustained attention markers differentiate atypical development: The case of Williams syndrome and Down's syndrome. *Neuropsychologia, 132*, 107148. doi:10.1016/j.neuropsychologia.2019.107148

Shin, M., Siffel, C., & Correa, A. (2010). Survival of children with mosaic Down syndrome. *American Journal of Medical Genetics, Part A, 152a*(3), 800–801. doi:10.1002/ajmg.a.33295

Stagni, F., Giacomini, A., Emili, M., Trazzi, S., Guidi, S., Sassi, M., . . . Bartesaghi, R. (2016). Short- and long-term effects of neonatal pharmacotherapy with epigallocatechin-3-gallate on hippocampal development in the Ts65Dn mouse model of Down syndrome. *Neuroscience, 333*, 277–301. doi:10.1016/j.neuroscience.2016.07.031

Stagni, F., Giacomini, A., Guidi, S., Ciani, E., & Bartesaghi, R. (2015). Timing of therapies for Down syndrome: The sooner, the better. *Frontiers in Behavioral Neuroscience, 9*, 265. doi:10.3389/fnbeh.2015.00265

Starbuck, J. M., Dutka, T., Ratliff, T. S., Reeves, R. H., & Richtsmeier, J. T. (2014). Overlapping trisomies for human chromosome 21 orthologs produce similar effects on skull and brain morphology of Dp(16)1Yey and Ts65Dn mice. *American Journal of Medical Genetics, Part A, 164A*(8), 1981–1990. doi:10.1002/ajmg.a.36594

Stiles, J., & Jernigan, T. L. (2010). The basics of brain development. *Neuropsychology Review, 20*(4), 327–348. doi:10.1007/s11065-010-9148-4

Stringer, M., Abeysekera, I., Dria, K. J., Roper, R. J., & Goodlett, C. R. (2015). Low dose EGCG treatment beginning in adolescence does not improve cognitive impairment in a Down syndrome mouse model. *Pharmacology, Biochemistry, and Behavior, 138*, 70–79. doi:10.1016/j.pbb.2015.09.002

Stringer, M., Goodlett, C. R., & Roper, R. J. (2017). Targeting trisomic treatments: Optimizing Dyrk1a inhibition to improve Down syndrome deficits. *Molecular Genetics & Genomic Medicine, 5*(5), 451–465. doi:10.1002/mgg3.334

Sullivan, K. D., Evans, D., Pandey, A., Hraha, T. H., Smith, K. P., Markham, N., . . . Blumenthal, T. (2017). Trisomy 21 causes changes in the circulating proteome indicative of chronic autoinflammation. *Scientific Reports, 7*(1), 14818. doi:10.1038/s41598-017-13858-3

Takashima, S., Becker, L., Armstrong, D., & Chan, F. (1981). Abnormal neuronal development in the visual cortex of the human fetus and infant with Down's syndrome. A quantitative and qualitative Golgi study. *Brain Research, 225*(1), 1–21.

Takebayashi, H., Yoshida, S., Sugimori, M., Kosako, H., Kominami, R., Nakafuku, M., & Nabeshima, Y. (2000). Dynamic expression of basic helix-loop-helix Olig family members: Implication of Olig2 in neuron and oligodendrocyte differentiation and identification of a new member, Olig3. *Mechanisms of Development, 99*(1–2), 143–148.

Taylor-Phillips, S., Freeman, K., Geppert, J., Agbebiyi, A., Uthman, O. A., Madan, J., . . . Quenby, S. (2016). Accuracy of non-invasive prenatal testing using cell-free DNA for detection of Down, Edwards and Patau syndromes: A systematic review and meta-analysis. *BMJ Open, 6*(1), e010002. doi:10.1136/bmjopen-2015-010002

Teipel, S. J., Alexander, G. E., Schapiro, M. B., Moller, H. J., Rapoport, S. I., & Hampel, H. (2004). Age-related cortical grey matter reductions in non-demented Down's syndrome adults determined by MRI with voxel-based morphometry. *Brain, 127*(Pt 4), 811–824.

Teipel, S. J., Schapiro, M. B., Alexander, G. E., Krasuski, J. S., Horwitz, B., Hoehne, C., . . . Hampel, H. (2003). Relation of corpus callosum and hippocampal size to age in nondemented adults with Down's syndrome. *The American Journal of Psychiatry, 160*(10), 1870–1878. doi:10.1176/appi.ajp.160.10.1870

Tramutola, A., Lanzillotta, C., Arena, A., Barone, E., Perluigi, M., & Di Domenico, F. (2016). Increased mammalian target of rapamycin signaling contributes to the accumulation of protein oxidative damage in a mouse model of Down's syndrome. *Neuro-Degenerative Diseases, 16*(1–2), 62–68. doi:10.1159/000441419

Vicari, S. (2004). Memory development and intellectual disabilities. *Acta Paediatrica Supplement, 93*(445), 60–63; discussion 63–64.

Vicari, S., Marotta, L., & Carlesimo, G. A. (2004). Verbal short-term memory in Down's syndrome: An articulatory loop deficit? *Journal of Intellectual Disability Research, 48*(Pt 2), 80–92.

Vicari, S., Pontillo, M., & Armando, M. (2013). Neurodevelopmental and psychiatric issues in Down's syndrome: Assessment and intervention. *Psychiatric Genetics, 23*(3), 95–107. doi:10.1097/YPG.0b013e32835fe426

Villar, A. J., Belichenko, P. V., Gillespie, A. M., Kozy, H. M., Mobley, W. C., & Epstein, C. J. (2005). Identification and characterization of a new Down syndrome model, Ts[Rb(12.1716)]2Cje, resulting from a spontaneous Robertsonian fusion between T(171)65Dn and mouse chromosome 12. *Mammalian Genome Society, 16*(2), 79–90.

Watson-Scales, S., Kalmar, B., Lana-Elola, E., Gibbins, D., La Russa, F., Wiseman, F., . . . Tybulewicz, V. L. J. (2018). Analysis of motor dysfunction in Down syndrome reveals motor neuron degeneration. *PLoS Genetics, 14*(5), e1007383. doi:10.1371/journal.pgen.1007383

Weitzdoerfer, R., Dierssen, M., Fountoulakis, M., & Lubec, G. (2001). Fetal life in Down syndrome starts with normal neuronal density but impaired dendritic spines and synaptosomal structure. *Journal of Neural Transmission Supplementum* (61), 59–70.

White, N. S., Alkire, M. T., & Haier, R. J. (2003). A voxel-based morphometric study of nondemented adults with Down syndrome. *Neuroimage, 20*(1), 393–403.

Whittle, N., Sartori, S. B., Dierssen, M., Lubec, G., & Singewald, N. (2007). Fetal Down syndrome brains exhibit aberrant levels of neurotransmitters critical for normal brain development. *Pediatrics, 120*(6), e1465–1471.

Wilcock, D. M., Hurban, J., Helman, A. M., Sudduth, T. L., McCarty, K. L., Beckett, T. L., . . . Head, E. (2015). Down syndrome individuals with Alzheimer's disease have a distinct neuroinflammatory phenotype compared to sporadic Alzheimer's disease. *Neurobiology of Aging, 36*(9), 2468–2474. doi:10.1016/j.neurobiolaging.2015.05.016

Winter, T. C., Reichman, J. A., Luna, J. A., Cheng, E. Y., Doll, A. M., Komarniski, C. A., . . . Uhrich, S. B. (1998). Frontal lobe shortening in second-trimester fetuses with trisomy 21: Usefulness as a US marker. *Radiology, 207*(1), 215–222. doi:10.1148/radiology.207.1.9530318

Wishart, J. G. (1993). The development of learning difficulties in children with Down's syndrome. *Journal of Intellectual Disability Research, 37 (Pt 4)*, 389–403.

Wisniewski, K. E. (1990). Down syndrome children often have brain with maturation delay, retardation of growth, and cortical dysgenesis. *American Journal of Medical Genetics Supplement, 7*, 274–281.

Wisniewski, K. E., & Kida, E. (1994). Abnormal neurogenesis and synaptogenesis in Down syndrome brain. *Dev Brain Dysfunct.*

Wisniewski, K. E., Laure-Kamionowska, M., & Wisniewski, H. M. (1984). Evidence of arrest of neurogenesis and synaptogenesis in brains of patients with Down's syndrome. *New England Journal of Medicine, 311*(18), 1187–1188.

Wisniewski, K. E., & Schmidt-Sidor, B. (1989). Postnatal delay of myelin formation in brains from Down syndrome infants and children. *Clinical Neuropathology, 8*(2), 55–62.

Witton, J., Padmashri, R., Zinyuk, L. E., Popov, V. I., Kraev, I., Line, S. J., . . . Jones, M. W. (2015). Hippocampal circuit dysfunction in the Tc1 mouse model of Down syndrome. *Nature Neuroscience, 18*(9), 1291–1298. doi:10.1038/nn.4072

Xing, L., Salas, M., Zhang, H., Gittler, J., Ludwig, T., Lin, C.-S., . . . Tycko, B. (2013). Creation and characterization of BAC-transgenic mice with physiological overexpression of epitope-tagged RCAN1 (DSCR1). *Mammalian Genome: Official Journal of the International Mammalian Genome Society, 24*(1–2), 30–43. doi:10.1007/s00335-012-9436-9

Xu, X., Roby, K. D., & Callaway, E. M. (2010). Immunochemical characterization of inhibitory mouse cortical neurons: Three chemically distinct classes of inhibitory cells. *The Journal of Comparative Neurology, 518*(3), 389–404. doi:10.1002/cne.22229

Yu, T., Li, Z., Jia, Z., Clapcote, S. J., Liu, C., Li, S., . . . Yu, Y. E. (2010). A mouse model of Down syndrome trisomic for all human chromosome 21 syntenic regions. *Human Molecular Genetics, 19*(14), 2780–2791. doi:10.1093/hmg/ddq179

Yu, T., Liu, C., Belichenko, P., Clapcote, S. J., Li, S., Pao, A., . . . Yu, Y. E. (2010). Effects of individual segmental trisomies of human chromosome 21 syntenic regions on hippocampal long-term potentiation and cognitive behaviors in mice. *Brain Research, 1366*, 162–171. doi:10.1016/j.brainres.2010.09.107

Zanin, M. P., Mackenzie, K. D., Peiris, H., Pritchard, M. A., & Keating, D. J. (2013). RCAN1 regulates vesicle recycling and quantal release kinetics via effects on calcineurin activity. *Journal of Neurochemistry, 124*(3), 290–299. doi:10.1111/jnc.12086

Zhang, L., Meng, K., Jiang, X., Liu, C., Pao, A., Belichenko, P. V., . . . Yu, Y. E. (2013). Human chromosome 21 orthologous region on mouse chromosome 17 is a major determinant of Down syndrome-related developmental cognitive deficits. *Human Molecular Genetics, 23*(3), 578–589. doi:10.1093/hmg/ddt446

Zhou, Q., & Anderson, D. J. (2002). The bHLH transcription factors OLIG2 and OLIG1 couple neuronal and glial subtype specification. *Cell, 109*(1), 61–73.

CHAPTER 22

Animal Models of Down Syndrome

Anna J. Moyer *and* Roger H. Reeves

Abstract

Is intellectual disability a treatable feature of persons with Down syndrome? Researchers have made tremendous progress in the last 30 years, from creating the first mouse model of Down syndrome to completing the first major clinical trial for cognitive impairment in people with Down syndrome. Until recently, normalizing brain development and function seemed too lofty a goal, and indeed, even proposing a candidate therapy requires answering a number of difficult questions. How does trisomy 21, a molecular diagnosis, cause the clinical phenotypes of Down syndrome? When, where, and how do trisomic genes act to disrupt normal development and which genes are involved with which outcomes? Which brain regions and behaviors are most impaired? Is there an early developmental window of time during which treatments are most effective? This article discusses how animal models such as laboratory mice can be used to understand intellectual disability and to develop new treatments for cognitive impairment.

Key Words: intellectual disability, Down syndrome, mouse models, development, cognitive impairment, animal models, trisomy 21, treatment

Introduction

The mechanisms by which trisomy 21 results in cognitive impairment remained largely mysterious until the Ts65Dn mouse model of Down syndrome was introduced 30 years ago (M. T. Davisson, Schmidt, & Akeson, 1990). Mouse models help to overcome some of the barriers to investigating developmental and functional phenotypes in people with Down syndrome, including access to neuronal tissues across the lifetime, practicality of longitudinal studies, and the ability to make chemical and genetic manipulations. Studying Ts65Dn mice led researchers to propose that an imbalance of excitatory and inhibitory synapses in the forebrain causes deficits in learning and memory (Hanson, Blank, Valenzuela, Garner, & Madison, 2007; Rissman & Mobley, 2011; Siarey, Stoll, Rapoport, & Galdzicki, 1997). These findings formed the basis for a phase II clinical trial of the drug basmisanil, which regulates inhibitory signaling by binding to $GABA_A$ receptors. Despite promising results in Ts65Dn mice and a general sense of optimism among scientists, clinicians, and the Down syndrome community following the phase I trial, basmisanil did not significantly improve the measures of cognitive function selected for the phase II trial, and an ongoing pediatric trial was discontinued (Fernandez et al., 2007; Reeves et al., 2019).

The failure of clinical trials based on mouse research is not unique to the Down syndrome field, but studying persons with Down syndrome does present some unique challenges (Perrin, 2014). Designing appropriate endpoints in people with intellectual disability is an issue requiring continued development, and correlating deficits in specific behavioral tasks between humans and mice requires understanding which brain regions are involved in those behaviors (Edgin et al., 2010; Edgin, Mason, Spano, Fernandez, & Nadel, 2012). Although the Ts65Dn mouse is the most well-characterized mouse model of Down syndrome, its chromosomal makeup does not precisely mirror the genetic etiology of trisomy 21 (Gupta, Dhanasekaran, & Gardiner, 2016). Initial investigation of a new model carrying 93% of chromosome 21 protein coding genes, the TcMAC21 mouse, holds promise but will require further characterization (Kazuki et al., 2020). A number of other mouse models are available, yet none has emerged as a definitive replacement for Ts65Dn mice. Some researchers assert the superiority of particular models, but attempts to compare models directly are few and far between (Aziz et al., 2018; O'Doherty et al., 2005; Yu, Li et al., 2010). More than twenty different drug treatments improve hippocampal function in mouse models of Down syndrome, and strategies for prioritizing which therapies should move forward to clinical trials are urgently needed (Gardiner, 2015).

As clinical trials to ameliorate intellectual disability become a reality, we propose that a critical analysis of Down syndrome models using a standardized framework could help to weigh the utility of data collected in diverse preclinical models. In this article, we consider the molecular causes of Down syndrome-associated phenotypes, establish six design principles for Down syndrome models, formalize a framework for assessing their validity, and discuss emerging trends in Down syndrome research.

The Molecular Basis of Down Syndrome Phenotypes

In 1959, a group led by Jérôme Lejeune and Marthe Gautier in Paris showed that Down syndrome is caused by trisomy for chromosome 21, and Patricia Jacobs in Edinburgh quickly confirmed this finding (Jacobs, Baikie, Court Brown, & Strong, 1959; Lejeune, Gautier, & Turpin, 1959). At around 48 million bases in length, chromosome 21 is the smallest chromosome and makes up only about 1.5% of the total genome (Hattori et al., 2000; Lander et al., 2001; Schneider et al., 2017). Recently, Gupta et al. (2016) reported that chromosome 21 contains 222 protein-coding genes and 325 nonprotein-coding genes, but this estimate is likely to evolve with our understanding of gene structure and function and the "telomere to telomere" (T2T) project to finish the human genome sequence (https://genomeinformatics.github.io/CHM13v1/).

In general, each copy of a gene produces 50% of the encoded product. Evidence from many experiments to quantify RNA and protein levels in tissues from individuals with trisomy 21 has indicated that *on average*, trisomic genes are expressed at 150% of the normal level (Kurnit, 1979; Olmos-Serrano et al., 2016; Williams et al., 2008). The overexpression of dosage-sensitive chromosome 21 genes could cause Down syndrome phenotypes, but trisomy for any chromosome may be detrimental regardless of the particular sequence (Potier et al., 2006; Roper & Reeves, 2006; Shapiro, 1983). This concept forms the basis for two overlapping hypotheses:

1. Aneuploidy stress (related concepts are sometimes referred to as "amplified developmental instability"): the mere presence of an extra chromosome causes phenotypes that are independent of the specific DNA sequence.
2. Gene dosage effect: specific trisomic genes cause specific phenotypes when overexpressed.

In fact, neither of these simplistic descriptions provides a complete conceptual platform for understanding the impact of trisomy. Single gene effects always occur on a genetic background that is already imbalanced by trisomy, which could cause, for example, small delays in cell division occasioned by the need to replicate the extra chromosome or to sort the extra pair of chromosomes during mitosis. Overexpression of a specific single gene may have a greater or lesser effect on a given trait, but perturbations due to this single gene occur in the context of overexpression of other chromosome 21 genes. For practical reasons, most research has focused on investigating the gene dosage effect model, but there is also some evidence for the role of aneuploidy stress, especially related to disruption of central molecular pathways such as protein synthesis and degradation (Beach et al., 2017). Thus, both aneuploidy stress and gene dosage effects may contribute to Down syndrome pathogenesis (Fig. 22.1).

Comparing shared features among individuals with gains or losses of chromosomes (aneuploidies) would be the most straightforward way to address the aneuploidy stress model. However, trisomy 21 is the only autosomal aneuploidy that is consistently survivable beyond infancy, and in fact, only about 20% of trisomy 21 conceptuses survive to term (Brewer, Holloway, Stone, Carothers, & FitzPatrick, 2002; Hassold & Jacobs, 1984; Hook, Mutton, Ide, Alberman, & Bobrow, 1995). The loss of all embryos with autosomal monosomies and most embryos with autosomal trisomies suggests that there is strong in-utero selection against aneuploidy,— that is, having a balanced genome with exactly two copies of every autosomal chromosome is important for survival. Although humans do not tolerate most aneuploidies, trisomic cells can be grown in culture. Cells isolated from mouse embryos with trisomy for chromosome 1, 13, 16, or 19 and skin cells from humans with trisomy 21 proliferate more slowly than normal cells (Segal & McCoy, 1974; B. R. Williams et al., 2008). Aneuploid cells also share common defects in protein turnover and degradation, DNA replication, cell division, and metabolism (Siegel & Amon, 2012; Zhu, Tsai, Gordon, & Li, 2018). The observation that aneuploidy activates

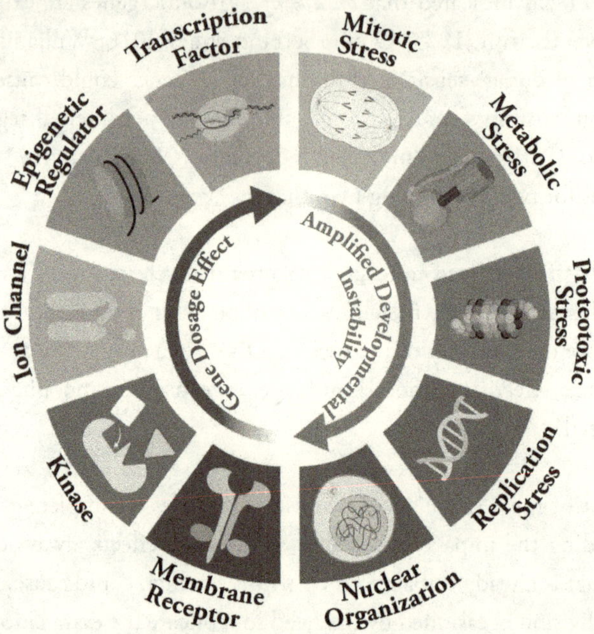

Figure 22.1. Evidence for the aneuploidy stress/amplified developmental instability model includes mitotic stress, metabolic stress, proteotoxic stress, replication stress, and changes in nuclear organization due to the presence of an extra chromosome (Kemeny et al., 2018; Siegel & Amon, 2012; Zhu et al., 2018). Five examples of how overexpression of a single trisomic gene could affect cellular function are shown. Proteins called transcription factors activate or inhibit the expression of other genes, and overexpression of the 31 transcription factors located on chromosome 21 could modulate the expression of genes on other chromosomes (Antonarakis, 2017; Lejeune et al., 1959). Overexpression of epigenetic regulators could remodel chromatin, overexpression of an ion channel could change the cell's electrical properties, overexpression of a kinase could activate signaling pathways, and overexpression of a membrane receptor could make a cell more sensitive to an environmental signal (Reeves et al., 2019; Roper & Reeves, 2006).

common stress pathways, independent of the particular chromosomes that are trisomic, lends credence to the aneuploidy stress model.

In contrast, most research of persons with Down syndrome has involved attempts to link specific trisomic genes with specific phenotypes. Geneticists typically divide conditions into two broad categories: monogenic and polygenic (Badano & Katsanis, 2002). Monogenic (Mendelian) disorders are caused by deleterious variants in single genes, whereas polygenic (complex) disorders are caused by a combination of environmental factors and common variants in multiple genes. Is Down syndrome more like a monogenic or a polygenic disorder? The underlying assumption of researchers who attempt to associate a single trisomic gene with a single phenotype is that features of persons with Down syndrome are caused by the sum of the effects of overexpressing single trisomic genes. In its simplest form, overexpression of Gene A alone could cause heart defects, Gene B alone could cause cerebellar hypoplasia, and Gene C alone could cause craniofacial abnormalities. Overexpression of Gene A, Gene B, and Gene C together would then cause heart defects, cerebellar hypoplasia, and craniofacial abnormalities.

This simplistic model would hold true in cases where the triplication of one chromosome 21 gene is sufficient to cause a Down syndrome-associated phenotype. For instance, all individuals with trisomy 21 develop neuropathology resembling Alzheimer's disease, which has been attributed to triplication of the *APP* gene (Glenner & Wong, 1984; Wisniewski, Wisniewski, & Wen, 1985). Researchers have also described rare individuals without Down syndrome who have three copies of the *APP* gene—and not the rest of chromosome 21—who develop early-onset Alzheimer's disease with cerebral amyloid angiopathy (Rovelet-Lecrux et al., 2006). Finally, individuals with trisomy for portions of chromosome 21 not including the *APP* gene do not show signs of dementia or Alzheimer's neuropathology (Doran et al., 2017; Prasher et al., 1998). These studies suggest that triplication of the *APP* gene is both *necessary* and *sufficient* to cause Alzheimer's neuropathology, but the story is not so simple. Variants in other genes that are not on chromosome 21, such as *APOE*, affect the age of onset and severity of Alzheimer's disease in people with or without Down syndrome (D'Souza et al., 2020). In a mouse model of Down syndrome, overexpression of chromosome 21 genes enhances the detrimental effects of *APP* overexpression, and more than 10 chromosome 21 genes may modify disease progression (Wiseman et al., 2015, 2018). Although the link between *APP* triplication and Alzheimer's disease is arguably the most straightforward example of a single gene dosage effect, many chromosome 21 genes likely participate in the development of Alzheimer's neuropathology. The reductionist view of "one trisomic gene per phenotype" is difficult to maintain in light of the complex network of trisomic genes that modify Alzheimer's disease in individuals with Down syndrome.

Moreover, if many trisomic genes contribute to each Down syndrome phenotype, the phenotype caused by overexpressing all trisomic genes together may not be the simple sum of the phenotypes caused by overexpressing trisomic genes one at a time. One way that trisomic genes could have nonadditive interactions is due to the cell's ability to overcome, or buffer, small changes in gene expression (Hartman, Garvik, & Hartwell, 2001). Likewise, overexpression of some trisomic genes may protect against the effects of other trisomic genes, such that the final phenotype results from the actions of all trisomic genes.

In practice, however, investigating nonadditive interactions between trisomic genes is enormously challenging. If a research group wished to study the individual effect of overexpressing each of the chromosome 21 protein-coding genes in mice, they would need to produce 222 mouse strains—one for each gene. To explore the effect of overexpressing any *two* genes at the same time would require 24,531 mouse strains, which is far beyond the bounds of possibility using current methods. As a result, most research studies adopt a hypothesis-driven approach to examine the effects of one gene or the interactions between a select few genes. More unbiased strategies for interrogating the effects of multiple trisomic genes will require the development of new experimental techniques and the reframing of Down syndrome as a complex, polygenic disorder.

Six Design Principles for Down Syndrome Models

If it were possible to remove the extra chromosome from every cell of an adult with Down syndrome, would it affect his or her congenital heart defect? Intellectual disability? Leukemia risk? Down syndrome is a developmental disorder, and researchers use a number of model systems to determine where, when, and how trisomic genes act to perturb normal developmental processes. Mice are the most commonly used model system for disease research, and they act as a stand-in for human subjects in cases where performing experiments on humans is unethical or technically infeasible (Justice & Dhillon, 2016; Rosenthal & Brown, 2007). But mice are not humans, and mouse models of Down syndrome are at best an approximation of the human condition. The recent failure of 80% of human clinical trials based on preclinical mouse research highlights the importance of choosing an appropriate model system—whether human cells, organoids, nematodes, fruit flies, zebrafish, mice, nonhuman primates, or mathematical models—and establishing that the model reflects the relevant features of Down syndrome (Perrin, 2014; Reeves et al., 2019).

We propose the following six design principles for Down syndrome models:

1. Models should be genetically representative of trisomy 21.
   - Overexpressing a single gene may not produce the same effect as overexpressing the same gene in the context of trisomy.
   - The presence of an extra, freely segregating chromosome may cause different phenotypes than those caused by internal duplications.
   - Outbred animals better reflect human genetic diversity than inbred, genetically identical animals but may show more individual variability.
   - Overexpressing human genes in nonhuman models relies on human genes functioning appropriately in those systems.
   - Mosaicism, the presence of the extra chromosome in some but not all cells, increases inter-individual variation.
   - Mapping panels will only identify gene-phenotype associations if a small number of trisomic genes have major effects on the phenotype or if multiple genes of small effect are physically contiguous on the chromosome.
2. Tissues containing the pertinent cell types should be accessible.
3. Models of developmental processes should be dynamic or develop in some way.
4. Models should be amenable to genetic or pharmacological manipulation.
5. Models should possess quantifiable phenotypes that resemble Down syndrome-associated phenotypes.
6. When choosing the best model for a given experiment, ethics, cost, practicality, and the ability to share models between labs should be considered.

Models Should Be Genetically Representative of Trisomy 21

Animals that are more closely related to humans are by definition more genetically similar to humans. This genetic similarity, called conservation, is evident at three different levels: gene order on the chromosome, DNA sequence, and protein sequence. The order of genes is roughly conserved between mouse and human, and one could reorganize the mouse genome into something resembling the human genome by making about 300 rearrangements (Mouse Genome Sequencing et al., 2002). Although mice have no chromosome 21, the mouse versions of human chromosome 21 genes, homologs, are located in three blocks on mouse chromosomes 10, 16, and 17 (Gupta et al., 2016). The conservation of DNA sequence between mouse and human is about 40% identical throughout the genome but about 85% identical within protein-coding genes (Makalowski, Zhang, & Boguski, 1996; Mouse Genome Sequencing et al., 2002). Some proteins are human- or mouse-specific, whereas other human and mouse proteins are nearly or 100% identical.

The conservation between human and mouse gene order, also called conservation of synteny, is critical because it has allowed researchers to create mice with trisomy for the chunks of the mouse genome that are homologous to human chromosome 21 (M. T. Davisson et al., 1993; Lana-Elola et al., 2016; Sago et al., 1998; Yu, Liu et al., 2010). Because overexpression of a single gene may have a different or more profound effect when overexpressed together with other trisomic genes, models that overexpress multiple homologs of chromosome 21 genes simultaneously are more genetically representative of Down syndrome than those overexpressing single chromosome 21 homologs.

The first major mouse model of Down syndrome took advantage of the fact that some chromosome 21 homologs are positioned near the end of mouse chromosome 16. In 1990, Muriel Davisson used radiation to induce rearrangements between mouse chromosomes. A screen of the resulting mice identified one in which the tip of chromosome 16 was fused to a small piece of chromosome 17, creating mice with trisomy for about half of the protein-coding mouse genes that have homologs on human chromosome 21 (M. T. Davisson et al., 1990, 1993). Although this mouse strain, called Ts65Dn, is trisomic for 90 protein-coding genes that are homologous to human chromosome 21 genes, it is also trisomic for 35 protein-coding genes that are not chromosome 21 homologs (Duchon et al., 2011; Gupta et al., 2016; Reinholdt et al., 2011). The Ts65Dn mouse has been the workhorse of Down syndrome research for nearly three decades, but concerns about its genetic content have prompted the creation of more genetically representative mouse models (Gupta et al., 2016). For example, chromosome engineering has been used to create duplications of the mouse genome regions homologous to human chromosome 21 to interrogate possible roles of genes in those segments for contributions to Down syndrome-like features (Herault et al., 2017).

What is the "perfect" mouse model? Choosing which model to use for a particular experiment is a critical decision, but every available model has strengths and weaknesses (Fig. 22.2).

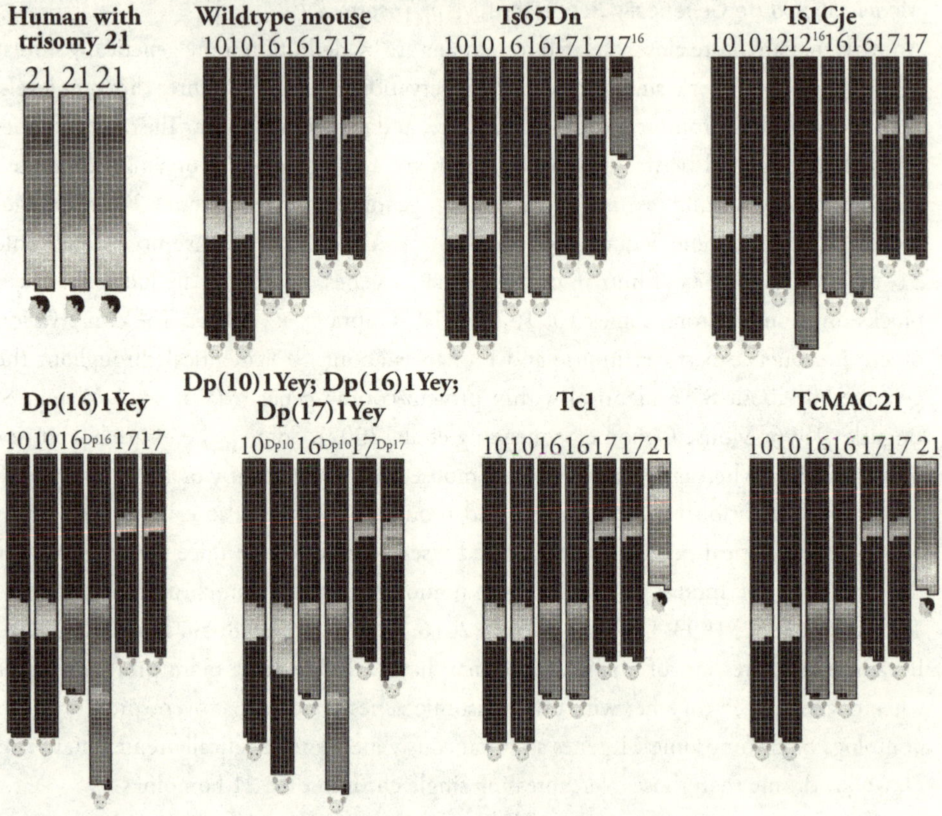

Figure 22.2. Genetic content of select Down syndrome mouse models. Each colored square represents one human chromosome 21 gene or homolog, and each black square represents ~500 kb of sequence that is not homologous to human chromosome 21. Ts65Dn and Ts1Cje mice are the results of translocations, whereas Dp(16)1Yey mice and Dp(10)1Yey; Dp(16)1Yey; Dp(17)1Yey mice contain tandem segmental duplications of mouse chromosome regions that are homologous to human chromosome 21. Tc1 and MAC21 mice possess portions of human chromosome 21 in addition to the normal complement of mouse chromosomes. Figure created with Biorender.com.

Ts65Dn mice have an extra freely segregating chromosome, but this chromosome contains genes that are not homologous to chromosome 21 genes (Duchon et al., 2011). It is the most well-established model, and labs may continue to study it because of the wealth of literature describing its phenotypes (Hardesty, 2018). Another popular model, Ts1Cje, is trisomic for a portion of chromosome 16 that is fused to chromosome 12 (Sago et al., 1998). Unlike Ts65Dn mice, Ts1Cje mice are not trisomic for genes on mouse chromosome 17, but they are monosomic for seven genes on chromosome 12 (Duchon et al., 2011). Because this model does not have an extra freely segregating chromosome, it cannot be used to study the general effects of aneuploidy, but having a normal chromosome number may also be why male Ts1Cje mice are more fertile than Ts65Dn mice (M. Davisson et al., 2007).

Another important consideration is genetic background. Except for monozygotic twins, humans are not genetically identical—a typical genome varies from the standard "reference" genome at four to five million sites (Genomes Project et al., 2015). Genetic variation throughout the genome may contribute to the wide range of phenotypic variability in people with Down syndrome (Epstein, 2014). However, many mouse strains commonly used for research are inbred, meaning that within a mouse strain, individual mice are more or less genetically identical (Festing, 2014). Genetic background also affects the severity of phenotypes in mouse models of Down syndrome. In one analysis, trisomic Ts1Rhr embryos possessed larger precursors of the mid and lower face than wild-type mice on an inbred genetic background, but they showed no difference on a mixed background with contributions from three inbred strains (Deitz & Roper, 2011). In another, genetic background affected the frequency of heart defects in trisomic Tc1 mice (Dunlevy et al., 2010). Moreover, the widely used Ts65Dn mouse model cannot be maintained as an inbred strain, which may complicate direct comparisons with trisomic models that are maintained as inbred strains (Aziz et al., 2018; Moore et al., 2010). The choice between studying a single inbred strain, comparing multiple inbred strains, or working with outbred stocks has practical significance. The genetic homogeneity of inbred mice may reduce variability, especially for behavioral phenotypes, which means that fewer mice are required to power statistical analyses (Chia, Achilli, Festing, & Fisher, 2005). A key consideration is whether the benefit of genetic homogeneity outweighs the poor correspondence to human genetic variation for a particular research question (Chia et al., 2005; Festing, 2014; Saul, Philip, Reinholdt, Center for Systems Neurogenetics of, & Chesler, 2019).

Researchers must also choose between overexpressing human chromosome 21 genes or overexpressing mouse homologs of chromosome 21 genes. New techniques in chromosome engineering have accelerated the pace of Down syndrome model development, but there is a fundamental limit to how well native mouse genes can mirror human trisomy 21. Human chromosome 21 contains nine protein-coding genes with no mouse homologs, and mouse chromosome 16 contains four protein-coding genes with no human homologs (Gupta et al., 2016). Dp(10)1Yey; Dp(16)1Yey; Dp(17)1Yey mice have direct duplications of all regions of the mouse genome that are homologous to human chromosome 21 and best represent the mouse orthologs in a model of Down syndrome currently available (P. V. Belichenko et al., 2015; Yu, Li et al., 2010). Despite the genetic similarity to human trisomy 21, these mice do not overexpress the nine human-specific chromosome 21 genes, and practical issues with breeding sufficient numbers of trisomic mice for many types of analyses have hampered its widespread use (Gupta et al., 2016).

O'Doherty et al. (2005) took a different tack by introducing human chromosome 21 into mouse cells. The resulting transchromosomic "Tc1" mice contain about 80% of human chromosome 21 as a freely segregating chromosome. Transchromosomic mice offer an approach for studying the effects of human-specific chromosome 21 genes, but there is no guarantee that human genes will functional appropriately when overexpressed in mouse cells. Additionally, more than fifty chromosome 21 genes are deleted or duplicated in Tc1 mice, and because mouse cells have a tendency to lose the human chromosome when dividing, adult Tc1 mice are mosaics—that is, they contain a mix of trisomic and wild-type cells (Gribble et al., 2013; O'Doherty et al., 2005). Because the random loss of chromosome 21 makes each Tc1 mouse a genetically distinct animal, this mosaicism may increase the phenotypic variability between trisomic animals.

Because human chromosomes propagate more faithfully in mouse cells when they are fused to small portions of mouse chromosomes, this technique can be used to create nonmosaic transchromosomic models (Takiguchi et al., 2014). A new mouse model, TcMAC21, contains most of the long arm of human chromosome 21 fused to a mouse artificial chromosome (Kazuki et al., 2020). Initial characterization indicates that the MAC21 chromosome is stable throughout mitosis and that TcMAC21 mice possess phenotypes relevant to Down syndrome. Although the long arm of chromosome 21 is nearly intact, TcMAC21 mice are not trisomic for the gene-poor short arm of chromosome 21.

Our discussion so far has focused on mouse models because the conservation of gene order between mouse and human supports the development of models that are trisomic for many genes. But does the low conservation of synteny in lower organisms mean that animal models like nematodes and fruit flies cannot be used to study Down syndrome? Is it ever useful to consider one or a few human chromosome 21 homologs at a time? Down syndrome is among the most complicated genetic perturbations compatible with life, and investigating one chromosome 21 homolog at a time can make studying gene-phenotype associations a more tractable problem. Screening individual chromosome 21 homologs in simple model organisms and characterizing the phenotypes of individuals with trisomy for part of chromosome 21 are two methods for simplifying the complexity of gene dosage effects in Down syndrome.

The first approach involves modulating the expression level of individual chromosome 21 homologs and screening for relevant phenotypes. Many types of large screens are not practical in mammalian models like mice, but they can be effective tools for characterizing chromosome 21 homologs in less complex systems. Nordquist, Smith, and Pierce (2018) examined simple behaviors in the microscopic nematode worm *C. elegans* and reported ten chromosome 21 homolog mutants with abnormal locomotion, exploration, or feeding. This screen may help to prioritize uncharacterized genes, but knockdown of genes may not produce the same phenotype as overexpression of the same genes. Edie et al. (2018) overexpressed 164 human chromosome 21 genes (cDNAs) in developing zebrafish embryos and identified eleven genes that cause gross morphological phenotypes when overexpressed. Although the extent to which *C. elegans* and zebrafish phenotypes apply to human trisomy 21 is unknown, these methods provide a first-pass evaluation of uncharacterized chromosome 21 genes and lend support for follow-up analysis of individual genes in mammalian systems.

The second method for simplifying the complex problem of assigning trisomic genes to particular phenotypes is to examine individuals who are trisomic for portions of chromosome 21, called partial trisomies (Lana-Elola, Watson-Scales, Fisher, & Tybulewicz,

2011). Mapping features to particular regions of chromosome 21 is challenging because individuals with partial trisomy are rare—a recent effort to integrate data from partial trisomy 21 cases identified only 107 individuals (Pelleri et al., 2017). This method is most powerful when many individuals are available for analysis, when the trait is defined quantitatively, when the exact trisomic region is known, when the trait occurs to a similar degree in most or all people with full trisomy 21, and when the trait is much more common in people with Down syndrome than in the general population (Korbel et al., 2009). In the laboratory, chromosome engineering techniques have facilitated the creation of high-resolution mouse "mapping panels" that are trisomic for small regions of the mouse chromosomes that are homologous to human chromosome 21 (Lana-Elola et al., 2016; Liu et al., 2014). Because the precise region of trisomy is controlled by the investigator and because a large number of mice can be bred and characterized in the lab, mouse mapping panels overcome some of the limitations of using human partial trisomies to associate phenotypes with particular trisomic genes.

The success of these strategies depends on the underlying genetic architecture of Down syndrome-associated traits. Mapping panels are most effective for traits that are caused primarily by trisomy for a single gene that has a major effect on the phenotype or by genes that are physically adjacent on the chromosome. However, we have no a priori knowledge of how many trisomic genes influence each phenotype or how these genes are distributed throughout the chromosome. Perhaps one or two trisomic genes have a large effect on the development of Hirschsprung disease in people with Down syndrome, whereas fifty trisomic genes of small effect could underlie intellectual disability. The complexity of the developmental processes involved in forming the brain suggests that many chromosome 21 genes may modulate brain development or physiology. Nevertheless, examinations of partial trisomy in humans and mapping panels in mice have identified candidate regions that are associated with phenotypes including congenital heart defects and leukemia risk (Korbel et al., 2009; Liu et al., 2014). Lana-Elola et al. (2016) concluded that at least two trisomic genes are required for the development of heart defects in mice. Another group used partial trisomy cases to prioritize chromosome 21 genes implicated in heart defects and overexpressed pairs of candidate genes in *Drosophila* to identify two genes that cooperate to disrupt heart development (Grossman et al., 2011). Determining which trisomic genes act to cause a given phenotype relies both on creating models that overexpress the hundreds of genes on chromosome 21 simultaneously and on establishing new methods for interrogating the complex interactions between chromosome 21 genes.

Tissues Containing the Pertinent Cell Types Should Be Accessible

Given that no animal model of Down syndrome is perfectly representative of trisomy 21, why not use human cells from individuals with Down syndrome? One obstacle is that two of the most salient features of Down syndrome, intellectual disability and Alzheimer's disease, affect tissues that are difficult to access in living people. Postmortem brain samples have provided important information about gene expression and morphological changes in brain structure, but they do not allow researchers to study single individuals longitudinally (Golden & Hyman, 1994; Olmos-Serrano et al., 2016; Pelleri et al., 2018; Schmidt-Sidor, Wisniewski, Shepard, & Sersen, 1990; Sylvester, 1983). And, although skin cells, blood, and cerebrospinal fluid can be collected from individuals with Down syndrome, their molecular similarity to differentiated neuronal tissues is less than ideal. Mouse models help to bridge this gap by providing access to tissues and organs across developmental stages. Induced pluripotent stem cells (iPSCs) are an exciting alternative that allow researchers to collect skin from individuals with Down syndrome and produce differentiated cell types like neurons and hematopoietic cells (Banno et al., 2016; Weick et al., 2013). When similarity to native tissues is validated, iPSCs could supplement or replace animal models of Down syndrome for some applications.

Models of Developmental Processes Should Be Dynamic or Develop in Some Way

During development of the human body, diverse cell types must coordinate processes like proliferation, migration, and differentiation to form properly organized tissues. This intricate operation relies on the ability of cells to communicate with one another via signaling pathways and other external cues. Because the phenotypes of Down syndrome change across the lifetime, determining the cause of particular developmental features requires studying a system that also develops in some way. In one such study, Roper et al. (2009) used both trisomic mouse embryos and cultured mouse cells to identify the early origins of craniofacial abnormalities in Down syndrome. The structure that eventually forms the mid and lower face contained fewer neural crest cells in trisomic Ts65Dn embryos than in wild-type embryos. When the source of neural crest cells was isolated and grown in culture, fewer neural crest cells migrated out of trisomic explants, and trisomic neural crest cells also responded less to an external proliferative signal. These experiments suggest that an insufficient number of cells is available to form the lower jaw because trisomic neural crest cells do not proliferate enough early in development. Because this deficit originates much earlier in development than the formation of the jaw, their discovery of the cause of craniofacial abnormalities depended on having access to an animal model across multiple stages of development.

Other recent efforts focus on modeling the complexity of brain development in persons with Down syndrome. Real et al. (2018) generated cortical neurons from human iPSCs with trisomy 21 and transplanted them into the mouse cortex, where the cells grew as grafts for several months. Similarly, Xu et al. (2019) produced 3D cerebral organoids from trisomic iPSCs and transplanted human neural progenitor cells into the brains of newborn mice, which impaired one form of memory in mice transplanted with trisomic cells but not in mice transplanted with control cells. As technologies for creating "mini-brain" organoids and transplanting trisomic neurons into mouse brains mature, they will provide much needed methods for examining early brain development in persons with Down syndrome.

Models Should Be Amenable to Genetic or Pharmacological Manipulation

The foundation of experimental research is the ability to measure the effect of manipulating treatment conditions on some phenotype of interest. Genetic research often involves mutating a gene and observing the phenotype that results. In studies of Down syndrome, genetic manipulations are helpful for associating trisomic genes with particular phenotypes. For example, data suggesting that reducing expression of the trisomic gene *SYNJ1* rescued an endosomal abnormality supports the hypothesis that *SYNJ1* plays a role in development of the endosomal phenotype (Cossec et al., 2012). Access to genomic sequence data from many organisms and new technologies for manipulating the genome have broadened the range of possible Down syndrome model systems (Birling et al., 2017; Ovchinnikov, Korn, Virshup, Wells, & Wolvetang, 2018). At the same time, treatments for Down syndrome phenotypes may prioritize drug treatments over genetic manipulations like gene therapy. Once a trisomic gene is associated with a feature of Down syndrome, a drug that inhibits the trisomic protein or a related pathway could be used to rescue the phenotype of interest. Drug screens have also been used to identify compounds that rescue the proliferation of trisomic cells and candidate drugs for treating acute myeloid leukemia (Nakano-Kobayashi et al., 2017; Wiggers et al., 2019). Model systems that allow easy genetic manipulation and drug treatment pave the way for the development of human therapies.

Models Should Possess Quantifiable Phenotypes That Resemble Down Syndrome-Associated Phenotypes

The appropriate criteria for validating Down syndrome models are not always obvious, but sharing phenotypic features with Down syndrome is an indisputable requirement. Extensive evidence from decades of research has confirmed that mouse models of Down syndrome do possess many Down syndrome-associated phenotypes, including heart defects, skeletal and craniofacial abnormalities, resistance to some forms of solid tumors, and impairments in learning and memory (Aziz et al., 2018; P. V. Belichenko et al., 2015; O'Doherty et al., 2005; Reeves et al., 1995; Richtsmeier, Baxter, & Reeves, 2000; Sussan, Yang, Li, Ostrowski, & Reeves, 2008; Williams, Mjaatvedt, & Moore, 2008). How well mouse behaviors resemble specific forms of cognitive impairment in individuals with Down syndrome remains an open question. As clinical trials in people with Down syndrome accelerate, determining the extent to which rodent behavioral assays predict analogous measures in humans will be essential.

Researchers hoping to translate mouse discoveries to the clinic have several questions to consider:

- Do human and mouse cognitive phenotypes share common developmental or functional origins?
- Is it possible to design tasks that target specific brain regions, or do all tasks require coordination between multiple brain regions?

- If we identify a specific cognitive phenotype in a mouse model, can we use that phenotype to design new endpoints for human clinical trials?
- Will a treatment that rescues a cognitive phenotype in a mouse model have the same effect in humans? Will it work via the same mechanism or during the same developmental period?
- How can we estimate whether a treatment that produces a *statistically* significant effect in mice will produce a *clinically* significant effect in humans?

Although some processes like speech and language development are uniquely human, a promising approach is to compare human and mouse measures that rely on the same brain regions (Fig. 22.3).

We will focus our discussion on two of the three brain regions assessed by the Arizona Cognitive Test Battery, which is comprised of a series of neuropsychological tasks designed specifically for persons with Down syndrome (Table 22.1; Edgin et al., 2010).

CEREBELLUM

Structure: Individuals with Down syndrome and the Ts65Dn mouse model share many cerebellar phenotypes, including a disproportional reduction in volume and reduced granule cell density (Aylward et al., 1997; Baxter, Moran, Richtsmeier, Troncoso, & Reeves, 2000; Roper et al., 2006). In contrast, the severity of the anatomical phenotypes varies among other Down syndrome mouse models (Olson et al., 2004; Olson et al., 2007; Powell et al., 2016; Starbuck, Dutka, Ratliff, Reeves, & Richtsmeier, 2014).

Physiology: A few changes in electrophysiology have been reported in the Ts65Dn cerebellum, including increased excitability, larger amplitude action potentials, and smaller tonic $GABA_A$ receptor currents in trisomic granule cells (Das et al., 2013; Szemes, Davies, Garden, & Usowicz, 2013; Usowicz & Garden, 2012).

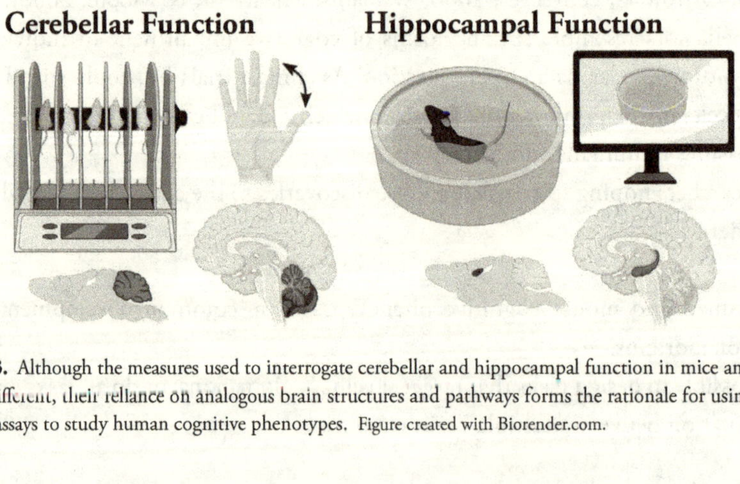

Figure 22.3. Although the measures used to interrogate cerebellar and hippocampal function in mice and humans may look different, their reliance on analogous brain structures and pathways forms the rationale for using mouse behavioral assays to study human cognitive phenotypes. Figure created with Biorender.com.

Table 22.1. Examples of Structural, Physiological, and Behavioral Measures of Regional Brain Phenotypes in Both Human and Mouse

Brain Region	Phenotype Level	Mouse Measures	Human Measures
Cerebellum	Structural	Volume (Olson et al., 2004; Olson et al., 2007; Powell et al., 2016; Starbuck et al., 2014), granule cell density (Baxter et al., 2000), granule cell precursor proliferation (Roper et al., 2006), Purkinje cell density (Baxter et al., 2000)	Volume (Aylward et al., 1997), granule cell density (Baxter et al., 2000)
	Physiological	Granule cell excitability (Usowicz & Garden, 2012), action potential amplitude, $GABA_A$ receptor current (Szemes et al., 2013)	
	Behavioral	Rotarod (Haydar & Reeves, 2012), gait analysis (Hampton et al., 2004), eyeblink conditioning (Kloth et al., 2015), vestibulo-ocular reflex adaptation (Gutierrez-Castellanos et al., 2013)	From the Arizona Cognitive Test Battery: CANTAB Simple Reaction Time task, Finger Sequencing Task, NEPSY Visuomotor Precision task (Edgin et al., 2010)
Hippocampus	Structural	Spine density (P. V. Belichenko et al., 2004), synaptic structure (Popov et al., 2011), interneuron number and composition (Chakrabarti et al., 2010)	Gray matter density (Menghini, Costanzo, & Vicari, 2011), dendritic architecture (Ferrer & Gullotta, 1990), size (Raz et al., 1995; Sylvester, 1983), myelination (Abraham et al., 2012), neurogenesis (Guidi et al., 2008)
	Physiological	Hippocampal LTP and LTD (Kleschevnikov et al., 2004; Siarey et al., 1999; Siarey et al., 1997)	
	Behavioral	Novel object recognition test (Hyde & Crnic, 2002; O'Doherty et al., 2005), object-in-place test (Fernandez & Garner, 2007), spontaneous alternation test (P. V. Belichenko et al., 2007), Morris water maze (Reeves et al., 1995), contextual fear conditioning (Costa et al., 2008)	From the Arizona Cognitive Test Battery: CANTAB Paired-Associates Learning task, spatial memory through navigation in computer-generated arena (Edgin et al., 2010)

Behavior: Despite the dramatic reduction in volume, identifying consistent impairments in cerebellum-specific behaviors has been challenging (Edgin et al., 2012). Traditional symptoms of cerebellar dysfunction highlight its role in motor control, such as ataxia, dysmetria, and tremor (Schmahmann, 2004). However, a growing appreciation for the cerebellum's involvement in higher-order cognitive processes like executive function, emotional processing, and language suggests that cerebellar hypoplasia could have far-reaching effects on cognitive impairment in persons with Down syndrome (Schmahmann, 2019). The following tasks are used to assess cerebellar function in mice:

- *Rotarod*: In this test of motor coordination, mice are trained to balance on a stationary or rotating rod (Carter, Morton, & Dunnett, 2001). The length of time that a mouse balances on the rod before falling is a measure of coordination and motor learning. The protocols for performing this test vary widely between labs, and reports of Rotarod impairment in trisomic mice are inconsistent (Haydar & Reeves, 2012).
- *Footprint analysis*: Walking and running gait can be assessed in mice with automated video recording or by coating the animal's feet in nontoxic paint and allowing it to walk along a strip of paper (Carter et al., 2001). Alterations in gait dynamics have been reported in Ts65Dn and Tc1 mice (Galante et al., 2009; Hampton, Stasko, Kale, Amende, & Costa, 2004).
- *Eyeblink conditioning*: Eyeblink conditioning is a type of classical conditioning that relies on the cerebellum, brainstem, and hippocampus (Boele, Koekkoek, & De Zeeuw, 2010; Reeb-Sutherland & Fox, 2015). It has been used to assess cerebellar function in people with Down syndrome and in mouse models of autism but not in mouse models of Down syndrome (Kloth et al., 2015; Ohlrich & Ross, 1968; Woodruff-Pak, Romano, & Papka, 1996).
- *Vestibulo-ocular reflex adaptation*: This test of cerebellar learning measures adaptation of the reflex that stabilizes images on the retina during head movement (Clopath, Badura, De Zeeuw, & Brunel, 2014). Abnormal vestibulo-ocular reflex learning has been reported in people with Down syndrome and in the Ts65Dn mouse model (Costa, 2011; Gutierrez-Castellanos et al., 2013).

Candidate treatments: Treatment with Smoothened Agonist (SAG), an activator of the Sonic hedgehog signaling pathway, rescued cerebellar morphology in Ts65Dn mice (Das et al., 2013; Roper et al., 2006). Although treatment with SAG improved performance on a hippocampal-dependent behavioral task, it did not affect subtle impairments in vestibulo-ocular reflex adaptation (Gutierrez-Castellanos et al., 2013). Because the Sonic hedgehog signaling pathway is central to many developmental processes, direct stimulation of the pathway may have unwanted effects on regions other than the cerebellum (Singh et al., 2015). However, these findings demonstrate that cerebellar hypoplasia can be ameliorated with a single perinatal treatment. The ability of SAG treatment to rescue a hippocampal-dependent task also raises questions about the involvement of the cerebellum in cognitive processes like spatial learning (Das et al., 2013; Gutierrez-Castellanos et al., 2013).

HIPPOCAMPUS

Structure: Given its essential role in learning and memory, the medial temporal lobe in mouse models of Down syndrome has been the subject of intense focus. Abnormalities in synaptic structure and cell-type composition in the hippocampus have been reported in Down syndrome mouse models, leading to the prominent hypothesis that overinhibition disrupts hippocampal synaptic plasticity (P. V. Belichenko, Kleschevnikov, Salehi, Epstein, & Mobley, 2007; P. V. Belichenko et al., 2004; Chakrabarti et al., 2010; Zorrilla de San Martin, Delabar, Bacci, & Potier, 2018). Ts65Dn mice possess small differences in CA1, CA3, and dentate gyrus cellularity (Insausti et al., 1998; Lorenzi & Reeves, 2006). Spine density is decreased in trisomic dentate gyrus granule cells, and hippocampal synaptic structure is also abnormal (P. V. Belichenko et al., 2004; P. V. Belichenko et al., 2007; Popov, Kleschevnikov, Klimenko, Stewart, & Belichenko, 2011). A study of cell-type composition linked an increased number of inhibitory interneurons in the CA1 region of Ts65Dn mice to overexpression of the trisomic genes *Olig1* and *Olig2* (Chakrabarti et al., 2010).

Physiology: Hippocampal long-term potentiation (LTP) and long-term depression (LTD) are thought to be the physiological bases for learning and memory, and the Galdzicki and Mobley groups characterized reduced LTP and increased LTD in hippocampal slices from Ts65Dn mice (Bliss & Lomo, 1973; Kleschevnikov et al., 2004; Neves, Cooke, & Bliss, 2008; Pastalkova et al., 2006; Siarey et al., 1999; Siarey et al., 1997). These findings have been replicated by numerous groups, but reports are difficult to compare given that the methods used to stimulate LTP vary (Costa & Grybko, 2005; Das & Reeves, 2011; Siarey et al., 1999). LTP is strongly correlated with learning and memory tasks, which makes electrophysiology a common endpoint in studies of behavioral evaluation based on genetic and pharmacological manipulations of mouse models (Jeffery & Morris, 1993; Moser, Krobert, Moser, & Morris, 1998). LTP and LTD have been assessed in hippocampal slices, but in vivo confirmation of altered synaptic plasticity using intact brains could provide further insight into hippocampal dysfunction in mouse models of Down syndrome (Blaise, 2013).

Behavior: The following behavioral tests are used to assess hippocampal function in mouse models.

- *Novel object recognition test:* This test takes advantage of the mouse's natural exploratory behavior and preference for novelty to probe object recognition memory (Antunes & Biala, 2012). The animal is first presented with two objects, then one object is replaced with an unfamiliar object. Mice tend to spend more time investigating the novel object than the familiar object. Modifications to the basic task shift reliance on environmental context and object position. For example, the object-in-place test requires mice to remember a familiar object when it is moved to a new location (Fernandez & Garner, 2007). Novel object recognition and object-in-place tests are frequently used to characterize hippocampal dysfunction in mouse models of Down syndrome, but reported deficits depend on mouse model and testing paradigm (N. P. Belichenko et al., 2009; Fernandez & Garner, 2007; Fernandez et al., 2007; Hyde & Crnic, 2002; O'Doherty et al., 2005).

- *Spontaneous alteration test:* When placed in a T- or Y-shaped maze, mice tend to explore a less recently visited arm of the maze (Conrad, Galea, Kuroda, & McEwen, 1996; Holter et al., 2015). The spontaneous alternation test has been used to measure short-term working memory in Ts65Dn, Ts1Cje, Ts1Rhr, and Tc1 mice (N. P. Belichenko et al., 2009; P. V. Belichenko et al., 2007; Fernandez et al., 2007; O'Doherty et al., 2005).
- *Morris water maze:* This test is used to quantify spatial navigation and memory by placing a mouse in a tank of opaque water and measuring its ability to learn the position of a hidden platform using contextual cues (Morris, 1984; Vorhees & Williams, 2006). The platform is removed, and the mouse continues to search for the platform in its former location. Deficits in the Morris water maze are robust in Ts65Dn mice as compared to control littermates, but other Down syndrome models are more variably affected (Morice et al., 2008; Olson et al., 2007; Reeves et al., 1995; Sago et al., 2000). The Morris water maze is one example of a test that has been adapted to study hippocampal function in people with Down syndrome with results in some tests that parallel those in mice (Edgin et al., 2010; Pennington, Moon, Edgin, Stedron, & Nadel, 2003).
- *Contextual fear conditioning:* Mice are trained to associate a context with an aversive stimulus, such as an electric shock. When exposed to the context, mice show freezing behavior even in the absence of the aversive stimulus (Fanselow & Poulos, 2005). Reduced freezing response has been observed in several Down syndrome mouse models (Costa, Scott-McKean, & Stasko, 2008; Salehi et al., 2009; Yu, Liu et al., 2010).

Candidate treatments: A striking number of pharmacological treatments are reported to rescue hippocampal function in the Ts65Dn mouse model (Gardiner, 2015). Several of these candidate drugs aim to correct the hippocampal excitation-inhibition imbalance by dampening the response to inhibitory signals (Braudeau et al., 2011; Fernandez et al., 2007; Martinez-Cue et al., 2013). On the basis of mouse preclinical data, one such drug targeting $GABA_A$ receptors reached phase II clinical trials (Reeves et al., 2019; Zorrilla de San Martin et al., 2018). Basmisanil's failure to significantly improve cognitive function in people with Down syndrome was a disappointing outcome, but it also offers the opportunity for a critical analysis of the mouse behavioral tests that supported development of the human trial.

A central unanswered question is why so many drug treatments rescue learning and memory via purportedly diverse mechanisms. Are there really so many ways to "fix" impairments in learning and memory, or could treatments somehow activate a common adaptive cellular stress response pathway (Brose, Savonenko, Devenney, Smith, & Reeves, 2019)? Another possibility is that the measures used to assess hippocampal function in mice are nonspecific, and the rescue of upstream processes improves hippocampal function indirectly. For example, treatment with the Sonic hedgehog agonist SAG was hypothesized to affect cerebellar morphology and function by stimulating granule cell precursor proliferation (Roper et al., 2006). SAG treatment indeed rescued cerebellar morphology, but performance on a hippocampal-dependent test was normalized while performance on a cerebellum-dependent test was not (Das et al., 2013; Gutierrez-Castellanos et al., 2013). On the basis of these experiments alone, it is not obvious whether SAG treatment improved performance on the Morris water maze by direct stimulation of the hippocampus or by rescue of cerebellar input to the forebrain.

Another obstacle to comparing the effects of candidate treatments is that the procedures for conducting behavioral experiments vary widely, and the same models are rarely assessed in the same lab at the same time. Even within a lab, results from behavioral tests may depend on the season and the sex of the experimenter (Drickamer, 1990; Ferguson & Maier, 2013; Sorge et al., 2014). Although consistent impairment on a task across labs and conditions provides an indication that the phenotype is robust, the lack of standardized protocols makes prioritizing which of the 20-plus candidate drugs should move forward to clinical trials a complicated undertaking.

The relationship between behavioral tasks and specific brain regions also merits further attention in people and in mice. Functional specialization of hippocampal subregions suggests that people with Down syndrome may possess relative impairments in some learning and memory tasks; however, most reports in which mouse behavioral tasks are referred to as "hippocampal-dependent" do not involve the examination of functional specialization within the hippocampus (Clark, Fernandez, Sakhon, Spano, & Edgin, 2017; Edgin et al., 2012; Fernandez & Garner, 2008; Smith, Kesner, & Korenberg, 2014; Sommer, Rose, Glascher, Wolbers, & Buchel, 2005). Behavioral tests are often too complex to assess one specific brain region in isolation, but tests also likely differ in the extent to which they rely on input from additional brain regions and phenotypes like body size and muscle strength. For example, measurements of learning and memory in the Morris water maze are more immune to hypo- or hyperactivity than mazes with land-based locomotion

(Vorhees & Williams, 2006). Similarly, eyeblink conditioning and vestibulo-ocular reflex adaptation depend less on musculoskeletal performance than measures like gait analysis and Rotarod (Boele et al., 2010; Gutierrez-Castellanos et al., 2013).

Given these challenges, thoughtful analysis of the implementation and interpretation of behavioral assays in Down syndrome mouse models may promote translation to human therapies. In particular, scientists should (a) make an effort to blind experimenters to genotype and treatment when possible, (b) standardize protocols between labs, (c) assess rescue of behaviors in multiple mouse models and multiple labs for candidate treatments, (d) communicate with researchers who design behavioral tasks for people with Down syndrome, and (e) probe subregion specialization using novel behavioral tests.

Researchers Should Consider Ethics, Cost, Practicality, and the Ability to Share Models Between Labs

The abstract merits of an ideal Down syndrome model can be delineated clearly, but in practice, technical constraints often limit the utility of otherwise optimal models. For example, the Dp(10)1Yey; Dp(16)1Yey; Dp(17)1Yey mouse model is trisomic for all regions of the mouse genome that are homologous to human chromosome 21, making it one of the most genetically representative mouse models currently available (Yu, Li et al., 2010). However, these mice are difficult to breed, and producing enough mice to conduct preclinical studies is challenging (Gupta et al., 2016). Chimpanzee trisomy 21 is likely the closest nonhuman model of Down syndrome, but using primates for Down syndrome research raises both ethical and practical concerns, and the NIH does not support the use of chimpanzees (Bloomsmith et al., 2019; Hirata, Hirai, Nogami, Morimura, & Udono, 2017). Given that funding for Down syndrome research is finite, scientists should aim to use the most simple and cost-effective model available for a particular research question. Recent studies in zebrafish and *C. elegans* highlight the advantages of using lower-model organisms for screens; however, evidence from rodent models will likely remain a key rationale for new human clinical trials in the near future (Edie et al., 2018; Nordquist et al., 2018).

A Framework for Integrating Design Principles and Measures of Validity

We have described six design principles to consider when choosing an experimental model of Down syndrome. Another way to discuss the usefulness of Down syndrome models is in the context of validity. Thirty years ago, Willner (1984) introduced three major criteria for assessing the validity of animal models for psychiatric conditions. More recently, Belzung and Lemoine (2011) reformulated Willner's original principles into a set of five criteria: homological, pathogenic, mechanistic, face, and predictive validity. Although

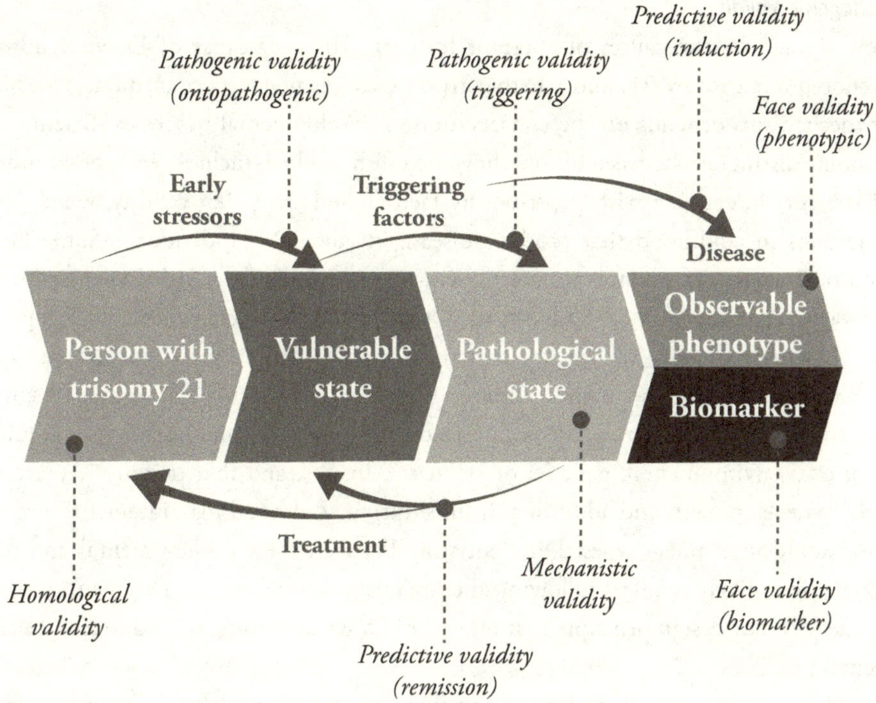

Figure 22.4. The similarity of disease development and progression at each of these stages forms the basis for assessments of model validity. Validity is divided broadly into whether the same factors cause disease in human and model, whether the mechanism of disease is similar between human and model, and whether the observable phenotypes in human and model resemble one another. Adapted from (Belzung & Lemoine, 2011). Figure created with Biorender.com.

Belzung and Lemoine's framework focuses on anxiety disorders and depression, we can use it to reorganize our design principles in terms of validity (Fig. 22.4).

This approach emphasizes the requirement that animal models reflect the process by which phenotypes develop in people with Down syndrome.

Homological Validity

Is the model genetically representative of human trisomy 21? Our first design principle is that models should reflect the human condition at the DNA level. Homological validity includes both similarity of the DNA sequence and conservation of gene order. A model with strong homological validity will have three copies of all chromosome 21 genes or of the model's endogenous chromosome 21 homologs. Moreover, the sequence similarity between the model's genes and human chromosome 21 genes should be high enough to imply shared function. Since many chromosome 21 genes act on genes elsewhere in the genome, homological validity extends to conservation across the genome.

Pathogenic Validity

How similar are the causes of aberrant features? The root cause of Down syndrome phenotypes is trisomy 21, and whether trisomy causes phenotypes in models via similar mechanisms depends on the conservation of developmental processes. Belzung and Lemoine distinguish between ontopathogenic validity, which includes early environmental stressors interacting with predisposing factors, and triggering validity, which refers to triggers in adulthood that produce disease in vulnerable individuals. Some Down syndrome-associated phenotypes are present in every individual with Down syndrome but vary in severity between individuals. Other phenotypes occur only in some people with Down syndrome. We suggest that trisomy 21 is sufficient to cause some Down syndrome-associated phenotypes without further stochastic or environmental effects; that trisomy 21 is a strong predisposing factor for developmental phenotypes requiring additional environmental, genetic, or stochastic insults; and that trisomy 21, stressors early in development, and additional insults during adulthood may interact to produce some adult-onset phenotypes. Differentiating between these developmental and functional effects likely requires following the organism throughout development, which is in line with our design principle that models of Down syndrome should reflect developmental processes.

Many assessments of pathogenic validity in animal models of Down syndrome focus on trisomy as a predisposing factor and assume that common phenotypes between humans and models share a common biological mechanism. Pathogenic validity also extends beyond trisomic chromosome 21 genes. For example, mutations in the disomic gene *CRELD1* are associated with congenital heart defects in families and in people with Down syndrome, and mutations in the mouse *Creld1* gene increase the frequency of congenital heart defects in Ts65Dn mice (Li et al., 2012, 2016). This finding suggests that *Creld1* mutations have good ontopathogenic validity with regard to congenital heart defects in Down syndrome.

Mechanistic Validity

Whereas pathogenic validity deals with the causes of Down syndrome-associated phenotypes, mechanistic validity refers to the similarity of the underlying disease pathogenesis at the cellular and molecular levels. Mechanistic validity is concerned with the way in which factors like trisomic genes and environmental insults actually generate the final phenotype and it is also the level at which therapeutics act—effective treatments targeting disease mechanisms at appropriate developmental periods will return the affected organism to the initial or vulnerable state. At the molecular level, models of Down syndrome show strong mechanistic validity if they overexpress trisomic genes to the same extent as people with Down syndrome and if the same developmental pathways or cellular processes are perturbed. We separate these molecular level phenotypes from organ- or organism-level phenotypes because a disease mechanism may not produce the same end phenotype in different model systems. For example, both Ts65Dn mice and people with Down syndrome show age-dependent loss of basal forebrain cholinergic neurons, but these neuronal changes may not produce comparable behavioral symptoms in humans and mice (Granholm, Sanders, & Crnic, 2000; Holtzman et al., 1996; Yates, Simpson, Maloney, Gordon, & Reid, 1980).

Face Validity

Face validity refers to the similarity of observed phenotypes between human and model systems, which corresponds to our design principle that models should possess quantitative phenotypes resembling Down syndrome-associated phenotypes (see "Models Should Possess Quantifiable Phenotypes That Resemble Down Syndrome-Associated Phenotypes " for a discussion of cerebellar and hippocampal phenotypes). Belzung and Lemoine partition face validity into ethological validity, or the similarity of behavioral phenotypes between humans and model systems, and biomarker validity (2011). For models of Down syndrome, face validity can include phenotypes other than behaviors, such as craniofacial abnormalities and congenital heart defects. For this reason, we include ethological validity in a broader category of phenotypic validity.

Predictive Validity

Predictive validity refers both to the likelihood that a model will develop phenotypes given the underlying disease triggers and to the likelihood that phenotypes will be rescued by appropriate treatments. The latter, called remission validity, is difficult to assess in animal models of Down syndrome because no effective therapeutic agents are currently available for most Down syndrome-associated phenotypes. One example of predictive validity is evidence that early intervention in humans and environmental enrichment in mice both improve cognitive phenotypes (Chakrabarti, Scafidi, Gallo, & Haydar, 2011; Mahoney, Perales, Wiggers, & Herman, 2006).

Scientists and clinicians who study persons with Down syndrome face the enormous challenge of choosing which potential therapies should move forward through the clinical pipeline. Conducting a clinical trial is extremely expensive, and identifying which model systems best reflect the human condition will benefit persons with Down syndrome, their families, researchers, and pharmaceutical companies alike. Ts65Dn is the most well-established mouse model of Down syndrome, but recent concerns about homological validity call into question whether Ts65Dn is the most appropriate model for human clinical trials (Gupta et al., 2016). Here we have formalized a series of design principles and adapted a framework of validity to assess the appropriateness of various Down syndrome models (Table 22.2). Considering this framework may help to estimate the value of data obtained from a given model system.

Table 22.2. Considering Five Categories of Validity to Determine Whether Ts65Dn Mice are a Valid Model for Down Syndrome-Associated Alzheimer's Disease

Type of validity	Similarity of . . .	Applied to Alzheimer's disease in Ts65Dn Down syndrome mouse model
Homological	Trisomic content, both in gene number and sequence conservation	The Ts65Dn mouse is trisomic for 90 protein-coding genes that are homologous to chromosome 21 genes and 35 protein-coding genes that are not chromosome 21 homologs (Duchon et al., 2011; Gupta et al., 2016). The mouse *App* and human *APP* genes are highly conserved but differ by three amino acids within the Aβ peptide region. One of these amino acid differences may make mouse Aβ less prone to forming aggregates than the human peptide (Hong et al., 2010).
Pathogenic (ontopathogenic)	Early factors that interact with trisomy to produce a vulnerable state	*APOE* allele affects amyloid burden in people with Down syndrome (Hyman, West, Rebeck, Lai, & Mann, 1995; Prasher et al., 2008). One test of ontopathogenic validity would be to assess whether mouse *Apoe* or a human *APOE* transgene affect neuropathology in Ts65Dn mice (Liao et al., 2015).
Pathogenic (triggering)	Triggers that shift the organism from a vulnerable to a disease state	Environmental triggers of Alzheimer's disease in Down syndrome are not well characterized, but age is a major contributing factor to disease development in people and in the Ts65Dn mouse model. Given that sleep fragmentation is associated with Alzheimer's risk in the general population and in a mouse model of Alzheimer's disease, one test of triggering validity would be to compare the effect of chronic sleep fragmentation on disease development in humans with Down syndrome and the Ts65Dn model (Macedo, Balouch, & Tabet, 2017; Minakawa et al., 2017).
Mechanistic	The assumed disease mechanism underlying phenotypes	People with Down syndrome and Ts65Dn mice both experience age-dependent loss of basal forebrain cholinergic neurons (Granholm et al., 2000). However, unlike people with Down syndrome, Ts65Dn mice do not develop amyloid plaques (Netzer et al., 2010).
Face (phenotypic)	Symptoms and features of the disease state	Ts65Dn mice display impairments in learning and memory that worsen with age (Granholm et al., 2000; Reeves et al., 1995).
Predictive (induction)	Progression to the disease state given exposure to etiological factors	The inductive validity measures the correspondence between etiological factors (trisomy, genetic background, environmental triggers, etc.) and the likelihood of developing symptoms.

Table 22.2. *Continued*		
Type of validity	Similarity of . . .	Applied to Alzheimer's disease in Ts65Dn Down syndrome mouse model
Predictive (remission)	Response to effective treatments	The NMDA receptor antagonist memantine improves learning and memory in people with Alzheimer's disease and in the Ts65Dn mouse model of Down syndrome, but *not* in people with Down syndrome (Costa et al., 2008; Hanney et al., 2012; Kishi et al., 2017).

Reasons for Optimism: Emerging Trends in Down Syndrome Research

Although the reality of clinical trials raises the stakes for the research of persons with Down syndrome, it is also an opportune time to reexamine which model systems provide the best path forward toward effective therapeutics. In response to critical discussions about the gene content of Ts65Dn mice, several groups have generated new models that better reflect the genetic basis of trisomy 21, including mice that are trisomic for all mouse homologs of chromosome 21 genes and mice that contain most of human chromosome 21 fused to a mouse artificial chromosome (Gupta et al., 2016; Kazuki et al., 2020; Yu, Li et al., 2010). New rat models could provide access to more sophisticated behavioral measures and permit procedures where the small size of mouse tissues is limiting (Birling et al., 2017). Organoids and transplantation of trisomic neurons into mouse brains are two new methods that may supplement traditional mouse models of brain development (Real et al., 2018; Xu et al., 2019). Continued research will reveal whether a consensus concerning the best replacement for Ts65Dn mice emerges in the scientific community.

In addition to creating models that are more genetically representative of trisomy 21, a current goal is to design new behavioral tests that better represent specific forms of cognitive impairment. Translational research often progresses from mouse to man, but a promising approach involves two-way collaboration between basic scientists and developmental psychologists to develop tasks that can be implemented equivalently in people and in rodents. For example, one group based a series of new measures of medial temporal lobe function in humans on a report that Ts65Dn mice exhibit specific deficits in dentate gyrus function (Clark et al., 2017; Smith et al., 2014). Identifying simple tasks that probe the same brain regions in humans and mice will support translation of mouse research to human studies.

Comparisons between mouse models are another useful way to demonstrate that findings are robust. Until recently, most research labs focused on one or two Down syndrome mouse models; however, comparing phenotypes between models may help to mask model-specific artifacts that are not relevant to human trisomy 21. Side-by-side examination of models using consistent methods in the same lab would promote the identification of subtle phenotypic differences between models. One effort to compare Ts65Dn, Ts1Cje, and Dp(16)1Yey mice across development revealed distinctive impairments in brain development, gene expression, and learning and memory between the three models (Aziz et al., 2018). Showing that a treatment is effective in multiple models provides further evidence that its effect is not due to a particular model's idiosyncrasies.

Studying all chromosome 21 genes individually remains technically challenging, but new screening methods should accelerate the annotation of uncharacterized chromosome 21 genes. A library of chromosome 21 cDNAs is publicly available, and a technique called CRISPR activation could be used to screen all chromosome 21 protein-coding and nonprotein-coding genes in a single pooled experiment (Edie et al., 2018; Joung et al., 2017; Ovchinnikov et al., 2018). In combination with a fluorescent reporter or single-cell RNA sequencing, CRISPR activation could rapidly profile the individual effects of chromosome 21 genes on cellular processes and gene expression (Dixit et al., 2016; Jaitin et al., 2016).

Another approach to simplifying the complexity of dosage imbalance is to search for "common denominator" pathways that are perturbed in multiple trisomic contexts. For example, disruption of the Sonic hedgehog signaling pathway could affect development of the cerebellum, heart, skull, and enteric nervous system (Currier, Polk, & Reeves, 2012). Chromosome 21 contains four interferon receptor genes, and upregulation of interferon signaling could contribute to the increased incidence of leukemia and autoimmune disorders in people with Down syndrome (Sullivan et al., 2016). Because comprehensively determining the actions of each individual chromosome 21 gene throughout the lifetime is a nearly intractable problem, examining common pathways may suggest new therapeutic avenues without knowledge of the specific mechanism underlying pathway disruption.

The convergence of new model systems, new behavioral assays, and new molecular techniques suggests that rational treatments for cognitive impairment in Down syndrome are near at hand, and lessons learned from these studies may also benefit research in related fields (see Box 22.1).

In the span of 30 years, research on persons with Down syndrome has progressed from the development of the first mouse model to completion of the first major clinical trials, and basic scientists, clinicians, and the Down syndrome community alike share a spirit of optimism for the future (M. T. Davisson et al., 1990; Reeves et al., 2019). Moving forward, prudent use of resources necessitates a critical analysis of Down syndrome models to determine which research strategies are most likely to identify effective therapies.

Box 22.1 What the Scientific Community Can Learn From Down Syndrome Research

Down syndrome is the most common genetic cause of intellectual disability, affecting an estimated 5 million individuals worldwide (GBD 2015 Disease and Injury Incidence and Prevalence Collaborators, 2016). Although Down syndrome research has the potential to improve the quality of life for people with Down syndrome, it also offers valuable insights for the scientific community at large. Because Down syndrome affects most body systems, successful investigation of Down syndrome-associated phenotypes has required a spirit of collegiality and collaboration between disparate disciplines, which is an increasingly recognized objective in other scientific fields. Down syndrome research may also benefit individuals without Down syndrome, including those with Alzheimer's disease, cancer, and type 2 diabetes (Hartley et al., 2015; Hasle, Friedman, Olsen, & Rasmussen, 2016; Peiris et al., 2016). Creating cognitive batteries for people with Down syndrome is challenging, and lessons learned from recent efforts could be applied to design valid endpoints for clinical trials in other populations with intellectual disability (Edgin et al., 2010; Liogier d'Ardhuy et al., 2015). Finally, Down syndrome serves as a model complex disease because phenotypes are caused by small increases in the expression of hundreds of genes, but unlike most complex diseases, the genetic cause of Down syndrome features is known. The complexity of Down syndrome pathogenesis makes identifying effective therapeutics a formidable task; however, in the last few decades, the research community has made encouraging progress toward unraveling the origins of intellectual disability in Down syndrome, and these advances may have far-reaching significance for other fields of study.

Acknowledgments

This work is supported in part by PHS awards HD038384, HD098540, and U54HD079123-01A1 (RHR); and by T32GM07814 and 1F31HD098826-01 (AJM). All conclusions are the authors' own and do not necessarily reflect those of the National Institutes of Health.

References

Abraham, H., Vincze, A., Veszpremi, B., Kravjak, A., Gomori, E., Kovacs, G. G., & Seress, L. (2012). Impaired myelination of the human hippocampal formation in Down syndrome. *Int J Dev Neurosci*, *30*(2), 147–158. doi:10.1016/j.ijdevneu.2011.11.005

Antonarakis, S. E. (2017). Down syndrome and the complexity of genome dosage imbalance. *Nat Rev Genet*, *18*(3), 147–163. doi:10.1038/nrg.2016.154

Antunes, M., & Biala, G. (2012). The novel object recognition memory: Neurobiology, test procedure, and its modifications. *Cogn Process*, *13*(2), 93–110. doi:10.1007/s10339-011-0430-z

Aylward, E. H., Habbak, R., Warren, A. C., Pulsifer, M. B., Barta, P. E., Jerram, M., & Pearlson, G. D. (1997). Cerebellar volume in adults with Down syndrome. *Arch Neurol*, *54*(2), 209–212. doi:10.1001/archneur.1997.00550140077016

Aziz, N. M., Guedj, F., Pennings, J. L. A., Olmos-Serrano, J. L., Siegel, A., Haydar, T. F., & Bianchi, D. W. (2018). Lifespan analysis of brain development, gene expression and behavioral phenotypes in the Ts1Cje, Ts65Dn and Dp(16)1/Yey mouse models of Down syndrome. *Dis Model Mech*, *11*(6). doi:10.1242/dmm.031013

Badano, J. L., & Katsanis, N. (2002). Beyond Mendel: An evolving view of human genetic disease transmission. *Nat Rev Genet*, *3*(10), 779–789. doi:10.1038/nrg910

Banno, K., Omori, S., Hirata, K., Nawa, N., Nakagawa, N., Nishimura, K., . . . Ozono, K. (2016). Systematic cellular disease models reveal synergistic interaction of trisomy 21 and GATA1 mutations in hematopoietic abnormalities. *Cell Rep, 15*(6), 1228–1241. doi:10.1016/j.celrep.2016.04.031

Baxter, L. L., Moran, T. H., Richtsmeier, J. T., Troncoso, J., & Reeves, R. H. (2000). Discovery and genetic localization of Down syndrome cerebellar phenotypes using the Ts65Dn mouse. *Hum Mol Genet, 9*(2), 195–202. doi:10.1093/hmg/9.2.195

Beach, R. R., Ricci-Tam, C., Brennan, C. M., Moomau, C. A., Hsu, P. H., Hua, B., . . . Amon, A. (2017). Aneuploidy Causes Non-genetic Individuality. *Cell, 169*(2), 229–242. e221. doi:10.1016/j.cell.2017.03.021

Belichenko, N. P., Belichenko, P. V., Kleschevnikov, A. M., Salehi, A., Reeves, R. H., & Mobley, W. C. (2009). The "Down syndrome critical region" is sufficient in the mouse model to confer behavioral, neurophysiological, and synaptic phenotypes characteristic of Down syndrome. *J Neurosci, 29*(18), 5938–5948. doi:10.1523/JNEUROSCI.1547-09.2009

Belichenko, P. V., Kleschevnikov, A. M., Becker, A., Wagner, G. E., Lysenko, L. V., Yu, Y. E., & Mobley, W. C. (2015). Down syndrome cognitive phenotypes modeled in mice trisomic for all Hsa 21 homologues. *PLoS One, 10*(7), e0134861. doi:10.1371/journal.pone.0134861

Belichenko, P. V., Kleschevnikov, A. M., Salehi, A., Epstein, C. J., & Mobley, W. C. (2007). Synaptic and cognitive abnormalities in mouse models of Down syndrome: Exploring genotype-phenotype relationships. *J Comp Neurol, 504*(4), 329–345. doi:10.1002/cne.21433

Belichenko, P. V., Masliah, E., Kleschevnikov, A. M., Villar, A. J., Epstein, C. J., Salehi, A., & Mobley, W. C. (2004). Synaptic structural abnormalities in the Ts65Dn mouse model of Down syndrome. *J Comp Neurol, 480*(3), 281–298. doi:10.1002/cne.20337

Belzung, C., & Lemoine, M. (2011). Criteria of validity for animal models of psychiatric disorders: Focus on anxiety disorders and depression. *Biol Mood Anxiety Disord, 1*(1), 9. doi:10.1186/2045-5380-1-9

Birling, M. C., Schaeffer, L., Andre, P., Lindner, L., Marechal, D., Ayadi, A., . . . Herault, Y. (2017). Efficient and rapid generation of large genomic variants in rats and mice using CRISMERE. *Sci Rep, 7*, 43331. doi:10.1038/srep43331

Blaise, J. H. (2013). Long-term potentiation of perforant pathway-dentate gyrus synapse in freely behaving mice. *J Vis Exp, 81*. doi:10.3791/50642

Bliss, T. V., & Lomo, T. (1973). Long-lasting potentiation of synaptic transmission in the dentate area of the anaesthetized rabbit following stimulation of the perforant path. *J Physiol, 232*(2), 331–356. doi:10.1113/jphysiol.1973.sp010273

Bloomsmith, M. A., Clay, A. W., Lambeth, S. P., Lutz, C. K., Breaux, S. D., Lammey, M. L., . . . Bourgeois, S. R. (2019). Survey of behavioral indices of welfare in research chimpanzees (Pan troglodytes) in the United States. *J Am Assoc Lab Anim Sci, 58*(2), 160–177. doi:10.30802/AALAS-JAALAS-18-000034

Boele, H. J., Koekkoek, S. K., & De Zeeuw, C. I. (2010). Cerebellar and extracerebellar involvement in mouse eyeblink conditioning: The ACDC model. *Front Cell Neurosci, 3*, 19. doi:10.3389/neuro.03.019.2009

Braudeau, J., Delatour, B., Duchon, A., Pereira, P. L., Dauphinot, L., de Chaumont, F., . . . Potier, M. C. (2011). Specific targeting of the GABA-A receptor alpha5 subtype by a selective inverse agonist restores cognitive deficits in Down syndrome mice. *J Psychopharmacol, 25*(8), 1030–1042. doi:10.1177/0269881111405366

Brewer, C. M., Holloway, S. H., Stone, D. H., Carothers, A. D., & FitzPatrick, D. R. (2002). Survival in trisomy 13 and trisomy 18 cases ascertained from population based registers. *J Med Genet, 39*(9), e54. doi:10.1136/jmg.39.9.e54

Brose, R. D., Savonenko, A., Devenney, B., Smith, K. D., & Reeves, R. H. (2019). Hydroxyurea improves spatial memory and cognitive plasticity in mice and has a mild effect on these parameters in a Down syndrome mouse model. *Front Aging Neurosci, 11*, 96. doi:10.3389/fnagi.2019.00096

Carter, R. J., Morton, J., & Dunnett, S. B. (2001). Motor coordination and balance in rodents. *Curr Protoc Neurosci, Chapter 8* , Unit 8 12. doi:10.1002/0471142301.ns0812s15

Chakrabarti, L., Best, T. K., Cramer, N. P., Carney, R. S., Isaac, J. T., Galdzicki, Z., & Haydar, T. F. (2010). Olig1 and Olig2 triplication causes developmental brain defects in Down syndrome. *Nat Neurosci, 13*(8), 927–934. doi:10.1038/nn.2600

Chakrabarti, L., Scafidi, J., Gallo, V., & Haydar, T. F. (2011). Environmental enrichment rescues postnatal neurogenesis defect in the male and female Ts65Dn mouse model of Down syndrome. *Dev Neurosci, 33*(5), 428–441. doi:10.1159/000329423

Chia, R., Achilli, F., Festing, M. F., & Fisher, E. M. (2005). The origins and uses of mouse outbred stocks. *Nat Genet, 37*(11), 1181–1186. doi:10.1038/ng1665

Clark, C. A. C., Fernandez, F., Sakhon, S., Spano, G., & Edgin, J. O. (2017). The medial temporal memory system in Down syndrome: Translating animal models of hippocampal compromise. *Hippocampus, 27*(6), 683–691. doi:10.1002/hipo.22724

Clopath, C., Badura, A., De Zeeuw, C. I., & Brunel, N. (2014). A cerebellar learning model of vestibulo-ocular reflex adaptation in wild-type and mutant mice. *J Neurosci, 34*(21), 7203–7215. doi:10.1523/JNEUROSCI.2791-13.2014

Conrad, C. D., Galea, L. A., Kuroda, Y., & McEwen, B. S. (1996). Chronic stress impairs rat spatial memory on the Y maze, and this effect is blocked by tianeptine pretreatment. *Behav Neurosci, 110*(6), 1321–1334.

Cossec, J. C., Lavaur, J., Berman, D. E., Rivals, I., Hoischen, A., Stora, S., . . . Potier, M. C. (2012). Trisomy for synaptojanin1 in Down syndrome is functionally linked to the enlargement of early endosomes. *Hum Mol Genet, 21*(14), 3156–3172. doi:10.1093/hmg/dds142

Costa, A. C. (2011). An assessment of the vestibulo-ocular reflex (VOR) in persons with Down syndrome. *Exp Brain Res, 214*(2), 199–213. doi:10.1007/s00221-011-2820-y

Costa, A. C., & Grybko, M. J. (2005). Deficits in hippocampal CA1 LTP induced by TBS but not HFS in the Ts65Dn mouse: A model of Down syndrome. *Neurosci Lett, 382*(3), 317–322. doi:10.1016/j.neulet.2005.03.031

Costa, A. C., Scott-McKean, J. J., & Stasko, M. R. (2008). Acute injections of the NMDA receptor antagonist memantine rescue performance deficits of the Ts65Dn mouse model of Down syndrome on a fear conditioning test. *Neuropsychopharmacology, 33*(7), 1624–1632. doi:10.1038/sj.npp.1301535

Currier, D. G., Polk, R. C., & Reeves, R. H. (2012). A Sonic hedgehog (Shh) response deficit in trisomic cells may be a common denominator for multiple features of Down syndrome. *Prog Brain Res, 197*, 223–236. doi:10.1016/B978-0-444-54299-1.00011-X

Das, I., Park, J. M., Shin, J. H., Jeon, S. K., Lorenzi, H., Linden, D. J., . . . Reeves, R. H. (2013). Hedgehog agonist therapy corrects structural and cognitive deficits in a Down syndrome mouse model. *Sci Transl Med, 5*(201), 201ra120. doi:10.1126/scitranslmed.3005983

Das, I., & Reeves, R. H. (2011). The use of mouse models to understand and improve cognitive deficits in Down syndrome. *Dis Model Mech, 4*(5), 596–606. doi:10.1242/dmm.007716

Davisson, M., Akeson, E., Schmidt, C., Harris, B., Farley, J., & Handel, M. A. (2007). Impact of trisomy on fertility and meiosis in male mice. *Hum Reprod, 22*(2), 468–476. doi:10.1093/humrep/del397

Davisson, M. T., Schmidt, C., & Akeson, E. C. (1990). Segmental trisomy of murine chromosome 16: A new model system for studying Down syndrome. *Prog Clin Biol Res, 360*, 263–280.

Davisson, M. T., Schmidt, C., Reeves, R. H., Irving, N. G., Akeson, E. C., Harris, B. S., & Bronson, R. T. (1993). Segmental trisomy as a mouse model for Down syndrome. *Prog Clin Biol Res, 384*, 117–133.

Deitz, S. L., & Roper, R. J. (2011). Trisomic and allelic differences influence phenotypic variability during development of Down syndrome mice. *Genetics, 189*(4), 1487–1495. doi:10.1534/genetics.111.131391

D'Souza, H., Mason, L., Mok, K. Y., Startin, C. M., Hamburg, S., Hithersay, R., . . . London Down Syndrome (LonDownS) Consortium. (2020). Differential associations of apolipoprotein E ε4 genotype with attentional abilities across the life span of individuals with Down syndrome. *JAMA Netw Open, 3*(9), e2018221. doi: 10.1001/jamanetworkopen.2020.18221.

Dixit, A., Parnas, O., Li, B., Chen, J., Fulco, C. P., Jerby-Arnon, L., . . . Regev, A. (2016). Perturb-seq: Dissecting molecular circuits with scalable single-cell RNA profiling of pooled genetic screens. *Cell, 167*(7), 1853–1866 e1817. doi:10.1016/j.cell.2016.11.038

Doran, E., Keator, D., Head, E., Phelan, M. J., Kim, R., Totoiu, M., . . . Lott, I. T. (2017). Down syndrome, partial trisomy 21, and absence of Alzheimer's disease: The role of APP. *J Alzheimers Dis, 56*(2), 459–470. doi:10.3233/JAD-160836

Drickamer, L. C. (1990). Seasonal variation in fertility, fecundity and litter sex ratio in laboratory and wild stocks of house mice (*Mus domesticus*). *Lab Anim Sci, 40*(3), 284–288.

Duchon, A., Raveau, M., Chevalier, C., Nalesso, V., Sharp, A. J., & Herault, Y. (2011). Identification of the translocation breakpoints in the Ts65Dn and Ts1Cje mouse lines: Relevance for modeling Down syndrome. *Mamm Genome, 22*(11–12), 674–684. doi:10.1007/s00335-011-9356-0

Dunlevy, L., Bennett, M., Slender, A., Lana-Elola, E., Tybulewicz, V. L., Fisher, E. M., & Mohun, T. (2010). Down's syndrome-like cardiac developmental defects in embryos of the transchromosomic Tc1 mouse. *Cardiovasc Res, 88*(2), 287–295. doi:10.1093/cvr/cvq193

Edgin, J. O., Mason, G. M., Allman, M. J., Capone, G. T., Deleon, I., Maslen, C., . . . Nadel, L. (2010). Development and validation of the Arizona Cognitive Test Battery for Down syndrome. *J Neurodev Disord, 2*(3), 149–164. doi:10.1007/s11689-010-9054-3

Edgin, J. O., Mason, G. M., Spano, G., Fernandez, A., & Nadel, L. (2012). Human and mouse model cognitive phenotypes in Down syndrome: Implications for assessment. *Prog Brain Res, 197*, 123–151. doi:10.1016/B978-0-444-54299-1.00007-8

Edie, S., Zaghloul, N. A., Leitch, C. C., Klinedinst, D. K., Lebron, J., Thole, J. F., . . . Reeves, R. H. (2018). Survey of human chromosome 21 gene expression effects on early development in *Danio rerio*. *G3 (Bethesda), 8*(7), 2215–2223. doi:10.1534/g3.118.200144

Epstein, C. J. (2014). Down syndrome (trisomy 21). In D. Valle, A. L. Beaudet, & B. Vogelstein (Eds.), *The Online Metabolic and Molecular Bases of Inherited Disease*. New York, NY: McGraw-Hill.

Fanselow, M. S., & Poulos, A. M. (2005). The neuroscience of mammalian associative learning. *Annu Rev Psychol, 56*, 207–234. doi:10.1146/annurev.psych.56.091103.070213

Ferguson, S. A., & Maier, K. L. (2013). A review of seasonal/circannual effects of laboratory rodent behavior. *Physiol Behav, 119*, 130–136. doi:10.1016/j.physbeh.2013.06.007

Fernandez, F., & Garner, C. C. (2007). Object recognition memory is conserved in Ts1Cje, a mouse model of Down syndrome. *Neurosci Lett, 421*(2), 137–141. doi:10.1016/j.neulet.2007.04.075

Fernandez, F., & Garner, C. C. (2008). Episodic-like memory in Ts65Dn, a mouse model of Down syndrome. *Behav Brain Res, 188*(1), 233–237. doi:10.1016/j.bbr.2007.09.015

Fernandez, F., Morishita, W., Zuniga, E., Nguyen, J., Blank, M., Malenka, R. C., & Garner, C. C. (2007). Pharmacotherapy for cognitive impairment in a mouse model of Down syndrome. *Nat Neurosci, 10*(4), 411–413. doi:10.1038/nn1860

Ferrer, I., & Gullotta, F. (1990). Down's syndrome and Alzheimer's disease: dendritic spine counts in the hippocampus. *Acta Neuropathol, 79*(6), 680–685.

Festing, M. F. (2014). Evidence should trump intuition by preferring inbred strains to outbred stocks in preclinical research. *ILAR J, 55*(3), 399–404. doi:10.1093/ilar/ilu036

Galante, M., Jani, H., Vanes, L., Daniel, H., Fisher, E. M., Tybulewicz, V. L., . . . Morice, E. (2009). Impairments in motor coordination without major changes in cerebellar plasticity in the Tc1 mouse model of Down syndrome. *Hum Mol Genet, 18*(8), 1449–1463. doi:10.1093/hmg/ddp055

Gardiner, K. J. (2015). Pharmacological approaches to improving cognitive function in Down syndrome: Current status and considerations. *Drug Des Devel Ther, 9*, 103–125. doi:10.2147/DDDT.S51476

GBD 2015 Disease and Injury Incidence and Prevalence Collaborators. (2016). Global, regional, and national incidence, prevalence, and years lived with disability for 310 diseases and injuries, 1990–2015: A systematic analysis for the Global Burden of Disease Study 2015. *Lancet, 388*(10053), 1545–1602. doi:10.1016/S0140-6736(16)31678-6

Genomes Project, C., Auton, A., Brooks, L. D., Durbin, R. M., Garrison, E. P., Kang, H. M., . . . Abecasis, G. R. (2015). A global reference for human genetic variation. *Nature, 526*(7571), 68–74. doi:10.1038/nature15393

Glenner, G. G., & Wong, C. W. (1984). Alzheimer's disease and Down's syndrome: sharing of a unique cerebrovascular amyloid fibril protein. *Biochem Biophys Res Commun, 122*(3), 1131–1135. doi:10.1016/0006-291x(84)91209-9

Golden, J. A., & Hyman, B. T. (1994). Development of the superior temporal neocortex is anomalous in trisomy 21. *J Neuropathol Exp Neurol, 53*(5), 513–520. doi:10.1097/00005072-199409000-00011

Granholm, A. C., Sanders, L. A., & Crnic, L. S. (2000). Loss of cholinergic phenotype in basal forebrain coincides with cognitive decline in a mouse model of Down's syndrome. *Exp Neurol, 161*(2), 647–663. doi:10.1006/exnr.1999.7289

Gribble, S. M., Wiseman, F. K., Clayton, S., Prigmore, E., Langley, E., Yang, F., . . . Carter, N. P. (2013). Massively parallel sequencing reveals the complex structure of an irradiated human chromosome on a mouse background in the Tc1 model of Down syndrome. *PLoS One, 8*(4), e60482. doi:10.1371/journal.pone.0060482

Grossman, T. R., Gamliel, A., Wessells, R. J., Taghli-Lamallem, O., Jepsen, K., Ocorr, K., . . . Bier, E. (2011). Over-expression of DSCAM and COL6A2 cooperatively generates congenital heart defects. *PLoS Genet, 7*(11), e1002344. doi:10.1371/journal.pgen.1002344 [doi] PGENETICS-D-11-01353 [pii]

Guidi, S., Bonasoni, P., Ceccarelli, C., Santini, D., Gualtieri, F., Ciani, E., & Bartesaghi, R. (2008). Neurogenesis impairment and increased cell death reduce total neuron number in the hippocampal region of fetuses with Down syndrome. *Brain Pathol, 18*(2), 180–197. doi:10.1111/j.1750-3639.2007.00113.x

Gupta, M., Dhanasekaran, A. R., & Gardiner, K. J. (2016). Mouse models of Down syndrome: Gene content and consequences. *Mamm Genome, 27*(11–12), 538–555. doi:10.1007/s00335-016-9661-8

Gutierrez-Castellanos, N., Winkelman, B. H., Tolosa-Rodriguez, L., Devenney, B., Reeves, R. H., & De Zeeuw, C. I. (2013). Size does not always matter: Ts65Dn Down syndrome mice show cerebellum-dependent motor learning deficits that cannot be rescued by postnatal SAG treatment. *J Neurosci, 33*(39), 15408–15413. doi:10.1523/JNEUROSCI.2198-13.2013

Hampton, T. G., Stasko, M. R., Kale, A., Amende, I., & Costa, A. C. (2004). Gait dynamics in trisomic mice: Quantitative neurological traits of Down syndrome. *Physiol Behav, 82*(2–3), 381–389. doi:10.1016/j.physbeh.2004.04.006

Hanney, M., Prasher, V., Williams, N., Jones, E. L., Aarsland, D., Corbett, A., . . . researchers, M. t. (2012). Memantine for dementia in adults older than 40 years with Down's syndrome (MEADOWS): A randomised, double-blind, placebo-controlled trial. *Lancet, 379*(9815), 528–536. doi:10.1016/S0140-6736(11)61676-0

Hanson, J. E., Blank, M., Valenzuela, R. A., Garner, C. C., & Madison, D. V. (2007). The functional nature of synaptic circuitry is altered in area CA3 of the hippocampus in a mouse model of Down's syndrome. *J Physiol, 579*(Pt 1), 53–67. doi:10.1113/jphysiol.2006.114868

Hardesty, R. A. (2018). Much ado about mice: Standard-setting in model organism research. *Stud Hist Philos Biol Biomed Sci, 68–69*, 15–24. doi:10.1016/j.shpsc.2018.04.001

Hartley, D., Blumenthal, T., Carrillo, M., DiPaolo, G., Esralew, L., Gardiner, K., . . . Wisniewski, T. (2015). Down syndrome and Alzheimer's disease: Common pathways, common goals. *Alzheimers Dement, 11*(6), 700–709. doi:10.1016/j.jalz.2014.10.007

Hartman, J. L., IV, Garvik, B., & Hartwell, L. (2001). Principles for the buffering of genetic variation. *Science, 291*(5506), 1001–1004. https://pubmed.ncbi.nlm.nih.gov/11232561

Hasle, H., Friedman, J. M., Olsen, J. H., & Rasmussen, S. A. (2016). Low risk of solid tumors in persons with Down syndrome. *Genet Med, 18*(11), 1151–1157. doi:10.1038/gim.2016.23

Hassold, T. J., & Jacobs, P. A. (1984). Trisomy in man. *Annu Rev Genet, 18*, 69–97. doi:10.1146/annurev.ge.18.120184.000441

Hattori, M., Fujiyama, A., Taylor, T. D., Watanabe, H., Yada, T., Park, H. S., . . . sequencing, c. (2000). The DNA sequence of human chromosome 21. *Nature, 405*(6784), 311–319. doi:10.1038/35012518

Haydar, T. F., & Reeves, R. H. (2012). Trisomy 21 and early brain development. *Trends Neurosci, 35*(2), 81–91. doi:10.1016/j.tins.2011.11.001

Herault, Y., Delabar, J. M., Fisher, E. M. C., Tybulewicz, V. L. J., Yu, E., & Brault, V. (2017). Rodent models in Down syndrome research: Impact and future opportunities. *Dis Model Mech, 10*(10), 1165–1186. doi:10.1242/dmm.029728

Hirata, S., Hirai, H., Nogami, E., Morimura, N., & Udono, T. (2017). Chimpanzee Down syndrome: A case study of trisomy 22 in a captive chimpanzee. *Primates, 58*(2), 267–273. doi:10.1007/s10329-017-0597-8

Holter, S. M., Garrett, L., Einicke, J., Sperling, B., Dirscherl, P., Zimprich, A., . . . Wurst, W. (2015). Assessing cognition in mice. *Curr Protoc Mouse Biol, 5*(4), 331–358. doi:10.1002/9780470942390.mo150068

Holtzman, D. M., Santucci, D., Kilbridge, J., Chua-Couzens, J., Fontana, D. J., Daniels, S. E., . . . Mobley, W. C. (1996). Developmental abnormalities and age-related neurodegeneration in a mouse model of Down syndrome. *Proc Natl Acad Sci U S A, 93*(23), 13333–13338. doi:10.1073/pnas.93.23.13333

Hong, L., Carducci, T. M., Bush, W. D., Dudzik, C. G., Millhauser, G. L., & Simon, J. D. (2010). Quantification of the binding properties of Cu2+ to the amyloid beta peptide: Coordination spheres for human and rat peptides and implication on Cu2+-induced aggregation. *J Phys Chem B, 114*(34), 11261–11271. doi:10.1021/jp103272v

Hook, E. B., Mutton, D. E., Ide, R., Alberman, E., & Bobrow, M. (1995). The natural history of Down syndrome conceptuses diagnosed prenatally that are not electively terminated. *Am J Hum Genet, 57*(4), 875–881.

Hyde, L. A., & Crnic, L. S. (2002). Reactivity to object and spatial novelty is normal in older Ts65Dn mice that model Down syndrome and Alzheimer's disease. *Brain Res, 945*(1), 26–30. doi:10.1016/s0006-8993(02)02500-3

Hyman, B. T., West, H. L., Rebeck, G. W., Lai, F., & Mann, D. M. (1995). Neuropathological changes in Down's syndrome hippocampal formation. Effect of age and apolipoprotein E genotype. *Arch Neurol, 52*(4), 373–378. doi:10.1001/archneur.1995.00540280059019

Insausti, A. M., Megias, M., Crespo, D., Cruz-Orive, L. M., Dierssen, M., Vallina, I. F., . . . Florez, J. (1998). Hippocampal volume and neuronal number in Ts65Dn mice: A murine model of Down syndrome. *Neurosci Lett, 253*(3), 175–178. doi:S0304394098006417 [pii]

Jacobs, P. A., Baikie, A. G., Court Brown, W. M., & Strong, J. A. (1959). The somatic chromosomes in mongolism. *Lancet*, *1*(7075), 710. doi:10.1016/s0140-6736(59)91892-6

Jaitin, D. A., Weiner, A., Yofe, I., Lara-Astiaso, D., Keren-Shaul, H., David, E., . . . Amit, I. (2016). Dissecting immune circuits by linking CRISPR-pooled screens with single-cell RNA-seq. *Cell*, *167*(7), 1883–1896 e1815. doi:10.1016/j.cell.2016.11.039

Jeffery, K. J., & Morris, R. G. (1993). Cumulative long-term potentiation in the rat dentate gyrus correlates with, but does not modify, performance in the water maze. *Hippocampus*, *3*(2), 133–140. doi:10.1002/hipo.450030205

Joung, J., Konermann, S., Gootenberg, J. S., Abudayyeh, O. O., Platt, R. J., Brigham, M. D., . . . Zhang, F. (2017). Genome-scale CRISPR-Cas9 knockout and transcriptional activation screening. *Nat Protoc*, *12*(4), 828–863. doi:10.1038/nprot.2017.016

Justice, M. J., & Dhillon, P. (2016). Using the mouse to model human disease: Increasing validity and reproducibility. *Dis Model Mech*, *9*(2), 101–103. doi:10.1242/dmm.024547

Kazuki, Y., Gao, F. J., Li, Y., Moyer, A. J., Devenney, B., Hiramatsu, K., . . . Reeves, R. H. (2020). A nonmosaic transchromosomic mouse model of down syndrome carrying the long arm of human chromosome 21. *Elife*, *9*. doi:10.7554/eLife.56223

Kemeny, S., Tatout, C., Salaun, G., Pebrel-Richard, C., Goumy, C., Ollier, N., . . . Gouas, L. (2018). Spatial organization of chromosome territories in the interphase nucleus of trisomy 21 cells. *Chromosoma*, *127*(2), 247–259. doi:10.1007/s00412-017-0653-6

Kishi, T., Matsunaga, S., Oya, K., Nomura, I., Ikuta, T., & Iwata, N. (2017). Memantine for Alzheimer's disease: An updated systematic review and meta-analysis. *J Alzheimers Dis*, *60*(2), 401–425. doi:10.3233/JAD-170424

Kleschevnikov, A. M., Belichenko, P. V., Villar, A. J., Epstein, C. J., Malenka, R. C., & Mobley, W. C. (2004). Hippocampal long-term potentiation suppressed by increased inhibition in the Ts65Dn mouse, a genetic model of Down syndrome. *J Neurosci*, *24*(37), 8153–8160. doi:10.1523/JNEUROSCI.1766-04.2004

Kloth, A. D., Badura, A., Li, A., Cherskov, A., Connolly, S. G., Giovannucci, A., . . . Wang, S. S. (2015). Cerebellar associative sensory learning defects in five mouse autism models. *Elife*, *4*, e06085. doi:10.7554/eLife.06085

Korbel, J. O., Tirosh-Wagner, T., Urban, A. E., Chen, X. N., Kasowski, M., Dai, L., . . . Korenberg, J. R. (2009). The genetic architecture of Down syndrome phenotypes revealed by high-resolution analysis of human segmental trisomies. *Proc Natl Acad Sci U S A*, *106*(29), 12031–12036. doi:10.1073/pnas.0813248106

Kurnit, D. M. (1979). Down syndrome: gene dosage at the transcriptional level in skin fibroblasts. *Proc Natl Acad Sci U S A*, *76*(5), 2372–2375. doi:10.1073/pnas.76.5.2372

Lana-Elola, E., Watson-Scales, S. D., Fisher, E. M., & Tybulewicz, V. L. (2011). Down syndrome: Searching for the genetic culprits. *Dis Model Mech*, *4*(5), 586–595. doi:10.1242/dmm.008078

Lana-Elola, E., Watson-Scales, S., Slender, A., Gibbins, D., Martineau, A., Douglas, C., . . . Tybulewicz, V. (2016). Genetic dissection of Down syndrome-associated congenital heart defects using a new mouse mapping panel. *Elife*, *5*. doi:10.7554/eLife.11614

Lander, E. S., Linton, L. M., Birren, B., Nusbaum, C., Zody, M. C., Baldwin, J., . . . International Human Genome Sequencing, C. (2001). Initial sequencing and analysis of the human genome. *Nature*, *409*(6822), 860–921. doi:10.1038/35057062

Lejeune, J., Gautier, M., & Turpin, R. (1959). Etude des chromosomes somatiques de neuf enfants mongoliens [Study of somatic chromosomes from 9 mongoloid children]. *C R Hebd Seances Acad Sci*, *248*(11), 1721–1722.

Li, H., Cherry, S., Klinedinst, D., DeLeon, V., Redig, J., Reshey, B., . . . Reeves, R. H. (2012). Genetic modifiers predisposing to congenital heart disease in the sensitized Down syndrome population. *Circ Cardiovasc Genet*, *5*(3), 301–308. doi:10.1161/CIRCGENETICS.111.960872

Li, H., Edie, S., Klinedinst, D., Jeong, J. S., Blackshaw, S., Maslen, C. L., & Reeves, R. H. (2016). Penetrance of congenital heart disease in a mouse model of Down syndrome depends on a trisomic potentiator of a disomic modifier. *Genetics*, *203*(2), 763–770. doi:10.1534/genetics.116.188045

Liao, F., Zhang, T. J., Jiang, H., Lefton, K. B., Robinson, G. O., Vassar, R., . . . Holtzman, D. M. (2015). Murine versus human apolipoprotein E4: Differential facilitation of and co-localization in cerebral amyloid angiopathy and amyloid plaques in APP transgenic mouse models. *Acta Neuropathol Commun*, *3*, 70. doi:10.1186/s40478-015-0250-y

Liogier d'Ardhuy, X., Edgin, J. O., Bouis, C., de Sola, S., Goeldner, C., Kishnani, P., . . . Khwaja, O. (2015). Assessment of cognitive scales to examine memory, executive function and language in individuals with Down syndrome: Implications of a 6-month observational study. *Front Behav Neurosci, 9*, 300. doi:10.3389/fnbeh.2015.00300

Liu, C., Morishima, M., Jiang, X., Yu, T., Meng, K., Ray, D., . . . Yu, Y. E. (2014). Engineered chromosome-based genetic mapping establishes a 3.7 Mb critical genomic region for Down syndrome-associated heart defects in mice. *Hum Genet, 133*(6), 743–753. doi:10.1007/s00439-013-1407-z

Lorenzi, H. A., & Reeves, R. H. (2006). Hippocampal hypocellularity in the Ts65Dn mouse originates early in development. *Brain Res, 1104*(1), 153–159.

Macedo, A. C., Balouch, S., & Tabet, N. (2017). Is sleep disruption a risk factor for Alzheimer's disease? *J Alzheimers Dis, 58*(4), 993–1002. doi:10.3233/JAD-161287

Mahoney, G., Perales, F., Wiggers, B., & Herman, B. (2006). Responsive teaching: Early intervention for children with Down syndrome and other disabilities. *Downs Syndr Res Pract, 11*(1), 18–28.

Makalowski, W., Zhang, J., & Boguski, M. S. (1996). Comparative analysis of 1196 orthologous mouse and human full-length mRNA and protein sequences. *Genome Res, 6*(9), 846–857. doi:10.1101/gr.6.9.846

Martinez-Cue, C., Martinez, P., Rueda, N., Vidal, R., Garcia, S., Vidal, V., . . . Hernandez, M. C. (2013). Reducing GABAA alpha5 receptor-mediated inhibition rescues functional and neuromorphological deficits in a mouse model of down syndrome. *J Neurosci, 33*(9), 3953–3966. doi:10.1523/JNEUROSCI.1203-12.2013

Menghini, D., Costanzo, F., & Vicari, S. (2011). Relationship between brain and cognitive processes in Down syndrome. *Behav Genet, 41*(3), 381–393. doi:10.1007/s10519-011-9448-3

Minakawa, E. N., Miyazaki, K., Maruo, K., Yagihara, H., Fujita, H., Wada, K., & Nagai, Y. (2017). Chronic sleep fragmentation exacerbates amyloid beta deposition in Alzheimer's disease model mice. *Neurosci Lett, 653*, 362–369. doi:10.1016/j.neulet.2017.05.054

Moore, C. S., Hawkins, C., Franca, A., Lawler, A., Devenney, B., Das, I., & Reeves, R. H. (2010). Increased male reproductive success in Ts65Dn "Down syndrome" mice. *Mamm Genome, 21*(11–12), 543–549. doi:10.1007/s00335-010-9300-8

Morice, E., Andreae, L. C., Cooke, S. F., Vanes, L., Fisher, E. M., Tybulewicz, V. L., & Bliss, T. V. (2008). Preservation of long-term memory and synaptic plasticity despite short-term impairments in the Tc1 mouse model of Down syndrome. *Learn Mem, 15*(7), 492–500. doi:10.1101/lm.969608

Morris, R. (1984). Developments of a water-maze procedure for studying spatial learning in the rat. *J Neurosci Methods, 11*(1), 47–60.

Moser, E. I., Krobert, K. A., Moser, M. B., & Morris, R. G. (1998). Impaired spatial learning after saturation of long-term potentiation. *Science, 281*(5385), 2038–2042. doi:10.1126/science.281.5385.2038

Mouse Genome Sequencing, C., Waterston, R. H., Lindblad-Toh, K., Birney, E., Rogers, J., Abril, J. F., . . . Lander, E. S. (2002). Initial sequencing and comparative analysis of the mouse genome. *Nature, 420*(6915), 520–562. doi:10.1038/nature01262

Nakano-Kobayashi, A., Awaya, T., Kii, I., Sumida, Y., Okuno, Y., Yoshida, S., . . . Hagiwara, M. (2017). Prenatal neurogenesis induction therapy normalizes brain structure and function in Down syndrome mice. *Proc Natl Acad Sci U S A, 114*(38), 10268–10273. doi:10.1073/pnas.1704143114

Netzer, W. J., Powell, C., Nong, Y., Blundell, J., Wong, L., Duff, K., . . . Greengard, P. (2010). Lowering beta-amyloid levels rescues learning and memory in a Down syndrome mouse model. *PLoS One, 5*(6), e10943. doi:10.1371/journal.pone.0010943

Neves, G., Cooke, S. F., & Bliss, T. V. (2008). Synaptic plasticity, memory and the hippocampus: A neural network approach to causality. *Nat Rev Neurosci, 9*(1), 65–75. doi:10.1038/nrn2303

Nordquist, S. K., Smith, S. R., & Pierce, J. T. (2018). Systematic functional characterization of human 21st chromosome orthologs in Caenorhabditis elegans. *G 3 (Bethesda)* , *8*(3), 967–979. doi:10.1534/g3.118.200019

O'Doherty, A., Ruf, S., Mulligan, C., Hildreth, V., Errington, M. L., Cooke, S., . . . Fisher, E. M. (2005). An aneuploid mouse strain carrying human chromosome 21 with Down syndrome phenotypes. *Science, 309*(5743), 2033–2037. doi:10.1126/science.1114535

Ohlrich, E. S., & Ross, L. E. (1968). Acquisition and differential conditioning of the eyelid response in normal and retarded children. *J Exp Child Psychol, 6*(2), 181–193.

Olmos-Serrano, J. L., Kang, H. J., Tyler, W. A., Silbereis, J. C., Cheng, F., Zhu, Y., . . . Sestan, N. (2016). Down syndrome developmental brain transcriptome reveals defective oligodendrocyte differentiation and myelination. *Neuron, 89*(6), 1208–1222. doi:10.1016/j.neuron.2016.01.042

Olson, L. E., Roper, R. J., Baxter, L. L., Carlson, E. J., Epstein, C. J., & Reeves, R. H. (2004). Down syndrome mouse models Ts65Dn, Ts1Cje, and Ms1Cje/Ts65Dn exhibit variable severity of cerebellar phenotypes. *Dev Dyn, 230*(3), 581–589. doi:10.1002/dvdy.20079

Olson, L. E., Roper, R. J., Sengstaken, C. L., Peterson, E. A., Aquino, V., Galdzicki, Z., . . . Reeves, R. H. (2007). Trisomy for the Down syndrome 'critical region' is necessary but not sufficient for brain phenotypes of trisomic mice. *Hum Mol Genet, 16*(7), 774–782. doi:10.1093/hmg/ddm022

Ovchinnikov, D. A., Korn, O., Virshup, I., Wells, C. A., & Wolvetang, E. J. (2018). The impact of APP on Alzheimer-like pathogenesis and gene expression in Down syndrome iPSC-derived neurons. *Stem Cell Reports, 11*(1), 32–42. doi:10.1016/j.stemcr.2018.05.004

Pastalkova, E., Serrano, P., Pinkhasova, D., Wallace, E., Fenton, A. A., & Sacktor, T. C. (2006). Storage of spatial information by the maintenance mechanism of LTP. *Science, 313*(5790), 1141–1144. doi:10.1126/science.1128657

Peiris, H., Duffield, M. D., Fadista, J., Jessup, C. F., Kashmir, V., Genders, A. J., . . . Keating, D. J. (2016). A syntenic cross species aneuploidy genetic screen links RCAN1 expression to beta-cell mitochondrial dysfunction in type 2 diabetes. *PLoS Genet, 12*(5), e1006033. doi:10.1371/journal.pgen.1006033

Pelleri, M. C., Cattani, C., Vitale, L., Antonaros, F., Strippoli, P., Locatelli, C., . . . Caracausi, M. (2018). Integrated quantitative transcriptome maps of human trisomy 21 tissues and cells. *Front Genet, 9*, 125. doi:10.3389/fgene.2018.00125

Pelleri, M. C., Gennari, E., Locatelli, C., Piovesan, A., Caracausi, M., Antonaros, F., . . . Cocchi, G. (2017). Genotype-phenotype correlation for congenital heart disease in Down syndrome through analysis of partial trisomy 21 cases. *Genomics, 109*(5–6), 391–400. doi:10.1016/j.ygeno.2017.06.004

Pennington, B. F., Moon, J., Edgin, J., Stedron, J., & Nadel, L. (2003). The neuropsychology of Down syndrome: Evidence for hippocampal dysfunction. *Child Dev, 74*(1), 75–93.

Perrin, S. (2014). Preclinical research: Make mouse studies work. *Nature, 507*(7493), 423–425. doi:10.1038/507423a

Popov, V. I., Kleschevnikov, A. M., Klimenko, O. A., Stewart, M. G., & Belichenko, P. V. (2011). Three-dimensional synaptic ultrastructure in the dentate gyrus and hippocampal area CA3 in the Ts65Dn mouse model of Down syndrome. *J Comp Neurol, 519*(7), 1338–1354. doi:10.1002/cne.22573

Potier, M. C., Rivals, I., Mercier, G., Ettwiller, L., Moldrich, R. X., Laffaire, J., . . . Dauphinot, L. (2006). Transcriptional disruptions in Down syndrome: A case study in the Ts1Cje mouse cerebellum during postnatal development. *J Neurochem, 97 Suppl 1* , 104–109. doi:10.1111/j.1471-4159.2005.03624.x

Powell, N. M., Modat, M., Cardoso, M. J., Ma, D., Holmes, H. E., Yu, Y., . . . Ourselin, S. (2016). Fully-automated muMRI Morphometric phenotyping of the Tc1 mouse model of Down syndrome. *PLoS One, 11*(9), e0162974. doi:10.1371/journal.pone.0162974

Prasher, V. P., Farrer, M. J., Kessling, A. M., Fisher, E. M., West, R. J., Barber, P. C., & Butler, A. C. (1998). Molecular mapping of Alzheimer-type dementia in Down's syndrome. *Ann Neurol, 43*(3), 380–383. doi:10.1002/ana.410430316

Prasher, V. P., Sajith, S. G., Rees, S. D., Patel, A., Tewari, S., Schupf, N., & Zigman, W. B. (2008). Significant effect of APOE epsilon 4 genotype on the risk of dementia in Alzheimer's disease and mortality in persons with Down syndrome. *Int J Geriatr Psychiatry, 23*(11), 1134–1140. doi:10.1002/gps.2039

Raz, N., Torres, I. J., Briggs, S. D., Spencer, W. D., Thornton, A. E., Loken, W. J., . . . Acker, J. D. (1995). Selective neuroanatomic abnormalities in Down's syndrome and their cognitive correlates: Evidence from MRI morphometry. *Neurology, 45*(2), 356–366. doi:10.1212/wnl.45.2.356

Real, R., Peter, M., Trabalza, A., Khan, S., Smith, M. A., Dopp, J., . . . De Paola, V. (2018). In vivo modeling of human neuron dynamics and Down syndrome. *Science, 362*(6416). doi:10.1126/science.aau1810

Reeb-Sutherland, B. C., & Fox, N. A. (2015). Eyeblink conditioning: A non-invasive biomarker for neurodevelopmental disorders. *J Autism Dev Disord, 45*(2), 376–394. doi:10.1007/s10803-013-1905-9

Reeves, R. H., Delabar, J., Potier, M. C., Bhattacharyya, A., Head, E., Lemere, C., . . . Busciglio, J. (2019). Paving the way for therapy: The Second International Conference of the Trisomy 21 Research Society. *Mol Syndromol, 9*(6), 279–286. doi:10.1159/000494231

Reeves, R. H., Irving, N. G., Moran, T. H., Wohn, A., Kitt, C., Sisodia, S. S., . . . Davisson, M. T. (1995). A mouse model for Down syndrome exhibits learning and behaviour deficits. *Nat Genet, 11*(2), 177–184. doi:10.1038/ng1095-177

Reinholdt, L. G., Ding, Y., Gilbert, G. J., Czechanski, A., Solzak, J. P., Roper, R. J., . . . Davisson, M. T. (2011). Molecular characterization of the translocation breakpoints in the Down syndrome mouse model Ts65Dn. *Mamm Genome, 22*(11–12), 685–691. doi:10.1007/s00335-011-9357-z

Richtsmeier, J. T., Baxter, L. L., & Reeves, R. H. (2000). Parallels of craniofacial maldevelopment in Down syndrome and Ts65Dn mice. *Dev Dyn, 217*(2), 137–145. doi:10.1002/(SICI)1097-0177(200002)217:2<137::AID-DVDY1>3.0.CO;2-N

Rissman, R. A., & Mobley, W. C. (2011). Implications for treatment: GABA(A) receptors in aging, Down syndrome and Alzheimer's disease. *J Neurochem, 117*(4), 613–622. doi:10.1111/j.1471-4159.2011.07237.x [doi]

Roper, R. J., Baxter, L. L., Saran, N. G., Klinedinst, D. K., Beachy, P. A., & Reeves, R. H. (2006). Defective cerebellar response to mitogenic Hedgehog signaling in Down [corrected] syndrome mice. *Proc Natl Acad Sci U S A, 103*(5), 1452–1456. doi:10.1073/pnas.0510750103

Roper, R. J., & Reeves, R. H. (2006). Understanding the basis for Down syndrome phenotypes. *PLoS Genet, 2*(3), e50. doi:10.1371/journal.pgen.0020050

Roper, R. J., VanHorn, J. F., Cain, C. C., & Reeves, R. H. (2009). A neural crest deficit in Down syndrome mice is associated with deficient mitotic response to Sonic hedgehog. *Mech Dev, 126*(3–4), 212–219. doi:10.1016/j.mod.2008.11.002

Rosenthal, N., & Brown, S. (2007). The mouse ascending: perspectives for human-disease models. *Nat Cell Biol, 9*(9), 993–999. doi:10.1038/ncb437

Rovelet-Lecrux, A., Hannequin, D., Raux, G., Le Meur, N., Laquerriere, A., Vital, A., . . . Campion, D. (2006). APP locus duplication causes autosomal dominant early-onset Alzheimer disease with cerebral amyloid angiopathy. *Nat Genet, 38*(1), 24–26. doi:10.1038/ng1718

Sago, H., Carlson, E. J., Smith, D. J., Kilbridge, J., Rubin, E. M., Mobley, W. C., . . . Huang, T. T. (1998). Ts1Cje, a partial trisomy 16 mouse model for Down syndrome, exhibits learning and behavioral abnormalities. *Proc Natl Acad Sci U S A, 95*(11), 6256–6261. doi:10.1073/pnas.95.11.6256

Sago, H., Carlson, E. J., Smith, D. J., Rubin, E. M., Crnic, L. S., Huang, T. T., & Epstein, C. J. (2000). Genetic dissection of region associated with behavioral abnormalities in mouse models for Down syndrome. *Pediatr Res, 48*(5), 606–613. doi:10.1203/00006450-200011000-00009

Salehi, A., Faizi, M., Colas, D., Valletta, J., Laguna, J., Takimoto-Kimura, R., . . . Mobley, W. C. (2009). Restoration of norepinephrine-modulated contextual memory in a mouse model of Down syndrome. *Sci Transl Med, 1*(7), 7ra17. doi:10.1126/scitranslmed.3000258

Saul, M. C., Philip, V. M., Reinholdt, L. G., Center for Systems Neurogenetics of, A., & Chesler, E. J. (2019). High-diversity mouse populations for complex traits. *Trends Genet, 35*(7), 501–514. doi:10.1016/j.tig.2019.04.003

Schmahmann, J. D. (2004). Disorders of the cerebellum: Ataxia, dysmetria of thought, and the cerebellar cognitive affective syndrome. *J Neuropsychiatry Clin Neurosci, 16*(3), 367–378. doi:10.1176/jnp.16.3.367

Schmahmann, J. D. (2019). The cerebellum and cognition. *Neurosci Lett, 688*, 62–75. doi:10.1016/j.neulet.2018.07.005

Schmidt-Sidor, B., Wisniewski, K. E., Shepard, T. H., & Sersen, E. A. (1990). Brain growth in Down syndrome subjects 15 to 22 weeks of gestational age and birth to 60 months. *Clin Neuropathol, 9*(4), 181–190.

Schneider, V. A., Graves-Lindsay, T., Howe, K., Bouk, N., Chen, H. C., Kitts, P. A., . . . Church, D. M. (2017). Evaluation of GRCh38 and de novo haploid genome assemblies demonstrates the enduring quality of the reference assembly. *Genome Res, 27*(5), 849–864. doi:10.1101/gr.213611.116

Segal, D. J., & McCoy, E. E. (1974). Studies on Down's syndrome in tissue culture. I. Growth rates and protein contents of fibroblast cultures. *J Cell Physiol, 83*(1), 85–90. doi:10.1002/jcp.1040830112

Shapiro, B. L. (1983). Down syndrome—A disruption of homeostasis. *Am J Med Genet, 14*(2), 241–269. doi:10.1002/ajmg.1320140206

Siarey, R. J., Carlson, E. J., Epstein, C. J., Balbo, A., Rapoport, S. I., & Galdzicki, Z. (1999). Increased synaptic depression in the Ts65Dn mouse, a model for mental retardation in Down syndrome. *Neuropharmacology, 38*(12), 1917–1920. doi:10.1016/s0028-3908(99)00083-0

Siarey, R. J., Stoll, J., Rapoport, S. I., & Galdzicki, Z. (1997). Altered long-term potentiation in the young and old Ts65Dn mouse, a model for Down syndrome. *Neuropharmacology, 36*(11–12), 1549–1554. doi:10.1016/s0028-3908(97)00157-3

Siegel, J. J., & Amon, A. (2012). New insights into the troubles of aneuploidy. *Annu Rev Cell Dev Biol, 28*, 189–214. doi:10.1146/annurev-cellbio-101011-155807

Singh, N., Dutka, T., Devenney, B. M., Kawasaki, K., Reeves, R. H., & Richtsmeier, J. T. (2015). Acute upregulation of hedgehog signaling in mice causes differential effects on cranial morphology. *Dis Model Mech, 8*(3), 271–279. doi:10.1242/dmm.017889

Smith, G. K., Kesner, R. P., & Korenberg, J. R. (2014). Dentate gyrus mediates cognitive function in the Ts65Dn/DnJ mouse model of Down syndrome. *Hippocampus, 24*(3), 354–362. doi:10.1002/hipo.22229

Sommer, T., Rose, M., Glascher, J., Wolbers, T., & Buchel, C. (2005). Dissociable contributions within the medial temporal lobe to encoding of object-location associations. *Learn Mem, 12*(3), 343–351. doi:10.1101/lm.90405

Sorge, R. E., Martin, L. J., Isbester, K. A., Sotocinal, S. G., Rosen, S., Tuttle, A. H., . . . Mogil, J. S. (2014). Olfactory exposure to males, including men, causes stress and related analgesia in rodents. *Nat Methods, 11*(6), 629–632. doi:10.1038/nmeth.2935

Starbuck, J. M., Dutka, T., Ratliff, T. S., Reeves, R. H., & Richtsmeier, J. T. (2014). Overlapping trisomies for human chromosome 21 orthologs produce similar effects on skull and brain morphology of Dp(16)1Yey and Ts65Dn mice. *Am J Med Genet A, 164A*(8), 1981–1990. doi:10.1002/ajmg.a.36594

Sullivan, K. D., Lewis, H. C., Hill, A. A., Pandey, A., Jackson, L. P., Cabral, J. M., . . . Espinosa, J. M. (2016). Trisomy 21 consistently activates the interferon response. *Elife, 5*. doi:10.7554/eLife.16220

Sussan, T. E., Yang, A., Li, F., Ostrowski, M. C., & Reeves, R. H. (2008). Trisomy represses Apc(Min)-mediated tumours in mouse models of Down's syndrome. *Nature, 451*(7174), 73–75. doi:10.1038/nature06446

Sylvester, P. E. (1983). The hippocampus in Down's syndrome. *J Ment Defic Res, 27 (Pt 3)*, 227–236.

Szemes, M., Davies, R. L., Garden, C. L., & Usowicz, M. M. (2013). Weaker control of the electrical properties of cerebellar granule cells by tonically active GABAA receptors in the Ts65Dn mouse model of Down's syndrome. *Mol Brain, 6*, 33. doi:10.1186/1756-6606-6-33

Takiguchi, M., Kazuki, Y., Hiramatsu, K., Abe, S., Iida, Y., Takehara, S., . . . Oshimura, M. (2014). A novel and stable mouse artificial chromosome vector. *ACS Synth Biol, 3*(12), 903–914. doi:10.1021/sb3000723

Usowicz, M. M., & Garden, C. L. (2012). Increased excitability and altered action potential waveform in cerebellar granule neurons of the Ts65Dn mouse model of Down syndrome. *Brain Res, 1465*, 10–17. doi:10.1016/j.brainres.2012.05.027

Vorhees, C. V., & Williams, M. T. (2006). Morris water maze: Procedures for assessing spatial and related forms of learning and memory. *Nat Protoc, 1*(2), 848–858. doi:10.1038/nprot.2006.116

Weick, J. P., Held, D. L., Bonadurer, G. F., 3rd, Doers, M. E., Liu, Y., Maguire, C., . . . Bhattacharyya, A. (2013). Deficits in human trisomy 21 iPSCs and neurons. *Proc Natl Acad Sci U S A, 110*(24), 9962–9967. doi:10.1073/pnas.1216575110

Wiggers, C. R. M., Govers, A., Lelieveld, D., Egan, D. A., Zwaan, C. M., Sonneveld, E., . . . Bartels, M. (2019). Epigenetic drug screen identifies the histone deacetylase inhibitor NSC3852 as a potential novel drug for the treatment of pediatric acute myeloid leukemia. *Pediatr Blood Cancer, 66*(8), e27785. doi:10.1002/pbc.27785

Williams, A. D., Mjaatvedt, C. H., & Moore, C. S. (2008). Characterization of the cardiac phenotype in neonatal Ts65Dn mice. *Dev Dyn, 237*(2), 426–435. doi:10.1002/dvdy.21416

Williams, B. R., Prabhu, V. R., Hunter, K. E., Glazier, C. M., Whittaker, C. A., Housman, D. E., & Amon, A. (2008). Aneuploidy affects proliferation and spontaneous immortalization in mammalian cells. *Science, 322*(5902), 703–709. doi:10.1126/science.1160058

Willner, P. (1984). The validity of animal models of depression. *Psychopharmacology (Berl), 83*(1), 1–16. doi:10.1007/bf00427414

Wiseman, F. K., Al-Janabi, T., Hardy, J., Karmiloff-Smith, A., Nizetic, D., Tybulewicz, V. L., . . . Strydom, A. (2015). A genetic cause of Alzheimer disease: Mechanistic insights from Down syndrome. *Nat Rev Neurosci, 16*(9), 564–574. doi:10.1038/nrn3983

Wiseman, F. K., Pulford, L. J., Barkus, C., Liao, F., Portelius, E., Webb, R., . . . LonDown, S. C. (2018). Trisomy of human chromosome 21 enhances amyloid-beta deposition independently of an extra copy of APP. *Brain, 141*(8), 2457–2474. doi:10.1093/brain/awy159

Wisniewski, K. E., Wisniewski, H. M., & Wen, G. Y. (1985). Occurrence of neuropathological changes and dementia of Alzheimer's disease in Down's syndrome. *Ann Neurol, 17*(3), 278–282. doi:10.1002/ana.410170310

Woodruff-Pak, D. S., Romano, S., & Papka, M. (1996). Training to criterion in eyeblink classical conditioning in Alzheimer's disease, Down's syndrome with Alzheimer's disease, and healthy elderly. *Behav Neurosci, 110*(1), 22–29.

Xu, R., Brawner, A. T., Li, S., Liu, J. J., Kim, H., Xue, H., . . . Jiang, P. (2019). OLIG2 drives abnormal neurodevelopmental phenotypes in human iPSC-based organoid and chimeric mouse models of Down syndrome. *Cell Stem Cell, 24*(6), 908–926 e908. doi:10.1016/j.stem.2019.04.014

Yates, C. M., Simpson, J., Maloney, A. F., Gordon, A., & Reid, A. H. (1980). Alzheimer-like cholinergic deficiency in Down syndrome. *Lancet, 2*(8201), 979. doi:10.1016/s0140-6736(80)92137-6

Yu, T., Li, Z., Jia, Z., Clapcote, S. J., Liu, C., Li, S., . . . Yu, Y. E. (2010). A mouse model of Down syndrome trisomic for all human chromosome 21 syntenic regions. *Hum Mol Genet, 19*(14), 2780–2791. doi:10.1093/hmg/ddq179

Yu, T., Liu, C., Belichenko, P., Clapcote, S. J., Li, S., Pao, A., . . . Yu, Y. E. (2010). Effects of individual segmental trisomies of human chromosome 21 syntenic regions on hippocampal long-term potentiation and cognitive behaviors in mice. *Brain Res, 1366*, 162–171. doi:10.1016/j.brainres.2010.09.107

Zhu, J., Tsai, H. J., Gordon, M. R., & Li, R. (2018). Cellular Stress Associated with Aneuploidy. *Dev Cell, 44*(4), 420–431. doi:10.1016/j.devcel.2018.02.002

Zorrilla de San Martin, J., Delabar, J. M., Bacci, A., & Potier, M. C. (2018). GABAergic over-inhibition, a promising hypothesis for cognitive deficits in Down syndrome. *Free Radic Biol Med, 114*, 33–39. doi:10.1016/j.freeradbiomed.2017.10.002

CHAPTER

23 Future Directions in Research on the Development of Persons With Down Syndrome

Leonard Abbeduto, Jacob A. Burack, *and* Jamie Edgin

Abstract

In this concluding chapter, the authors identify important areas for future research. Some areas reflect gaps in understanding the development of persons with Down syndrome, whereas others reflect special opportunities in which the field is poised to make scientifically and clinically important advances. In studying co-occurring conditions, the authors believe that research must move beyond diagnostic labels to understand the ways in which co-occurring conditions are manifested in Down syndrome. There is a need to move beyond studying problems of development and decline as distinct and instead, conceptualizing age-related decline as part of the developmental process and as subject to the same types of influences. Researchers also need to determine the efficacy of different methods of educating providers about the outcomes that are possible for individuals with Down syndrome and their families and about the optimal patterns of interaction among providers and family members. Although there has been an explosion in the use of digital technology to deliver services and support to individuals with intellectual and developmental disabilities, the efficacy of even well-validated interventions in this format is not guaranteed and thus, research on these extensions is needed. Down syndrome is typically associated with a high degree of dependence in the adult years. However, there is considerable within-syndrome variation in this regard and thus, it is important to identify the factors that promote greater independence, particularly those factors that are amenable to change though intervention. Addressing these research areas will lead to improved quality of life for persons with Down syndrome.

Key Words: Down syndrome, stem cells, gene therapy, telehealth, comorbid conditions, autism spectrum disorder, Alzheimer's disease, neurodegeneration, adult transition

Introduction

As we reflect on the completion of this volume, we begin by noting two historical points relevant to its publication. First, the publication of this volume occurs more than three decades after the first edited collection devoted to the development of persons with Down syndrome (Cicchetti & Beeghly, 1990), and, as would be expected, the volume reflects considerable advances in this area of research over the years. Most strikingly, the range of topics and available data covered here far exceeds that of the earlier seminal volume, and the technologies used in the research mirror the vast technological progress both in research and society at large. Second, since the idea for this volume was originally conceived, we have lost three eminent scholars, each of whom contributed uniquely to the study of the development of persons with Down syndrome—Janet Carr, through her more than half-century longitudinal program of research with persons with Down syndrome and family members; Edward Zigler, through his articulation of the developmental approach to the study of persons with intellectual disability that was eventually extended to the study of persons with Down syndrome; and Annette Karmiloff-Smith, through her application of a developmental neuroconstructivist approach to the study of persons with Down syndrome (for a discussion of early developmental approaches to the study of persons with Down syndrome, please see Burack et al., this volume). The ideas and influence of these three scholars are evident in many of the chapters in this volume. Although the authors of the chapters differ in their foci and methodologies, they all extend and expand on the earlier pioneering work and contribute meaningful pieces to the still incomplete mosaic of our understanding of the development of persons with Down syndrome.

This collection of chapters of state-of-the-art research and knowledge reflects much of the considerable progress in research about persons with Down syndrome over the last few decades. Another indicator of the growth in the field is that a search of PubMed for articles with Down syndrome in the title shows that 169 such articles were published in 1990, 162 in 2000, 383 in 2010, and 935 in 2020. This positive trajectory since 2000 is likely to increase even more dramatically because of shifts in interest among research funders. In 2018, for example, the National Institutes of Health, the largest funder of health-related research in the world, launched a trans-institute initiative called INCLUDE (INvestigation of Co-occurring conditions across the Lifespan to Understand Down syndromE) in response to a U.S. Congress directive. INCLUDE, which is supported by a large infusion of funds, has the goal of better health and quality of life for people with Down syndrome through research. A special emphasis of INCLUDE is research on conditions that, although disproportionately affecting people with Down syndrome, are likely to provide insights relevant to the general population—conditions such as Alzheimer's disease, autism, congenital heart disease, and diabetes. Private foundations throughout the world, such as the Lejeune Foundation, Global Down Syndrome Foundation, National Down Syndrome Society, and LuMIND IDSC Foundation, are growing as well, and collectively they have developed research funding programs of varying size and focus. In this concluding chapter, *The Oxford Handbook of Down Syndrome and Development*, we consider areas of research in which this renewed interest is likely to, or should, focus.

Treatment and Prevention of Adverse Conditions and Symptoms

The neurodiversity movement, which has largely been associated with issues surrounding persons with autism spectrum disorder (ASD; Happé & Frith, 2020), has also emerged in relation to persons with Down syndrome and other conditions associated with intellectual disability. The movement has many facets and nuances, but at its core it is a call to respect and value all humans equally regardless of their characteristics or abilities (Pellicano & Stears, 2011). In the case of persons with Down syndrome, the movement has led to a shift in thinking about the goal of treatment and prevention. In particular, the goal is not to cure or prevent Down syndrome but rather to reduce or prevent the disabilities or challenges associated with Down syndrome that reduce quality of life or prevent the individual from living an independent life of their choosing. On this latter view, valid goals would be to improve the rate of learning; reduce speech articulation difficulties to improve intelligibility; alleviate the symptoms of anxiety or ASD that serve as barriers to social interaction; prevent cardiac or sleep problems; and forestall or prevent the onset of dementia. These goals can be met both by working to promote adaptive change within the individual (e.g., encouraging the acquisition of new skills, encouraging a more physically active lifestyle) through behavioral or biomedical intervention and changing the environment in ways that better support the individual (e.g., providing a speech generating device for individuals with limited language or very reduced speech intelligibility). Interestingly, the neurodiversity view is entirely consistent with the developmental perspective championed decades earlier by Zigler and others, who argued that individual differences, including those embodied in the concept of intellectual disability, should be understood in terms of variations on a single developmental process. We, the editors of this volume, endorse extension of the neurodiversity perspective to conceptualizing approaches to treatment for people with Down syndrome.

Treatments to reduce or prevent the disabilities that can be associated with Down syndrome are likely to take many forms. Pharmacological treatments have and will continue to be developed. These are likely to be both based on symptoms (e.g., targeting depression in young adults with Down syndrome) and focused on core challenges (e.g., drugs with hypothesized localized impact on the balance of excitatory and inhibitory neurons in the hippocampus). Despite the promise of efficacy in preclinical studies of various pharmacological treatments for Down syndrome, however, results from human clinical trials to date have largely been disappointing with regard to the improvement of learning in people with Down syndrome. The same is true regarding other genetic conditions, most notably fragile X syndrome, with well more than two dozen "failed" trials to date (Erickson et al., 2017). We hope that researchers in the field of Down syndrome can learn lessons from, and not repeat the mistakes of, those in the field of fragile X syndrome research. These lessons include the following:

- Treatment should begin at the youngest ages possible while ensuring safety rather than, as is typically done now, beginning with adults or older adolescents (Hessl et al., 2016) and preceding to pediatric trials only if the trials with older individuals show efficacy (Erickson et al., 2018).

- The duration of the trials should extend beyond the 3 to 6 months that is the current standard in the field so that there is adequate time for treatment-induced behavioral change to be incorporated into the individual's repertoire in meaningful and measurable ways (Berry-Kravis et al., 2018).
- Outcome measures must have adequate psychometric properties, relate to functioning in meaningful, real-world contexts, and be sensitive to change even in short-term treatment trials (Berry-Kravis et al., 2013; Budimirovic et al., 2017; Hessl et al., 2016).
- Drug treatments should be combined with other nonmedical interventions such as behavioral therapies targeting the same outcomes as the drug but in ways that allow the combined and separate contributions to change to be determined (Thurman et al., 2020).

From the perspective of Down syndrome, the approach to clinical trials would benefit from being embedded within a developmental framework that recognizes the importance of the likely differential effects of an intervention at different developmental periods, the difficulty of changing a well-established developmental trajectory, the need to focus on long-term outcomes that are meaningful to the individual (rather than short-term transitory improvements), and the multiple factors that shape development.

Other biomedical treatment approaches are also on the horizon, including stem cell technologies (Zhao & Bhattacharyya, 2018). Induced pluripotent stem cells (iPSCs) are grown from tissue (e.g., skin) taken from affected individuals and provide a tool to study the development of a variety of cell types in comparison to similar cell types from typically developing individuals. Once grown and their properties understood, iPSCs can be used in vitro to study the efficacy of pharmaceutical treatments and other biological manipulations of the cells to learn about the potential promise of those therapeutics. There is also the hope that the stem cells themselves may provide therapeutic options when injected, implanted, and so forth, into healthy (e.g., nontrisomic) cells in circumscribed areas of the body, including the nervous system, perhaps leading to improved learning. Such therapies are already being tested for neurogenerative disorders such as Huntington's disease (Ebrahimi et al., 2020; Yoon et al., 2020; Yousefi, Abdollahii, Kouhbanani, & Hassanzadeh, 2020), and could be extended to Down syndrome (Bhattacharyya, 2020; Zhao & Bhattacharyya, 2020), which could entail shutting off genes that are overexpressed, bringing more balance to neurotransmitter systems or even fully silencing the extra chromosome.

We are hopeful that more behavioral and educational interventions will also be developed and tested for efficacy. There are surprisingly few such evidence-based interventions, and most involve an integration of operant behavioral and developmental principles with delivery by a trained clinician directly to the individual with Down syndrome. Arguably, most of these interventions have targeted language or prelinguistic precursors and focus on early development. We would encourage researchers to expand the range of targets to, for example, memory, executive function, and attention skills and to develop modules specific to age or developmental levels that ensure that treatment is delivered over the life course and in contexts that are functional and meaningful for the individual with Down syndrome (Crocker et al., 2013; Fidler & Nadel, 2007; Lemons et al., 2018; Yoder & Warren, 1998; Yoder, Woynaroski, Fey, & Warren, 2014). We would also hope to see a shift away from exclusively clinician-delivered approaches toward approaches in which individuals important to the individual with Down syndrome can be trained to provide some form of therapy. Parent-implemented interventions, for example, entail training parents, generally through didactics and real-time coaching, to deliver therapies in naturalistic contexts and interventions (McDuffie et al., 2016, 2018; Venker, McDuffie, Ellis Weismer, & Abbeduto, 2012). These latter interventions have the potential advantages of being delivered in multiple naturally occurring contexts rather than the clinic, which may promote generalization of learned skills, and at a higher "dose" than is possible in clinician delivery. In light of the important challenges documented for parents of people with Down syndrome, parent-implemented intervention are particularly promising. Other individuals, such as siblings and peers, can also be recruited into some interventions in light of the important roles that they naturally play in the lives of people with Down syndrome. Within the context of the developmental approach outlined in the Burack et al. chapter in this volume, changing the behavior of parents and siblings offers the potential of sustained change; that is, those individuals can continue to provide a more supportive and optimal environment for the person with Down syndrome even after the clinician or research withdraws. In addition, these supportive behaviors of parents and siblings are likely to be reinforced by improvements in the learning and behavior of the person with Down syndrome, thereby further supporting a positive developmental cascade.

As individuals with Down syndrome experience a range of formal educational programs at different points in the life course and with variability across countries, states, districts, and schools, we need to learn more about the most effective educational programs or approaches in terms of teaching basic academic skills such as reading and writing. We need to better understand how educational settings can support optimal social and emotional development and, ultimately, high quality of life and some degree of independence in adulthood. The optimal educational experiences will likely not be dramatically different for people with Down syndrome relative to individuals with disabilities due to other causes. Conversely, no single program or approach will work best for all individuals with Down syndrome.

Co-Occurring Conditions

As highlighted in other chapters of this volume, many individuals with Down syndrome also are diagnosed with other conditions, such as autism or depression. Indeed, considerable effort has been directed toward documenting the prevalence of these various co-occurring conditions among individuals with Down syndrome. We believe that an additional important task for research is to move beyond diagnostic labels to understand the ways in which these conditions are manifested in Down syndrome and the consequences of the challenges embodied in those diagnostic labels for everyday function. The basic idea is that there are likely to be differences in the symptomatology, consequences, and underlying mechanisms in conditions such as autism in Down syndrome compared to the idiopathic case or other neurodevelopmental conditions associated with intellectual disability (e.g., fragile X syndrome). These differences, which are hidden by the failure to delve deeper into the diagnostic label, may well have important consequences for treatment. Again, fragile X syndrome is illustrative (Abbeduto, McDuffie, & Thurman, 2014). As many as 60% of individuals with fragile X syndrome meet diagnostic criteria for ASD. However, once differences in cognitive ability are controlled, individuals with fragile X syndrome relative to those with idiopathic ASD have a less severe symptom presentation, fail to display some of the core symptoms of the disorder (e.g., pronoun reversal), and manifest symptoms that seem more closely related to cognitive and language ability and anxiety (Abbeduto et al., 2019; McDuffie, Thurman, Hagerman, & Abbeduto, 2015). Differential patterns of brain anomalies are also evidenced among persons with ASD and fragile X syndrome relative to those with only ASD cases (Hoeft et al., 2011). Clinically and mechanistically important differences may also be hidden by diagnostic labels such as attention-deficit/hyperactivity disorder (ADHD), anxiety, and depression in persons with Down syndrome. Thus, we encourage research designed to create more nuanced characterizations of these broad co-occurring diagnostic categories for individuals with Down syndrome.

Development Versus Degeneration

As illustrated in this volume, individuals with Down syndrome and their families face challenges during development as well as the likelihood of the early onset of Alzheimer's disease (AD) and dementia. In large measure, these problems of development and decline have been treated as separate problems, studied through different lenses and with different methodological and theoretical approaches. This specialization is seen even among researchers, with some focused only on development into early adulthood and others only on the neuropathology and symptoms of decline, with relatively few researchers bridging both. However, we believe that there would be value in conceptualizing age-related decline as part of the developmental process and as subject to the same types of influences. Indeed, although the roots of the decline of AD are changes in the brain, environmental factors, such as lifestyle, social support from family, and access to health care and related resources are likely to play a role in the progression of the disease at the individual level as well. In addition, there may be early indicators of risk and protection for the decline of AD or perhaps even early precipitating events, including environmental exposures, that would help explain the variability in AD symptom onset, profile, and course (Conners, Tungate, Abbeduto, Merrill, & Faught, 2018). Thus, following the developmental approach exemplified by Zigler and others, there is value in understanding age-related declines in terms of individual variation in the typical processes of development. Such a developmental approach would also offer the possibility of developing strategies for the prevention or at least the forestalling of symptoms. These interventions need not be exclusively biomedical; they could include physical activity, engagement in meaningful employment, and an active social life. Implementing such a developmental approach would require the long-term follow up of large, well-characterized cohorts of individuals with Down syndrome from childhood into adolescence and through adulthood. Such studies would be costly in terms of time and resources, but they are likely to offer the most promise of changing the trajectory of inevitable decline for so many individuals with Down syndrome.

Diagnostic Processes and Professional Interaction

There is a need for research focused on understanding and improving the interactions between individuals with Down syndrome and their families, on the one hand, and the professionals who serve them, on the other. For example, physicians and other health care professionals continue to generally paint the expected outcomes and options surrounding the birth of a child with Down syndrome in highly negative, nearly catastrophic terms (Crombag, Page-Christiaens, Skotko, & de Graaf, 2020; Schimmel, Mimouni, Yosef, & Wasserteil, 2020). Moreover, families suffer psychological hurt from this initial portrayal not only in the short term, but for many years to come (Poehlmann, Clements, Abbeduto, & Farsad, 2005). Many advocacy and support groups, therefore, have developed materials to assist professionals and families in "interpreting" the birth and diagnosis of a child with Down syndrome. What is needed from researchers, though, is evidence of the efficacy of different methods of educating providers about the actual outcomes for individuals with Down syndrome and their families, as well as evidence about the optimal patterns of interaction among providers and family members in terms of sharing accurate information and setting families along a better path of development. More generally, these issues arise predictably at various points in the life course, although the particular professionals involved may change, such as occurs at the transition into school and the transition from a pediatric to an adult healthcare system. In all cases, there is a need for research on ways of optimizing interactions to create professional-family partnerships (Head & Abbeduto, 2007). And, finally, professionals from all disciplines could benefit from an evidence-based approach on how to interact with individuals with Down syndrome in ways that are not only respectful but also honor the agency of the individual with Down syndrome.

Technology

In the past decade, there has been an explosion in the use of digital technology to deliver services and support to people in need of assistance, including individuals with intellectual and developmental disabilities (Abbeduto, 2020; Valentine et al., 2020). Video teleconferencing has made telehealth delivery of care commonplace in most larger health care systems. This same technology is being used to provide and monitor a range of behavioral treatments delivered into the home, most of which involve the parent as therapeutic agent and with various degrees of synchronous or asynchronous training of parents (Bullard, McDuffie, & Abbeduto, 2017; McDuffie et al., 2018; Vismara, McCormick, Shields, & Hessl, 2019). However, the efficacy of even well-validated interventions in this format is not guaranteed, and numerous iterative adaptations for digital delivery are necessary. In fact, research evaluating the efficacy of telehealth interventions is only beginning, and thus far applications to the treatment of the challenges associated with persons with Down syndrome are few and small in scope. More sophisticated digital technologies, such as virtual and augmented reality to improve everything from attention to vocational skills, and robots to support the acquisition of social skills, are now being tested for efficacy among persons with ASD, ADHD, and other conditions (Burke, Li, Grudzien, & Garcia, 2020; Levac, Dumas, & Meleis, 2018; Zheng et al., 2020). These technologies have the potential to extend the opportunity for intervention well beyond what is possible in the traditional model of the clinician delivering directly to the participant; to provide services in a way that is convenient, less, costly, and more accessible to individuals with Down syndrome and their families; and to do so in ways that may better support generalization of learned skills.

Technology also allows researchers to address previously intractable questions. Perhaps most notable in this regard is the advent of machine learning (i.e., artificial intelligence) that allows the processing of large amounts of data to discern patterns that lead to predictive algorithms. These algorithms are being used to make diagnostic determinations in behavioral conditions such as ASD and to identify the downstream consequences of genes in human development through the construction of genes based on developmental function (Iakovidou, Lanzarini, Singh, Fiori, & Santosh, 2020; Park, 2020; Ruan, Webster, Li, & Wang, 2020). Machine learning can likely help parse and identify the determinants of the phenotypical variability among individuals with Down syndrome.

Transition to an Independent Adult Life

Although Down syndrome is typically associated with a high degree of dependence in the adult years, there is considerable within-syndrome variation in this regard (Karmiloff-Smith et al., 2016). Identifying the factors that promote greater independence, particularly those that are amenable to change though intervention, is important to ensure optimal quality of life. Researchers of persons with ASD have focused considerable effort on identifying the skills and experiences that adults with ASD require to achieve maximum independence and positive outcomes in education, employment, socialization, and habitation (DaWalt, Usher, Greenberg, & Mailick, 2019; Friedman, Sterling, DaWalt, & Mailick, 2019; Laxman, Taylor, DaWalt, Greenberg, & Mailick, 2019). As a result, we are beginning to see the emergence of evidence-based interventions and calls for policy changes to promote greater independence, improved access to educational and vocational opportunities, and a richer, more inclusive, social life for the adult with ASD (DaWalt, Greenberg, & Mailick, 2018). Unfortunately, the factors that lead to lesser or greater independence in areas such as vocational functioning among individuals with Down syndrome have not been adequately investigated. Understandably, perhaps, this may reflect the emphasis on Alzheimer's disease in research on the lives of adults with Down syndrome. Nonetheless, many adults with Down syndrome are free of the phenotypic symptoms of Alzheimer's disease for decades, and thus an interest in promoting their independence is warranted. Moreover, based on the literature on healthy aging in the general populations, positive benefits of enhanced independence and an active lifestyle could be expected to forestall the onset of neurodegeneration in individuals with Down syndrome. We would encourage more such research and hope that it would be informed by collaborations with, and attention to the perspectives of, adults with Down syndrome.

References

Abbeduto, L. (2020). Presidential address, 2020—Using technology to deliver services and supports in homes, neighborhoods, and communities: Evidence and promise. *Intellectual and Developmental Disabilities, 58*(6), 525–531. doi:10.1352/1934-9556-58.6.525

Abbeduto, L., McDuffie, A., & Thurman, A. J. (2014). The fragile x syndrome–autism comorbidity: What do we really know? *Frontiers in Genetics, 5*, 355. https://doi.org/10.3389/fgene.2014.00355

Abbeduto, L., Thurman, A. J., McDuffie, A., Klusek, J., Feigles, R. T., Ted Brown, W., . . . Roberts, J. E. (2019). ASD Comorbidity in fragile X syndrome: Symptom profile and predictors of symptom severity in adolescent and young adult males. *Journal of Autism and Developmental Disorders, 49*(3), 960–977. https://doi.org/10.1007/s10803-018-3796-2

Berry-Kravis, E., Hessl, D., Abbeduto, L., Reiss, A. L., Beckel-Mitchener, A., & Urv, T. K. (2013). Outcome measures for clinical trials in fragile X syndrome. *Journal of Developmental and Behavioral Pediatrics, 34*(7), 508–522. https://doi.org/10.1097/DBP.0b013e31829d1f20

Berry-Kravis, E. M., Lindemann, L., Jønch, A. E., Apostol, G., Bear, M. F., Carpenter, R. L., . . . Jacquemont, S. (2018). Drug development for neurodevelopmental disorders: Lessons learned from fragile X syndrome. *Nature Reviews Drug Discovery, 17*(4), 280–299. https://doi.org/10.1038/nrd.2017.221

Bhattacharyya, A. (2020). Advancing knowledge of Down syndrome brain development and function with human stem cells. *American Journal on Intellectual and Developmental Disabilities, 25*(2), 90–92. https://doi.org/10.1352/1944-7558-125.2.90

Budimirovic, D. B., Berry-Kravis, E., Erickson, C. A., Hall, S. S., Hessl, D., Reiss, A. L., . . . Kaufmann, W. E. (2017). Updated report on tools to measure outcomes of clinical trials in fragile X syndrome. *Journal of Neurodevelopmental Disorders, 9*(1), 14. https://doi.org/10.1186/s11689-017-9193-x

Bullard, L., McDuffie, A., & Abbeduto, L. (2017). Distance delivery of a parent-implemented language intervention for young boys with fragile X syndrome. *Autism & Developmental Language Impairments, 2*, 239694151772869. https://doi.org/10.1177/2396941517728690

Burke, S. L., Li, T., Grudzien, A., & Garcia, S. (2020). Brief report: Improving employment interview self-efficacy among adults with autism and other developmental disabilities using Virtual Interactive Training Agents (ViTA). *Journal of Autism and Developmental Disorders, 51* (2), 741–748. https://doi.org/10.1007/s10803-020-04571-8

Cicchetti, D., & Beeghly, M. (Eds.). (1990). *Children with Down syndrome: A developmental perspective.* Cambridge University Press. https://doi.org/10.1017/CBO9780511581786

Conners, F. A., Tungate, A. S., Abbeduto, L., Merrill, E. C., & Faught, G. G. (2018). Growth and decline in language and phonological memory over two years among adolescents with down syndrome. *American Journal on Intellectual and Developmental Disabilities, 123*(2), 103–118. https://doi.org/10.1352/1944-7558-123.2.103

Crocker, L. D., Heller, W., Warren, S. L., O'Hare, A. J., Infantolino, Z. P., & Miller, G. A. (2013). Relationships among cognition, emotion, and motivation: Implications for intervention and neuroplasticity in psychopathology. *Frontiers in Human Neuroscience, 7*, 261. https://doi.org/10.3389/fnhum.2013.00261

Crombag, N. M. T. H., Page-Christiaens, G. C. M. L., Skotko, B. G., & de Graaf, G. (2020). Receiving the news of Down syndrome in the era of prenatal testing. *American Journal of Medical Genetics, Part A, 182*(2), 374–385. https://doi.org/10.1002/ajmg.a.61438

DaWalt, L. S., Greenberg, J. S., & Mailick, M. R. (2018). Transitioning together: A multi-family group psychoeducation program for adolescents with ASD and their parents. *Journal of Autism and Developmental Disorders, 48*(1), 251–263. https://doi.org/10.1007/s10803-017-3307-x

DaWalt, L. S., Usher, L. V., Greenberg, J. S., & Mailick, M. R. (2019). Friendships and social participation as markers of quality of life of adolescents and adults with fragile X syndrome and autism. *Autism, 23*(2), 383–393. https://doi.org/10.1177/1362361317709202

Ebrahimi, T., Abasi, M., Seifar, F., Eyvazi, S., Hejazi, M. S., Tarhriz, V., & Montazersaheb, S. (2020). Transplantation of stem cells as a potential therapeutic strategy in neurodegenerative disorders. *Current Stem Cell Research & Therapy, 15*, 133–144. https://doi.org/10.2174/1574888X15666200628141314

Erickson, C. A., Davenport, M. H., Schaefer, T. L., Wink, L. K., Pedapati, E. V, Sweeney, J. A., . . . Berry-Kravis, E. (2017). Fragile X targeted pharmacotherapy: Lessons learned and future directions. *Journal of Neurodevelopmental Disorders, 9*(1), 7. https://doi.org/10.1186/s11689-017-9186-9

Erickson, C., Kaufmann, W., Budimirovic, D., Lachiewicz, A., Haas-Givler, B., Miller, R., . . . Berry-Kravis, E. (2018). Best practices in fragile X syndrome treatment development. *Brain Sciences, 8*(12), 224. https://doi.org/10.3390/brainsci8120224

Fidler, D. J., & Nadel, L. (2007). Education and children with Down syndrome: Neuroscience, development, and intervention. *Mental Retardation and Developmental Disabilities Research Reviews, 13*(3), 262–271. https://doi.org/10.1002/mrdd.20166

Friedman, L., Sterling, A., DaWalt, L. S., & Mailick, M. R. (2019). Conversational language is a predictor of vocational independence and friendships in adults with ASD. *Journal of Autism and Developmental Disorders, 49*(10), 4294–4305. https://doi.org/10.1007/s10803-019-04147-1

Happé, F., & Frith, U. (2020, March 1). Annual research review: Looking back to look forward—changes in the concept of autism and implications for future research. *Journal of Child Psychology and Psychiatry and Allied Disciplines, 61*(3), 218–232. https://doi.org/10.1111/jcpp.13176

Head, L. S., & Abbeduto, L. (2007). Recognizing the role of parents in developmental outcomes: A systems approach to evaluating the child with developmental disabilities. *Mental Retardation and Developmental Disabilities Research Reviews, 13*(4), 293–301. https://doi.org/10.1002/mrdd.20169

Hessl, D., Sansone, S. M., Berry-Kravis, E., Riley, K., Widaman, K. F., Abbeduto, L., . . . Gershon, R. C. (2016). The NIH Toolbox Cognitive Battery for intellectual disabilities: Three preliminary studies and future directions. *Journal of Neurodevelopmental Disorders, 8*(1), 35. https://doi.org/10.1186/s11689-016-9167-4

Hoeft, F., Walter, E., Lightbody, A. A., Hazlett, H. C., Chang, C., Piven, J., & Reiss, A. L. (2011). Neuroanatomical differences in toddler boys with fragile X syndrome and idiopathic autism. *Archives of General Psychiatry, 68*(3), 295–305. https://doi.org/10.1001/archgenpsychiatry.2010.153

Iakovidou, N., Lanzarini, E., Singh, J., Fiori, F., & Santosh, P. (2020). Differentiating females with Rett syndrome and those with multi-comorbid autism spectrum disorder using physiological biomarkers: A novel approach. *Journal of Clinical Medicine, 9*(9), 2842. https://doi.org/10.3390/jcm9092842

Karmiloff-Smith, A., Al-Janabi, T., D'Souza, H., Groet, J., Massand, E., Mok, K., . . . Strydom, A. (2016). The importance of understanding individual differences in Down syndrome. *F1000Research, 5*, 389. doi: 10.12688/f1000research.7506.1.

Laxman, D. J., Taylor, J. L., DaWalt, L. S., Greenberg, J. S., & Mailick, M. R. (2019). Loss in services precedes high school exit for teens with autism spectrum disorder: A longitudinal study. *Autism Research, 12*(6), 911–921. https://doi.org/10.1002/aur.2113

Lemons, C. J., King, S. A., Davidson, K. A., Puranik, C. S., Al Otaiba, S., & Fidler, D. J. (2018). Personalized reading intervention for children with Down syndrome. *Journal of School Psychology, 66*, 67–84. https://doi.org/10.1016/j.jsp.2017.07.006

Levac, D., Dumas, H. M., & Meleis, W. (2018). A Tablet-based interactive movement tool for pediatric rehabilitation: Development and preliminary usability evaluation. *JMIR Rehabilitation and Assistive Technologies, 5*(2), e10307. https://doi.org/10.2196/10307

McDuffie, A., Banasik, A., Bullard, L., Nelson, S., Feigles, R. T., Hagerman, R., & Abbeduto, L. (2018). Distance delivery of a spoken language intervention for school-aged and adolescent boys with fragile X syndrome. *Developmental Neurorehabilitation, 21*(1), 48–63. https://doi.org/10.1080/17518423.2017.1369189

McDuffie, A., Machalicek, W., Bullard, L., Nelson, S., Mello, M., Tempero-Feigles, R., . . . Abbeduto, L. (2016). A spoken-language intervention for school-aged boys with fragile X syndrome. *American Journal on Intellectual and Developmental Disabilities, 121*(3), 236–265. https://doi.org/10.1352/1944-7558-121.3.236

McDuffie, A., Thurman, A. J., Hagerman, R. J., & Abbeduto, L. (2015). Symptoms of Autism in Males with Fragile X Syndrome: A Comparison to Nonsyndromic ASD Using Current ADI-R Scores. *Journal of Autism and Developmental Disorders, 45*(7), 1925–1937. https://doi.org/10.1007/s10803-013-2013-6

Park, D. I. (2020). Genomics, transcriptomics, proteomics and big data analysis in the discovery of new diagnostic markers and targets for therapy development. *Progress in Molecular Biology and Translational Science, 173*, 61–90. https://doi.org/10.1016/bs.pmbts.2020.04.017

Pellicano, E., & Stears, M. (2011). Bridging autism, science and society: Moving toward an ethically informed approach to autism research. *Autism Research, 4*(4), 271–282. https://doi.org/10.1002/aur.201

Poehlmann, J., Clements, M., Abbeduto, L., & Farsad, V. (2005). Family experiences associated with a child's diagnosis of fragile X or Down syndrome: Evidence for disruption and resilience. *Mental Retardation, 43*(4), 255–267. https://doi.org/10.1352/0047-6765(2005)43[255:FEAWAC]2.0.CO;2

Ruan, M., Webster, P. J., Li, X., & Wang, S. (2020). Deep neural network reveals the world of autism from a first-person perspective. *Autism Research, 4*(2), 333–342. https://doi.org/10.1002/aur.2376

Schimmel, M. S., Mimouni, F. B., Yosef, T. M., & Wasserteil, N. (2020). "Your baby has Down syndrome": What is the preferable way to inform parents? *Journal of Perinatology, 40*(8), 1163–1166. https://doi.org/10.1038/s41372-020-0701-6

Thurman, A. J., Potter, L. A., Kim, K., Tassone, F., Banasik, A., Potter, S. N., . . . Abbeduto, L. (2020). Controlled trial of lovastatin combined with an open-label treatment of a parent-implemented language intervention in youth with fragile X syndrome. *Journal of Neurodevelopmental Disorders, 12*(1), 12. https://doi.org/10.1186/s11689-020-09315-4

Valentine, A. Z., Brown, B. J., Groom, M. J., Young, E., Hollis, C., & Hall, C. L. (2020, August 1). A systematic review evaluating the implementation of technologies to assess, monitor and treat neurodevelopmental disorders: A map of the current evidence. *Clinical Psychology Review, 80*, 101870. https://doi.org/10.1016/j.cpr.2020.101870

Venker, C. E., McDuffie, A., Ellis Weismer, S., & Abbeduto, L. (2012). Increasing verbal responsiveness in parents of children with autism: A pilot study. *Autism, 6* (6), 568–585. https://doi.org/10.1177/1362361311413396

Vismara, L. A., McCormick, C. E. B., Shields, R., & Hessl, D. (2019). Extending the parent-delivered Early Start Denver Model to young children with fragile X syndrome. *Journal of Autism and Developmental Disorders, 49*(3), 1250–1266. https://doi.org/10.1007/s10803-018-3833-1

Yoder, P. J., & Warren, S. F. (1998). Maternal responsivity predicts the prelinguistic communication intervention that facilitates generalized intentional communication. *Journal of Speech, Language, and Hearing Research, 41*(5), 1207–1219. https://doi.org/10.1044/jslhr.4105.1207

Yoder, P., Woynaroski, T., Fey, M., & Warren, S. (2014). Effects of dose frequency of early communication intervention in young children with and without Down syndrome. *American Journal on Intellectual and Developmental Disabilities, 119*(1), 17–32. https://doi.org/10.1352/1944-7558-119.1.17

Yoon, Y., Kim, H. S., Jeon, I., Noh, J. E., Park, H. J., Lee, S., . . . Song, J. (2020). Implantation of the clinical-grade human neural stem cell line, CTX0E03, rescues the behavioral and pathological deficits in the quinolinic acid-lesioned rodent model of Huntington's disease. *Stem Cells, 38*(8), 936–947. https://doi.org/10.1002/stem.3191

Yousefi, N., Abdollahii, S., Kouhbanani, M. A. J., & Hassanzadeh, A. (2020). Induced pluripotent stem cells (iPSCs) as game-changing tools in the treatment of neurodegenerative disease: Mirage or reality? *Journal of Cellular Physiology*, *235*(12), 9166–9184. https://doi.org/10.1002/jcp.29800

Zhao, X., & Bhattacharyya, A. (2018). Human models are needed for studying human neurodevelopmental disorders. *American Journal of Human Genetics*, *103*(6), 829–857. https://doi.org/10.1016/j.ajhg.2018.10.009

Zhao, X., & Bhattacharyya, A. (2020). Advances in human stem cells and genome editing to understand and develop treatment for fragile X syndrome. *Advances in Neurobiology*, *25*, 33–53. https://doi.org/10.1007/978-3-030-45493-72

Zheng, Z., Nie, G., Swanson, A., Weitlauf, A., Warren, Z., & Sarkar, N. (2020). A Randomized controlled trial of an intelligent robotic response to joint attention intervention system. *Journal of Autism and Developmental Disorders*, *50*(8), 2819–2831. https://doi.org/10.1007/s10803-020-04388-5

CHAPTER 24

Future Directions: The Voices of Persons With Down Syndrome and Their Relatives

Jacob A. Burack *and* Emily Stubbert

Abstract

This epilogue presents a collection of testimonials from a group of individuals whose lives have all been affected by Down syndrome. It provides a voice to the mothers, fathers, siblings, and to individuals with Down syndrome themselves, allowing them to recount their journeys with the condition. These real-life narratives also provide insight into different familial views on systemic supports, educational resources, and methods of diagnosis, among other things. Some of these individuals founded organizations to advocate for persons with Down syndrome, such as the Down Syndrome Information Alliance, Down Syndrome International, and the Down Syndrome Research Institute. These perceptions reflect the experiences of a very small number of people whose lives are affected by the condition. Nevertheless, these accounts can be sources of awareness and inspiration.

Key Words: Down syndrome, persons with Down syndrome, Down syndrome diagnosis, educational resources, systemic supports, Down Syndrome Information Alliance, Down Syndrome International, Down Syndrome Research Institute

In this epilogue, we present a collection of testimonials from a group of individuals sharing one thing in common: their lives have all been touched by Down syndrome. The purpose of this chapter is to provide a voice to this group of mothers, fathers, siblings, and individuals with Down syndrome themselves, allowing them to discuss their journeys in connection with the condition of Down syndrome. These messages bring us one step closer to these families and their experiences of understanding, fulfillment, heartbreak, and joy. These real-life narratives also provide insight into familial views on systemic supports, educational resources, methods of diagnosis, and more. In presenting these accounts, we note that these perceptions reflect the experiences of a very small number of people whose lives are affected by Down syndrome, but we hope that they will be sources of awareness and inspiration for the readers of this volume.

Martin and Pamela Chasen

Dr. Martin and Pamela Chasen were born in South Africa and came to Canada with their two daughters in 2004. Presently residing in Toronto with Tikvah, they are committed parents and advocates for people with special needs and inclusion.

A Child Is Born

The excitement and suspense mounts whilst living through the final weeks of any pregnancy. Will the baby be a boy, with a healthy weight, or a girl with golden hair? What does the future hold for this gift, this miracle? A sportsman? An actress? Loved by others? Tall and handsome? and so on and on the dreams go.

Are there any parents, grandparents and family members who ever really imagine any other course of life for themselves and their new family member? Surely very few! Perhaps those who know antenatally of possible consequences of the pregnancy, but these are exceptions. For most people, who could or would ever imagine a child who will develop leukemia, or another who will become a drug addict, and yet another who will be injured from whatever cause. If only families could plan for the future, then they could be partially prepared for the event. Forewarned is forearmed.

And so we began our journey together with Tikvah—a beautiful child born with Down syndrome. Armed with an expectation that we can have input into her destiny and equipped with the documented experiences and anticipation of world experts, we took the first few steps and moved forward. With enthusiasm to make this child a giver to the community, and a solid citizen, living a meaningful life. We chose to rise to the challenge and opportunity presented to us. We had a small inkling that the road ahead would not be the one well walked, but rather we would be beating the path open for our family and others. A privilege indeed! We were being given a task, but we could arrange and organize for the expedition.

And so it has been an exciting life with Tikvah, she has led us to meet a whole new group of "family and friends." We have experienced highs and lows, and each stage of the journey has enriched our existence—not at the time, but when we reflect afterwards, and so we now know that it will work out. Our faith has intensified when we see this young woman dancing and singing without shame. When she clearly expresses her need for friendship and her desire to do acts of kindness. We appreciate her sincerity and her value within our family and the community.

In kindergarten she first learned to play with peers and to take turns. In elementary school, she had dedicated teachers who taught her patiently and with love how to read and write. In high school she has mastered the art of extracurricular activities such as dancing and singing, in addition to exceling at her scholarly subjects, which include English, art, math, and nature studies, with inclusion in these classes at a regular school. With help from "shadows" who diligently pre-teach and mediate her learning and evaluation, Tikvah has been able to attend regular classes with children of all abilities. She also volunteers regularly on weekends, as do most students of her age at all Canadian schools.

And next year and the year after and the year after that? We look forward to helping this young woman achieve her maximum potential in every sphere in which she applies herself. Whilst the waters are still muddy at times, they do flow consistently and in the right direction; at times they gush and at other times they trickle.

And so a child is born: a miracle, a gift, and a potential in every child. The birth of such a child is our birth as well. We all grow; we all require nourishment and light and company. It happens that sometimes one sees a flash of light ahead and the path forward is clear and bright. But that light can disappear very quickly and all we are left with is the memory of what the path ahead looked like when it was illuminated. This is the inspiration that we seek and find.

Thank you, Tikvah, for coming into our life with light and hope.

Heather Scott

In 2001, Heather had her first child, Gabby, who was born with Down syndrome. In 2004, along with two other families, Heather founded the Down Syndrome Information Alliance, where she is currently the Program Director. Heather previously worked for Sacramento County as a Deputy Sheriff and now also works at the Sacramento County Office of Education Infant Development Program as an Infant Educator. She is also a committee member of the National Scientific Advisory Committee for the MIND Institute and the California Government Affairs Committee, as well as a member of the Denver Down Syndrome Clinic Task Force Group. In addition, she coaches for the Special Olympics. Together, she and her husband Andrew have six children.

In October of 2001, I gave birth to my first daughter, Gabriella. My labor with her was long and difficult and there were a few complications during her birth. None of these complications were serious or long term, but I assumed they were the reason for the room to all of a sudden fill up with many doctors. It took a bit of time for someone to tell me I had a daughter. I kept asking "Do I have a boy or a girl?" After a long while, the doctor told me that he thought my daughter had Down syndrome. He told me we had many options and that we could even have her placed in an institution. I cried—a lot. I don't ever remember crying that much in my whole life. I was so shocked. There was no prenatal indication that she had Down syndrome. I was so scared. I kept thinking I let my family down. I literally thought to myself "But she's too cute to have Down syndrome" Of course, in hindsight, I loathe myself for that thought. Of course, babies with Down Syndrome are just as cute as other babies! I wondered if we would still use the name we picked out for her. As if her disability made her unworthy of our perfect name. I was so ignorant then. I blame my lack of knowledge about disabilities, my fear, my complete exhaustion mixed with hormones and my medical team's misguided words—their offer for taking her and putting her somewhere else. Their telling me all the things she would never do.

I called my Godmother who has a daughter with a disability. She was the only person I knew at the time who had a child with a disability. She rushed to my hospital room and said, "Sweetheart, you can do this. Of all the disabilities, I'd pick Down syndrome. You have no idea how great your life is going to be."

Gabby had a few issues with learning how to suck and breastfeed and ended up spending a few days in the NICU with jaundice. I spent all my time with her in the NICU holding her and trying to feed her. We took her home after a total of 5 days in the NICU. We spent a lot of time with the lactation nurses and working on feeding. We finally decided to pump breast milk and feed Gabby with a bottle. We did this so we could get her the nutrients she needed while working on her oral motor strength for feeding. Once that was all worked out, we settled into a great routine. I loved being a Mommy to her. I loved sleeping with her and taking her on walks and errands. Our life was typically normal and lovely.

Gabby's younger sister joined our family in December of 2003. Being in the hospital also meant staying my first night ever away from Gabby. My favorite memory is when she came the next day to meet her sister and she just laid in bed with me and held Lucy for as long as she could. I knew instantly that having more children was such a good thing for Gabby. She matured so much wanting to help do everything for her sister.

Gabby started preschool in the fall of 2004 and it started the road to her inclusive education. Around the same time, I also worked with two other families to start the Down Syndrome Information Alliance, a local resource and support group for families who have children with Down syndrome as well as the professionals that served them. A big part of our mission is to support newly diagnosed families with information and guidance as they navigate this new road. In addition, we provide medical professionals training on how to give a diagnosis of Down syndrome. This is an especially important training for me given how I was given the news. In addition, about 90% of the new parents that I have talked to over the past 13 years have similar experiences.

Gabby's father and I divorced when she was about 5. To be honest it had nothing to do with her disability—just two people wanting different things out of life. I have since remarried and our family has expanded to a total of six kids, Gabby being the oldest. My husband will often say, "I don't know what it was like, I don't know what it must have felt that to get a diagnosis" I remind him often' "Yes, but you CHOOSE this. You knew I had a daughter with a disability and you said yes to it all." He has never balked at any hard situation. He has held my hand through the hard times and great times. And he is so thankful for the gift of Gabby and Down syndrome and what it has taught our family.

As I sat down to type this, I could not get through reliving these memories without crying. Remembering her birth is just too much sometimes. I am so mad that I ever felt that sad. I am ashamed of how sad I was to have a child with Down syndrome. On the day that should have been the happiest of my life, I was made to feel the saddest I have ever felt. I feel frustration that the doctor made it sound like it was the worst thing ever, when really it was a little glitch in the plan. I can only try to forgive myself little by little and understand that I didn't have the knowledge and insight that I do now.

Our life with Gabby is pretty amazing. I have made friends that I never would have had, I have found a passion in disability awareness and I have learned many life lessons that I don't think I would have been exposed to if it weren't for her. She is a fantastic young lady who is a sophomore at her local high school and is looking forward to moving out and going to college. She is also a die hard Justin Beiber and One Direction fan and loves going to music concerts. She runs track for her high school team, beating her personal record again and again last year and swims for Special Olympics, bringing home 4 gold medals in the Summer Games this past summer. Gabby is the oldest of six in our family, and loves being a big sister. She has dreams of working in a fire department or police department and getting married. Our family life is full and rewarding because of Gabby and the life lessons that loving someone with a disability has taught us.

My hope, as information becomes more easily available and accessible, is that the medical community starts to see people with Down syndrome, or any disability as people of value, worthy of a great life and all the chances, resources and support to meet their dreams. Families of loved ones with disabilities need a medical team that supports the whole family, wishes and dreams included, not just fixing a medical ailment. I've talked to hundreds of new families over the years, and their joy of having a new baby should not have been stolen because of the way a doctor views a disability. We want our children to be seen as babies and children first, and then take into consideration the disability. There are so many times I wish that the Doctor that gave us the news could see her now—happy, smart, thriving young lady with big goals and dreams."

Elaine Linn

Elaine Linn is the parent of two young adults with disabilities and complex health needs, including a son with Down syndrome. Elaine works as a public affairs and community engagement specialist, uniting partners in health and disability policy initiatives. She co-founded the Down Syndrome Information Alliance in Sacramento and serves on several advisory and leadership groups.

When my son Toby was diagnosed with Trisomy 21 a day after his birth it was a complete shock. I had no exposure to people with disabilities, much less Down syndrome. My only awareness of the condition came from a 1980s TV show, "Life Goes On," and while I was somewhat aware of the cognitive delays, I was completely unaware of the myriad health problems associated with the Down syndrome.

I suddenly found myself thrust into situation I had never imagined. My husband and I had a 3-year-old son, lived comfortably in a suburban neighborhood, and worked full time. I entered the hospital full of anticipation and emerged full of grief and dread. My newborn son was unable to eat normally, had an unexplained infection, faced a life-threatening congenital heart defect, and more tests were pending. And this was just this week. Who knew what the future held? I was handed a book, "Babies with Down Syndrome: A New Parents Guide," which was thoroughly overwhelming. I couldn't read for more than 5 minutes without breaking into sobs. In fact, I didn't stop crying for 4 full days.

"This isn't happening," was my overwhelming thought, followed by, "What does this mean for Jake (my older son)." As an only child, I was thrilled my son would have a sibling, who I imagined to be a companion and supporter through life. This vision was upended and I was living in a fog of despair, uncertainty, and stress during a time when my family should have been at home, embracing and celebrating a new addition to our family.

Multiple specialists would visit my son in the NICU, yet we never knew when, so we couldn't plan to be there for a report. They provided a private place where I could pump breastmilk, but wouldn't allow me to lock the door, creating immense stress. Every hour or so they would close the NICU, so we had approximately 45 minutes at a time to feed, change, and hold our baby, talk with doctors and nurses, and pump. This was a rigorous schedule, especially since Toby was still developing feeding skills and ingesting a few grams could take most of that time. Meanwhile, other family members yearned to visit the baby. My family was extremely supportive through this time. They would wait for hours until I was willing to give up my rotation for them to go in. Of course, because I wanted to spend every minute with Toby, and be there for any doctor visits, I didn't want to leave. I was unable to mother my baby, unable to care for my frightened and confused toddler, unable to fully comprehend the medical situation, and anxious about pleasing my family. The stress, on top everything, was insufferable.

This would become the recurrent theme for our lives.

What should we do? Were we doing it correctly? Were we doing enough? I researched ways to heighten the senses through movement, sound, scent, and play, and instituted a daily regimen of "therapy" within days of Toby's homecoming. When we requested clinic-based therapy soon after, providers thought we should "just enjoy our baby," but I quickly realized I never wanted to look back and regret not trying an intervention or a treatment. I became conditioned to meet resistance at every turn.

Through multiple procedures, surgeries, and hospitalizations, providers visited unpredictably and gave a report to whoever happened to be in the room at any given time. Although we requested reports only be given to us, providers would report to anyone in the room. Now it was a game of telephone, and we had to hope that the family member who came to provide half an hour's respite got the story straight. Providers would frequently give contradicting recommendations, and we were not allowed to join rounds or group conferences. I have learned to become a sophisticated healthcare consumer and advocate, and consequently often find providers making assumptions about my level of knowledge and leaving out information.

Before Toby was 6 months old he had spent time at four hospitals, had three surgical procedures, and his immune system was compromised. We had to isolate ourselves from family and friends, and even take extended leave of absences from work. This strained us emotionally, financially, and from a practical standpoint. Someone always had to stay home with the baby so, for nearly 2 years, we never went anywhere as a family.

As Toby grew and developed, things simultaneously became easier and more difficult. Services were available, but Toby required up to six clinic-based therapy sessions a week. How would we work and be involved in Toby's care, much less the healthy growth and development of our other child? Every therapist provided critical "homework," all of which could never be completed, creating a constant feeling of failure. Hospitalizations faded only if we could keep infection at bay.

Fortunately, Toby's medical conditions have mostly resolved, and he is now a healthy, active, well-behaved teenager. He has a moderate intellectual disability and is very athletic, verbal, and social. However, he does not communicate feelings, and is not able to report well on his experiences. We constantly wonder about his emotional well-being and hope no one is mistreating him in any way.

We continue to fight health plans for access to specialists, and school districts for inclusive opportunities, as we also navigate the complex system of public policies seemingly intended to leave our son isolated, unemployed, and in poverty. We are told to travel across multiple counties to see a pediatric subspecialist when there is one a few miles away, although in a different medical group. We are forced to prepare for and endure hours long meetings with school officials every year, where we must be prepared to negotiate an equitable education for our son. We must inform family members not to give Toby cash for his birthday or write him into their will, so that he doesn't own anything that would jeopardize his benefits. We must proactively learn federal and state health care and education laws so we can protect what should be provided without hurdles.

We face assumptions, stigma, and barriers every single day. Providers almost always avoid engaging Toby directly, and instead defer to us. People stare everywhere we go. Rarely a week passes when I don't have to repair a breakdown in communication among healthcare providers or school officials. I don't just get to be Toby's mother. I must be an advocate, defender, social worker, service coordinator, and case manager for every aspect of his life, all while managing the regular competing demands of life.

The demands are high and the rewards colossal. But I often think, "Why does it have to be so *hard*?" If providers would consider the competing demands on our family and provide more inclusive environments for communication, many conflicts could be averted. I am not a medical professional or a trained educator, but I would appreciate being treated as a respected equal. I would much rather be a powerful partner than adversary, and fostering positive relationships is critical. Let's each assume each other's competence as a foundation for collaboration, and together we can achieve greatness.

Efrat Dotan

Efrat Dotan has been volunteering and working as a teacher's assistant at Shalva's inclusive preschool for 11 years. Previously, during her teenage and young adult years, she participated in Shalva's After School Activity Center, a rehabilitative recreational program for children and teens with disabilities.

To Fly Far and High

EMBRACING INDEPENDENCE

My name is Efrat Dotan and I am thirty-three and a half years old. I live in an independent living apartment for women with Down syndrome in the Givat Shaul neighborhood of Jerusalem. From the time I was born until the age of thirty I lived at home with my family, meaning with my parents and my siblings. I am the youngest of four children, two boys and two girls, and I am very close with my sister. At home, I received lots of love, patience, and good care, but as I got older, I felt a desire to be more independent and to advance in different areas. I understood that I was living in a bubble.

My parents are amazing. They are really the best in the world. They did everything for me when I was younger and taught me how to be independent; and independent life is not simple—every day there are so many decisions to make. For example, when you get dressed, should I wear winter clothes or summer clothes? My parents taught me how to make all of those decisions. And, most importantly, through all of these decisions I learned to be flexible with changes in my life. Life goes on in a routine and there is a lot to do, but if something changes then I change with it. If I am in the middle of doing something and somebody tells me to do something else, then I change direction on my own without getting frazzled.

MOVING TO AN INDEPENDENT LIVING APARTMENT

My first reaction to the idea of moving to an independent living apartment was sadness. All of a sudden everything that identified me for my whole life until now came into question. I was full of tension about how to live with people who are not my family members. How should I relate to my friends? How will they relate to me? How will they speak with me? Will they be polite and friendly? I am a very sensitive person. This is something that I know about myself and it can be frightening for me if people do not treat me politely. Then I got nervous about leaving my community. How will the community surrounding the independent living apartment relate to me? What will they say about me? Will they say that I'm retarded, or fat? But I was just imagining things. After meeting my apartment counsellors and my roommate I understood that we will never hurt one another. We will always accept our differences and treat each other as equals. My friends in the apartment are good to me and they have a positive influence on me. We have learned a lot from living together with friends, especially how to compromise. I have to compromise and be flexible to changes even if it is difficult for me. Life in the apartment opens me up to so many new opportunities that I enjoy, but one day I might like to marry someone and have a family of my own.

HOW I RELATE TO HAVING DOWN SYNDROME

I noticed that, for the most part, people who do not know me do not treat me nicely. People who do know me are nice to me and are usually impressed with my achievements and my development. I know that my life is not so simple because I have Down syndrome, but I don't have a choice in the matter; this is how I was born. I can't take out my extra chromosome, but I can overcome it. I tell myself, "Efrat, keep advancing, put forth all of your effort to move forward and learn new things. Even if it looks difficult for you, don't give up. *If it looks difficult it just means that you have to try harder but it doesn't mean that you can't do it.* " Sometimes, difficult tasks have an emotional toll for me as well because I'm so sensitive. I deal with this by allowing myself to engage with those emotions instead of pretending that they are not there. I know that I really am capable of being independent. I know how to spread my wings to reach places, to fly far and high. I can achieve my goals and do anything that I put my mind to. Life is like a stream of water, it keeps on flowing and I flow with it no matter what challenges may arise because I am larger than life.

Lital Shkibay

Lital Shkibay is a mother of four. Or is her third child and is fully integrated in their local, mainstream school system. Lital operates her own interior design and home-styling business. Lital is an inspirational speaker who lectures about the acceptance of children with disabilities in their families, communities, and society at large.

My Light

THE PREGNANCY AND BIRTH

We'll start with the fact that I was married with two children. I got pregnant with my third child and during the third month of the pregnancy, I did a nuchal translucency scan. The results came back saying that I had a 1/17 chance of giving birth to a child with Down syndrome. I thought that the world had come to an end. At that point, I began a series of different tests, and with each one, I came to understand more profoundly that this was really happening. The following days and months were far from simple. In fact, they were full of tears and worries. And then the big day came when I went into labor. As soon as she was born, I anxiously lifted my head to look at her. I slowly returned to a laying position, turned to my husband who was by my side, and I said to him, "It's true."

THE FIRST MONTHS POSTPARTUM

The first month after Or was born was very challenging for me. I remember crying while I nursed her. This difficult image is seared into my memory. It was very hard for me to deal with all of the questions and pity from other people, and I am grateful that my family was so supportive. When I would walk down the street with Or, I would close the stroller visor so no one could see her in an effort to avoid the stares and questions from other people. But my husband, Oded, was very strong and supportive. He told me something that I will never forget: "The way that we will accept her and show her to the world is the way that the world will see her."

Today, I am in a different place in terms of my relationship with Or. My acceptance is at 100% and I love her in ways that are beyond words. She has blessed our family with so much happiness and light. Sometimes I am angry with myself about that first month of her life, frustrated that it took me so long to wipe away those first tears, but I understand that this was part of the process that I had to go through as her mother. Since then, we've left that month in the past and moved on.

OUR NEW FAMILY DYNAMIC

When Or was born, my oldest daughter Shay was 5 years old and my son Ilay was 3 years old. When I came home from the hospital we all sat together as a family and I explained to them, mustering up all of my confidence and using simple words that children their age could understand, that they have a sweet new baby sister and that she has Down syndrome. They asked me about Down syndrome and it was important for me to be the one to explain this concept to them. The relationship between my four children is so special, and thankfully so normal. My children are all so sensitive to Or, yet they are not afraid to get upset with her as all siblings do. She is treated like a regular child in the family and I think this has been very helpful in developing Or's ability to interact so naturally in inclusive social situations.

ISRAEL'S FIRST MODEL WITH DOWN SYNDROME

When Or was in preschool, a representative of a support organization for parents of children with Down syndrome approached me about the idea of Or auditioning for a fashion modeling opportunity. Even with her unmistakable Down syndrome look, Or is very beautiful and I agreed to be open to this opportunity. The modeling agent accepted her; and at the age of four-years-old my daughter became Israel's first model with Down syndrome. It turned out that Or loved the camera and her captivating smile made her an instant superstar. She participated in television shows, commercials, and fashion magazines.

I am constantly reminded of my husband's words during those difficult times when I tried to hide Or under the stroller visor: "The way that we will accept her and show her to the world is the way that the world will see her." For me, still today, the modeling is very much a personal healing process, a kind of compensation for that difficult first month. It is my ultimate chance to show her to the world in the most positive way. Moreover, Or's modeling has been very instrumental in raising social awareness and acceptance of children with disabilities in general, and Down syndrome specifically. The modeling has allowed Or to become included in different social and cultural areas that were previously inaccessible to these special children. That being said, the road ahead is still long. There remains a fair amount of rejection for them to overcome.

CONCLUSIONS

Our family loves Or unconditionally and we are proud of every step she takes in her journey. We show her to the world with pride and embody the message that children with disabilities can equally participate in society.

Pat Clarke

Pat is president of the European Down Syndrome Association and vice president of the European Disability Forum. His son David, who has Down syndrome, has been his inspiration and he has served as chairman and chief executive of Down Syndrome Ireland. Pat is a passionate advocate for the inclusion of persons with Down syndrome in society, particularly in education and employment, and he has led many successful initiatives on both these issues, nationally and internationally. Presently his work is on broader disability issues at a European and international level but hopes to "retire" soon.

Great Expectations

"10 March 1981 our son David was born with Down syndrome (DS). He was not expected to survive the first few days and in the event that he did survive, Madeline and I were informed that we should not expect him to live past 25 years of age. Survive he did, and is now a fine man of 36 who leads a full and productive life, contributing to his family and to the broader society in Ireland and Europe. While we were not advised directly, others whom we have met over the years were advised to find a good home for their child, start again, and have more children to replace the child with DS. We did have two more daughters to join David's older sibling, but David stayed with us and was as much a part of our family as any of the rest of us.

At this point, David was a baby and needed all the care that any baby needs, just like his siblings, and we reckoned that as his disability appeared we, as a family, would grow with him and all would be natural in the normal course of events. We had expectations for David fueled not only from natural instinct as parents but also fueled by David's siblings who expected David to do the same things as they did (albeit David ultimately drew the line at playing with Barbies). He participated in all aspects of family life, the chores, the sport and games, the leisure time and travel and entertainment—it was normal and natural.

When it came to the Education System it was an entirely different story. There were no expectations on the part of the professionals that we as a family were dealing with on David's behalf. I cannot emphasize enough that there NONE. It was a fight to get the special school system to even realize that David and his peers could be educated—could be taught to read and write or could have a level of education that would give them independence.

Over 30 years ago a pilot project of Mainstream Education for children with DS began in Dublin with 10 children getting a place in their local school with their siblings and peers. These parents who had an expectation for their children paid for the resource teacher with assistance from the National DS organization. Today 80% of children with DS attend their local school with educational and other supports provided by the State. It is acknowledged from within the sector that this Initiative by DS Ireland opened the door for other disabilities to seek mainstream education as an option for their children. Because of geography at the time David was not able to avail of this service and continued in segregated special education until he was 18. We as parents kept pushing his teachers to offer more to David than just a babysitting service and give him the skills he would need in the future to live a good and independent life. It was a struggle, however, as they held the old stereotypical expectations for a person with DS. But David crossed the frontier of expectations. He had the ambition, his family had expectations and with some work David enthusiastically plotted and participated in the journey—his resilience being nothing short of admirable. While there were many set-backs, bureaucracy etc., along the way David successfully attended college gaining a diploma, went abroad on a few occasions with friends as part of an organized program, secured a meaningful job and broke a few hearts along the way. He is currently and reluctantly single!

David is not so unique, he is in all ways exactly the same as all other individuals in society. He likes nothing better than a beer or two after work, following football, listening to his music and having a chance to hang out with others. David has employs an inspiring philosophy on life regularly advising his sisters to "trust yourself..be kind to others . . . and just get on with it and pass no remarks". Family means a lot to David and he loves hanging out with his two little nieces, although is more than happy to hand them back!

David has a passion for many things that involve people. One of his passions is motorbikes and he loves being part of a gang that travels around Ireland raising money for charity. He loves his job, has a post of responsibility, is part of the team and makes a meaningful contribution to the organization. David continuously challenges preconceived notions about what people with DS can do. His siblings watched in awe when attending an international conference in Asia, he was invited on stage and spoke confidently and perfectly to people with DS and their parents about his life and his expectations. In later years David became somewhat of a mentor to others with DS and acted as a delegate leader and presenter when attending conferences.

While David and his family have a long way to go in overcoming the societal, familial apathy, social and political boundaries preventing full independence, David, daily exercises independence where he can whether that is travelling to his job and navigating various transport systems, engaging in social media, going to work and growing in his job, keeping in touch with friends and attending various social activities.

The frontier is there but you don't need a passport or a visa—just ambition and expectation."

Penny Robertson

Penny Robertson is the mother of Shona, a wonderful daughter who has inspired and delighted everyone around her for the 39 years of her life. "Shona's Down syndrome changed the direction of my life, taking me away from my profession as a geology teacher to learn about early intervention, lobbying, advocacy, and disability rights." Penny's passion and dedication to improving the world for those like her daughter led her to set up the Australian International School, a totally inclusive school with campuses in Jakarta and in Bali; the Australian Down Syndrome Association; the Asia-Pacific Down Syndrome Association; and, along with colleagues from Mexico and Canada, Down Syndrome International. She was made a Member of the Order of Australia for her services to the education of the intellectually disabled, and in 2020 she coauthored "International Guidelines for Education Learners with Down Syndrome," published by Down Syndrome International.

The following is a transcript of the speech given by Robertson in 2014 at the World Down Syndrome Day at United Nations Head Quarters in New York, United States.

"In the five minutes allocated to me, I thought it best to share the lessons I have learned from my experience of what works best as a parent and as a manager of education programs for people with disabilities.

Firstly, successful programs require a strong group of parents, united in their desires and goals for their children. In 1994 I went to live in Indonesia and when I went to enroll my daughter in school I found myself one of a group of parents whose children had been locked out of the existing international schools. Demand for places in these schools allowed the exclusion students with disabilities. The schools considered it too much trouble to cater for children in need of additional learning support. As concerned parents, we acted to challenge those views of social responsibility and today the Australian International School offers inclusive education from preschool to Year 12 in Jakarta, Bali, and Kalimantan.

Secondly, inclusive education requires a clearly articulated and agreed statement of educational outcomes and teaching methodologies. Long-term as well as short-term goals are important. Timelines and reporting procedures are very necessary. Individualized tasks are essential. Tailored programs require clearly enunciated learning goals and a baseline against which to assess progress for all those concerned in the child's education. It is important that parents are involved and that they feel empowered to question what is offered. It is the responsibility of schools to ensure that they commit to best practice and that they implement the conclusions of sound research. Your teachers will all be overworked and probably underpaid, but that does not mean that they need not be interested in new findings. Approached in the right way, they will be delighted to have new information presented to them and to become partners in managing, monitoring and celebrating the achievements of their students with their individual learning programs.

Thirdly, it is important to have a staff which is receptive and led by leaders who are committed to inclusive education. Research has repeatedly identified this as the most important aspect of all in determining how successful the child's education experience will be. The most productive practices involve a close and collaborative relationship between parents and all staff involved in a student's education. This relationship is extremely important. A number of years ago in Jakarta, we had parents enrolling their student without making us aware of all the issues they had faced with their child. This was usually because they were scared their child would be refused admission if we did know. Trust and good communication between the school and the family is essential.

My aim has been to make Australian Independent School the center of excellence and a model for other schools in Indonesia and the world! This is a central to our school's mission and it is written into our founding document. We take seriously the "fit" of staff as our agents of change to deliver the schools' founding principles.

In Indonesia children with disabilities were routinely hidden away. We have taken a quantum leap to gain bureaucratic acceptance of an education system which Indonesian bureaucrats had no experience. My daughter was the first person with Down syndrome that most of the authorities with whom I had to deal had ever met. I should pay a tribute to them as, almost to a person, they showed interest and understanding of the need to foster a more progressive and humanitarian approach to special education, and they assisted me through the processes of registration, licensing, etcetera from go to whoa. That was 15 years ago and, even then, more dedicated and visionary bureaucrats could see benefits for Indonesian families. Today we have schools committed to some form of inclusive education, but clearly not enough. The World Down Syndrome Day video features children from 68 countries in education. Our goal is to make it 193 countries.

Fourthly, the parents and educators must have the ability to lobby effectively at every level of administration and government. As parents, we need to engage in lobbying the moment we encounter unfairness and discrimination, whether it be in your neighborhood school, or in government policies and practices such as those which deprive people with Down syndrome of their vote in elections. Today, it is a matter of intense pride to parents that we can leave some of that lobbying to our self-advocates.

Finally, I want to urge every parent to believe in their child's ability to achieve and in the importance of normalizing the environment for the child's development as an independent adult. Patience, perseverance and humor will be needed to meet that goal. We have a big task ahead of us to get every country to accept what we know to be the right of every person with a disability, namely, the right to an inclusive, individualized education. It is of crucial importance that we not lose sight of that goal because of our frustration with the pace of progress. Parents of my generation only need to look back at the availability and quality of the information and services 30 years ago to see what can be achieved by advocating, lobbying, and direct action.

Just as we celebrated the progress of the early intervention we provided for our babies with DS, we now need to celebrate their achievements throughout the course of their school and post-school education, and we must continue to insist on the ultimate acceptance of the Convention on the Rrights for People with Disabilities (CRPD) by every country on earth. We are especially grateful for the acknowledgment of World Down

Syndrome Day by the United Nations because we know it will greatly assist our world-wide community to achieve rights and recognition for people with DS the world over."

Andy Loebus and Jennifer Shields

Andy Loebus was a high school teacher and the founder of the Down Syndrome Research Institute. He died in 2022, still fully convinced that the effort to create appropriate educational spaced for people with Down syndrome is important and indeed transformative work. Jennifer Shields is a lecturer in Disability Studies at King's University College, London, Ontario.

Our fourth son Kristov Loebus was born on November 3, 1996. Because he has Down syndrome, he had to go through two heart surgeries and a few hospital stays that made us very anxious, but then he got on with school and sports and work and appears to be living a pretty good life.

It would be great to report that Kristov has taught us, his family members, to live in the moment and to treasure the small things, but we don't seem to be particularly gifted at either of those. The biggest lesson we seem to have learned from living with Kristov has been about personal responsibility and the necessity of taking action rather than waiting for external assistance.

Having a family member with Down syndrome exposes the holes in the way society is organized. When the school system is clearly not built for your child, when doctors and therapists are not educated about the details of the particular syndrome that you deal with every day, when the inadequacies of transit mean that you must drive your young person everywhere, when work opportunities are few and far between, and when housing options seem out of reach, it becomes apparent that many things must change if people with Down syndrome and others are to live interdependent, fulfilling lives.

Kristov's birth and life prompted us to follow the example of the great Jo Mills, who founded the Down Syndrome Research Foundation in British Columbia, Canada, and to start the Down Syndrome Research Institute Summer School (DSRI), which ran for 12 summers in London, Ontario. My husband and I are teachers, so we chose to do what we could with the skills that we had in the area that we knew best. DSRI was a training ground for many people in the education system (teachers, educational assistants, speech language pathologists, occupational therapists, physiotherapists, researchers) to become more acquainted with the intricacies of Down syndrome. It also provided an opportunity to test support models that had not yet made their way into the mainstream.

It took excruciating, recurring personal effort each year to fundraise; hire and train the staff; plan the instruction and special events; and lead, supervise, and evaluate each summer's activities, but over time. the DSRI team also learned and modeled many key findings, such as:

- The initial assessment of the skills of students with Down syndrome can assist greatly in the design of appropriate instruction.

- Integrated supports are superior to siloed supports.
- Attention to communication across the curriculum is an effective approach for students with Down syndrome, whose life trajectories can be positively affected by improved language and communication skills.
- Behavior is a bigger factor than many people want to acknowledge in students with Down syndrome, and it should be incorporated in educational planning.

We have also learned that while the inclusion of people with Down syndrome in all walks of life is an important and valid goal, their particular constellations of characteristics are more salient and can be addressed in a more targeted fashion when they are grouped (at least for some time, for select activities) with other young people with the same exceptionality.

DSRI and the learning that emerged from it would not have happened if we had opted to wait for "the authorities" or "the Ministry" to intervene. We understood that there was no substitute for individual initiative and action, and instead of waiting for the cavalry to ride over the hill and save us, there was great value in building the structures that we needed. Efforts for change must involve government ministries, boards of education, and numerous other agencies, but it is also true that the impetus for change can come from affected individuals and their allies, who can use their skills in the sectors they know best to try out the approaches they would like to see in the mainstream.

The American historian, Jill Lepore, has studied the most effective defenders of democracy and the attitudes that motivate them. Their confidence that "political problems are not external forces beyond our control: they are forces within our control" compels them to act without hesitation: "Don't ask whether you need an umbrella. Go outside and stop the rain."[1]

Without our son Kristov in our lives, we might still be waiting for meteorological information. But because of our love for him and the clarity of purpose he gave us, we started DSRI. The work itself and the wonderful families and activists we met along the way have taught us that civil society is not an abstraction: it functions and thrives when all of us contribute our modest, varied efforts to transform the social landscape.

Angela, Jackie, and Valerie Nyhout

Valerie is a self-advocate and a two-time Special Olympics World Games Silver medalist in alpine skiing who enjoys her job at a social media company. Jacqueline is a speech-language pathologist who currently works with children with disabilities and their families. Angela is a researcher and lecturer who studies language comprehension and hypothetical thinking in development.

As two siblings of a person with Down syndrome, as well as the self-advocate herself, we believe between the three of us we understand quite well the potential of people with Down syndrome. We have spent the better part of our lives advocating for equality and respect. We have presented together at a national conference sharing what we believe to be the keys to building a meaningful life for people with Down syndrome.

Perhaps to better understand why we felt equipped to share such advice, we'll share a bit about ourselves. The oldest, Angela, is a postdoctoral fellow at the University of Toronto, where she does research on cognitive development in childhood. She has been a volunteer for Special Olympics for the past 14 years, having coached cross-country skiing, athletics, and soccer. In the middle, Jackie is a speech–language pathologist currently working in Calgary, Alberta. She works with children with intellectual disabilities (including people with Down syndrome) and their families. Jackie is also a former Special Olympics soccer coach. Finally, Val. Val happens to have Down syndrome but that certainly doesn't define who she is. She works full-time at an internet company, is writing a book, maintains a blog, plays seven Special Olympics sport, and is a World Games Silver Medalist in alpine skiing. The three of us have spent a fair bit of time with other people with Down syndrome in a variety of settings.

AS SIBLINGS OF A PERSON WITH DOWN SYNDROME, HERE IS WHAT WE THINK RESEARCHERS, PRACTITIONERS, AND POLICY-MAKERS SHOULD KNOW

People with Down syndrome have dreams and goals just like the typical population, and, like the typical population, they may need help determining what those goals are (think how many people you have met who have changed majors in university, or altered their career path). However, they may face a number of obstacles to realizing their goals.

First, people with Down syndrome are often underestimated. From the moment parents receive a diagnosis for their baby with Down syndrome, they are often told what their child will not be able to do. What many people do not realize is that people with Down syndrome can enjoy many of the same successes and experiences that the typical population does. Families of young children with Down syndrome are often surprised when we tell them that Val works at a job she loves, competed in Austria at the Special Olympics World Games, and was prom queen in high school. Being underestimated can become a self-fulfilling prophecy. A student will not achieve their potential in school if their teacher focuses only on their limitations, or their potential on the field if their coach thinks they are physically limited. Worse yet, a belief in the physical limitations of people with Down syndrome may lead to health problems if they are encouraged into a sedentary lifestyle. Val competes in a range of individual and team sports, from alpine skiing and golf to basketball and soccer. While it is important to be realistic when setting goals, we must be sure not to set unnecessary barriers to people with Down syndrome by signaling to them that we do not believe in them. Focusing on strengths rather than on limitations can support people with Down syndrome to achieve success and work towards their goals. We've seen Val's strengths turn into achievements numerous times throughout her life.

Second, people with Down syndrome often lack the necessary access to achieve their goals. This may be a lack of access to reliable transportation, financial resources, or the emotional support needed to stick with their goals. Professionals can help by connecting them with community resources and encouraging family members, support workers, and friends to speak to them about and encourage their goals.

We think it is important to recognize that every individual one encounters in life has a unique set of goals, skills, and character traits to be admired. By recognizing, respecting, and encouraging these talents, we can help the other person to feel valued, and perhaps they will do the same in return.

People with Down syndrome can teach. The three of us have learned valuable lessons from one another. Often when individuals speak of learning from people with disabilities, they speak of lessons in patience and compassion. Although this may be true in many cases, this is not what we are talking about here. Val has a number of admirable skills and character traits of her own. Val has taught us skills in her areas of expertise. She is an expert downhill skier, and has taken us skiing and helped us refine our technique. Shifting from the role of learner to the role of teacher can be empowering and helps to create equality. In terms of character traits, Val approaches life's challenges with persistence and a sense of humor. Watching Val overcome odds and expectations through hard work and persistence—for example, learning to ride a bicycle after being told she would not be able to by doctors—has been inspiring, and encourages us to persevere in the face of obstacles.

AS A PERSON WITH DOWN SYNDROME, HERE IS WHAT I THINK RESEARCHERS, PRACTITIONERS, AND POLICY-MAKERS SHOULD KNOW

See me as a person. When someone sees me, I hope they do not just see Down syndrome. If someone looked at you and decided they knew everything about you just by your face, you wouldn't like that. Respect me enough to get to know me. And please, if there is something about me that you want to talk about, talk to me. I don't like it when people talk about me like I am not in the room.

Give me time and I will learn. Sometimes, it takes me a little longer to learn things. That doesn't mean I can't learn. For example, when I was learning how to do my job, I had a job coach. He didn't just walk around and talk about what I should do, he showed me. If you talk and show me what you want me to do, I will learn it. You may have to give me time but I will learn it. I will stick with something until I know how to do it and then I will get better and better at it. For example, right now I am trying to become a better golfer. I am listening to my coaches and watching what they show me and I will practice and practice and I will get better. Also, let me try things. You don't know if I can do something or not, if I am not given a chance to try. If someone told you that they did not think you could learn to swim so you should not bother trying, you wouldn't like that. Neither do I. For example, there are people who thought I wouldn't be able to take the train by myself. Well, I take the train all the time now to Union Station in Toronto to visit my sister. It's about a 2-hour train ride and I do this on my own.

Finally, *include me.* I am really fun. I love sports. I love to travel (so far I have been to 14 countries). I like to play games and watch movies. I love my job. You see? I bet there is something we have in common that we could talk about. I am just like everyone else and I want to be part of what is happening. My website/blog is called "Downright **Val**uable." Do you know why? Because I am.

In summary, our recommendations? Let people with Down syndrome discover their own talents and strengths; demonstrate genuine interest in them; and treat them with the same respect you would afford anyone else.

Note

1. Lepore, Jill. "The Last Time Democracy Almost Died," *The New Yorker*, February 3, 2020.

INDEX

Tables, figures, and boxes are indicated by *t*, *f*, and *b* following the page number

B

C

D

G

H

Q

R

X

Y

Z